ACUTE ASTHMA
ASSESSMENT AND MANAGEMENT

EDITORS

JESSE B. HALL, MD
Professor of Medicine and of Anesthesia and Critical Care
Chief, Section of Pulmonary and Critical Care Medicine
Director, Medical Intensive Care Unit and Respiratory Therapy
Pritzker School of Medicine
University of Chicago
Chicago, Illinois

THOMAS C. CORBRIDGE, MD
Associate Professor of Medicine
Director, Medical Intensive Care Unit
Northwestern University Medical School
Chicago, Illinois

CARLOS RODRIGO, MD
Centro de Tratamiento Intensivo
Asociación Española Primera de Socorros Mutuos
Montevideo, Uruguay

GUSTAVO J. RODRIGO, MD
Departmento de Emergencia
Hospital Central de las FF AA
Montevideo, Uruguay

McGRAW-HILL
Medical Publishing Division

New York   St. Louis   San Francisco   Auckland   Bogotá
Caracas   Lisbon   London   Madrid   Mexico City   Milan   Montreal
New Delhi   San Juan   Singapore   Sydney   Tokyo   Toronto

McGraw-Hill

*A Division of The **McGraw·Hill** Companies*

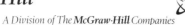

ACUTE ASTHMA: ASSESSMENT AND MANAGEMENT

1234567890 DOCDOC 09876543210

ISBN 0-07-026026-5

This book was set in Times Roman by The PRD Group.
The editors were Michael Medina, Susan R. Noujaim,
and Peter J. Boyle.
The production supervisor was Richard Ruzycka.
The index was prepared by Tony Greenberg, MD.

R. R. Donnelley and Sons was printer and binder.

This book is printed on acid-free paper.

Library of Congress Cataloging-in-Publication Data

Asthma : assessment and management / [edited by] Jesse B. Hall . . . [et al].
    p. ; cm.
  Includes bibliographical references and index.
  ISBN 0-07-026026-5
    1. Asthma.   I. Hall, Jesse B.
  [DNLM: 1. Asthma—diagnosis.   2. Asthma—therapy. WF 553 A85223 2000]
RC591 .A753 2000
616.2'38—dc21

                                             99-088571

Jesse B. Hall:
> *For Barbara, Aaron, Daniel, and Nora*

Thomas C. Corbridge:
> *To Susan*

Gustavo J. Rodrigo:
> *To my parents, my wife, Mabel, and my children Federico, Maria Florencia, and Marina.*

Carlos Rodrigo:
> *To my parents, my wife, Lilián, and my children Ana and Carlos.*

CONTENTS

CONTRIBUTORS

MICHAEL B. ANDERSON
Alfred Hospital
Victoria, Australia
Chapter 13

VITO BRUSASCO, MD
Associate Professor, Respiratory Medicine
Cattedra di Fisiopatologia Respiratoria
Dipartimento di Scienze Motorie e Riabilitative
Università di Genova
Genova, Italy
Chapter 5

WILLIAM W. BUSSE, MD
Professor of Medicine
Head, Section of Allergy and Clinical
Immunology
Department of Medicine
University of Wisconsin Medical School
Madison, Wisconsin
Chapter 18

PERE CASAN, MD
Professor, Respiratory Department
Hospital Santa Creu i Sant Pau
Barcelona, Spain
Chapter 17

GIUSEPPE N. COLASURDO, MD
Division of Pulmonary and Critical Care Medicine
Department of Pediatrics
University of Texas-Houston Medical School
Houston, Texas
Chapter 15

THOMAS C. CORBRIDGE, MD
Associate Professor of Medicine
Director, Medical Intensive Care Unit
Northwestern University Medical School
Chicago, Illinois
Chapter 9

OKAN ELIDEMIR, MD
Pediatric Pulmonary Division
Department of Pediatrics
Baylor College of Medicine
Houston, Texas
Chapter 15

LELAND L. FAN, MD
Professor of Pediatrics
Baylor College of Medicine
Houston, Texas
Chapter 15

ANNA GANASSINI, MD
Chief Assistant, Respiratory Division
Servizio di Fisiopatologia Respiratoria
Divisione di Pneumologia
Ospedale Maggiore di Verona
Verona, Italy
Chapter 5

JESSE B. HALL, MD
Professor of Medicine and of Anesthesia and Critical
Care
Chief, Section of Pulmonary and Critical Care Medicine
Director, Medical Intensive Care Unit and Respiratory
Therapy
Pritzker School of Medicine
University of Chicago
Chicago, Illinois
Chapter 11

JAMES W. LEATHERMAN, MD
Hennepin County Medical Center
Minneapolis, Minnesota
Chapter 14

HÉCTOR LITVAN, MD
Chief of Cardiac Anesthesia and Post-Operative
Intensive Care Unit
Hospital Santa Creu i Sant Pau
Universitat Autònoma de Barcelona
Barcelona, Spain
Chapter 17

CONSTANTINE A. MANTHOUS, MD
Assistant Clinical Professor of Medicine
Pulmonary and Critical Care Division
Yale University School of Medicine
Bridgeport Hospital
Bridgeport, Connecticut
Chapter 11

WILLIAM A. MARINELLI, MD
Assistant Professor of Medicine
Division of Pulmonary and Critical Care
University of Minnesota
Hennepin County Medical Center
Minneapolis, Minnesota
Chapter 14

G. UMBERTO MEDURI, MD
Professor of Medicine
Division of Pulmonary and Critical Care Medicine
University of Tennessee, Memphis
Veterans Affairs Medical Center
Memphis, Tennessee
Chapter 12

NESTOR A. MOLFINO, MD
Adjunct Professor of Medicine
Department of Medicine
McGill University
Vice-President, Scientific Affairs
Theratechnologies, Inc.
Montreal, Canada
Chapter 3

PATRICK T. MURRAY, MD
Assistant Professor of Anesthesia, Critical Care
Medicine, and Clinical Pharmacology
University of Chicago
Chicago, Illinois
Chapter 9

LUIS J. NANNINI, JR., MD, FCCP
Hospital de G. Baigorria
Facultad de Ciencias Médicas
Universidad Nacional de Rosario
Rosario, Argentina
Chapter 2

RITU NAYAR, MD
Assistant Professor of Pathology
Northwestern University Medical School
Chicago, Illinois
Chapter 4

MICHAEL R. PINSKY, MDCM, FCCP, FCCM
Director of Research
Division of Critical Care Medicine
Professor of Anesthesiology and Critical Care Medicine
University of Pittsburgh School of Medicine
Pittsburgh, Pennsylvania
Chapter 7

CARLOS RODRIGO, MD
Centro de Tratamiento Intensivo
Asociación Española Primera de Socorros Mutuos
Montevideo, Uruguay
Chapters 8, 10

GUSTAVO J. RODRIGO, MD
Departmento de Emergencia
Hospital Central de las FF AA
Montevideo, Uruguay
Chapters 8, 10

R. RODRIGUEZ-ROISIN, MD, FRCP
Professor of Medicine
Chairman, Department of Medicine
Universitat de Barcelona
Barcelona, Spain
Chapter 6

ANDREA ROSSI, MD
Divisione di Pneumologia
Ospedale Civile Maggiore di Borgo Trento
Azienda Opedaliera di Verona
Verona, Italy
Chapter 5

MICHAEL SCHATZ, MD
Department of Allergy
Kaiser Permanente Medical Center
San Diego, California
Chapter 16

CARLOS D. SCHEINKESTEL
Clinical Associate Professor
Monash University
Alfred Hospital
Victoria, Australia
Chapter 13

DAVID H. SMITH, PhD
University of Washington Visiting Research Fellow
Centre of Health Economics
University of York
York, England
Chapter 1

SEAN D. SULLIVAN, PhD
Associate Professor
Departments of Pharmacy and Health Services
University of Washington
Seattle, Washington
Chapter 1

DAVID V. TUXEN, MD, FRACP, DHM
Honorary Clinical Associate Professor
Director of Intensive Care and Hyperbaric Medicine
Alfred Hospital
Prahran, Victoria, Australia
Chapter 13

KEVIN WEISS, MD
Associate Professor of Internal Medicine
Rush Medical College
Director, Center for Health Services Research
Rush Primary Care Institute
Rush-Presbyterian-St. Luke's Medical Center
Chicago, Illinois
Chapter 1

ROBERT A. WISE, MD
Professor of Medicine
Johns Hopkins Asthma Center
Baltimore, Maryland
Chapter 16

ANJANA V. YELDANDI, MD
Associate Professor
Department of Pathology
Northwestern University Medical School
Chicago, Illinois
Chapter 4

KARI J. ZAHORIK, MD
Clinical Fellow in Allergy
Section of Allergy and Clinical Immunology
Department of Medicine
University of Wisconsin Hospital and Clinics
Madison, Wisconsin
Chapter 18

PREFACE

The idea for this book originated in South America, but through close friendship and professional collaboration it traveled quickly north to Chicago. The four editors, all engaged in the study and care of acutely ill asthmatics, recognized a need for a textbook devoted to the care of these patients. The primary purpose of this text, we felt, should be the delivery of state-of-the-art information to practicing clinicians.

We decided that a definitive text of acute severe asthma must accomplish two distinctly different goals—both quite analogous to good patient care. First, it must provide constructive information on the assessment and management of the acute attack—with the goal of restoring the patient, without complication, to a state of quiet breathing. This required comprehensive chapters on assessing the acutely ill patient, acute care pharmacology, bronchodilator delivery, face-mask ventilation, and intubation and mechanical ventilation.

But that was not enough. We recognized that many cases of acute asthma represent failure of outpatient management and its fundamental components of education, communication, environmental control, pharmacotherapy, and an acute action plan. We therefore felt strongly that we should review key elements of these issues, believing that they should be addressed in the acute care setting whenever possible to prevent future exacerbation. We think it is no longer acceptable to discharge a patient home with the hope that another healthcare provider will address these issues at some later date. That happens all too infrequently.

No discussion of acute asthma would be complete without an analysis of the alarming trends in asthma prevalence and mortality that have occurred in many parts of the world over the last several decades. We have therefore included chapters on epidemiology, morbidity, and mortality and hope emphatically to make the point that we must support sound epidemiologic research as well as practice good outpatient care to turn the tide. We must understand the basis for worsening asthma and the "asthma paradox" (i.e., increasing asthma morbidity and mortality despite advances in the understanding and treatment of asthma), or we can expect to see more and more cases of acute asthma and death from asthma in the years to come.

We attempted to appeal to a wide range of clinicians, realizing that most, at some point in their careers, are faced with the challenges of assessing and managing the acutely ill asthmatic. Most chapters contain information important to all, while others, such as those on pediatric asthma, pregnancy, anesthesia, and mechanical ventilation, may be better suited to the specialist. If we have done our job, practitioners of family practice, general practice, obstetrics, pediatrics, internal medicine, emergency medicine, anesthesia, intensive care, allergy, and pulmonology will all find this text useful.

One of the advantages of having editors on both sides of the equator is that we have had access to an incredibly talented, international set of authors. Of this we are most proud. We asked our contributors to write state-of-the-art, extensively referenced, and evidence-based reviews for the clinician. They have produced superb contributions. We apologize to them for delays along the way and a zealous review process; these efforts were necessary to produce a book that is homogeneous in style and readily accessible to the reader.

In addition to chapter authors, we wish to thank Dr. Alan Leff, Professor of Medicine at the University of Chicago, for writing the Introduction and for his tireless devotion to academic scholarship and basic asthma investigation, which has yielded many successes. We also wish to thank our publisher, McGraw-Hill, for its support of this project. Without the patience and persistence of McGraw-Hill editors Susan Noujaim, Peter Boyle, Michael Medina, Joe Hefta, and Martin Wonsiewicz, this project would not have been so easy and enjoyable. Finally, we wish to thank Eileen Brendel for her steadfast commitment and unsurpassed secretarial support.

Jesse B. Hall, MD
Thomas C. Corbridge, MD
Carlos Rodrigo, MD
Gustavo J. Rodrigo, MD

INTRODUCTION

During the past decade, there has been remarkable progress in the elucidation of the pathogenesis of asthma. The understanding of asthma as an inflammatory process of the conducting airways has focused on therapeutic interventions that have led us into the era of designer drugs. A new generation of high potency inhaled corticosteroids has freed many patients from the requirements for oral corticosteroids, thus avoiding potentially devastating side effects. In addition, the development of long-acting β_2-adrenergic agonists, also administered by inhalation, has improved substantially the quality of life for asthma patients. New classes of drugs currently in use, such as the anti-leukotriene agents, have provided therapy targeted at specific inflammatory pathways. In the near future, other compounds directed at cytokines and ligands associated with inflammatory cell activation and migration promise to afford even better therapies for the tens of millions of patients afflicted with asthma.

These exciting new developments, and the promise they hold forth, also pose a perverse danger. The battle is not won, and asthma therapy—even when administered optimally—may still fail. About 7–10% of all patients with asthma have severe asthma. To date, there is no convincing evidence that this phenotype can be distinguished early in life or that progression to severe asthma can be prevented by current therapies. What is clear is that the 20% of asthma patients who are the most severely affected consume 80% of the total cost of asthma care. While poor adherence and suboptimal treatment regimens often account for failed therapy, asthma treatment for the severely affected is complex and expensive. And for some, even the best therapies do not bring the disease under full control.

Thus, while we can expect asthma therapies to continue to improve into this millenium, epidemiological trends suggest that we can also expect the number of asthma patients to continue to increase and, with this, the number of severe asthmatics who will fail therapy for various reasons. At best, this will lead to weeks of missed work or school each year—at worst, to hospitalization or, increasingly, fatal asthma. The danger of the optimism spawned by the new therapies, which unquestionably have improved the lives of millions of asthma patients, is that acute asthma, which occurs most often in the minority of severely affected patients, will become an orphan disease. Indeed, the proportion of severe asthma patients has not decreased in recent decades, despite improved therapies, and costs and incidence continued to increase. It is thus particularly important that we are not lulled into complacency by the pharmacological progress made to date. Indeed, the demand for care of acute asthma is greater than ever.

It therefore is with particular excitement that I introduce this new textbook by Hall, Corbridge, Rodrigo, and Rodrigo, *Acute Asthma: Assessment and Management*. This multidisciplinary approach addresses the problem of acute asthma head-on, beginning with the epidemiological and economic impact of acute asthma and progressing to description of the characteristics of these patients that separate them clinically from the more fortunate majority of asthma patients whose disease can be controlled reasonably well. The treatment arena for patients with severe acute asthma is different. Acutely ill asthma patients often do not see their usual treating physicians. They appear in emergency settings to physicians unfamiliar with the patient, a patient who may be too dyspneic to relate a clear history. There may be little time for decision making, respiratory failure may ensue quickly, and failure to support ventilation of these patients in a timely way is the ultimate disaster.

Even when intervention is timely, an entirely new set of problems must be addressed. These problems that often accompany severe acute asthma—need for mechanical ventilation, sedation, and paralysis; hypercapnea and acidosis; and barotrauma—are never encountered in the routine management of asthma. It is with great interest and anticipation that I note that each of these concerns is addressed by outstanding authors in this textbook. Finally, *Acute Asthma: Assessment and Management* culminates in a discussion of educational intervention and chronic asthma. An understanding of both is offered to the clinician so that he or she may prevent the patient from experiencing another frightening encounter with severe acute asthma.

Viewed in another way, acute asthma is a different disease than even severe stable asthma. For reasons not fully defined, patients lose their ability to respond to bronchodilator medications. Issues of muscle fatigue and barotrauma emerge as imminent life-threatening events. Mechanical ventilation and refractoriness to massive pharmacological therapy occur in patients who only days previously may have been reasonably stable on self-administered medications. This is a special disease process, requiring special skills and a carefully contemplated therapeutic approach. It is the ultimate hope that if acute asthma is managed well, all asthma patients, even those most severely affected, will live to see the day when novel therapies insure that these events occur no longer. Until then, we are fortunate to have a reference such as *Acute Asthma: Assessment and Management* so that our sickest patients will come to enjoy these better days.

Alan R. Leff, MD
Chicago, IL

ACUTE ASTHMA

ASSESSMENT AND MANAGEMENT

Chapter 1

EPIDEMIOLOGY AND COSTS OF ACUTE ASTHMA

David H. Smith
Kevin Weiss
Sean D. Sullivan

INTRODUCTION

Asthma is currently viewed as a chronic inflammatory disease of the airways. This view is based on pathophysiologic observations, but to fully characterize this disease, the social impact on individuals, their family and friends, or within their community also needs to be understood. From the perspective of the asthmatic patient, this condition is often characterized by long periods without asthma symptoms (mild subclinical inflammatory disease state) interspersed with shorter periods of highly variable acute exacerbations, during which these patients would consider themselves to have active asthma. To affected individuals, these acute exacerbations cause important disruptions in their daily activities that, not infrequently, lead to the need for urgent care. Periods of acute exacerbations similarly impact on their family and friends. For children with asthma, acute exacerbations lead to disruptions in their parents' or other caretakers' daily work or recreational activities. For adults, acute exacerbations can lead to significant work loss and possibly affect career or family decisions. From a societal perspective, these acute episodes, which often lead to emergency department (ED) visits, hospitalizations, and rarely, to death, have substantial health economic impact in both public and private health sectors.

The purpose of this chapter is to explore what is known about the epidemiology and socio-economic burden of acute asthma. Using epidemiologic and health economic information, the authors present an overview of the social burden of acute asthma. The first section of this overview explores how the epidemiologic literature contributes to our understanding of the burden of acute asthma. The second section examines what is known about the health economic impact of acute asthma.

Since the focus of this book is on acute rather than chronic asthma, a number of interesting issues relating to the comprehensive social burden of asthma is beyond the scope of this review. However, a number of interesting comprehensive reviews of asthma epidemiology,[1-5] and health economics[6,7] are available for the reader. Also, whenever possible, the authors have included a multinational perspective. However, owing to the limited availability of national population-based health data, much of the information presented will draw heavily on the United States experience, where comprehensive national health surveillance data is maintained by the National Center for Health Statistics (NCHS) and the Agency for Health Care Policy and Research (AHCPR).

EPIDEMIOLOGY OF ACUTE ASTHMA

It seems most useful to begin an examination of the epidemiology of acute asthma with a perspective of the overall prevalence of the disease. Asthma is currently estimated to afflict 14 to 15 million people in the United States,[8] more than 5% of the population. About 4.8 million (33%) of those with asthma are less than 18 years of age, based on data from the U.S. National Health Interview Survey (NHIS).[8] From 1982 to 1992, the overall annual U.S. age-adjusted self-reported prevalence increased from 34.7 per 1000 to 49.4 per 1000 population (42% increase). Among those 5 to 34 years of age, the prevalence increased from 34.6 per 1000 to 52.6 per 1000 (52% increase). The prevalence rate for males increased from 39.7 to 51.4 per 1000 (29% increase), while the rate for females increased from 29.4 to 53.6 per 1000 (82% increase).[9] In 1984, the overall age-adjusted self-reported prevalence rate was approximately 37 per 1000 and the rate for African Americans was approximately 32 per 1000. By 1992, African Americans had a higher prevalence rate, approximately 58 per 1000, while the overall rates had increased to 52 per 1000.[9] These data also indicate that, in recent years, the increase in asthma prevalence in the United States has occurred more dramatically among: 1) females, 2) those who are less than 35 years of age, and 3) blacks.

Because international surveys on both adults[10] and children[11] have recently been conducted, more is now known about the international variations in asthma prevalence. Worldwide, over 100 million people are estimated to be afflicted with asthma.[7] The prevalence of asthma varies significantly from country to country, however. For example, in 1990, asthma prevalence was estimated at 3% in Sweden, 4% in the United States, 6% in the United Kingdom and 8.5% in Australia.[7] Physician-diagnosed asthma in New Zealand and Australia has been estimated at 11% to 13%, 1.2% in Erfurt, Germany, and 1.5% to 3% in Spain.[12] It is well known, however, that the data regarding prevalence of asthma is highly dependent on the definition used. The rate of self-reported asthma appears to vary substantially depending on the exact wording of the questions asked, as well as how the survey is administered.[5,10] For example, United States estimates of asthma prevalence can vary from 3 to 10.5% depending on the questions employed to ascertain asthma prevalence.

While there is much literature available on the general burden of asthma, it is more difficult to characterize the specific epidemiology of acute asthma. With the waxing and waning of symptoms, the burden of this illness is not easy to clearly estimate. To our knowledge, while there are several longitudinal cohort studies of the *natural* history of asthma, there are no population-based longitudinal studies examining the burden of asthma. Therefore, any description of the burden of acute asthma will be limited to information based on cross-sectional population studies. Also, there are no commonly used definitions of "acute asthma." Without a clear definition, investigators are limited to devising proxy measures for acute asthma, using *acute asthma events*. Perhaps the most common acute asthma events in epidemiologic literature are based on health care utilization (e.g., the number of times a patient sought urgent care, including unscheduled doctor visits; visits to an ED; or hospital admissions). Asthma mortality, although infrequent, is also commonly viewed as a measure of the burden of acute asthma, independent of any type of health care utilization.

Hospitalizations For Asthma

In 1994 there were an estimated 450,000 hospital admissions for asthma in the United States.[13] From 1980 to 1993, the annual U.S. hospital admission rate for patients 0 to 24 years of age increased from 16.8 per 10,000 to 21.4 per 10,000 population (28%).[14] Age-adjusted annual rates of hospital discharge with asthma as the primary diagnosis decreased slightly during 1982 to 1992 from 18.4 per 10,000 to 17.9 per 10,000.[14] Among those 5 to 34 years of age, the rate remained stable during 1982 and 1993 at 12.8 per 10,000. However, rates for females were consistently higher than for males, and rates for blacks were consistently higher than for whites.[9] In 1993, among those patients 0 to 24 years of age, blacks were 3.4 times more likely to be hospitalized for asthma. Boys 0 to 14 years of age were more likely to be hospitalized than girls in the same age range, but in the 15- to 24-year-old range, girls were 2.1 times more likely than boys to be hospitalized for asthma.[14]

In the United Kingdom, there were almost 94,000 hospitalization episodes for asthma totalling over 3.2 million bed days in National Health Service (NHS) hospitals during the 1994 to 1995 fiscal year.[15] One study done in New South Wales, Australia,[16] estimated that there were 16,223 hospital admissions in 1986, an increase of 30% between 1979 and 1986. The greatest relative increases during this period occurred for patients less than 15 years of age; patients more than 45 years of age maintained stable admission rates during this same period. One study reported that there were 281,000 bed days of inpatient asthma care throughout Canada in 1990.[17]

While hospitalizations represent an important aspect of acute asthma, ED or dispensary use may be a better proxy of acute asthma because hospitalizations for asthma are often preceded by an ED visit and ED visits do not frequently end in hospitalizations.

Emergency Department Visits for Asthma

In the United States, asthma represents the eleventh most frequent diagnosis (illness or injury) in the ED, and adolescents and young adults are the most likely age groups to visit the ED for treatment.[18] Unfortunately, there is little data on the characteristics of those who use the ED for acute episodes of asthma.[19] There are however, some small hospital-based studies that have examined the epidemiology of ED use for acute asthma. One recent study[20] compared the characteristics of two groups of age- and gender-matched patients with recurrent visits to the ED at a large medical center in Chicago, Illinois. One group of 26 patients with recurrent ED visits had one hospital admission for asthma per year, and another group of 28 patients had two or more hospital admissions per year for asthma. The researchers found that patients with multiple hospital admissions were more likely to be African American, have been prescribed inhaled corticosteroids, and have had asthma onset before 11 years of age. Patients with multiple admissions also had a greater average length of stay

(3.3 days versus 2.4 days, p < .05) than did those with one or less hospitalizations per year.

There is little population-based international data available regarding the use of emergency care for asthma. Much of the literature on this subject reflects information based on small geographic areas, or from individual health care institutions. One study reported 182,000 emergency visits for asthma in Canada in 1990.[17] Data from New South Wales show that asthma accounted for 12.3% of all emergency visits at the Royal Alexandra Hospital for Children in 1990, and that, at the Royal Prince Alfred Hospital, asthma accounted for 2% of all adult emergency care visits.[16] The authors estimate that there were over 55,000 total emergency care visits due to asthma between 1988 and 1989. A study in Greenwich, England, showed that of patients who had an exacerbation of asthma in the last 6 months of the study, 50% sought urgent medical help.[21]

Asthma Mortality

Unlike the hospital admissions and ED visits, asthma mortality is a rare event that has been well studied. Deaths from asthma are especially troubling, given that they are often considered to be preventable. In the United States, from 1982 through 1991, the overall annual age-adjusted death rate for asthma increased from 13.4 per million population to 18.8 per million (40% increase). Interestingly, the rate for males increased by 34%, while the rate for females increased by 59%.[9] During this same period, the age-adjusted death rate among those 5 to 34 years of age increased by 42%, similar to the overall annual increase of 40%.[14] However, among those patients 0 to 24 years of age, the age-adjusted death rate increased by 118% from 1980 to 1993, and in 1993, of those in this age group, blacks and males were much more likely to die from asthma.[8]

As shown in Figure 1.1, the long-term trends in asthma mortality in the United States have consistently demonstrated higher rates for blacks than for other races. In 1994, the death rate for blacks was more than double the rate for other races. Sly and O'Donnell found that the U.S. age-adjusted

**Age Adjusted US Death Rate From Asthma
per 100,000 Population, 1984 - 1994**

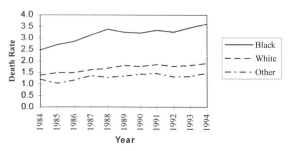

Figure 1-1

Age-adjusted U.S. death rate from asthma, 1984–1994 (per 10,000 persons). (From Office of Analysis and Epidemiology: Mortality Statistics, National Center for Health Statistics. Atlanta, Center for Disease Control, 1998.)

rates for asthma mortality increased significantly (p < 0.0001) for blacks versus whites between 1980 and 1990.[22]

There are also geographic variations in the pattern of asthma mortality in the United States. In children and young adults, for example, one study showed that Cook County, Illinois, had death rates as high, and New York City had death rates three times as high as the United States over-all.[23] Other work has shown that extremely high rates of death from asthma appear to be concentrated in inner city areas and in small areas of high poverty.[24–26]

Internationally, there are also differences in patterns of asthma mortality. In the 1960s, for example, England and Wales, Scotland, Ireland, New Zealand, Australia, and Norway experienced dramatic increases in asthma mortality rates, while the United States, Germany, and Canada had relatively stable rates.[1] As shown in Figure 1-2, the relatively high death rates in New Zealand and Australia in the late 1980s and early 1990s converged in the mid-1990s with the death rates seen in the United States, England and Wales, and Canada.[27,28]

ECONOMIC BURDEN OF ACUTE ASTHMA

The previous section explored the social impact of asthma from an epidemiologic perspective. While this perspective is important in determining the sheer numbers of individuals experiencing acute episodes of asthma, it presents only a unidimensional view of the true social impact. Another important perspective of the social burden of asthma that has recently been receiving increasing attention relates to its economic burden. This next section attempts to characterize the current understanding of the economic burden of acute asthma.

Burden Of Illness Studies

Burden of illness studies enumerate and quantify the pain and suffering, quality of life changes, lost productivity, premature mortality, and direct financial (medical and nonmedical) costs resulting from disease. These studies estimate illness burden by using standard economic evaluation methods that value disease morbidity and mortality as lost opportunity. The results of these studies are used

Figure 1-2

International patterns of asthma mortality (deaths per 100,000 persons), 1960–1994 in persons 5 to 34 years of age, showing the different trends. ■–■, New Zealand; ●–●, England and Wales; △–△, Australia; ○–○, Canada; □–□, United States. (With permission, from Beasley, et al[27])

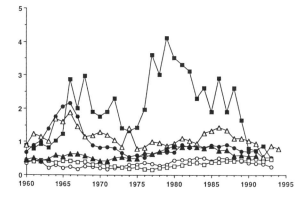

Table 1-1
Components of the costs of acute asthma

Societal Perspective	
Health system perspective *(direct expenditures)*	*Patient perspective* *(indirect expenditures)*
Urgent office visits	Work loss
Emergency department visits	School loss
Hospitalization	Housekeeping loss
Medications, equipment, and supplies	Days of restricted activity
	Mortality

to inform policy makers about the relative societal health and economic impact of a specific illness.

Recently, there have been several prevalence-based burden of illness studies of asthma, both in the United States[29,30] and internationally.[16,17] The United States studies estimated that the total burden of asthma was approximately $6 billion per year, between 1992 and 1994 ($600 to $700 per asthmatic).[29,30] These reports considered a wide range of social and medical care costs of asthma, but failed to differentiate between acute and nonacute disease.

Acute asthma occurs when the patient has an asthma exacerbation. These acute attacks and their sequela are viewed differently, from a burden of illness viewpoint, depending on the perspective of the analyst. Table 1-1 lists key components of the cost of asthma from both the patient and the health system perspective. The societal perspective takes both of these perspectives (patient and health system) into account in the same estimate.

From the perspective of patients, an acute event includes the immediate pain and suffering involved, as well as the period of disability that may follow as they begin to stabilize. The entire period of disability would include time spent receiving emergency treatment as well as the recovery time. Recovery time from an acute episode of asthma includes the time spent both at work and home when activities are restricted to less than their usual level. Estimating the burden from the

patient's perspective also includes consideration of other patient-related expenses, such as the cost of travelling to and from the health care provider or out-of-pocket expenses for nonprescribed medications and health care equipment.

The health system perspective draws specific attention to elements of utilization and the incurred cost of medical resources. These factors may include: 1) frequency and use of emergency care (hospital and ED treatments), 2) additional ambulatory visits, 3) telephone consultations, 4) medications and tests as a consequence of the acute event; and 5) cost of medical and nonmedical personnel involved in the treatment and subsequent posttreatment period. Also, costs to society include the loss of work productivity and increased amount of time necessary for the care of a sick child. Health economics also estimate the costs of premature mortality, which is estimated as the lifetime loss of earnings due to loss of productivity.

It is worth noting at least one caveat in the above assessment of the costs of acute asthma: this approach is to assume that the impact of acute asthma on societal, health system, and individual costs can be linked back to the acute event itself. This assumption may not be accurate. An additional concern of illness burden determination has to do with measurement of nonmedical economic impact. The loss of worker productivity (time lost from work, school and housekeeping) *may or may not be associated with an acute event*. It is possible

Table 1-2

Annual health system use and expenditures for acute asthma in the United States (in millions)

	Weiss, et al[a] (1985 data)	Smith, et al[a] (1987 data)	NHDS,[b] NAMCS[b] (1994 data)
Emergency Department (ED)			
Number of visits	1.8	1.2	1.6
Expenditures	$200	$187	$483
Hospitalizations			
Number of visits	0.46	0.45	0.45
Expenditures	$1,059	$1,534	$1,694
Total ED and Hospital Expenditures	$1,259	$1,721	$2,177

[a]NOTE: From Weiss, et al[29]; Smith, et al.[30]

[b]ABBREVIATIONS: NHDS, The 1994 National Hospital Discharge Survey; NAMCS, The 1994 National Ambulatory Medical Care Survey (*From Sullivan and Weiss.*[13])

that asthma patients lose a day from work or school when they are seeking preventive maintenance care (i.e., not necessarily care for an acute exacerbation). The problem becomes, in part, one of definition of acute asthma. To the extent that this misattribution occurs, the data presented here are an overestimate of the impact of acute asthma. The data from burden of illness studies do not contain information about the circumstances surrounding loss of productivity, and thus do not define the state of the patient's asthma on the day of lost work. Because of these issues, the use of burden of illness studies to characterize acute asthma should be viewed with appropriate caution.

Patient Perspective Burden of illness studies can give some insight into the valuation of the components of acute asthma that are important from the patient's perspective. As shown in Table 1-1, it can be seen that the indirect factors that are important in assessing the impact of asthma from the patient's perspective are days lost from work, school and housekeeping; days of restricted activity at work, school or home; and the impact to society and family because of premature mortality. In the United States, the annual number of workdays lost because of asthma has been estimated to be from 2.1 to 3 million at an estimated

cost between $222 million and $346.3 million. School-loss estimates in the United States, for children less than 18 years of age, have ranged from 3.6 to 10 million days. The economic value assigned to these days is the value of the caregiver time when the child must stay at home. This value has a wide range of estimates, from $195 to $900 million. Housekeeping loss in the United States has been estimated at 769,000 days, and also has a wide range of economic impact, estimated from $21 to $503 million. These estimates for housekeeping and school-loss days are complicated by the use of data from different surveys, and the differing assumptions regarding the value of a lost day.[29,30] In Australia, asthma has been ranked as the sixteenth most common cause of illness at home, accounting for 400,000 to 500,000 days of lost work, valued at Aus$48 million in 1990.[16] The same study estimated that Aus$850,000 was forgone in 1990 because of waiting-time associated with accident and emergency care visits.

Restricted activity days, defined as a day when asthma causes the patient to be unable to engage in normal activities for at least one-half day, have been estimated to be 218 million days annually, at a cost of $18.3 million, in the United States.[30] With children 0 to 4 years of age who need a caregiver when asthma causes them to stay in bed, the caregiver also has lost productivity. Bed days for this group of children has been estimated at 369,000 days, with the lost productivity for the caregiver valued at $19 million annually.[30]

United States mortality associated with asthma in the late 1980s has been estimated to cause an economic loss of approximately $700 million annually.[29] However, asthma mortality in the United States has slowly increased since the 1980's, from less than 4000 deaths in 1985 to more than 5400 deaths in 1994. Thus, current costs related to asthma mortality most likely represent over $1 billion in lost productivity annually in the United States.

Health System Perspective   Table 1-2 lists the U.S. direct health system expenditure estimates for 1985, 1987, and 1994. The estimates are derived from two studies, [29,30] as well as recent analyses of the 1994 National Ambulatory Medical Care Survey (NAMCS), and the 1994 National Hospital Discharge Survey (NHDS).[13] One study, by Weiss and colleagues, used the 1985 NHDS and the 1985 NHIS,[29] while the Smith study used estimates from the 1987 National Medical Expenditure Survey.[30]

As shown in Table 1-2, annual ED visits for asthma have been estimated to cost from $200 million in 1985 to $483 million in 1994. The estimates also demonstrate that ED visits for asthma have decreased slightly from 1.8 million visits in 1985 to 1.6 million in 1994. Hospitalization expenditure estimates range from $1 billion in 1985 to $1.7 billion in 1994. The number of asthma hospitalizations has stayed relatively constant at 450,000 during the 10-year period from 1985 to 1994. Total expenditures for the direct costs of acute asthma range from $1.3 to $2.1 billion. These data suggest that the direct medical expenditures for acute asthma have increased by 86% during this period, with very little change in the number of hospital visits or ED use. Since there were no appreciable changes in the use of services, the increase may be the result of medical care inflation and the use of costly new technologies.

Regardless of the causes, it is interesting that despite sharp rises in the prevalence of asthma, overall use of ED and hospital care has remained relatively constant. Some of this apparent lack of

rise in hospital use may be the reflection of a decreased propensity to admit patients with acute asthma to the hospital due to improved ED management, especially considering the increased prevalence of managed care. One recent study on the use of the ED for accelerated diagnostic protocols for chest pain showed that increased ED management can reduce hospitalization rates, length of stay and total cost.[31]

Modest hospitalization rate changes may also be the result of better management of asthma with maintenance medications. For example, in the United States during 1985 and 1987, theophylline was the most frequently prescribed medication for those with asthma, followed by β_2 agonists.[29,30] From 1988 to 1991, there is evidence that inhaled β_2 agonists were the most frequently prescribed medications, followed by oral corticosteroids; theophylline was the third most frequently prescribed medication.[32] This shift in treatment patterns was expected in light of recommendations from the U.S. National Treatment Guidelines for Diagnosis and Treatment of Asthma released during 1991.[3,33]

Acute asthma, as measured by hospitalization and ED visits, was responsible for almost 60% of the overall annual direct costs of asthma in 1987. However, less than 25% of people with asthma were ever admitted to an ED or were hospitalized, indicating that although few people with asthma may have an acute episode requiring intensive intervention, in terms of health care utilization, the impact of acute asthma episodes on asthma-related health care costs is great.

Recognizing the shortcomings of a single measure to gauge the impact of acute asthma, Vollmer and colleagues summarized an episode of acute asthma by taking into account both inpatient and outpatient care for patients with asthma.[19] Using this approach, these researchers examined health care utilization in a large health care plan in the United States. They demonstrated that the rate of hospitalization for an acute asthma episode declined by approximately 5% for those 0 to 14 years of age, between the periods 1974 to 1980 and 1981 to 1987.[19] The study included all episodes of acute asthma occurring from 1967 to 1987. A consistent pattern of increased annual episodes of care was found for children less than 14 years of age. For boys, acute asthma episodes increased by 469%, from 230 per 100,000 population to 1310 per 100,000, while episodes for girls of the same age increased 200%, from 120 per 100,000 to 360 100,000. The differential increase was even more dramatic for children less than 5 years of age. In this group, acute asthma episodes increased for boys from 285 episodes per 100,000 population to 2025 per 100,000, and for girls, from 272 episodes per 100,000 to 432 per 100,000.

One distinct advantage in the interpretation of episode data versus data that look solely at hospitalization or ED admissions is that the episode data are less sensitive to changes in health care management. For example, decreased hospitalizations may occur because patients are less likely to be admitted over time for any disease, not because acute asthma is becoming less severe or less of a health concern. This issue is particularly germane given that almost 50% of all Americans are now enrolled in some kind of managed care plan,[34] a health care system with an incentive to reduce costs by reducing hospitalizations of any type and delivering more care in the outpatient setting.

Societal Perspective   The societal perspective of the costs of acute asthma is a combination of the patient and health system perspectives, and is therefore a quantification of the overall impact of acute asthma on society. The overall valuation of the indirect costs (patient perspective) of acute asthma was estimated at $1.7 billion in 1990, with mortality costs contributing an additional $819 million.[29] This estimate reflects 1985 data inflated to 1990 dollars. 1987 data inflated to 1994 dollars estimated that the indirect costs of acute asthma, excluding mortality costs, was $673 million.[30] These two studies were done using differing assumptions and datasets, so a range in the estimation is to be expected. Considering these estimates together, the indirect costs of acute asthma range from $1.5 to $2.6 billion. The direct costs (health system perspective) of acute asthma were $2.2 billion in 1994 (Table 1-2). These studies suggest that,

from a societal perspective, a reasonable estimate of the total costs of acute asthma range from $3.7 to $4.8 billion annually.

CONCLUSION

There are currently no well-defined methods for determining the true burden of asthma in its acute phase. Population-based longitudinal studies of the natural history of asthma would be useful; however, they are not readily available. Therefore, much of our understanding of the epidemiology of acute asthma rests on proxy measures, such as emergency care visits, hospital admissions, and mortality.

The economic burden of acute asthma is significant, with U.S. direct expenditures accounting for over $2.1 billion annually. The indirect burden of asthma is also impressive, with mortality accounting for almost $1 billion annually in the United States. Other indirect losses, such as lost productivity owing to missed work, school, and housekeeping are also important in the assessment of the burden of acute asthma (from the patient perspective). It is important to note that, at least for the United States, almost 60% of the direct expenditures for asthma are a result of ED visits and hospitalization, indicating that the majority of dollars spent for the treatment of asthma is used to control acute asthma rather than for early secondary prevention.

Epidemiologic and health economic literature suggests that there is a significant international burden of asthma, in general, and much of the costs of asthma may be due to acute care rather than preventive care. Based on recommendations from various national and international expert panels, asthma, when well treated, should be an illness with very little acute care needs. The data on the social burden of acute asthma may therefore suggest an important failure of various health care systems to efficiently allocate the necessary health care resources toward preventive care interventions that would reduce the social and economic burden of acute asthma.

REFERENCES

1. Weiss KB, Gergen PJ, et al: Breathing better or wheezing worse? The changing epidemiology of asthma morbidity and mortality. *Annu Rev Public Health* 14:491–513, 1993.
2. Moore BB, Sullivan SD, et al: Epidemiology and socioeconomic impact of severe asthma, in Szefler SJ, Leung DYM (eds): *Severe Asthma: Pathogenesis and Clinical Management.* New York, Marcel Dekker, 1995, pp 1–34.
3. National Heart, Lung and Blood Institute, World Health Organization: *Global Strategy for Asthma Management and Prevention; Workshop Report.* Bethesda, National Institutes of Health, 1995.
4. Pearce P, Beasley R, et al: *Asthma Epidemiology: Principles and Methods.* New York, Oxford University Press, 1998.
5. Gergen PJ, Weiss KB: in Busse WW, Tholgate S (eds): *Epidemiology of Asthma. Asthma and Rhinitis.* Boston, Blackwell Scientific, 1994, pp 15–31.
6. Weiss KB, Sullivan SD: The economic costs of asthma: a review and conceptual model. *Pharmacoeconomics* 4(1):14–30, 1993.
7. National Heart, Lung and Blood Institute, World Health Organization: Global Initiative for Asthma: *Global Strategy for Asthma Management and Prevention: Workshop Report, Socioeconomics.* Bethesda, National Institutes of Health, 1995, Chapt. 6.
8. Adams PF, Marano MA: Current estimates from the national health interview survey, 1994. *Vital Health Stat* 10:193, 1995.
9. Asthma—United States, 1982–1992. *MMWR* 43(51–52):952–955, 1995.
10. Chinn S, Burney P, et al: Variation in bronchial responsiveness in the European Community Respiratory Health Survey (ECRHS). *Eur Respir J* 10:2495–2501, 1997.
11. The ISAAC Steering Committee: Worldwide variation in prevalence of symptoms of asthma, allergic rhinoconjunctivitis, and atopic eczema. *Lancet* 352:1225–1232, 1998.
12. Janson C, Chinn S, et al: Physician-diagnosed asthma and drug utilization in the European Community Respiratory Health Survey. *Eur Respir J* 10(8):1795–1802, 1997.
13. Sullivan SD, Weiss KB: Unpublished Data: Estimates from the National Hospital Discharge Survey and the National Ambulatory Medical Care Survey, 1998.
14. Asthma mortality and hospitalization among children and young adults—United States, 1980–1993. *MMWR* 45(17):350–353, 1996.
15. Government Statistical Service: *Hospital Episode Statistics: Finished consultant episodes by diagnosis and operative procedure; injury/poisoning by external causes. England: Financial Year 1994–1995.* London, Government Statistical Service, 1996.
16. Mellis CM, Peat JK, et al: The cost of asthma in New South Wales. *Med J Aus* 155:522–528, 1991.
17. Krahn MD, Berka C, et al: Direct and indirect costs of asthma in Canada, 1990. *Can Med Assoc J* 154(6):821–831, 1996.
18. Burt CW, Knapp DE: Ambulatory care visits for asthma: United States, 1993–1994. *Adv Data* 277:1, 1996.
19. Vollmer WM, Osborne ML et al: Temporal trends in hospital based episodes of asthma care in a health maintenance organization. *Am Rev Respir Dis* 147:347–353, 1993.
20. Olopade CO, Alikakos Z, et al: Characteristics of predominantly nonwhite patients with frequent hospitalizations for acute asthma in Chicago. *J Asthma* 34(3):243–248, 1997.
21. Marks GB, Burney PG, et al: Asthma in Greenwich, UK: Impact of the disease and current management practices. *Eur Respir J* 10(6):1224–1229, 1997.
22. Sly RM, O'Donnell R: Stabilization of asthma mortality. *Ann Allergy Asthma Immunol* 78:347–354, 1997.
23. Weiss KB, Wagener DK: Changing patterns of asthma mortality: Identifying target populations at high risk. *JAMA* 264:1683–1687, 1990.
24. Wissow LS, Gittelsohn AM, et al: Poverty, race, and hospitalization for childhood asthma. *Am J Public Health* 78(7):777–782, 1988.
25. Carr W, Zeitek, et al: Asthma hospitalization and mortality in New York City. *Am J Public Health* 82:59–65, 1992.
26. Marder D, Targonski P, et al: Effect of racial and socioeconomic factors on asthma mortality in Chicago. *Chest* 101(6 suppl.):426S–429S, 1992.
27. Pearce P, Beasley R, et al: Studying time trends in asthma deaths, in *Asthma Epidemiology: Principles and Methods.* New York, Oxford University Press, 199), pp 203–224.
28. Beasley, R, Pearce N, et al: International trends in asthma mortality. *CIBA Foundation Symposium* 206:140–150, 1997.
29. Weiss KB, Gergen PJ, et al: An economic evaluation

of asthma in the United States [see comments]. *N Engl J Med* 326:862–866, 1992.

30. Smith DH, Malone DC, et al: A national estimate of the economic costs of asthma. *Am J Respir Crit Care Med* 156:787–793, 1997.

31. Roberts RR, Zalenski RJ, et al: Costs of an emergency department accelerated diagnostic protocol vs. hospitalization in patients with chest pain: A randomized controlled trial. *JAMA* 278(20):1670–1676, 1997.

32. Lanes SF, Birmann BM, et al: Characterization of asthma management in the Fallon Community Health Plan from 1988 to 1991. *Pharmacoeconomics* 10:378–385, 1996.

33. National Asthma Education Program; Guidelines for the Diagnosis and Treatment of Asthma. Bethesda, National Institutes of Health, 1991.

34. Office of the Actuary: Data from the Office of National Health Statistics. Washington, DC, *Health Care Financing Administration,* 1997.

Chapter 2

MORBIDITY AND MORTALITY FROM ACUTE ASTHMA

Luis J. Nannini, Jr.

INTRODUCTION

Review articles[1-3] and editorials[4-6] have discussed the paradox of the increased morbidity and mortality from asthma, despite the increased knowledge about this disease and the increased availability of new and effective medications. Fortunately, a downward trend in mortality from asthma has been observed in the last few years in some countries, particularly in New Zealand, a country in which asthma death has been of epidemic proportions. The purpose of this chapter is to review trends in asthma mortality, to discuss circumstances surrounding asthma deaths and to offer suggestions to reduce asthma morbidity and mortality.

INTERNATIONAL TRENDS IN ASTHMA MORTALITY

A summary of international trends in asthma mortality can be found in Table 2-1.

New Zealand

The United Kingdom, Australia, and New Zealand all experienced an increase in mortality in the late 1960s. Interestingly, although mortality decreased slightly throughout the 1970s in both the United Kingdom and Australia, it did not do so in New Zealand and, in fact, continued to rise (Fig. 2-1)[7,8] This second epidemic of death from

asthma in New Zealand has been extensively studied. Investigators in Wellington, New Zealand, conducted three consecutive case-control studies[9-11] designed to evaluate the hypothesis that unsupervised self-administration of fenoterol by inhalation increases the risk of death from asthma. In short, these studies suggested that use of fenoterol was associated with an increased risk of asthma death. They also attempted to distinguish a causal effect from the confounding variable that patients with severe disease received more medication, and their mortality rate increased not because of a specific drug effect but because of the severity of their disease. This "confounding" is substantial in nonrandomized epidemiological studies of asthma medications.[12]

Similarly, a group of investigators in Dunedin, New Zealand, believed it highly plausible that the increased mortality in the two New Zealand epidemics was due to a relatively rapid increase in asthma severity associated with the use of the more potent agents, isoproterenol and fenoterol, respectively.[13] Factor(s) that may be responsible for the deleterious effects of these agents are listed in Table 2-2. Whatever the mechanism, the frequent use of these agents appears to have increased the asthma severity and, consequently, morbidity and mortality.[22]

The rapid reversal of the epidemic of asthma deaths in young people in New Zealand following withdrawal of fenoterol in 1990 represents additional strong evidence for a causal link of fenoterol

Table 2-1
International trends in asthma mortality at a glance

Country	Period	Last trend	Mean rate per 100,000
Argentina	1980–1994	down	3.36
Australia	1960–1990	down	
Brazil	1980–1991	down	2.04
Canada	1927–1987	stable	
Chile	1980–1990		1.08
Costa Rica	1982–1991		3.76
Colombia	1979–1994	down	1.6
Cuba	1983–1992		4.09
Czech Republic	1990–1994	down	1.58
Denmark	1969–1988	up	
England/Wales	1960–1990	down	
Greece	1979–1991	down	
France	1925–1989	down	
France	1970–1990	up until 1986	
Ireland	1970–1991	up (25–34 yr group)	
Israel	1971–1990	up in <35 yr group	
Italy	1974–1988	stable	4.17
Japan	1979–1988	downward	
Mexico	1960–1988	down	
Zealand	1976–1992	down	
Paraguay	1991		0.8
Peru	1986–1991		3.7
Switzerland	1969–1993	downward	
Uruguay	1984–1990	down	5.63
United States	1941–1989	doubling	
United States	1980–1993	up in <25 yr group	
Venezuela	1980–1989		3.1

to increased mortality. In 1989, the epidemiological studies from the Wellington group led to a warning from the New Zealand Department of Health that fenoterol should not be used by patients with severe asthma. Fenoterol sales subsequently fell from a stable 30% of the β agonist market between 1983 to 1988 to 6% in 1990. During the same period, the mortality in the 5- to 34-year-old group fell from 2.3 per 100,000 to 1.1 per 100,000 in 1989, and .73 per 100,000 (a mortality rate lower than before the 1960s) in 1990. Thus, the end of the epidemic occurred after the withdrawal of fenoterol in 1990, just as it had commenced when fenoterol was introduced in 1976. By contrast, the increased use of β agonist drugs as a class occurred after the epidemic began; sales

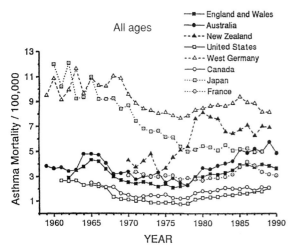

Figure 2-1

International trends in asthma mortality for all ages. 1960–1990. Deaths per 100,000. (From National Institute of Health)

continued to rise as mortality fell. These time-trend observations were sufficiently impressive to implicate fenoterol in the second mortality epidemic in New Zealand, but not β agonists as a class.[23,24]

However, outside New Zealand, asthma mortality has increased in countries where there is little use of fenoterol (e.g., Australia) and in countries in which fenoterol is not used at all (United States). Conversely, fenoterol use in Argentina increased considerably between 1983 and 1990, at which time it had more than 30% of the

market share, just as in New Zealand.[25] However, mortality rates in Argentina remained stable (albeit high) in the 1980s, with a range, for all ages, of 3 to 4 per 100,000, while in the 5- to 34-year-old group the mortality rate was less than 1 per 100,000.[26,27] Similarly, fenoterol has been used extensively in Germany, Austria, and Belgium without an associated epidemic of asthma deaths.[28,29]

Another factor in New Zealand that must be considered is the use of anti-inflammatory agents, and in particular, the use of inhaled steroids. The increased use of these drugs paralleled the mortality trend until 1979. Interestingly, higher dose beclomethasone formulations were used for the first time in 1979, just before the start of the decline of the mortality rate.[30]

Differences in native New Zealanders also confound the analysis. Mortality rates of the Maoris (18.9/100,000) and Pacific Island Polynesians (9.4/100,000) were, respectively, 5.5 and 2.8 times higher than the rate for Europeans (3.4/100,000) in New Zealand. However, the asthma mortality rate in European New Zealanders between the ages of 15 and 64 was 4.2 per 100,000, more than twice the rate of 1.84 per 100,000 found in the same age and racial group in the United Kingdom.[31] The majority of asthma deaths in New Zealand and the United Kingdom were judged to be preventable. In the United Kingdom, 11% of deaths were regarded as unavoidable compared to 27% in New Zealand, in the same age and race group.[7,32]

Overall, asthma is a more common and difficult problem in New Zealand. Many patients who die have suffered from a previous severe attack,[33] and acute asthma is responsible for 12% of admissions to intensive care units as compared with less than 3% in the United States.[34] Furthermore, there was a greater per capita consumption of anti-asthma medication in New Zealand in 1980 than in the United Kingdom and Australia.[35] Also, the therapeutic strategies differed: in the United Kingdom, none of the patients in the study group had a home nebulizer, while in New Zealand, 75 deaths (27%) occurred in asthmatics who had been prescribed domiciliary nebulizers.[36] In this regard, a recent study from Canada demonstrated an in-

Table 2-2

Questionable factors that relate mortality to β_2 agonists

- Cardiac events (pro-arrhythmic factor)[14]
- Hypokalemia and hypomagnesemia[15]
- Inducing poorer control of asthma[16,17]
- Tachyphylaxis of the preventive effects[18,19]
- Tachyphylaxis of the bronchodilator effect[17a,19a]
- Promoting corticosteroid resistance[20,21]
- More use in more severe patients

creased risk of cardiovascular death (not related to asthma) in users of β agonists taken orally or by nebulizer (but not by MDI), especially in patients with acute coronary insufficiency and congestive cardiomyopathy.[37] However, in another study, cardiac arrhythmias could not be demonstrated in patients treated with high doses of nebulized salbutamol.[38]

United States

In 1986, Woolcock questioned why asthma mortality was so low in the United States.[39] However, since then the rate of death from asthma has increased steadily in the United States, as it has in many other countries since the late 1970s.[40–42] In 1988 only 4580 death certificates in the United States listed asthma as the primary cause of death. Consequently, it might be said that mortality from asthma is not itself a major problem in the United States; however, asthma-related mortality rates may be underestimated by death certificate data.[43] An alternative approach to using death certificate data was to do a study in which the outcome of interest was survival from the onset of asthma. Silverstein and colleagues conducted such a study of 2499 residents of Rochester, Minnesota in whom asthma was diagnosed (definite or probable) between January 1, 1964 and December 31, 1983. There were 140 deaths during 14 (range, 0–29) years of follow-up.[44] Four percent of all deaths in the study cohort were due to asthma and survival among patients with asthma and no other lung disease did not differ from expected survival rates. The survival rate of patients over the age of 35 who had asthma and chronic obstructive lung disease was lower than expected. However, it is misleading to extrapolate data from primarily white, average income patients to other groups. As reported by Lang and Polansky, asthma deaths are disproportionately common in minority groups in inner cities and are inversely proportional to the percentage of high-school diplomas.[45] Small-area analyses of asthma hospitalization and mortality rates in New York City,[46] Chicago,[47,48] Baltimore,[49] and the State of California[50] have demonstrated that asthma morbidity and mortality

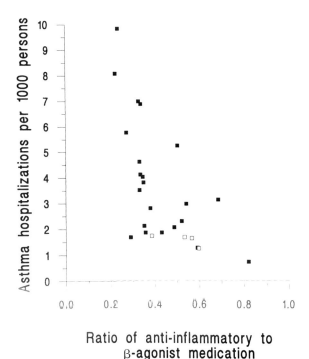

Figure 2-2
Relationship between age- and gender-adjusted asthma hospitalization rate and the ratio of inhaled anti-inflammatory medication (steroid plus cromolyn) to inhaled β agonist dispensed within each small geographic area. Each point represents a single small area: closed squares, *small areas within Boston;* open squares, *small areas in the suburbs adjacent to Boston where >86% of inhabitants are white and only 3 to 9% live in poverty. (From Gottlieb[51])*

are concentrated in inner city neighborhoods characterized by poverty and large minority populations. The reasons for this discrepancy are not completely understood. Possible explanations include lack of access to medical care and underuse of therapy. In other cities, such as Boston, a smaller population and consequently, smaller number of asthma deaths preclude a meaningful comparison of asthma mortality rates among the neighborhoods. However, Boston had an asthma hospitalization rate in 1992 that was twice the statewide rate and among neighborhoods within Boston there was a large variation in asthma hospi-

Table 2-3

Hospital discharges[a] and average length of stay for patients with asthma as first-listed diagnosis and ICD-9CM Code[b] in United States, 1993

	Discharges		
Age groups, yrs	No. of patient (×1000)	Rate per 10,000 population	Length of stay/days
All ages	458	18.3	4.4
Under 15	159	28.0	3.4
15–1944	128	10.9	3.5
45–64	94	19.0	5.4
65 and over	87	26.5	6.7

[a]NOTE: Discharges from nonfederal hospitals; excludes newborn infants.
[b]NOTE: Diagnostic groupings and code number inclusions are based on the International Classification of Diseases, 9th revision, Clinical Modification (ICD-9-CM).[52]

talization rates.[51] The areas with the highest asthma hospitalization rates were concentrated in Boston's inner city; these areas are characterized by high rates of poverty, low per capita income, fewer well-educated people, and large African American and Hispanic populations. Similar findings have been reported for New York City and Chicago.[46–48] In Boston, areas with high asthma hospitalization rates also had a lower ratio of inhaled anti-inflammatory medication (steroids plus cromolyn) to inhaled β agonist dispensed than did areas with low hospitalization rates (Fig. 2-2).[51] These data suggest that underuse of inhaled anti-inflammatory medication contributes to excess asthma morbidity.

Data regarding the number of asthma discharges, rates of asthma per 10,000 individuals, and length of stay, by age, for the entire United States, can be found in Table 2-3.[52]

Canada

Mortality from asthma in Canada has been reported to be highest in the prairie provinces and appears to be narrowly concentrated in patients over the age of 65, but there is a great variation between jurisdictions.[53] Alberta and Saskatchewan shared an overall mortality rate, from 1980 to 1989, of .7 per 100,000 per year among residents

less than 35 years of age, compared to a national rate of .4 per 100,000 for the same age group. Hospitalization for asthma in Alberta increased between 1980 and 1988 by 35% for individuals less than 15 years of age and by 48% for patients 15 to 34 years of age. In Saskatchewan, hospitalization declined by 2% in the younger group and increased by 35% in the older group. Manitoba, the third prairie province, is highly urbanized, as is Alberta, and has a large grain industry (as does Alberta and Saskatchewan). However, the mortality rate in Manitoba from asthma is .3 per 100,000 for residents under the age of 35 (one of the lowest in Canada).[53] In a 6-year study, asthma deaths in Manitoba varied from 13 to 32 per calendar year in 1988 in 1989, respectively. From 1982 to 1984 there were, on average, 17 deaths per year compared with 22 deaths per year from 1987 to 1989. More than 80% of deaths ascribed to asthma occurred in patients 65 years of age or older. However, there was no significant increase in deaths in Manitoba (or, in fact, in all of Canada) in the 1980s, despite an increase in prevalence.[54] This is likely because asthma severity did not increase during that same period of time.[55] Thus, despite an increase of 36.4% in the number of patients diagnosed with asthma between 1983 and 1988 in Manitoba, fewer patients were hospitalized in 1988 than in 1983. The duration of hospitalization and the number of emergency room visits decreased as well. The reason(s) for this encouraging trend in the decrease of hospital use, in the face of increased prevalence, is not clear; however it is possible that increased referral to specialists may have influenced this trend.

Barcelona and Soybean Dust

Twenty-six epidemics of asthma occurred in Barcelona, Spain, from 1981 to 1987. A collaborative research team including physicians, epidemiologists, and meteorologists can be credited for discovering a link between the atmospheric conditions during the unloading of ships in the harbor and outbreaks of asthma.[56,57] They observed that, when ships unloaded soybean under conditions of high barometric pressure and low wind speed, enough soybean dust was blown from the harbor to affect the atmosphere in the city, triggering widespread exacerbations of asthma.[58] The tiny soybean particles were thought to be small enough to enter through sealed windows, bypass the nose, and affect airways, thus explaining why even patients indoors suffered severe attacks.

A serologic case-control study showed that the serum of 64 of 86 (74.4%) epidemic cases had IgE antibodies against soybean antigens by radio-immunoadsorbent testing, compared to 4 of 86 (4.7%) controls.[59] The major allergen causing the epidemics was found to be a glycopeptide with a molecular mass of less than 14 kD, which is abundant in soybean dust.[60] As a result of this multidisciplinary study, bag filters were placed at the top of previously open storage silos, resulting in complete resolution of epidemic asthma. This experience in Barcelona is not similar to the experience in other cities with epidemic asthma, including New Orleans, Brisbane, New York, and Birmingham, mainly because in these cities the specific causes are controversial. However, it is likely that many of these cases (which are often classified as idiopathic) will prove to be caused by airborne allergens.

England and Wales

The total number of hospital admissions with a discharge diagnosis of asthma rose considerably through the 1970s and 1980s in England and Wales. Data from the early 1990s show that the number of hospital admissions stabilized at approximately 100,000 per year, 50% of whom were children. Mortality decreased in the latter half of the 1980s and, although changes were small, they clearly indicated a reversal of previous trends.[61,62]

Latin and South America

Several reports have shown that there was a 95% accuracy rate in the diagnosis of asthma as the underlying cause of death for persons 5 to 34 years of age,[63,64] but only a 61% accuracy rate for those over the age of 54. These data should be taken into account when observing mortality rates in Latin America, since the accuracy of death certificates has not been validated in this region. One study analyzed the accuracy of death certificates in a small geographic area and found a net overestimation of asthma deaths due to registration and coding procedures.[27]

Between 1980 and 1990, the mortality rate for all ages was highest (per 100,000) in Uruguay and Mexico (5.63), and the lowest rates were in Chile (1.86) and Paraguay (0.8). However, in the 5- to 34-year-old group, Costa Rica had the highest mortality rate (1.38 per 100,000).[65]

In Mexico, mortality rates from asthma decreased between 1960 and 1988 despite an increase in hospitalization for asthma from 10 to 140 per 100,000 inhabitants. The states in Mexico with the highest rates were Morelos, Sur Baja California, Nuevo León, Durango and Tamaulipas.[66]

In Cuba, the average asthma mortality rate in 1985 to 1987 was 3.8 per 100,000, while in Havana the rate was 4.3 per 100,000.[67]

Twenty-seven asthma patients in Tarma, Peru, a city situated more than 3000 meters above sea level, and a control group of asthma patients from Lima (situated 150 meters above sea level) were followed for 6 years. At the end of the study, five patients in the high altitude of Tarma died, while there were no deaths in the group from Lima, leading to speculation that hypoxia played a role.[68] In contrast, one Italian study showed that after staying at least 72 hours at high altitude, bronchial responsiveness to hypotonic challenge was significantly reduced in lowland asthmatics.[69] Furthermore, exposure to pollutants and allergens, including house dust mites, was reduced at high altitude.[70]

Between 1984 and 1994 the mortality rate from asthma in Uruguay was 5.45 per 100,000 (inhabitants of all ages), but only 0.52 for inhabitants 5 to 34 years of age.[71] Similarly, in Argentina the official unpublished mortality rates for 1994 were 2.17 and .39 per 100,000 for all ages, and the 5- to 34-year-old group, respectively. Mortality rates in both Mexico and Uruguay have declined slightly in the last decade.[26] Similarly, asthma death rates declined in Sao Paulo, Brazil between 1970 to 1992.[72]

Other Geographic Locations

Between 1970 and 1990 mortality in France increased, peaking in 1986 among those between 5 and 34 years of age.[73] The influenza epidemics in the winter of 1985 and 1986 appear to have been responsible for some of these mortality variations.[74]

In Greece, where the prevalence of asthma is about the same as other European countries, bronchodilator consumption increased dramatically between 1979 and 1991. Despite this increase, annual deaths from asthma decreased continuously from 84 deaths in 1979 to 11 deaths in 1991.[75]

In Switzerland, asthma mortality has decreased in the last several years, particularly in middle-aged males. In the early 1990s, 250 deaths per year were attributed to asthma.[76]

In Denmark, however, asthma mortality rates increased between 1969 and 1988, an increase that could not be explained by coding practices.[77]

In Italy, asthma mortality increased from .3 per 100,000 people in 1978 to 4.17 per 100,000 people in 1985. During that time, the sale of xanthines and β_2 agonists similarly increased. However, between 1985 and 1988 asthma mortality leveled, which may have been related to an increase in the sale of anti-inflammatory medications.[78]

In Yokkaichi, Japan, the recent remarkable improvement in air quality was followed by a decrease in mortality from asthma.[79] Interestingly, in Nagasaki, Japan, the number of deaths due to asthma increased between 1990 and 1992.[80]

Another interesting phenomenon occurred in the South Fore area of the Eastern Highlands of Papua, New Guinea.[81,82] In that area, the rise in prevalence of adult asthma from .1 to 7.3% was not matched by a similar increase in asthma in the adjacent Asaro Valley. Although living conditions in these two areas are comparable, the mean density of house dust mite in the blankets of residents in the South Fore area was found to be significantly higher, suggesting an important role for house dust mites in the pathogenesis of asthma in this area.

THE RELATIONSHIP BETWEEN MORTALITY AND PREVALENCE

Though mortality is closely related to prevalence,[39] high prevalence is not necessarily associated with high mortality, likely due to changes in disease treatment or disease severity.[53,54] Indeed, prevalence and mortality can trend in opposite directions. For instance, in south Australia, childhood wheeze increased significantly from 24% in 1984 to 36% in 1992,[83] but mortality rates have been decreasing since 1989.[84] At this time, mortality and prevalence are probably trending in opposite directions, but this has not yet been confirmed.

On the other hand, a study of Israeli military recruits (which makes up a large percentage of young Jewish adults) demonstrated an increase in asthma prevalence of 21.7% (from 5.3 to 6.5%) between 1986 and 1988.[85] There were no significant changes between 1987 and 1989. During this same period, there was no indication that asthma severity had changed. However, asthma mortality increased in the 5- to 34-year-old group from 0.18 per 100,000 between 1976 to 1980 to .4 per 100,000 between 1980 and 1990.[86]

Another example of the confusing relationship between prevalence and mortality is seen on Tristan da Cunha, a tiny volcanic island with 300 inhabitants, in the middle of the South Atlantic Ocean. Likely because of gene enrichment, there is a high prevalence of asthma on this island. Of

282 islanders tested with methacholine, 46.9% had a positive challenge defined by the provocative dose of methacholine required to drop FEV_1 by 20% being $< 8mg/mL$ ($PC_{20} < 8mg/mL$), with 23% of the population having a $PC_{20} < 4mg/mL$. Despite this incredibly high prevalence of asthma, there is no evidence of excessive mortality. In fact, for the past 50 years the island population has been stable.[87]

PRACTICAL IMPLICATIONS

Death From Asthma

Where   Many asthma deaths occur at home or during transport to the hospital, and the concomitant delays in receiving care have not been adequately addressed by most published guidelines.[88–91] In the United States, between 1979 and 1987, 52.3% of all deaths in the 5- to 34-year-old group occurred outside the hospital.[92] Greater numbers have been reported in other countries. In the United Kingdom, 86% of deaths occurred at home or at work,[32,93–95] and in Argentina more than 70% of deaths occurred outside the hospital.[27] Many (but not all) of these patients had severe chronic asthma, a history of hospitalization and frequent acute episodes.

Why   It must be emphasized that the severity of an asthma attack and the speed with which deterioration occurs are often not appreciated by the patient, relatives, or physicians,[32] in part because of lack of education.[96] In addition, a reduced chemosensitivity to hypoxia and blunted perception of dyspnea during resistive loading in patients who have had a near-fatal asthma attack has been confirmed by Kikuchi and colleagues.[97] Similarly, reduced awareness of bronchoconstriction induced by methacholine has been described in elderly asthmatic patients, also possibly contributing to a lack of appreciation of disease severity and asthma mortality.[98a,b] Whatever the reasons, it is clear that delay in instituting therapy is a crucial contributing factor to asthma deaths.

There are some well-known causes of potentially fatal asthma, including hypersensitivity to aspirin,[99–101] inadvertent β blocker administration (even in eye drops),[102–104] hypersensitivity to sulfites[90,105] and other food preservatives, alcohol,[106] respiratory tract viral infections,[107] exposure to aeroallergens, such as *Alternaria alternata*,[108] soybean dust,[109] strong emotions,[110] and illicit drug use.[111] However, these triggers have been identified in less than 10% of cases of near-fatal asthma, suggesting that there is a lack of education regarding the triggers and mechanism of acute severe disease.[112] It is possible that the epidemic use of inhaled illicit drugs such as "crack" cocaine and heroin will result in increasing morbidity and mortality, at least based upon early anecdotal reports.[112a]

How   1.   *Patients with both asthma and irreversible airflow obstruction* (i.e., "fixed" asthma) are at risk for death when a superimposed attack further increases airflow obstruction and lung hyperinflation, similar to patients with chronic obstructive pulmonary disease (COPD).[113]

2.   *Slow-onset fatal asthma* may occur in any patient, even those with normal lung function between attacks, when airflow obstruction progresses over the course of hours to days. This occurs when there is a delay in initiating appropriate therapy (and occasionally in spite of appropriate therapy).[113a,113b] These patients are often young and have a long history of asthma.[32,114,115]

3.   *Sudden-onset fatal asthma* occurs in less than 3 hours and appears to be pathologically distinct from slow-onset disease. Sudden-onset disease is characterized by a paucity of eosinophils and more neutrophils in the mucosa of the airway, compared with slow-onset attacks.[116] Sudden deaths often occur outside the hospital and may mimic a cardiac event. They are often considered unavoidable deaths because the attacks can occur so suddenly and severely that there is insufficient time for help to arrive.[32,117,118] However, it is possible that a better outpatient program, attention to minimizing triggers, and rapid treatment (such as

Table 2-4
Circumstances surrounding death from asthma

Failure to recognize deteriorating clinical condition[32,36,112,115,118,122–128,129]

Over reliance on β_2 inhalers and nebulizers[10,32,36,94,96,112,114,115,121–131]

High β_2 consumption: more than 1.4 canister per month[131] and less than one inhaled corticosteroid aerosol[132]

A recent hospital admission[122]

Previous near-fatal attack[96,99,118,124–128,133–137]

Lack of access to medical care or delay in seeking help[32,36,46–50,112,124–129,133–137]

Lack of assessment of the severity of the attack[32,90,96,112,124–128,129,133–137]

Poorly perceived asthma[96,97]

Administration of hyperoxic mixtures[5,96]

Unadvertised exposure to precipitating allergens (alternaria alternata,[108] soybean dust),[109] or drugs (β blockers,[102–104] aspirin),[99–101] or conservatives (sodium metabisulfite)[90,105]

Extreme bronchial lability[99,112,116,118,121,123–128,135]

Daily variability in PEFR of greater than 50%[121,123–128]

Psychiatric or psychosocial factors (malignant form)[118,137,138]

access to an emergency syringe for administration of parenteral epinephrine) may prevent some deaths.

Who Although all patients with asthma are at risk[96] of a fatal attack, more women are treated for acute asthma in emergency departments (EDs),[119] and generally there has been an increase in asthma deaths in middle-aged women.[42,73] This observation is not universal; in Hong Kong, between 1976 and 1985, mortality from asthma has increased annually for males in the 5- to 34-year-old group, but not for females.[120]

The presence of eosinophilia, a high degree of reversibility following bronchodilator, advanced age, poor baseline pulmonary function, and smoking are all risk factors for mortality in asthma.[121] Table 2-4 lists those, and other factors associated with asthma death.

When Deaths from asthma occur with increased frequency on the weekends, particularly on Sundays.[33] In the United Kingdom, 41% of deaths occurred between Friday night and Monday, in one study,[32] and an increase in the severity of attacks was reported during weekends.[139]

Seasonal Variations Seasonal variation in asthma mortality has been reported in many countries[108,140] although this is not universally true. In New Zealand, there has been no seasonal pattern in asthma death (or in admission to the ICU) in patients more than 25 years of age.

Seasonal patterns in asthma morbidity have long been recognized and have been linked to seasonal exposure to specific antigens,[108,109,141,142] infections,[143] and high levels of air pollutants.[144,145] For example, analysis of the medical records of a large health maintenance organization (HMO) in the northwestern region of the United States between 1979 and 1987, demonstrated a modest increase in hospitalizations in the spring season and a larger increase in the fall season, in the 0- to 14-year-old group.[146] The 15- to 65-year-old group showed only an increase in spring season hospitalizations, while the over 64-year-old group exhibited a single peak in the late winter/early spring months. Similar patterns for hospitalization have been reported by Weiss, drawing on the National Hospital Discharge Survey.[147] These studies were not designed to identify the cause(s) of seasonal variation.

Unexplained increases in hospital admissions for asthma have been reported in other countries, including Canada, England, and Wales. Dales and colleagues found that among preschool children in metropolitan Toronto, Canada, between 1981 and 1989, respiratory infection was the major identifiable risk factor for the large autumnal increase of asthma hospitalizations.[148] On the other hand, in older epidemiologic studies of viral infections and exacerbations of asthma, virus detection rates have been low, possibly owing to methodologic problems in detecting and identifying respiratory viruses.[149] Through the development of polymerase chain reaction (PCR) assays, Johnston and colleagues[150] reported that viral upper respiratory infections were associated with >80% of asthma exacerbations in children in the Southampton area of the United Kingdom. They also demonstrated a strong correlation between seasonal patterns of upper respiratory infections and hospital admissions for asthma. This relationship was stronger for pediatric admissions than for adult admissions. Not surprisingly, school attendance is a major factor in transmitting respiratory viruses (especially rhinoviruses) and there are more asthma admissions when school is in session than during holidays.[143] In adults, the role of respiratory viruses is less clear.[151]

SOLUTIONS

The outcome of patients with potentially fatal asthma who do not delay treatment and who arrive at the hospital before respiratory arrest,[130,134,152] or even in respiratory arrest,[153] is generally good.[32] In these patients, it is also critical to maintain an adequate circulation to avoid anoxic brain injury. These data stress the importance of education and healthcare access in the earliest stages of acute asthma. Also crucial to the outcome is appropriate

pharmacotherapy (see Chap. 9) and avoidance of premature hospital discharge.[154]

Acute asthma attacks signal the need for education and follow-up to establish an appropriate outpatient program and an acute asthma action plan. Indeed, key elements of such a plan should be addressed in the acute care setting because there is a low participation rate in outpatient education programs among asthmatics recently discharged from the hospital.[155] Also of interest is the fact that the use of emergency room asthma treatment guidelines can decrease monthly asthma relapse rates and monthly asthma admission rates in an inner-city patient population.[156]

Despite the multiple barriers associated with poverty, appropriate outpatient management can diminish morbidity and mortality due to asthma. In this regard, the promotion of education programs or preferably, the creation of an asthma center that provides education, free access, and free inhaled and systemic corticosteroids, could dramatically reduce asthma hospitalization within a few years, despite poverty and low income.[157] Prevention is always better than the best treatment. (Table 2-5)

Attempts to teach self-management skills without addressing whether there are financial and practical concerns (e.g., patients who could not purchase the prescribed drug) are unlikely to suc-

Table 2-5
Solutions

- Access to expert-based care systems
- Education in the acute care setting and in the outpatient setting
- Increased use of anti-inflammatory medications
- Monitoring accuracy of death certificates
- Confidential inquiry into asthma deaths to provide feedback regarding quality care to healthcare providers
- Free treatment for residents in the populations at high risk
- Epidemiologic research regarding trends in prevalence and mortality

---

ceed. There are marked differences between the knowledge of self-management that patients have and their actual behavior, particularly in terms of potentially life-saving actions such as seeking medical help when appropriate or calling for an ambulance. Some factors associated with this knowledge-behavior gap are: 1) being non-European, 2) anxiety, 3) concerns about medical costs, and 4) sole reliance on Social Security for household income.[158]

Concurrent with education and healthcare access must be the appropriate use of anti-inflammatory medications.[152a,b,c] Indeed, sales of medium- and high-dose inhaled corticosteroids are a marker of good overall management.[30,77,159] Fortunately, recommendations for early use of anti-inflammatory therapy have been generally accepted but ensuring adequate patient compliance remains a challenge.[159a,b]

Follow-up programs (using the appropriate language) are crucial. In one study of 12 asthmatics who were followed for 18 months after near-fatal asthma with respiratory arrest, two of five patients who refused to participate in an outpatient program died, compared to no patient deaths in the group of 13 compliant patients.[126] Although a number of models are likely to be effective, there are data demonstrating better outcome with an expert based system.[160] Similarly, expert care improves hospital management.[161] Although expert consultation or care may not always be available, or desirable, for ongoing management, a reasonable goal is for all patients admitted for acute asthma to be seen at least once by a specialist.[162]

Many prospective studies suggest that physician expertise is correlated with outcome and overall cost. In two similar prospective studies, patients were randomly assigned to an expert asthma clinic center or to routine care (control group).[163–164] Control group patients received no formal education, were seen only at predetermined intervals, and were encouraged to follow-up with their family physicians or go to the ED when symptoms became troublesome. These patients had significantly more hospitalizations, more ED visits, and more days lost from work compared with patients assigned to the asthma centers. Interestingly, how-

ever, there was no relationship between regional density of asthma specialists and asthma mortality,[165] probably reflecting poor access of high risk patients to specialist care. A summary of suggestions to improve asthma outcome are included in Table 2-5.

CONCLUSION

In this chapter, some of the alarming trends in asthma prevalence worldwide, the circumstances that surround asthma death have been reviewed and some suggestions to reduce asthma morbidity and mortality have been suggested. The hope is that continued epidemiologic research, combined with education, increased use of inhaled corticosteroids, and improved access to quality healthcare will eliminate the asthma paradox in the years to come.

REFERENCES

1. Barnes PJ: A new approach to the treatment of asthma. *N Engl J Med* 321:1517–1527, 1989.
2. Kemp JP: Approaches to asthma management. *Arch Intern Med* 153:805–812, 1993.
3. Skorodin MS: Pharmacotherapy for asthma and chronic obstructive pulmonary disease. *Arch Intern Med* 153:814–828, 1993.
4. Cochrane GM: Acute severe asthma:oxygen and high dose beta agonist during transfer for all? *Thorax* 50:1–2, 1995.
5. McFadden ER Jr: Fatal and near-fatal asthma. *N Engl J Med* 324:409–411, 1991.
6. Banner AS: The increase in asthma prevalence. *Chest* 108:301–302, 1995.
7. Sears MR: Why are deaths from asthma increasing? *Eur Respir J* 69(Suppl 147):175–181, 1986.
8. Jackson R, et al: International trends in asthma mortality: 1970 to 1985. *Chest* 94:914–919, 1988.
9. Crane J, Pearce NE, Flatt A, et al: Prescribed fenoterol and death from asthma in New Zealand, 1981–1983: Case-control study. *Lancet* 1:917–922, 1989.
10. Pearce NE, Grainger J, Atkinson M, et al: Case-control study of prescribed fenoterol and death from asthma in New Zealand, 1977–1981. *Thorax* 45:170–175, 1990.

11. Grainger J, Woodman K, Pearce N, et al: Prescribed fenoterol and death from asthma in New Zealand, 1981–1987:a further case-control study. *Thorax* 46:105–111, 1991.

12. Rea HH, Garret JE, Lanes SF: The association between asthma drugs and severe life-threatening attacks. *Chest* 110:1446–1451, 1996.

13. Adcock IM, Stevens DA, Barnes PJ: Interactions of glucocorticoids and beta 2-agonists. *Eur Respir J* 9:160–168, 1996.

14. Wilson JD, Sutherland DC, Thomas AC: Has the change to beta-agonists combined with oral theophylline increased cases of fatal asthma? *Lancet* 1:1235–1237, 1981.

15. Bodenhamer J, Bergstrom R, Brown D, et al: Frequently nebulized β agonists for asthma: Effects on serum electrolytes. *Ann Emerg Med* 21:1337–1342, 1992.

16. Sears MR, Taylor DR, Print CG, et al: Regular inhaled beta-agonist treatment in bronchial asthma. *Lancet* 336:1391–1396, 1990.

17. Wang ZL, Bramley AM, McNamara A: Chronic fenoterol exposure increases in vivo and in vitro airway responses in guinea pigs. *Am J Respir Crit Care Med* 149:960–965, 1994.

18. Cockcroft DW, McParland CP, Britto S, et al: Regular inhaled salbutamol and airway responsiveness to allergen. *Lancet* 342:833–837, 1993.

19. O'Connor BJ, Aikman SL, Barnes PJ: Tolerance to the nonbronchodilator effects of inhaled Beta$_2$ agonists in asthma. *N Engl J Med* 327:1204–1208, 1992.

19a. Tan S, Hall IP, Dewar J, Dow E, Lipworth B: Association between beta 2-adrenoceptor polymorphism and susceptibility to bronchodilator desensitisation in moderately severe stable asthmatics. *Lancet* 350:995–999, 1997.

19b. Weir TD, Mallek N, Sandford AJ, Bai TR, et al: β2-adrenergic receptor haplotypes in mild, moderate and fatal/near fatal asthma. *Am J Respir Crit Care Med* 158:787–791, 1998.

20. Woolcock AJ: Corticosteroid-resistant asthma. *Am J Respir Crit Care Med* 154:S45–S48, 1996.

21. Taylor DR, Sears MR: Regular beta-adrenergic agonists. *Chest* 106:552–559, 1994.

22. Sears MR: Changing patterns in asthma morbidity and mortality. *J Allergy Clin Immunol* 5:66–72, 1995.

23. Beasley R, Pearce N, Crane J, Burgess C: Withdrawal of fenoterol and the end of the New Zealand asthma mortality epidemic. *Int Arch Allergy Immunol* 107:325–327, 1995.

24. Pearce N, Beasley R, Crane J, et al: End of the New Zealand asthma mortality epidemic. *Lancet* 345:41–44, 1995.

25. Molfino NA, Nannini LJ Jr, Chapman KR, Slutsky AS: Trends in pharmacotherapy for chronic airflow limitation in Argentina: 1983–1990. *Medicina Bs As* 54:103–109, 1994.

26. Neffen H, Baena Cagnani C, Malka S, et al: Asthma mortality in Latin America. *J Investig Allergol Clin Immunol.* 7:249–253, 1997.

27. Nannini LJ: Mortalidad asociada al asma en el Municipio de Rosario. *Medicina* 55:647–651, 1995.

28. Haas JF, Staudinger HW, Schuijt C: Asthma deaths in New Zealand. *Br Med J* 304:1634, 1992.

29. Lanes SF, Birmann B, Raiford D, Walker AM: International trends in sales of inhaled fenoterol, all inhaled beta agonists, and asthma mortality, 1970–1992. *J Clin Epidemiol* 50:321–328, 1997.

30. Garrett J, Kolbe J, Richards G, et al: Major reduction in asthma morbidity and continued reduction in asthma mortality in New Zealand: What lessons have been learned? *Thorax* 50:303–311, 1995.

31. Sears MR, Rea HH, Rothwell RPG, O'Donnell TV, et al: Asthma mortality: comparison between New Zealand and England. *Br Med J* 293:1342–1345, 1986.

32. British Thoracic Association: Death from asthma in two regions of England. *Br Med J* 285:1251–1255, 1982.

33. Sears MR, Rea HH, Beaglehole R, et al: Asthma mortality in New Zealand: a two year national study. *N Z Med J* 98:271–275, 1985.

34. Zimmerman J, Knaus WA, Judson J, et al: Patient selection for intensive care: A comparison of New Zealand and United States hospitals. *Crit Care Med* 16:318–326, 1988.

35. Keating G, Mitchell EA, Jackson R, et al: Trends in sales of drugs for asthma in New Zealand, Australia and the United Kingdom, 1975–1981. *Br Med J* 289:348–351, 1984.

36. Sears MR, Rea HH, Fenwick J, et al: 75 deaths in asthmatics prescribed home nebulizers: *Br Med J* 294:477–480, 1987.

37. Suissa S, Hemmelgarn B, Blais L, Ernst P: Bronchodilators and acute cardiac death. *Am J Respir Crit Care Med* 154:1598–1602, 1996.

38. Martelli NA, Nannini LJ, Menga G, Molfino NA:

High doses of salbutamol nebulized in air in acute severe asthma. *Am J Respir Crit Care Med* 155:935, 1997. Abstract

39. *National Institutes of Health*. National Heart, Lung, and Blood Institute: Global strategy for asthma management and prevention. #95-3659. January 1995:13–16.

40. Woolcock AJ: Worldwide differences in asthma prevalence and mortality *Chest* 90:S40–S45, 1986.

41. Weiss KB, Gergen PJ, Wagener DK: Breathing better or wheezing worse? The changing epidemiology of asthma morbidity and mortality. *Annu Rev Public Health* 14:491–513, 1993.

42. Roberts C, Mayer JD, Henderson WR Jr: Asthma deaths in Washington state, 1980–1989: geographic and demographic distributions *Ann Allergy Asthma Immunol* 76:20–26, 1996.

43. Hunt LW, Silverstein MD, et al: Accuracy of the death certificate in a population-based study of asthma patients. *JAMA* 269:1947–1952, 1993.

44. Silverstein MD, Reed CE, O'Connell JE, et al: Long-term survival of a cohort of community residents with asthma. *N Engl J Med* 331:1537–1541, 1994.

45. Lang DM, Polansky M: Patterns of asthma mortality in Philadelphia from 1969–1991. *N Engl J Med* 331:1542–1546, 1994.

46. Carr W, Zeitel L, Weiss K: Variations in asthma hospitalizations and deaths in New York City. *Am J Public Health* 82:59–65, 1992.

47. Targonski PV, Persky VW, Orris P, Addington W: Trends in asthma mortality among African Americans and whites in Chicago, 1968 through 1991. *Am J Public Health* 84:1830–1833, 1994.

48. Marder D, Targonski P, Orris P, et al: Effect of racial and socioeconomic factors on asthma mortality in Chicago. *Chest* 101:426S–429S, 1992.

49. Malveaux FJ, Houlihan D, Diamond EL: Characteristics of asthma mortality and morbidity in African-Americans. *J Asthma* 30:431–437, 1993.

50. Schenker MB, Gold EB, Lopez RL, Beaumont JJ: Asthma mortality in California, 1960–1989. Demographic patterns and occupational associations. *Am Rev Respir Dis* 147:1454–1460, 1993.

51. Gottlieb DJ, Beiser A, O'Connor GT: Poverty, race, and medication use are correlates of asthma hospitalization rates. *Chest* 108:28–35, 1995.

52. Headrick L, Crain E Evans D, et al: National Asthma Education and Prevention Program Working Group Report on the quality of asthma care. *Am J Respir Crit Care Med* 154:S96–S118, 1996.

53. Wilkins K, Mao Y: Trends in rates of admission to hospital and death from asthma among children and young adults in Canada during the 1980s. *Can Med Assoc J* 148:185–190, 1993.

54. Manfreda J, Becker AB, Wang PZ, et al: Trends in physician-diagnosed asthma prevalence in Manitoba between 1980 and 1990. *Chest* 103:151–157, 1993.

55. Erzen D, Roos LL, Manfreda J, Anthonisen NR: Changes in asthma severity in Manitoba. *Chest* 108:16–23, 1995.

56. Antó JM, Sunyer J, Rodríguez Roisin R, et al: Community outbreaks of asthma associated with inhalation of soybean dust. *N Engl J Med* 320:1097–1102, 1989.

57. Picado C: Barcelona's asthma epidemics: clinical aspects and intriguing findings. *Thorax* 47:197–200, 1992.

58. Aceves M, Grimalt JO, Sunyer J et al: Identification of soybean dust as an epidemic asthma agent in urban areas by molecular marker and RAST analysis of aerosols. *J Allergy Clin Immunol* 88:124–134, 1991.

59. Sunyer J, Antó JM, Rodrigo MJ, Morell F: Clinical and toxicoepidemiological Committee. Case-control study of serum IgE antibodies reactive with soybean in epidemic asthma. *Lancet* 1:179–182, 1989.

60. Swanson MC, Li JT, Wentz Murtha PE, et al: Source of the aeroallergen of soybean dust: a low molecular mass glycopeptide from the soybean tela. *J Allergy Clin Immunol* 87:783–788, 1991.

61. *Lung & Asthma Information Agency*: Factsheet 96/2.

62. Hyndman SJ, Williams DRR, Merrill SL, et al: Rates of admission to hospital for asthma. *Br Med J* 308:1596–1600, 1994.

63. Wright SC, Evans AE, Sinnamon DG, Mac Mahon J: Asthma mortality and certification in Northern Ireland. *Thorax* 49:141–143, 1994.

64. Subcommittee of the British Thoracic Association Research Committee: Accuracy of death certificates in bronchial asthma. *Thorax.* 39:505–509, 1984.

65. Carrasco E: Epidemiology of asthma in Latin America, in Neffen HE, Baena Cagnani CE.(eds): *Proceedings Interasma 1995 Congress.* Buenos Aires, 1995, pp 135–139.

66. Salas Ramírez M, Segura Méndez NH, Martínez

Cairo Cueto S: Tendencias de la mortalidad por asma en México 116:298–306, 1994.

67. Batule Batule M, García Castañeda OM, Toledo Vila H, Vidaillet Rodríguez J: Mortality by bronchial asthma and relation to atmospheric conditions in Havana City. *Rev cuba. Med* 29:473–484, 1990.

68. Accinelli R: Mortalidad por asma bronquial en residentes de la altura. *Acta Andin* 2:191–200, 1993.

69. Allegra L, Cogo A, Legnani D, et al: High altitude exposure reduces bronchial responsiveness to hypo-osmolar aerosol in lowland asthmatics. *Eur Respir J* 8:1842–1846, 1995.

70. Boner AL, Comis A, Schiassi M, et al: Bronchial reactivity in asthmatic children at high and low altitude. *Am J Respir Crit Care Med* 151:1194–1200, 1995.

71. Baluga JC, Spagna F, Ceni M: Mortalidad por asma en Uruguay. Período 1984–1994. *Rev Med Uruguay* 13:12–22, 1997.

72. Lotufo PA, Benseñor IJ, de Lolio CA: Mortality from asthma in the state of S. Paulo, Brazil (1970–1992). *Rev Saude Publica* 29:434–439, 1995.

73. Cooreman J, Segala C, Henry C, Neukirch F: Trends in asthma-induced mortality in France from 1970–1990. *Tuber Lung Dis* 75:182–187, 1994.

74. Cadet B, Robine JM, Leibovici D: Dynamics of asthma mortality in France: seasonal fluctuations and peak mortality in 1985–1987. *Rev Epidemiol Sante Publique* 42:103-118, 1994.

75. Melissinos C G, Gourgoulianis K: Inhaled drug consumption and asthma mortality in Greece. *Chest* 107:1771–1772, 1995. Letter

76. La Vecchia C, Levi F, Lucchini F: Trends in mortality from bronchial asthma in Switzerland, 1969–1993. *Rev Epidemiol Sante Republique* 44:155–161, 1996.

77. Juel K, Pedersen PA: Increasing asthma mortality in Denmark 1969–1988. Not because of changed coding practices. *Ugeskr Laeger* 155:3986–3988, 1993.

78. Mormile F, Chiappini F, Feola G, Ciappi G: Death from asthma in Italy (1974–1988): Is there a relationship with changing pharmacological approaches? *J Clin Epidemiol* 49:1459–1466, 1996.

79. Kitabatake M, Manjurul H, Feng-yuan P, et al: Trends of air pollution versus those of consultation rate and mortality rate for bronchial asthma in individuals aged 40 years and above in the Yokkaichi region. *Nippon Eiseigaku Zasshi* 50:737–747, 1995.

80. Matsuse H, Shimoda T, Kohno S, et al: A clinical study of mortality due to asthma. *Ann Allergy Asthma Immunol* 75:267–272, 1995.

81. Turner KJ, Stewart GA, Woolcock AJ, et al: Relationship between mite densities and the prevalence of asthma: comparative studies in two populations in the Eastern Highlands of Papua New Guinea. *Clin Allergy* 18:331–340, 1988.

82. Turner KJ, Dowse GK, Stewart GA, Alpers MP: Studies on bronchial hyperreactivity, allergic responsiveness, and asthma in rural and urban children of the highlands of Papua New Guinea. *J Allergy Clin Immunol* 77:558–566, 1986.

83. Crockett AJ, Cranston JM, Alpers JH: The changing prevalence of asthma-like respiratory symptoms in South Australian rural school children. *J Pediatr Child Health* 31:213–217, 1995.

84. Sly RM: Changing asthma mortality. *Ann Allergy* 73:259–268, 1994.

85. Kivity S, Shochat Z, Bressler R, et al: The characteristics of bronchial asthma among a young adult population. *Chest* 108:24–27, 1995.

86. Livne M, Weissgarten J, Stav D, et al: Asthma mortality in Israel 1971–1990. *Ann Allergy Asthma Immunol* 76:261–265, 1996.

87. Zamel N, McClean PA, Sandell PR, et al: Asthma on Tristan da Cunha: looking for the genetic link. *Am J Respir Crit Care Med* 153:1902–1906, 1996.

88. Woolcock AJ, Rubinfield A, Seale P, et al: Asthma management plan, 1989. *Med J Aust* 151:650–653, 1989.

89. Hargreave FE, Dolovich J, Newhouse MT: The assessment and treatment of asthma: A conference report. *J Allergy Clin Immunol* 85:1098–1111, 1990.

90. *National Heart, Lung, and Blood Institute*: Guidelines for the diagnosis and management of asthma. *J Allergy Clin Immunol* 88(Suppl 3, part 2):497, 1991.

91. Guidelines on the management of asthma. *Thorax* 48(Suppl 1):24,1993.

92. Weiss KB, Wagener DK: Changing patterns of asthma mortality. Identifying target populations at high risk. *JAMA* 264:1683–1687, 1990.

93. Mohan G, Harrison BD, Badminton RM, et al: A confidential enquiry into deaths caused by asthma in an English health region: implications for general practice. *Br J Gen Pract* 46:529–532, 1996.

94. Sears MR, Rea HH, Rothwell RPG, et al: Asthma mortality: comparison between New Zealand and England. *Br Med J.* 293:1342–1345, 1986.

95. Wareham NJ, Harrison BDW, Jenkins PF, et al: A district confidential enquiry into deaths due to asthma. *Thorax* 48:1117–1120, 1993.

96. McFadden ER Jr, Warren EL: Observations on asthma mortality. *Ann Intern Med* 127:142–147, 1997.

97. Kikuchi Y, Okabe S, Tamura G, Hida W, et al: Chemosensitivity and perception of dyspnea in patients with a history of near-fatal asthma. *N Engl J Med* 330:1329–1334, 1994.

98. Connolly MJ, Crowley JJ, Charan NB, et al: Reduced subjective awareness of bronchoconstriction provoked by methacholine in elderly asthmatic and normal subjects as measured on a simple awareness scale. *Thorax* 47:410–413, 1992.

98a. Chetta A, Gerra G, Foresi A, et al: Personality profiles and breathlessness perception in outpatients with different gradings of asthma. *Am J Respir Crit Care Med.* 157:116–122, 1998.

98b. Veen JC, Smits HH, Ravensberg AJ, et al: Impaired perception of dyspnea in patients with severe asthma. *Am J Respir Crit Care Med.* 158:1134–1141, 1998.

99. Marquette CH, Saulnier F, Leroy O, et al: Long term prognosis of near-fatal asthma. *Am Rev Respir Dis* 146:76–81, 1992.

100. Slepian IK, Mathews KP, McLean JA: Aspirin-sensitive asthma. *Chest* 85:386–391, 1985.

101. Picado C, Castillo JA, Montserrat JM, Agustí Vidal A: Aspirin-intolerance as a precipitating factor of life-threatening attacks of asthma requiring mechanical ventilation. *Eur Respir J* 2:127–129, 1989.

102. Songür N, Fujimura M, Mizuhashi K, et al: Involvement of thromboxane A$_2$ in propranol-induced bronchoconstriction after allergic bronchoconstriction in guinea pigs. *Am J Respir Care Med* 149:1488–1493, 1994.

103. Toogood JH. Beta-blocker therapy and the risk of anaphylaxis. *Can Med Assoc J* 136:929–933, 1987.

104. Mc Neill RS: Effect of beta-adrenergic-blocking agent, propranolol, on asthmatics. *Lancet* 2:1101–1102, 1964.

105. Wright W, Zhang YG, Salome CM, Woolcock AJ: Effect of inhaled preservatives on asthmatic subjects. I. Sodium metabisulfite. *Am Rev Respir Dis* 141:1400–1404, 1990.

106. Shimoda T, Kohno S, Takao A, et al: Investigation of the mechanism of alcohol induced bronchial asthma. *J Allergy Clin Immunol* 97:74–84, 1996.

107. Cheung D, Dick EC, Timmers MC, et al: Rhinovirus inhalation causes long-lasting excessive airway narrowing in response to methacholine in asthmatic subjects *in vivo*. *Am J Respir Crit Care Med* 152:1490–1496, 1995.

108. O'Hollaren MT, Yuninger JW, Offord KP, et al: Exposure to an aeroallergen as a possible precipitating factor in respiratory arrest in young patients with asthma. *N Engl J Med* 324:359–363, 1991

109. Ferrer A, Torres A, Roca J, et al: Characteristics of patients with soybean dust-induced acute severe asthma requiring mechanical ventilation. *Eur Respir J* 3:429–433, 1990.

110. Busse WW, Kiecolt-Glaser JK, Coe C, et al: Stress and asthma. *Am J Respir Crit Care Med* 151:249–252, 1995.

111. Levenson T, Greenberger P, Donoghue ER, Lifschultz BD: Asthma deaths confounded by substance abuse. An assessment of fatal asthma. *Chest* 110:604, 1996.

112. Nannini LJ Jr: Asma potencialmente fatal. *Arch Bronconeum (Barcelona)* 33:462–471, 1997.

112a. Cygan J, Trunsky M, Corbridge T: Inhaled heroin-induced status asthmaticus. *Chest* 117:272–275, 2000.

113. Brown PJ, Greville HW, Finucane KE: Asthma and irreversible airflow obstruction. *Thorax* 39:131–136, 1984.

113a. Veen JC, Smits HH, Hiemstra PS, et al: Lung function and sputum characteristics of patients with severe asthma during an induced exacerbation by double-blind steroid withdrawal. *Am J Respir Crit Care Med* 160:93–99, 1999.

113b. Wenzel SE, Schwartz LB, Langmack EL, et al: Evidence that severe asthma can be divided pathologically into two inflammatory subtypes with distinct physiologic and clinical characteristics. *Am J Respir Crit Care Med* 160:1001–1008, 1999.

114. Macdonald JB, Seaton A, Williams DA: Asthma deaths in Cardiff in 1963–1974: 90 deaths outside hospital. *Br Med J* i:1493–1495, 1976.

115. Johnson AJ, Nunn AJ, Somner AR, et al: Circumstances of deaths from asthma. *Br Med J* 288:1870–1872, 1984.

116. Sur S, Crotty TB, Kephart GM, et al: Sudden-onset fatal asthma. A distinct entity with few eo-

sinophils and relatively more neutrophils in the airway submucosa? *Am Rev Respir Dis* 148:713–719, 1993.

117. Barger LW, Vollmer WM, Felt R, Buist AS: Further investigation into the recent increase in asthma death rates: a review of 41 asthma deaths in Oregon in 1982. *Ann Allergy* 60:31–39, 1988.

118. Kallenbach JM, Frankel AH, Lapinsky SE, et al: Determinants of near fatality in acute severe asthma. *Am J Med* 95:265–272, 1993.

119. Goodman DE, Israel E, Rosenberg M, Johnston R, et al: The influence of age, diagnosis, and gender on proper use of metered-dose inhalers. *Am J Respir Crit Care Med* 150:1256–1261, 1994.

120. So SY, Ng MMT, Ip MSM, Lam WK: Rising asthma mortality in young males in Hong Kong, 1976–85. *Respir Med* 84:457–461. 1990.

121. Ulrik CS, Frederiksen J: Mortality and markers of risk of asthma death among 1075 outpatients with asthma. *Chest* 108:10–15. 1995.

122. Rea HH, Scragg R, Jackson R, et al: A case-control study of death from asthma. *Thorax* 41:833–839, 1986.

123. Hetzell MR, Clark TJH, Branthwaite MA: Asthma: Analysis of sudden deaths and ventilatory arrests in hospital. *Br Med J* 1:808–811, 1977.

124. Benatar S: Fatal asthma. *N Engl J Med* 314:423–429, 1986.

125. Leatherman J. Life-threatening asthma. *Clin Chest Med* 15:453–479, 1994.

126. Molfino NA, Nannini LJ, Rebuck A, Slutsky AS: The fatality-prone asthmatic patient. Follow-up study after near-fatal attacks. *Chest* 101:621–623, 1992.

127. Molfino NA, Slutsky AS: Near-fatal asthma. *Eur Respir J* 7:981–990, 1994.

128. Barriot P, Riou B: Prevention of fatal asthma. *Chest* 92:460–466, 1987.

129. Corbridge TC, Hall JB: The assessment and management of adults with status asthmaticus. *Am J Respir Crit Care Med* 151:1296–1316, 1995.

130. Darioli R, Perret C: Mechanical controlled hypoventilation in status asthmaticus. *Am Rev Respir Dis* 129:385–387, 1984.

131. Spitzer WO, Suissa S, Ernst P, et al: The use of beta-agonists and the risk of death and near death from asthma. *N Engl J Med* 326:501–506, 1992.

132. Ernst P, Spiltzer WO, Suissa S, et al: Risk of fatal and near-fatal asthma in relation to inhaled corticosteroids use. *JAMA* 268:3462–3464, 1992.

133. Boulet LP, Deschesnes F, Turcotte H, Gignac F:

Near-fatal asthma: Clinical and physiologic features, perception of bronchoconstriction, and psychologic profile. *J Allergy Clin Immunol* 88:838–846, 1991.

134. Crompton GK, Grant IWB, Bloomfield P: Edinburgh emergency asthma admission service; report on 10 years' experience. *Br Med J* 2:1199–1201, 1979.

135. Wasserfallen JB, Schaller MD, Feihl F, Perret CH: Sudden asphyxic asthma: A distinct entity? *Am Rev Respir Dis* 142:108–111, 1990.

136. Westerman DE, Benatar SR, Potgieter PD, Ferguson AD: Identification of the high-risk asthmatic patient. *Am J Med* 66:565–572, 1979.

137. Campbell DA, McLennan G, Coates JR, et al: A comparison of asthma deaths and near-fatal asthma attacks in South Australia. *Eur Respir J* 7:490–497, 1994.

138. Joseph KS, Blais L, Ernst P, Suissa S: Increased morbidity and mortality related to asthma among patients who use major tranquilizers. *Br Med J* 312:79–83, 1996.

139. Richards GN, Kolbe J, Fenwick J, Rea HH: Demographic characteristics of patients with severe life threatening asthma: comparison with asthma deaths. *Thorax* 48:1105–1109, 1993.

140. Knot A, Burn R: Seasonal variation and time trend in asthma mortality in England and Wales. *Br Med J* 289:233–234, 1984.

141. Packe GE, Ayres JG: Asthma outbreak during a thunderstorm. *Lancet* 2:199–204, 1986.

142. Bauman A: Asthma associated with thunderstorms. Grass pollen and the fall in temperature seem to be to blame. *Br Med J* 312:590–591, 1996.

143. Johnston SL, Pattmore PK, Sanderson G, et al: The relationship between upper respiratory infections and hospital admissions for asthma: a time-trend analysis. *Am J Respir Crit Care Med* 154:656–660, 1996.

144. Bates DV, Baker-Anderson M, Sizto R: Asthma attack periodicity: a study of hospital emergency visits in Vancouver. *Environ Res* 51:51–70, 1990.

145. Schwartz J, Slater D, Larson TV, et al: Particulate air pollution and hospital emergency room visits for asthma in Seattle. *Am Rev Respir Dis* 147:826–831, 1993.

146. Osborne ML, Vollmer WM, Buist AS: Periodicity of asthma, emphysema and chronic bronchitis in a northwest health maintenance organization. *Chest* 110:1458–1462, 1996.

147. Weiss KB: Seasonal trends in US asthma hospital-

izations and mortality. *JAMA* 263:2323–2328, 1990.

148. Dales RE, Schweitzer I, Toogood JH, et al: Respiratory infections and the autumn increase in asthma morbidity. *Eur Respir J* 9(1): 72–77, 1996.

149. Horn MEC, Reed SE, Taylor P: Role of viruses and bacteria in acute wheezy bronchitis in childhood: a study of sputum. *Arch Dis Child* 54:587–592, 1979.

150. Johnston SL, Pattemore PK, Sanderson G, et al: Community study of role of viral infections in exacerbations of asthma in 9-11 year old children. *Br Med J* 310:1225–1228, 1995.

151. Sokhandan M, McFadden ER Jr, Huang YT, Mazanee MB: The contribution of respiratory viruses to severe exacerbations of asthma in adults. *Chest* 107:1570–1575, 1995.

152. Mountain RD, Sahn SA: Clinical features and outcome in patients with acute asthma presenting with hypercapnia. *Am Rev Respir Dis* 138:535–539, 1988.

152a. Donahue JG, Weiss ST, Livingston JM, et al: Inhaled steroids and the risk of hospitalization for asthma. *JAMA* 277:887–891, 1997.

152b. Blais L, Suissa S, Boivin JF, Ernst P: First treatment with inhaled corticosteroids and the prevention of admissions to hospital for asthma. *Thorax* 53:1025–1029, 1998.

152c. Blais L, Ernst P, Boivin JF, Suissa S: Inhaled corticosteroids and the prevention of readmission to hospital for asthma. *Am J Respir Crit Care Med* 158:126–132, 1998.

153. Molfino NA, Nannini LJ, Martelli AN, Slutsky AS: Respiratory arrest in near-fatal asthma. *N Engl J Med* 324: 285–288, 1991.

154. Rodrigo G, Rodrigo C: A new index for early prediction of *hospitalization in patients with acute asthma. Am J Emerg Med* 15:8–13, 1997.

155. Yoon R, McKenzie DK, Miles DA, Bauman A: Characteristics of attenders and non-attenders at an asthma education program. *Thorax* 46:886–890, 1991.

156. Akerman MJ, Sinert R: A successful effort to improve asthma care outcome in an inner city emergency department. *J Asthma* 36:295–303, 1999.

157. Nannini LJ Jr: Asthma educational program including free treatment reduced hospitalizations for asthma. *Eur Respir J* 1997;10 suppl 25:1015. Abstract.

158. Kolbe J, Vamos M, Fergusson W, et al: Differential influences on asthma self-management knowledge and self-management behavior in acute severe asthma. *Chest* 110:1463–1468, 1996.

159. Kolbe J, Garrett J, Vamos M, Rea HH: Influences on trends in asthma morbidity and mortality: The New Zealand experience. *Chest* 106:211S–215S, 1994.

159a. Apter AJ, Reisine ST, Affleck G, et al: Adherence with twice-daily dosing of inhaled steroids. *Am J Respir Crit Care Med* 157:1810–1817, 1998.

159b. Côté J, Cartier A, Robichaud P, et al: Influence on asthma morbidity of asthma education programs based on self-management plans following treatment optimization. *Am J Respir Crit Care Med* 155:1509–1514, 1997.

160. Bartter T. Pratter MR: Asthma: better outcome at lower cost? The role of the expert in the care system. *Chest* 110:1589–1596, 1996.

161. Bucknall CE, Robertson C, Moran F, Stevenson RD: Differences in hospital asthma management. *Lancet* i:748–750, 1988.

162. Tattersfield AE: Who should look after asthma? *Thorax* 50:597–599, 1995.

163. Mayo PH, Richman J, Harris WH: Results of a program to reduce admissions for adult asthma. *Ann Intern Med* 112:864–871, 1990.

164. Ignacio-García JM, González Santos P: Asthma self-management education program by home monitoring of peak expiratory flow. *Am J Respir Crit Care Med* 151:353–359, 1995.

165. Sly RM, O'Donnell R: Association of asthma mortality with medical specialist density. *Ann Allergy* 68:340–344, 1992.

Chapter 3

NEAR-FATAL ASTHMA

Néstor A. Molfino

INTRODUCTION

The first description of asthma as a life-threatening condition is attributed to Arateus Di Cappadocia (81–131 A.D.).[1] Subsequently, the potentially fatal nature of asthma was described by Moises Maimonides in his Treatise on Asthma.[2] Following these original descriptions of the clinical features of acute near-fatal asthma attacks, Osler summarized some fundamental notions of the pathophysiology of severe fatal asthma.[3] The hypotheses as posed by Osler in 1892 included 1) the notion that asthma was due to spasm of bronchial muscles, 2) the possibility that the attack could be due to bronchial mucous membrane hyperemia (as proposed by Traube), vasomotor turgescence (as proposed by Webber), and/or diffuse hyperemic swelling (as proposed by Clark), and 3) the concept that inflammation of the small bronchioles was present in many cases (as proposed by Curschmann). Interestingly, these hypotheses have not been tested until recently in subjects with stable asthma. Consequently, the specific role of these pathophysiologic findings in fatal asthma remains poorly understood.[4] Because of this lack of complete understanding of the pathogenesis of asthma and despite the development of new therapeutic modalities, morbidity and mortality rates have not decreased as expected.[5]

The fundamental questions of how and why some patients die from asthma have occupied an important chapter in the history of asthma research. Difficulties encountered in this research have included the complex and partially understood pathophysiology of fatal asthma and the complex interactions and influences of factors such as patient and physician education, asthma medications, gene-environment relationships, and socioeconomic status of affected populations.

Major efforts are ongoing to increase patient and physician education, to develop better asthma therapies, and to improve asthma management regardless of the socioeconomic status of patients. Research is mandatory in order to improve the poor prognosis of patients who suffer from episodes of near-fatal asthma and who are unable to control the condition on an ambulatory basis.[6]

IDENTIFICATION OF ASTHMA PATIENTS AT RISK OF DYING

Although death from asthma is relatively rare in both ambulatory[7] and hospitalized patients[8] and only approximately 5% of all asthma patients need hospitalization[9,10] every physician must be able to identify high-risk patients. Proper identification of such patients,[11] rapid admission,[12] and relatively simple therapeutic measures[13] can avert or reverse respiratory failure in most cases.

The most specific epidemiologic marker associated with an increased risk of dying from asthma is hospitalization in the year preceding the near-fatal or fatal event.[14–17] This is particularly true if admissions are recurrent and patients require ventilatory assistance during admissions.[16] Nevertheless, a history of recurrent admissions is found in only 36% of fatal cases and ventilatory

Table 3-1

Demographic and epidemiologic markers found in subjects who suffer from near-fatal asthma attacks

- Age
- Ethnicity
- Previous life-threatening exacerbation
- Hospital admission within the last year[14–16]
- Inadequate general management
- Psychological and social problems[43–47]
- Lack of access to medical care
- Adrenoreceptor polymorphisms?[57–59]
- Use of high-dose inhaled β_2 agonists[52]
- Use of major tranquilizers[47]

SOURCE: From National Heart, Lung, and Blood Institute.[18]

assistance in only 6% of such cases." Thus, the specific disease characteristics that place patients at risk are still inadequately defined.

A number of useful characteristics known so far to identify fatality-prone asthmatics are summarized in Table 3-1.[18,19] Although previous occurrence of life-threatening events and hospitalization within the last year have a high positive predictive value, there are also many patients who require multiple drugs, have large variations in lung function, or exhibit associated psychological disorders, but never experience respiratory failure. Furthermore, many asthma patients attend an emergency department (ED) frequently as the primary source of care due to meager resources, but such visits do not constitute a major risk factor. Indeed, at least one study has shown that there is no increased usage of EDs after near-fatal asthma if equal access to medical care exists.[20] In this regard, risk factors such as age and ethnicity[21] may be indicative of socioeconomic barriers to adequate medical care in some parts of the world.[22] For example, Apter and colleagues have shown that the most influential factor predicting asthma treatment site was insurance status.[23] On the other hand, when existing socioeconomic differences do not influence access to medical help, it is still possible that inappropriate indoor air quality[24–26] plays

a role in the severity of asthma in patients with a low socioeconomic status.[27] Thus, either because of poor access to medical care or poor indoor air quality, a low socioeconomic status indicates a greater risk of developing near-fatal or fatal asthma.

Not surprisingly, lack of appropriate control of asthma has also been shown to be an important factor in deteriorating asthma that ultimately leads to death.[16,28–30] It is possible that an expanding group of patients who do not respond and/or comply completely to conventional therapy represent the population at the highest risk of near-fatal and fatal asthma attacks.[16] The reasons for lack of treatment compliance are numerous and range from the socioeconomic status of a patient to particular personality profiles.

Using data provided by a medical history, patients who have an increased risk of dying from asthma can be classified into two disparate groups:[29] those suffering from sudden severe overwhelming deterioration of airway function (*brittle asthma*) and those with long-standing asthma crises. This classification into two groups is supported by studies that monitored peak expiratory flow rates on a regular basis.[31,32] Although in some asthma patients the characteristics of the two groups overlap, it has been reported that near-fatal asthma attacks can be triggered by two different pathophysiologic mechanisms: 1) marked diurnal variations in peak flow rate,[32] and 2) severe airflow limitation with abnormal physiologic responses to airway narrowing.[33,34] Those patients with marked diurnal variations in peak flow rate may have normal peak flow rates on intermittent testing, but large fluctuations in flow may provoke sudden catastrophic attacks of asthma (*brittle asthma*). In these patients, near-fatal asthma attacks represented a more pure form of smooth muscle bronchoconstriction, and large oscillations in peak flow rates respond, in general (albeit not always), to the administration of inhaled bronchodilators.[14,16] Among the group of patients with severe airflow limitation and abnormal physiologic responses to airway narrowing, one subset showed blunted hypoxic ventilatory drive and did not respond to the development of bronchial narrowing and hypoxia with hyperventilation during acute attacks.[33] These patients may present with hypercapnia, even with moderate airway obstruction, and have an increased incidence of near-fatal episodes.[35] A second subset did not perceive the development of airway obstruction and was relatively symptom-free even with severe obstruction.[34,36] Although this condition is rare, it has been confirmed in both clinic[35] and laboratory[36] settings. It is important to identify patients in these groups, using appropriate questionnaires[37] and pulmonary function testing, because when they do report symptoms, albeit minimal, they may be at much greater risk of death than other asthma patients.

In one study of mechanically ventilated asthma patients, the characteristics of the two groups described above[29] were confirmed.[38] In this study, clinical features of patients with sudden asphyxic asthma were different from those who developed gradual deterioration, suggesting different pathophysiologic mechanisms leading to these near-fatal events. As described by many authors,[29,32,38,39] and demonstrated in epidemiologic studies of asthma deaths,[40–42] these most severely ill patients (and those who die) did not reach the hospital expeditiously. However, some deaths may be unavoidable due to rapid and overwhelming airflow deterioration.

Individuals with asthma and their relatives exhibit a higher incidence of panic disorders[43] and denial, which may be associated with a higher risk of life-threatening asthma.[44] Moreover, there are marked psychological differences between patients with *brittle asthma* and those with non-brittle asthma.[45] Miles and colleagues conducted a case-control study on patients with *brittle asthma* and non-brittle asthma to assess psychological profile and degree of family support by means of questionnaires.[45] They found that patients with *brittle asthma* thought they would delay seeking medical help and would use more self-medication during an asthma attack, and also would receive less family support during the attack. In addition, the personality profiles of individuals with asthma may be related to breathlessness perception, and more severe asthma may be related to poor perception and hypochondriasis.[46] Psychological factors may also explain the recently reported deadly association between the use of major tranquilizers and

death from asthma.[47] Indeed, the greatest risk of dying from asthma is present when subjects discontinue the use of major tranquilizers. Thus, it seems that special attention must be paid to the personality traits in any individual who suffers from asthma.

The possible increased risk of death from asthma due to the chronic use of β_2 agonists has been debated in the past few years. Although there is evidence that suggests β_2 agonists should be used on demand rather than on a regular basis,[48–50] the mechanisms by which β_2 agonists cause asthma deterioration have remained speculative. In addition, whether any putative deleterious effect applies to all β_2 agonists,[48,49] particularly the long-lasting formoterol and salmeterol, has not been demonstrated. Drazen and co-workers have reported no differences in asthma control in patients with mild asthma who were treated with salbutamol on a regular or as-needed basis and monitored for 16 weeks using peak flow meters.[50] Most likely, when mild asthma deteriorates into a moderate or severe stage, the need to increase the dose of inhaled β_2 agonists becomes a marker of uncontrolled asthma[51] and indirectly becomes a marker of risk of dying from asthma. Although the association between the use of inhaled β_2 agonists by metered-dose inhaler and the risk of fatal or near-fatal asthma has been clearly demonstrated,[52] patients with more severe asthma who are at risk of dying or developing near-fatal episodes are more prone to use β_2 agonists to alleviate their symptoms.[53,54] In this regard, patients who use more than one canister per month exhibit twice the risk of fatal or near-fatal asthma,[52] but this does not prove an actual causative association. Indeed, some investigators have suggested that the association of morbidity and mortality rates with sale of β_2 agonists can lead to a wrong conclusion regarding causative association.[55] When data generated in New Zealand that demonstrated a higher relative risk of dying from asthma in patients who were prescribed a β_2 agonist, fenoterol, by metered-dose inhaler, were reassessed using quantitative statistical methods of analysis, Suissa and Ernst[55] reached the exact opposite conclusion (i.e., inhaled steroids gave a greater association with asthma mortality than fenoterol). This indicates that relating sales of a medication to incidence of adverse events may lead to an inaccurate interpretation of data. This is particularly problematic if such conclusions are used for health care policy decisions.

On the other hand, a real risk of cardiovascular death in asthma patients has been suggested when oral or nebulized solutions of β_2 agonists and oral theophyllines are given to certain predisposed ambulatory asthmatic populations.[56] In this same study, no association was found between risk of death and use of inhaled β_2 agonists delivered via metered-dose inhalers.[56] Although the association of treatment of bronchospasm with inhaled β_2 agonists and cardiovascular death has been suggested in a number of studies,[56] the existence of such an association during the treatment of acute asthma in the ED is unlikely.[8,13,14]

Recently, pharmacogenetic studies have suggested that an association exists between polymorphisms of the β_2-adrenoreceptors and the severity of asthma and its response to inhaled β_2 agonists.[57-59] The interpretation of the results from these studies may have tremendous influence on asthma treatment in the future. It is known that the amino acid substitution ARG to GLY16 is more prevalent in patients with steroid-dependent asthma and nocturnal asthma, and that in children with and without asthma, homozygotes for ARG16 respond better to inhaled salbutamol.[57] The substitution GLN27 to GLU is associated with less bronchial hyperresponsiveness and it is not associated with response to inhaled bronchodilator, in children.[57] In addition, at least one report on the prevalence of specific polymorphisms in near-fatal asthma demonstrated a greater prevalence for GLY16 than for ARG16 and no differences in the prevalence of the substitution GLN27/GLU.[60] This supports recent findings demonstrating that homozygotes for GLY16 were more prone to bronchodilator desensitization than ARG16 homozigotes.[58] It appears that β_2-adrenoreceptor polymorphisms act as disease modifiers and are one of many genetic alterations involved in the pathophysiology of asthma.[59]

Some conclusions regarding treatment of asthma with inhaled β_2 agonists and its relationship to near-fatal asthma can be drawn from the available evidence: 1) the majority of patients presenting with near-fatal asthma are undertreated with anti-inflammatory medications,[37,61] 2) up-to-date asthma control is best achieved with inhaled steroids,[62] 3) inhaled β_2 agonists should be prescribed first and used on demand, but may be indicated on a regular basis to achieve asthma control,[50] 4) short-acting inhaled β_2 agonists are, by far, the best treatment in acute severe asthma owing to their potent bronchodilator effect,[13,14,63] 5) the need to use regular β_2 agonists indicates lack of asthma control,[51] greater severity, and higher risk of developing near-fatal or fatal asthma,[49] 6) there is evidence of a causative effect implicating inhaled solutions of these drugs in fatal outcome,[56] and 7) genotype in some patients can influence the severity of asthma and the response to treatment.[59]

In summary, proper identification of subjects at risk can be accomplished using appropriate asthma questionnaires that explore the factors involved in asthma deterioration for each individual patient.[37,64] Use of appropriate drug regimens to achieve asthma control, education, and use of peak flow recordings constitute the armamentarium available to manage patients with moderate and severe asthma; their use is mandatory in patients admitted to the hospital in the preceding year, or in whom life-threatening attacks have occurred in the past.[19] Peak flow rates may change prior to the development of symptoms and detection of these changes should lead to a modification of therapy to prevent sudden asthma attacks.[15] Molecular screening of affected populations may provide more specific pharmacogenetic data to guide asthma therapy in the near future.[59]

FACTORS THAT CAN PRECIPITATE NEAR-FATAL ASTHMA

There are factors that increase asthma symptoms and increase the need for reassessment of habits and medications.[19] Some of these factors can precipitate near-fatal asthma.[15,17] In order to prevent subsequent episodes of near-fatal asthma, it is important to thoroughly question patients and/or relatives[37,64] to pinpoint, if possible, a predominant

Table 3-2
Precipitating factors of near-fatal asthma episodes

- Allergens[38,68,70]
- Infections[38]
- Lack of appropriate assessment or treatment[29,91,138]
- Indoor/outdoor air pollution[80,139–141]
- Weather changes[67,79]
- Emotional upsets[38]
- Drugs[71,75,75a]

SOURCE: From Molfino and Slutsky[17]; National Heart, Lung and Blood Institute.[19]

cause for that particular episode.[38] In addition, the amount of time during which symptoms develop gives an indication of the development of airflow inflammation with rapid deterioration suggesting predominant airway smooth muscle contraction.[65]

Arnold and colleagues prospectively evaluated 261 episodes of acute asthma and found that 46% occurred within 24 hours prior to presentation, whereas 13% occurred less than 1 hour prior to presentation.[66] This time period may vary depending on a number of different factors, but clearly these data confirmed the existence of a group of patients in whom rapid and overwhelming deterioration of asthma can develop.[14,38,39]

Near-fatal asthma is more common in young people,[38] but can occur at any age and without gender distribution[14,18,29,39] and, although there are seasonal variations,[67] these episodes can occur at any time of the day or any day of the week.[14] However, Weiss has reported that death rates from asthma in the United States were higher during weekends.[67] Possible explanations for this finding include more time spent outdoors by asthmatics, reduced patient's compliance with therapy, and/or reduced efficiency of EDs.

Factors that can trigger near-fatal episodes are summarized in Table 3-2. Wasserfallen and co-workers found that those patients with asthma who developed sudden asphyxia had a massive exposure to allergens (3 of 10) or emotional upsets (4 of 10) as precipitating factors.[38] By contrast, the majority of patients (15 of 24) who required mechanical ventilation after gradual impairment of

respiratory function had a respiratory infection as the precipitating factor.[38]

The importance of allergens as triggering factors for near-fatal and fatal asthma has been demonstrated by O'Hollaren and colleagues.[68] They have reported that, for the patients in their study, all respiratory arrests due to asthma occurred during the Alternaria season and that these patients had markers of atopy that was significantly higher than the control group (asthmatics without respiratory arrest). These findings lend support to a previous British Thoracic Society study[69] that found that death from asthma was more frequent in atopic than in non-atopic patients. They also support results of a study by Polart and colleagues that demonstrated a more frequent rate of ED visits for acute asthma in atopic asthma patients.[70]

β blockers, aspirin, and/or nonsteroidal anti-inflammatory drugs (NSAIDs) can also precipitate near-fatal or fatal asthma. Picado and co-workers reviewed 92 asthma patients who required mechanical ventilation and found that aspirin had been the precipitating factor in 8% of the cases.[71] There are more than 200 compounds that contain aspirin and, in addition, cross-reactions with NSAIDs have been reported. These adverse reactions apparently are linked to the ability of such compounds to block the cyclooxygenase pathway with a shift towards the production of leukotrienes. The exact mechanism(s), however, remain unclear.[72] Unfortunately, in aspirin-sensitive patients even hydrocortisone can, on rare occasions, provoke a severe asthma attack that requires intubation.[73] It is well known that β blockers can trigger asthma decompensation.[74] They have been reported to cause exacerbations that persist for prolonged periods of time after the withdrawal of the drug and have, although rarely, caused death in patients with a known history of reversible bronchospasm.

Illicit drug use and alcohol may confound asthma morbidity and mortality. Levenson and colleagues reported an association between substance abuse and asthma deaths in Chicago.[75] By reviewing asthma deaths from the Cook County Office of the Medical Examiner, these investigators showed that 32% of asthma deaths were confounded by substance abuse (mainly cocaine, opioids, and alcohol), and concluded that some of the reported rise in asthma mortality is secondary to this abuse. Cygan and colleagues have collected five cases of near-fatal asthma in Chicago (four required mechanical ventilation) that were triggered by inhaled heroin.[75a] These cases emphasize the importance of considering substance abuse among the factors that can precipitate near-fatal and fatal asthma.

Certain foods can also provoke rare episodes of near-fatal and fatal asthma in children.[76] Sampson and colleagues identified six children and adolescents who died of anaphylactic reactions to foods and seven others who nearly died and required intubation.[76] Of these 13 children and adolescents, 12 had well-controlled asthma. The reactions were to peanuts (four patients), nuts (six patients), eggs (one patient), and milk (two patients), all of which were contained in foods such as candy, cookies, and pastry. The six patients who died had symptoms within 3 to 30 minutes of the ingestion of the allergen, but only two received epinephrine in the first hour. All patients who survived had symptoms within 5 minutes of allergen ingestion, and all but one received epinephrine within 30 minutes.

The number of episodes of acute near-fatal asthma[77] as well as the number of asthma admissions[78] have increased in the recent years, in certain parts of the world. The reasons for this increased incidence of cases of severe asthma, despite apparently improved management and better medications are unknown, but environmental factors may play a definite role. Weiss has demonstrated that between 1982 through 1986 the admission rates for asthma in the United States, on a yearly basis, oscillated seasonally and paralleled the mortality rates.[67] Asthma admissions reached a high in November, and deaths reached a high in February. This "uncoupling" of such curves strongly suggests that, at least in the United States, different environmental factors may be involved in the determination of admissions and fatalities from asthma. Whether this is also true in other countries who have experienced an increase in asthma morbidity and mortality is not known, but

seasonal trends in near-fatal asthma have been identified in other regions of the world.[79] For example Roux and colleagues found that children with fatality-prone characteristics represented a "seasonal" group, thus lending support to other reports[68] of seasonal, near-fatal attacks of asthma.[79]

The role of air pollution in precipitating near-fatal asthma is not yet clear. It is unlikely that relatively low levels of pollutants per se would precipitate an acute severe asthma attack, but thermal inversions with massive accumulation of pollutants can trigger severe asthma attacks.[15,31,80] Pollution might also act as an adjuvant factor in certain circumstances. In this regard, Molfino and colleagues have reported potentiation of the allergic bronchial response when resting asthma patients were exposed to a relatively low level of ozone (0.12 ppm) for 1 hour prior to the allergen challenge.[81] Of note, these levels of ozone are lower than levels commonly observed in large urban centers in summer months. Since ozone is the major component of photochemical pollution derived from traffic-related NO_2, the association found between high prevalence of asthma symptoms and NO_2[82] lends support to the possible causal association between inner city traffic-related pollution and asthma severity. More recently, evidence has been provided that suggests pollution and outdoor allergens are only important factors in the spring and summer months, at least in New York City.[83] Overnight hospital admissions for asthma there are significantly related to air masses that are meteorologically homogeneous and exert their influence predominantly during the fall and winter.[83] Air pollution had little influence on hospital admissions during fall and winter as air masses contained low concentrations of pollutants, even though this was exactly the converse in the spring and summer. Thus, there appears to be a differential seasonal response to weather and air pollution in individuals with asthma, in New York City. If these results can be replicated elsewhere, an asthma weather-watch warning system could be developed. Whether these results can be extrapolated to episodes of near-fatal and fatal asthma is not yet known, but reducing the magnitude of the stimulus is an obvious goal and all known precipitating factors should be minimized or eliminated in an effort to reduce both airway inflammation and responsiveness.[15]

The role of airway hyperresponsiveness in determining the risk of near-fatal and fatal asthma is controversial. In a group of patients who survived respiratory arrests[14,16] the author found increased airway responsiveness to methacholine within the range described as very severe[84] (i.e., PC_{20} FEV_1 <0.1 mg/mL when the patients were challenged 8 to 16 weeks after discharge).[17] This supports the data from Woolcock and colleagues who examined histamine challenges 3 to 10 weeks after near-fatal events.[84] In a longitudinal study of near-fatal asthma, Ruffin and colleagues demonstrated a geometric mean PC_{20} FEV_1 value of 0.23 mg/mL histamine (n = 45).[85] This value increased to 0.83 mg/mL after appropriate anti-inflammatory therapy. Although it has been suggested that reducing bronchial hyperresponsiveness to methacholine or histamine may be beneficial in all patients with asthma,[15,84] the importance of this approach in decreasing the likelihood of a fatal or near-fatal asthmatic attack has not yet been demonstrated. More recent evidence reported by Crimi and colleagues[86] has raised doubts regarding the importance of the relationship between bronchial hyperresponsiveness and airway inflammation in asthma. Their study strongly suggests that other as yet undefined factors different from inflammation may affect bronchial hyperresponsiveness. Nonetheless, the epidemiologic evidence suggests that use of inhaled steroids, which improve bronchial hyperresponsiveness, seem to decrease the risk of near-fatal and fatal attacks of asthma.[87]

A panel of experts from the U.S. National Institutes of Health have described the fundamental factors that can make asthma worse.[19] The factors that most frequently trigger near-fatal asthma attacks are summarized in Table 3-2.[17]

RECOGNITION OF NEAR-FATAL ASTHMA ATTACKS

In general, an asthma crisis can be easily recognized as life threatening. Patients may exhibit ei-

Table 3-3

Recognition of near-fatal asthma attacks

Potentially life-threatening indicators[a]
- Increasing wheeze and breathlessness. Patient unable to complete sentences in one breath or unable to get up from a chair or bed.
- Respiratory rate, ≥25 breaths/min
- Heart rate persistently ≥110 beats/min
- Peak expiratory flow <40% of predicted or best obtained <200 L/min
- Pulsus paradoxus ≥10 mm Hg

Imminently life-threatening indicators[b]
- Silent chest on auscultation
- Cyanosis
- Bradycardia
- Exhaustion, confusion or consciousness

[a,b]NOTE: Only one indicator necessary for a diagnosis of a severe asthma attack.
SOURCE: From Ernst, et al.[87]

ther respiratory arrest or, more frequently, a combination of severe dyspnea, difficulty in speaking, use of accessory muscles of respiration, silent chest on auscultation, and a Pa_{CO_2} value greater than 50 mm Hg (6.66 kPa) and/or an altered state if consciousness.[13,14,40,85] The acute signs and symptoms that indicate a potential or imminent near-fatal asthma attack are listed in Table 3-3.[18,88,89] When the patient is known to have suffered from similar previous episodes, rapid admission and treatment can be lifesaving.[12,28,90]

Crompton has defined the "catastrophic asthmatic" as the patient who develops a sudden severe attack of asthma despite receiving treatment that controls symptoms in most other patients.[39] Emphasis is put on the observation that many asthma patients of this type have a rapid decline in ventilatory function, making these episodes very difficult to predict. Other patients develop progressive airflow deterioration despite treatment in the ED setting, with increasing dyspnea, *decreasing* wheezing, normal or high Pa_{CO_2} values and fall of Pa_{O_2} and FEV_1 measurements.[14] Hetzel and colleagues studied the incidence of unexpected ventilatory arrest, some of which led to sudden death, in 1169 consecutive hospital admissions for asthma.[91] Accepted clinical criteria of a severe attack were not present in some of the episodes that appeared mild. In two studies, the risk of sudden death in some patients could not always be related to the severity of the attack.[14,91] However, it did correlate with the presence of excessive diurnal variation in peak expiratory flow rates (PEFR).[32] A number of other studies examining near-fatal asthma[38,39] clearly demonstrated that these near-fatal episodes were associated with more severe or more rapid deterioration than that seen in attacks that were not life-threatening. This suggests that the time it takes from onset of symptoms until the patient receives appropriate medical help may be critical in averting fatal asthma[16,28] since the severity of the obstruction, albeit not initially present, can increase suddenly. This rapid deterioration can also occur after the patient is admitted to the hospital[91,92] and sometimes following discharge, even with an FEV_1 level of >70%.[14] Criteria for hospital admission of patients with acute severe asthma treated at the ED have been published previously[18,88,89] and are updated on a continuous basis.[19]

Lack of recognition of life-threatening asthma can have devastating consequences. A number of recent reports continue to emphasize that despite the dissemination of guidelines to treat acute asthma,[11,19] inefficient implementation still exist in some settings[93] even among specialists.[94] A recent Canadian survey of ED physicians[93] found that 46% occasionally or never assessed FEV_1 and 27% occasionally, or never assessed PEFR. Although 97% of respondents used nebulized β agonists always or often, more than 25% used β agonist doses that were less than recommended. Oral steroids were prescribed at time of discharge occasionally by 51%, seldom by 19%, and never by 7% of responding physicians. Inhaled steroids were prescribed at time of discharge occasionally by 35%, seldom by 13%, and never by 16% of responding physicians, respectively.[93] The reasons for not providing proper care to patients presenting with acute asthma in the ED are only speculative and may include lack of perception of the relative severity of asthma as

compared with other acute emergency conditions and the fact that, when treated, the overall prognosis of most patients with asthma who are treated in the ED is good.[13,14] Thus, it is likely that quick, incomplete evaluations and undertreatment are common,[11,92,93] despite existing data on the importance of proper recognition and assessment of near-fatal asthma.[95]

PATHOPHYSIOLOGY OF LIFE-THREATENING ASTHMA

In the past few years, two major advances have occurred in the understanding of near-fatal asthma attacks. First, it has been determined that asphyxia is the predominant contributing factor in patients dying from asthma and second, the mechanisms by which airflow limitation develops and leads to asphyxia are now better understood.

Asphyxia and/or cardiac arrhythmias have always been thought to be the major pathophysiologic events directly implicated in fatal asthma. Because most deaths occur outside the hospital setting, little data examining the pathophysiologic mechanisms leading to death from asthma have been collected. However, studies of patients suffering from near-fatal asthmatic episodes can serve as surrogates, if we assume that the predominant pathophysiologic mechanisms found in near-fatal asthma are similar to those found in patients dying from asthma. Molfino and colleagues studied 10 patients who arrived at the hospital in respiratory arrest or in whom respiratory arrest developed within 20 minutes after admission.[14] These patients had characteristics similar to those described previously for patients at high risk of death from asthma, including a long history of disease (in young to middle-aged patients), previous near-fatal attacks or hospitalizations, delay in obtaining medical treatment, and sudden-onset of a rapidly progressive crisis.[41,42] They also exhibited marked hypercapnia evidenced by a mean ±1 SD Pa_{CO_2} value of 97.1 ± 31.1 mm Hg (12.9 ± 4.1 kPa) and acidemia (pH = 7.01 ± 0.11) before mechanical ventilation was begun. In addition, four patients were hypokalemic on admission. Despite marked severe respiratory acidosis, no patient had a serious cardiac arrhythmia during resuscitation or during hospitalization. Although one patient had atrial fibrillation and another had relative sinus bradycardia, both arrhythmias reverted to sinus rhythm after the initiation of ventilation with hyperoxic gas mixtures, demonstrating the secondary nature of such disturbances. The effects of hypoxemia on cardiac arrhythmias was previously described in dogs by Collins and colleagues, who demonstrated that cardiac disturbances were induced by lower doses of isoprenaline, if hypoxemia was present.[96] On the other hand, Steinhart and colleagues have reported that severe hypercapnia (>400 mm Hg or 53.3 kPa) in dogs resulted in heart failure that could be reversed by administration of catecholamines or worsened by administration of β blockers.[97] In patients with acute severe asthma, however, Douglas and colleagues reported no detectable cardiac arrhythmias in the presence of mild hypoxemia after administration of 1.25, 2.5, or 5 mg of air-nebulized salbutamol.[98] Similar results were reported by Bremner and colleagues in mildly hypoxic healthy volunteers treated with 800 μg of inhaled fenoterol[99] and by Newhouse and colleagues who administered 1600 μg of fenoterol or 3200 μg of salbutamol (albuterol) without supplemental oxygen, in acute asthmatics patients with mild hypoxemia.[55] Considered together, these animal[96,97] and human[55,98,99] studies suggest that mild hypoxemia does not pose a risk for the development of cardiac disturbances. Severe airflow limitation per se is the cause of death in the majority of cases. Patients with severe airway obstruction often have labile airways,[65,100,101] severe or partially reversible preexisting obstruction,[102] a provoking stimulus,[65,68] and impaired response to alterations in airway geometry.[35,36] Excess bronchial muscle shortening appeared to be the cause of sudden decompensation and death in some cases of asthma. This is likely to be true in asthma patients who die of severe airway obstruction and in whom no mucus plugging or submucosal edema of the airways is found postmortem.[103] Bai has reported an increased maximal response to contractile agonists such as histamine, electric field stimulation and acetylcho-

line in airway smooth muscle obtained from patients who died form asthma attacks.[100] In addition, this author reported a diminished relaxation response to β_2 agonists and theophylline in these tissues. Whether this is a result of a change in smooth muscle activation, in loading of the airway muscle, or in smooth muscle shortening is not clear.[103] On the other hand, many patients who suffer from near-fatal asthma often have airways filled with mucus plugs. This may indicate an excessive inflammatory process in the submucosa and lumen of the airways that results in severe airway narrowing, when coupled with normal or excessive airway smooth muscle contraction.[103] In this regard, it has been shown that in patients with fatal asthma, eosinophils are more abundant around central airway smooth muscle than in intraepithelial spaces.[104] In addition, Sur and colleagues reported that patients dying after crises of more than 2.5 hours had more eosinophils and less neutrophils compared to patients dying with crises of less than 1 hour duration.[65] The question of how much hypoxemia, hypercapnia, and acidosis humans can tolerate and if present, the effect of anti-asthmatic therapy (specifically β_2 agonists) on arrhythmias has been investigated by a number of researchers. Cardiac arrhythmias may still occur despite adequate oxygenation because of direct cardiotoxicity of the drugs or because of hypokalemia.[14,105] Hypokalemia can be the result of anti-asthmatic therapy[106,107] and can be associated with muscle weakness,[108] but its role in acute severe asthma is not yet clear. An increased mortality rate in asthma patients using inhaled solutions containing β_2 agonists has been found, suggesting that cardiovascular deaths may occur in predisposed patients treated with this therapeutic modality in the absence of supplemental oxygen.[56]

The most common acid-base disturbances in mild to moderate acute asthma are hypoxemia, hypocapnia, and respiratory alkalosis.[109] However, as the acute attack becomes more severe, major alterations in gas exchange with hypercapnia and respiratory acidosis (with[110] or without metabolic acidosis[110]) are generally found.[14,38,109,111–114] Hypoxemia is closely related to the degree of airway obstruction but rarely is severe (Pa_{O_2} <60 mm Hg

[<8 kPa]), although occasionally it can be aggravated by administration of β_2 agonists.[114] Hypoxemia is the result of severe ventilation-perfusion inequalities and must be corrected immediately.[109] Respiratory acidosis always indicates a potentially life-threatening asthma attack that requires urgent intervention. The presence of respiratory acidosis does not, however, necessarily mean that mechanical ventilation is required, since airway obstruction and hypercapnia can be reversed by conventional medical therapy.[13] In addition, a number of reports suggest that healthy humans can tolerate extremely severe respiratory acidosis if they are adequately oxygenated. Frumin and colleagues studied eight patients who were subjected to apneic oxygenation for periods ranging from 18 to 55 minutes during routine operative procedures.[115] All patients maintained their oxygen saturations at greater than 98%. However, at the end of the apneic period, Pa_{CO_2} values ranged from 130 to 250 mm Hg (17.3 to 33.3 kPa) and pH ranged from 6.97 to 6.72. Despite these extremely severe derangements, six of the eight patients maintained normal sinus rhythm, only two had occasional premature ventricular contractions and all recovered without obvious sequelae. Similarly, Clowes and colleagues studied subjects who breathed gas mixtures containing high concentrations of carbon dioxide.[116] Arterial pH decreased to values as low as 6.8, yet all subjects had uneventful recoveries. Thus, if hypoxemia is avoided, severe respiratory acidosis seems to be well tolerated. However, it is important to point out that patients outside the hospital setting who develop severe respiratory acidosis are likely to be hypoxemic since they are not breathing oxygen-enriched gas mixtures. Although the effects of inhaled β_2 agonists in the presence of severe hypoxemia are not known, epidemiologic evidence suggests that cardiac deaths seem more frequent in patients receiving inhaled solutions of β_2 agonists in a domiciliary setting where oxygen supplementation is unlikely to happen.[56]

Hyperinflation is a constant finding in acute asthma as a result of the prolonged time constant of the respiratory system leading to a positive alveolar pressure at the end of expiration, a phenomenon referred to as intrinsic PEEP ($PEEP_i$) or auto-PEEP.[117] The magnitude of auto-PEEP and alveolar pressure is directly related to the minute ventilation, the mechanical time constant of the respiratory system, and is inversely related to expiratory time.[117] There is also regional hyperinflation owing to a lack of homogeneity in the time constants of various alveolar regions. These factors increase the risk of barotrauma and hemodynamic deterioration and have important implications regarding mechanical ventilation of patients with asthma, and will be described below. In addition, hyperinflation has been shown to be an important factor that produces respiratory muscle impairment in asthma patients.[118,119] Although it appears that muscle fatigue does not play an important role, by itself, during acute bronchospasm,[118] one of the beneficial effects of β agonists in acute asthma may be related to the reduction of lung volume, which in turns improves diaphragmatic function and endurance.[119]

TREATMENT

Even though there are some differences from one country to another and between ED settings in the same country,[18,88,89] all initial therapeutic measures for acute severe asthma aim to avoid death from asphyxia. Conscious patients presenting with life-threatening asthma must immediately receive β_2 agonists (either by nebulizer or MDI), oxygen as indicated, and systemic steroids.[19] While β_2 agonists treat the bronchospastic component of the attack,[13] steroids are used for their anti-inflammatory effects. However, steroids do not act immediately and no alleviation of life-threatening bronchospasm should be expected due to steroids until 4 to 6 hours of administration.[120] For this reason steroids should be administered on arrival or as soon as possible.

The use of intravenous theophylline and/or inhaled ipratropium is controversial. The overall population of acute asthmatics receives more benefit from inhaled β_2 agonists than it does from intravenous theophylline;[121] however, theophylline may prove to have a role in select patients.[122] Inhaled ipratropium bromide has been shown to offer a statistically significant bronchodilator effect, providing it is combined with inhaled β_2 agonists in some studies[123,124] but not in others.[125,126] Furthermore, the clinical relevance of the use of ipratropium bromide in acute asthma is uncertain.[126]

Many patients with severe asthma respond satisfactorily to inhaled β_2 agonists and intravenous steroids in a few hours,[13] yet no patient recovering from a life-threatening event should be discharged[14] before an in-hospital monitoring period of at least 24 hours. Home monitoring may be sufficient for most patients discharged from the ED,[120,127] but patients with life-threatening events can have sudden overwhelming fluctuations in pulmonary function and require close supervision in-hospital.[32]

The use of noninvasive positive pressure ventilation is discussed fully in Chapter 12. Occasionally, respiratory arrest and/or unconsciousness,[14] development of confusion and agitation, or a rising Pa_{CO_2} are indications for endotracheal intubation and mechanical ventilation. Because of a better understanding of the pathophysiology of barotrauma in the past few years, there has been a change in the approach to ventilating severe acute asthma patients based on the concepts of controlled mechanical hypoventilation.[128] The aim of this technique is to restore normal oxygenation while minimizing dynamic hyperinflation and alveolar pressures. This approach consists of ventilation with small tidal volumes, low respiratory rates, and relatively high inspiratory flow rates.[129] Sedation and paralysis of the patient are required and the initial ventilatory settings are adjusted as needed to maintain low peak lung distention pressures and adequate oxygenation. This approach is likely the reason for the decrease in mortality in mechanically ventilated asthmatics in the past decade,[14,128] and indeed in some studies the mortality rate of ventilated patients has been zero.[14,38,128,130] It also acknowledges a state of temporary hypercapnia and does not appear to prolong the duration of mechanical ventilation.[38,128,130] Williams

and colleagues examined the factors associated with hypotension, pulmonary barotrauma, and cardiac arrhythmias in all patients admitted to their ICU with severe asthma.[131] They found that hypotension and barotrauma occurred at a much higher rate in patients who had greater dynamic hyperinflation, as quantified by V_{EI}, the end-inspiration lung volume above FRC.[131] A detailed discussion of mechanical ventilation can be found in Chapter 13.

PREVENTION, OUTCOMES-RESEARCH, AND PHARMACOECONOMICS OF NEAR-FATAL ASTHMA

By using simple questionnaires it is possible to detect ambulatory asthma patients who may be at risk of having to attend an ED.[37] Wakefield and colleagues developed a practical screening questionnaire with a sensitivity of 90% and a specificity of 80% that identified adult patients highly likely to attend an ED within 1 year.[37] To do this, they retrospectively studied asthma patients who did and did not attend the ED due to asthma in the preceding year. The results confirmed that in the 437 patients studied, five variables were related to ED attendance: awakening with nocturnal asthma symptoms, admission to a hospital due to asthma in the past year, visiting more than one general practitioner for asthma in the past year, self-rating of asthma from moderate to severe, and having received oral steroids for asthma in the past month.[37]

A special at-home follow-up program should be implemented for patients suffering from life-threatening asthma. Patients with severe asthma have a 10% mortality rate in the year after the event.[6] Both rapid admission to specialized services[12] and improved patient compliance with therapy and follow-up programs appear to reduce mortality.[16] It is evident that subjects who comply with regular follow-up programs have a better survival rate than the ones who do not comply. One study consisted of 18-month follow-up visits in 12 patients who had been discharged following admission with near-fatal asthma attacks.[16] Only 7 of the 12 subjects consented to a strict monthly follow-up schedule. Whereas two of the patients in the noncompliant group died within 18 months of discharge, none of the compliant patients died within that same period. This study lends support to previous reports regarding the benefits of intensive follow-up of these patients.[12] Moreover, it appears that the most reasonable approach in patients discharged after near-fatal events is to provide adequate doses of inhaled anti-inflammatory therapy, regular peak flow monitoring,[132,133] and good communication with the physician or specialized service during the follow-up period.[12,15,16,134] Measures that should be taken by the patient during an acute attack of asthma at home and en route to hospital have been well defined and have been published following international consensus.[19,89] Another study in which 75 children who suffered from near-fatal asthma were followed for 8 years,[134] has demonstrated that aggressive and timely intervention prevented asthma deaths and provided reassurance to relatives and patients. However, although structured asthma education can significantly improve short-term compliance with treatment and knowledge about asthma, it seems that if appropriate therapy is provided, additional knowledge and education may not add extra benefits with regard to morbidity.[62]

Deficiencies in the ambulatory management of near-fatal asthma have been reported by several investigators. Campbell and colleagues found that, prior to a near-fatal asthma attack, 79% of patients reported weekly symptoms, 27% were using regular β_2 agonists, and 41% of them reported increasing the dose of such treatment when suffering a near-fatal event.[61] In addition, less than 50% of patients used inhaled steroids and only 7% reported increasing or adding oral steroids to the treatment regimen in response to the near-fatal event. In this regard, Kolbe and colleagues conducted a study to determine if asthma education changed patient knowledge and modified their behavior.[135] In 137 patients admitted with severe slow-onset asthma (>6 hours in 96% of patients), it was found that both knowledge and behavior

surrounding the acute attack were inadequate. There were discrepancies between knowledge and behavior in 1) seeking medical help [i.e., 82% knew what to do (knowledge) vs 52% who actually did it (behavior)], and 2) calling an ambulance (61% who knew what to do vs 23% who actually did it, respectively). Factors associated with this knowledge-behavior gap were mostly socioeconomic and included being non-European, anxiety, pessimism, stigmatization, concern about the medical costs, and being the only income for the household. Factors that correlated with both high knowledge and adequate behavior included physician-patient relationship, previous asthma morbidity, existence of an action plan, use of oral steroids, and availability of a peak flow meter. To determine the best action plan to prevent acute exacerbations in subjects with poor asthma control, Cowie and colleagues randomized 150 asthma-educated subjects who received no action plan, a symptom-based action plan, and a peak flow–based action plan.[136] At 6 months only the group who followed the peak flow–based action plan had a significantly decreased attendance to the ED. However, whether these positive results can be maintained with a more prolonged follow-up cannot be determined from this study.

With an emphasis on proper diagnosis, early treatment of acute asthma and strict follow-up plans, some health-economic variables are likely to improve. For example, Levenson and colleagues[137] have replicated and extended results described above[16] by implementing a comprehensive program for severe, fatality-prone, noncompliant asthma patients. These researchers evaluated the effects of the treatment protocol on asthma outcome and on in-patient costs. The protocol consisted of regularly scheduled visits with the same physician, 24-hour telephone access, adequate doses of inhaled anti-inflammatory drugs and psychiatric referral, if indicated. The number of hospitalizations declined markedly with no ICU admissions or fatalities in 4 years. Before the treatment protocol, the mean cost per patient per year was $US23,000 which fell to a postintervention mean of $US1,100. Therefore, these type of programs[16,138] allow successful and cost-effective management of near-fatal asthma. These results also support the contention that if patients are compliant, even with a history of previous episodes of near-fatal asthma, they tend to use the health care system as much as those without near-fatal asthma.[20] Every effort must be made, however, to avoid unnecessary asthma hospitalizations in patients with a history of near-fatal asthma, particularly if the patient, once stabilized, can be monitored in a special unit for a period of hours during which objective measurement of airflow obstruction can be made. These units, an intermediate step between the ED and the hospital ward, can be very helpful. For example, a prospective evaluation of the role of emergency diagnostic and treatment units as an alternative to hospitalization of asthma patients who did not respond to conventional ED treatment was conducted in 222 subjects presenting with an asthma attack.[138] The end points were medical outcome and cost-effectiveness; patient satisfaction; and quality of life in patients treated in the unit as compared to those receiving in-patient care. After 3 hours of treatment in the ED, patients were randomized to hospital admission and routine therapy or to a 9-hour treatment in the unit. Sixty-five patients (59%) were discharged from the unit and their rate of relapse was no different than patients discharged after regular hospital admission, during 8 weeks of follow-up. The length of stay, patient satisfaction, and quality of life parameters favored treatment at the unit, and the mean cost per patient was 50% less than an in-hospital stay. Thus, emergency assessment and treatment for acute asthma are safe and cost-effective.

CONCLUSIONS

The rates of death have stabilized yet remain higher than expected particularly in nonwhites and females. The persistence of high mortality rates may be explained by differences in severity of asthma or accuracy of diagnosis. Irrespective of the causes, improvements in overall management should reduce asthma mortality.[5] Near-fatal asthma is the penultimate step in patients with catastrophic asthma.[14] Identification of fatality-prone patients and recognition of the features of near-fatal asthma and understanding its pathophysiology, may lead to further reduction of these episodes.[65] The predominant pathophysiologic findings are the result of severe airway obstruction with severe alterations in acid-base status.[14] Respiratory arrest and coma upon admission, or severe dyspnea with silent chest on auscultation and use of accessory muscles of respiration, constitute the basic clinical picture.[88] Respiratory acidosis associated with hypoxemia and metabolic acidosis are the result of gross ventilation-perfusion alterations; hypoxemia is the principal factor that must be corrected immediately. Cardiac arrhythmias are rarely present.[14] Although difficult,[14,32] every effort must be made by physicians to identify the principal inciter(s) of a life-threatening attack of asthma; airway inflammation is not always the predominant finding in acute onset near-fatal and fatal asthma.[65]

Conventional treatment of acute attacks with high doses of inhaled β_2 agonists, oxygen, and intravenous steroids should occur without delay. Physicians should be very aggressive under these circumstances since severe asphyxia, as the result of massive airway obstruction, seems to be the important determinant of death during these episodes.[14] Mechanical ventilation is occasionally required as a last resort and, if instituted, it should be done using a strategy of controlled hypoventilation, to avoid barotrauma.

Objective measurement of pulmonary function (PEFR or FEV_1) must be obtained to monitor treatment in-hospital as soon as possible. Admission or in-hospital supervision for at least 24 hours is desirable in patients for whom relapses can be fatal. Upon discharge, patient education, close patient-physician communication, anti-inflammatory medications, inhaled β_2 agonists on demand, and regular peak flow monitoring are mandatory.

It has been determined that the inability, by the patient or the physician, to recognize asthma severity is a major risk factor in near-fatal and fatal asthma attacks.[11] The use of an intermediate stop between the ED and the hospital ward for rapid diagnosis and treatment, probably reduces morbidity and costs.

REFERENCES

1. Siegel SC: History of asthma death from antiquity. *J Allergy Clin Immunol* 80:458–462, 1987.
2. Maimonides M: *Treatise on Asthma*. Philadelphia, Lippincott, 1963.
3. Osler W: *The Principles and Practice of Medicine*. New York, Appleton and Co, 1892.
4. Dunnill MS: The pathology of asthma, with special references to changes in the bronchial mucosa. *J Cardiovasc Pharmacol* 13:27–49, 1960.
5. Sly RM, O'Donnell R: Stabilization of asthma mortality. *Ann Allergy Asthma Immunol* 78(4): 347–354, 1997.
6. McFadden ER Jr, Warren EL: Observations on asthma mortality. *Arch Intern Med* 127(2):142–147, 1997.
7. Silverstein MD, Reed CE, O'Connell EJ, et al: Long-term survival of a cohort of community residents with asthma. *N Engl J Med* 331:1537–1541, 1994.
8. Raimondi AC, Molfino NA: The impact of changing disease management on the in-hospital morbidity and mortality of 725 episodes of life-threatening asthma (abstr.). *Eur Respir J* 10(Suppl 25):118s, 1997.
9. Donahue JG, Weiss ST, Livingston JM, et al: Inhaled steroids and the risk of hospitalization for asthma. *JAMA* 277:887–891, 1997.
10. Stempel DA, Durcannin-Robbins JF, Hedblom EC, et al: Drug utilization evaluation identifies costs associated with high use of beta-adrenergic agonists. *Ann Allergy Asthma Immunol* 76:153–158, 1996.
11. Stableforth DE: Asthma mortality and physician competence. *J Allergy Clin Immunol* 80(3 pt 2):463–466, 1987.
12. Crompton GK, Grant IW, Chapman BJ, et al: Edinburgh Emergency Asthma Admission Service: Report on 15 years' experience. *Eur J Resp Dis* 70:266–271, 1987.
13. Raimondi AC, Schottlender J, Lombardi D, Molfino NA: Treatment of acute severe asthma with inhaled albuterol delivered via jet nebulizer, metered dose inhaler with spacer, or dry powder. *Chest* 112:24–28, 1997.
14. Molfino NA, Nannini LJ, Martelli AN, Slutsky AS: Respiratory arrest in near-fatal asthma. *N Engl J Med* 324:285–288, 1991.
15. McFadden ER Jr: Fatal and near-fatal asthma. *N Engl J Med* 324:409–410, 1991.
16. Molfino NA, Nannini LJ, Rebuck AS, Slutsky AS: The fatality-prone asthmatic patient. Follow-up study after near-fatal attacks. *Chest* 101:621–623, 1992.
17. Molfino NA, Slutsky AS: Near-fatal asthma. *Eur Respir J* 7:981–990, 1994.
18. National Heart, Lung, and Blood Institute: National Asthma Education Program, Expert Panel Report: Guidelines for the diagnosis and management of asthma. *J Allergy Clin Immunol* 88(3)2: 425–534, 1991.
19. National Heart, Lung, and Blood Institute: *Guidelines For The Diagnosis and Management of Asthma*. National Heart, Lung, and Blood Institute 1997 Publ No. 97-4051A.
20. Kesten S, Chew R, Hanania NA: Health-care utilization after near-fatal asthma. *Chest* 107:1564–1569, 1995.
21. Richards GN, Kolbe J, Fenwick J, Rea HH: Demographic characteristics of patients with severe life threatening asthma: Comparison with asthma deaths. *Thorax* 48:1105–1109, 1993.
22. Lang DM, Polansky M: Patterns of asthma mortality in Philadelphia from 1969 to 1991. *N Engl J Med* 331:1542–1546, 1994.
23. Apter AJ, Reisine ST, Kennedy DG, et al: To identify the demographic predictors of asthma treatment site: Outpatient clinic, emergency department, or hospital. *Ann Allergy Asthma Immunol* 79 (4):353–361, 1997.
24. Nelson HS, Hirsch SR, Ohman JL, et al: Recommendations for the use of residential air-cleaning devices in the treatment of allergic respiratory diseases. *J Allergy Clin Immunol* 82:661–669, 1988.
25. Platts-Mills TA, Chapman MD, Pollart S, et al: Specific allergens evoking immune reactions in the lung: Relationship to asthma. *Eur Respir J* 13(Suppl):68s–77s, 1991.
26. Sporik R, Holgate St, Platts-Mills TA, Cogswell

JJ: Exposure to house-dust mite allergen (Der p I) and the development of asthma in childhood. A prospective study [see comments]. *N Engl J Med* 323:502–507, 1990.

27. Ernst P, Demissie K, Joseph L, et al: Socioeconomic status and indicators of asthma in children. *Am J Respir Crit Care Med* 152:570–575, 1995.

28. Barriot P, Riou B: Prevention of fatal asthma. *Chest* 92:460–466, 1987.

29. Strunk RC: Identification of the fatality-prone subject with asthma. *J Allergy Clin Immunol* 83(2):477–484, 1989.

30. Riou B, Barriot P, Duroux P: Fatal asthma. *Rev Mal Respir* 5(4):353–361, 1988.

31. Benatar SR: Fatal asthma. *N Engl J Med* 314:423–429, 1986.

32. Turner-Warwick M: On observing patterns of airflow obstruction in chronic asthma. *Br J Dis Chest* 71:73–86, 1977.

33. Rubinfeld AR, Pain MC: Perception of asthma. *Lancet* 1:882–884, 1976.

34. Hudgel DW, Weil JV: Asthma associated with decreased hypoxic ventilatory drive: A family study. *Arch Intern Med* 80:623–625, 1974.

35. Kikuchi Y, Okabe S, Tamura G, et al: Chemosensitivity and perception of dyspnea in patients with a history of near-fatal asthma. *N Engl J Med* 330:1329–1334, 1994.

36. Kifle Y, Seng V, Davenport PW: Magnitude estimation of inspiratory resistive loads in children with life-threatening asthma. *Am J Respir Crit Care Med* 156 (5):1530–1535, 1997.

37. Wakefield M, Ruffin R, Campbell D, et al: A risk screening questionnaire for adults asthmatics to predict attendance at hospital emergency departments. *Chest* 112:1527–1533, 1997.

38. Wasserfallen J-B, Schaller M-D, Feihl F, Perret CH: Sudden asphyxic asthma: A distinct entity? *Am Rev Respir Dis* 142:108–111, 1990.

39. Crompton G: The catastrophic asthmatic. *Br J Dis Chest* 81:321–325, 1987.

40. Sears MR, Rea HH, Beaglehole R, et al: Asthma mortality in New Zealand: A two-year national study. *N Z Med J* 98:271–275, 1985.

41. Rea HH, Sears MR, Beaglehole R, Fenwick J: Lessons from the national asthma mortality study: circumstances surrounding death. *N Z Med J* 100(816):10–13, 1987.

42. Sears MR: Epidemiology of asthma, in O'Byrne

PM (ed): *Asthma as an Inflammatory Disease.* New York: Marcel Dekker, 1990, pp 15–48.

43. Perna G, Bertani A, Politi E, et al: Asthma and panic attacks. *Biol Psychiatry* 42(7):625–630, 1997.

44. Campbell DA, Yellowlees PM, McLennan G, et al: Psychiatric and medical features of near fatal asthma. *Thorax* 50(3):254–259, 1995.

45. Miles JF, Garden GM, Tunnicliffe WS, et al: Psychological morbidity and coping skills in patients with brittle and non-brittle asthma: A case-control study. *Clin Exp Allergy* 27(10):1151–1159, 1997.

46. Chetta A, Gerra G, Foresi A, et al: Personality profiles and breathlessness perception in outpatients with different gradings of asthma. *Am J Respir Crit Care Med* 157:116–122, 1998.

47. Joseph KS, Blais L, Ernst P, Suissa S: Increased morbidity and mortality related to asthma among asthmatic patients who use major tranquillisers. *Br Med J* 312 (7023):79–82, 1996.

48. Sears MR, Taylor DR, Print CG, et al: Regular inhaled beta-agonist treatment in bronchial asthma. *Lancet* 336:1391–1396, 1990.

49. Spitzer WO, Suissa S, Ernst P, et al: The use of beta-agonists and the risk of death and near death from asthma [see Comments]. *N Engl J Med* 326:501–506, 1992.

50. Drazen JM, Israel E, Boushey HA, et al: Comparison of regularly schedule with as-needed use of albuterol in mild asthma. *N Engl J Med* 335:841–847, 1996.

51. Suissa S, Blais L, Ernst P: Patterns of increasing beta-agonist use and the risk of fatal or near-fatal asthma. *Eur Respir J* 7(9):1602–1609, 1994.

52. Spitzer WO, Suissa S, Ernst P, et al: The use of β-agonists and the risk of death and near death from asthma. *N Engl J Med* 326:501–506, 1992.

53. Garrett JE, Lanes SF, Kolbe J, Rea HH: Risk of severe life-threatening and beta agonist type: an example of confounding by severity. *Thorax* 51 (11):1093–1099, 1997.

54. Rea HH, Garrett JE, Lanes SF, et al: The association between asthma drugs and severe life-threatening attacks. *Chest* 110(6):1446–1451, 1996.

55. Suissa S, Ernst P: Optical illusions from visual data analysis: Example of the New Zealand asthma mortality epidemic. *J Clin Epidemiol* 50(10):1079–1088, 1997.

56. Suissa S, Hemmelgarn B, Blais L, Ernst P: Bron-

chodilators and acute cardiac death. *Am J Respir Crit Care Med* 154(6 Pt 1):1598–1602, 1996.

57. Martinez FD, Graves PE, Baldini M, et al: Association between genetic polymorhisms of the beta2-adrenoceptor and response to albuterol in children with and without a history of wheezing. *J Clin Invest* 100(12):3184–3188, 1997.

58. Tan S, Hall IP, Dewar J, et al: Association between beta2-adrenoceptor polymorphisms and susceptibility to bronchodilator desensitisation in moderately severe stable asthmatics. *Lancet* 350(9083):995–999, 1997.

59. Liggett SB: Polymorphisms of the β_2-adrenergic receptor and asthma. *Am J Respir Crit Care Med* 156(4)pt 2:S156–S162, 1997.

60. Weir TD, Malleck N, Sandford AJ, et al: Genetic polymorphisms of the β_2-adrenergic receptor in fatal and near-fatal asthma (abstr.). *Am J Respir Crit Care Med* 155(4):A256, 1997.

61. Campbell DA, Luke CG, McLennan G, et al: Near-fatal asthma in South Australia: Descriptive features and medication use. *Aust N Z J Med* 26(3):356–362, 1996.

62. Cote J, Cartier A, Robichaud P, et al: Influence on asthma morbidity of asthma education programs based on self-management plans following treatment optimization. *Am J Respir Crit Care Med* 155(5):1509–1514, 1997.

63. Newhouse MT, Chapman KR, McCallum AL, et al: Cardiovascular safety of high doses of inhaled fenoterol and albuterol in acute severe asthma. *Chest* 110:595–603, 1996.

64. Campbell DA, McLennan G, Coates JR, et al: Near fatal asthma attacks: the reliability of descriptive information collected from close acquaintances. *Thorax* 48:1099–1104, 1993.

65. Sur S, Crotty TB, Kephart GM, et al: Sudden-onset fatal asthma. *Am Rev Respir Dis* 148:713–719, 1993.

66. Arnold AG, Lane DJ, Zapata E: The speed of onset and severity of acute severe asthma. *Br J Dis Chest* 76:157–163, 1982.

67. Weiss KB: Seasonal trends in US asthma hospitalizations and mortality. *JAMA* 263(17):2323–2328, 1991.

68. O'Hollaren MT, Yunginger JW, Offord KP, et al: Exposure to an aeroallergen as a possible precipitating factor in respiratory arrest in young patients with asthma. *N Engl J Med* 324:359–363, 1991.

69. British Thoracic Society: Comparison of atopic and non-atopic patients dying of asthma. *Br J Dis Chest* 81:30–34, 1987.

70. Pollart SM, Chapman MD, Fiocco GP, et al: Epidemiology of acute asthma: IgE antibodies to common inhalant allergens as a risk factor for emergency room visits. *J Allergy Clin Immunol* 83:875–882, 1989.

71. Picado C, Castillo JA, Montserrat JM, Agusti-Vidal A: Aspirin-intolerance as a precipitant factor of life-threatening attacks of asthma requiring mechanical ventilation. *Eur Respir J* 2(2):127–129, 1989.

72. Szczeklik A: Aspirin-induced asthma as a viral disease. *Clin Allergy* 18(1):15–20, 1988.

73. Partridge MR, Gibson GJ: Adverse bronchial reactions to intravenous hydrocortisone in two aspirin-sensitive asthmatic patients. *Br Med J* 1(6126):1521–1522, 1978.

74. Hunt LWJr, Rosenow III EC: Drug-induced asthma, in Weiss EB, Stein M (eds): *Bronchial Asthma*, 2d ed. Toronto, Little, Brown, 1993, pp 621–631.

75. Levenson T, Greenberger PA, Donoghue ER, Lifshultz BD: Asthma deaths confounded by substance abuse: An assessment of fatal asthma. *Chest* 110(3):604–610, 1996.

75a. Cygan J, Trunsky M, Corbridge T: Inhaled heroin-induced status asthmaticus: Five cases and a review of the literature. *Chest* 117:272–275, 2000.

76. Sampson HA, Mendelson L, Rosen JP: Fatal and near-fatal anaphylactic reactions to food in children and adolescents. *N Engl J Med* 327:380–384, 1992.

77. Williams MH Jr: Increasing severity of asthma from 1960 to 1987. *N Engl J Med* 320(15):1015–1016, 1989.

78. Costello JF: Asthma-A United Kingdom view: Treatment and its implications, in Piper PJ, Krell RD (eds): *Advances in the Understanding and Treatment of Asthma*. New York, Ann NY Acad Sci, 1991, pp 7–14.

79. Roux P, Smit M, Weinberg EG: Seasonal and recurrent intensive care unit admissions for acute severe asthma in children. *S Afr Med J* 83:177–179, 1993.

80. Piccolo MC, Perillo GME, Ramon CG, DiDio V: Outbreaks of asthma attacks and meteorologic parameters in Bahia Blanca, Argentina. *Ann Allergy* 60:107–110, 1988.

81. Molfino NA, Wright SC, Katz I, et al: Effect of low concentrations of ozone on inhaled allergen

responses in asthmatic subjects. *Lancet* 338:199–203, 1991.

82. Studnika M, Hackl E, Pischinger J, et al: Traffic-related NO2 and the prevalence of asthma and respiratory symptoms in seven year olds. *Eur Respir J* 10(10):2275–2278, 1997.

83. Jamason PF, Falkstein LS, Gergen PJ: A synoptic evaluation of asthma hospital admisions in New York city. *Am J Respir Crit Care Med* 156:1781–1788, 1997.

84. Drazen JM, Boushey HA, Holgate St, et al: The pathogenesis of severe asthma: A consensus report from the workshop on pathogenesis. *J Allergy Clin Immunol* 80(3, pt 2):428–437, 1991.

85. Ruffin RE, Latimer KM, Schembri D: Longitudinal study of near-fatal asthma. *Am Rev Respir Dis* 139:A68, 1989.

86. Crimi E, Spanevello A, Neri M, Ind PW, Rossi GA, Brusasco V: Dissociation between airway inflammation and airway hyperresponsiveness in allergic asthma. *Am J Respir Crit Care Med* 157:4–9, 1998.

87. Ernst P, Spitzer WO, Suissa S, et al: Risk of fatal and near-fatal asthma in relation to inhaled corticosteroid use. *JAMA* 268:3462–3464, 1992.

88. British Thoracic Society, Research Unit of the Royal College of Physicians of London: National Asthma Campaign Guidelines for the management of asthma in adults: II-acute severe asthma. *Br Med J* 301:797–801, 1990.

89. National Heart Lung, and Blood Institute: International consensus report on diagnosis and treatment of asthma. *Eur Respir J* 5:601–641, 1992.

90. Crompton G, Grant IWB, Bloomfield P: Edinburgh Emergency asthma admission service: Report of ten years experience. *Br Med J* 2:1199–1201, 1979.

91. Hetzel MR, Clark TJ, Branthwaite MA: Asthma: Analysis of sudden deaths and ventilatory arrests in hospital. *Br Med J* 1:808–811, 1977.

92. Rothwell RPG, Rea HH, Sears MR, et al: Lessons from the national asthma mortality study: Deaths in hospital. *N Z Med J* 100:199–202, 1987.

93. Grunfeild A, Beverage RC, Berkowitz J, Fitzgerald JM: Managment of acute asthma in Canada: An assessment of emergency physicians behavior. *J Exp Med* 15(14):547–556, 1997.

94. Rogado MC, de Diego A, ed la Cuadra P, Perpina M, Compte L, Leon M: Treatment of asthmatic crises at a hospital emergency service. Are the protocols followed? Anal Biochem 33(4):179–184, 1997.

95. Shalley MJ, Cross AB: Which patients are likely to die in an accident and emergency department. *Br Med J* 289:419–421, 1984.

96. Collins JM, McDevitt DG, Shanks RG, Swanton JG: The cardiotoxicity of isoprenaline during hypoxia. *Br J Pharmacol* 36:35–45, 1969.

97. Steinhart CR, Permutt S, Gurtner GH, Traystman RJ: Beta-adrenergic activity and cardiovascular response to severe respiratory acidosis. *Am J Physiol* 244:H46–H54, 1983.

98. Douglas JG, Rafferty P, Ferguson RJ, Prescott RJ, Crompton GK, Grant IWB: Nebulised salbutamol without oxygen in severe acute asthma: How effective and how safe? *Thorax* 40:180–183, 1985.

99. Bremner P, Woodman K, Beasley R, et al: Hypoxaemia increases the cardiovascular effects of fenoterol (abstr.). *Am Rev Respir Dis* 143(4):A648, 1991.

100. Bai TR: Abnormalities in airway smooth muscle in fatal asthma. *Am Rev Respir Dis* 141:552–557, 1990.

101. Bramley AM, Thomson RJ, Roberts CR, Schellenberg RR: Hypothesis: Excessive bronchoconstriction in asthma is due to decreased airway elastance. *Eur Respir J* 7:337–341, 1994.

102. Hudon C, Turcotte H, Laviotte M, Carrier G, Boulet LP: Characteristics of bronchial asthma with incomplete reversibility of airflow obstruction. *Ann Allergy Asthma Immunol* 78(2):195–202, 1997.

103. Hogg JC: Varieties of airway narrowing in severe and fatal asthma. *J Allergy Clin Immunol* 80(3 pt 2):417–419, 1987.

104. Synek M, Beasley R, Frew AJ, et al: Cellular infiltration of the airways in asthma of varying severity. *Am J Respir Crit Care Med* 154:224–230, 1996.

105. Laaban JP, Iung B, Chauvet JP, Psychyos I, Proteau J: Cardiac arrhythmias during the combined use of aminophylline and terbutaline in status asthmaticus. *Chest* 94(3):496–502, 1988.

106. Swenson ER, Aitken ML: Hypokalemia occurs with inhaled albuterol (abstract). *Am Rev Respir Dis* 131: A99, 1985.

107. Martelli A, Otero C, Gil B, Gonzalez S: Fenoterol and serum potassium. *Lancet* 1:1197, 1989.

108. Knochel JP: Neuromuscular manifestations of electrolyte disorders. *Am J Med* 72:521–535, 1982.

109. McFadden ER Jr, Lyons HA: Arterial-blood gas tension in asthma. *N Engl J Med* 278:1027–1032, 1968.

110. Roncoroni AJ, Adrogue JHA, DeObrutsky CW, Marchisio ML, Herrera MR: Metabolic acidosis in status asthmaticus. *Respiration* 33:85–94, 1976.

111. Mountain RD, Heffner JE, Brackett NC, Shann SA: Acid-base disturbances in acute asthma. *Chest* 98:651–655, 1990.

112. Permutt S: Physiologic changes in the acute asthmatic attack, in Austen KF, Lichtenstein LM (eds): *Asthma: Physiology, Immunopharmacology and Treatment.* New York, Academic Press, 1973, pp 15–27.

113. Palmer KN, Diamant ML: Hypoxaemia in bronchial asthma. *Lancet* 1:318, 1968.

114. Palmer KN, Diamant ML: Effect of salbutamol on spirometry and blood-gas tensions in bronchial asthma. *Br Med J* 1:31–32, 1969.

115. Frumin MJ, Epstein RM, Cohen G: Apneic oxygenation in man. *Anesthesiology* 20:789–798, 1959.

116. Clowes GHAJr, Hopkins AL, Simeone FA: Comparison of physiological effects of hypercapnia and hypoxia in production of cardiac arrest. *Ann Surg* 142:446–460, 1952

117. Pepe PE, Marini JJ: Occult positive end-expiratory pressure in mechanically ventilated patients with airflow obstruction: the auto-PEEP effect. *Am Rev Respir Dis* 126(1):166–170, 1982.

118. Lavietes MH, Grocela JA, Maniatis T, Potulski F, Ritter AB, Sunderam G: Inspiratory muscle strenght in asthma. *Chest* 93(5):1043–1048, 1988.

119. Weiner P, Suo J, Fernadez E, Cherniack RM: The effect of hyperinflation on respiratory muscle strenght and efficiency in healthy subjects and patients with asthma. *Am Rev Respir Dis* 141(6): 1501–1505, 1990.

120. Chapman KR, Verbeek PR, White JG, Rebuck AS: Effect of a short course of prednisone in the prevention of early relapse after the emergency room treatment of acute asthma. *N Engl J Med* 324:788–794, 1991.

121. McFadden ER Jr: Methylxantines in the treatment of asthma: The rise, the fall, and the possible rise again. *Arch Intern Med* 115(4):323–324, 1991.

122. Wrenn K, Slovis CM, Murphy F, Greenberg RS: Aminophylline therapy for acute bronchospastic disease in the emergency room. *Arch Intern Med* 115:241–247, 1991.

123. Teale C, Morrison JF, Muers MF, Pearson SB: Response to nebulized ipratropium bromide and terbutaline in acute severe asthma. *Respir Med* 86:215–218, 1992.

124. Whyte KF, Gould GA, Jeffrey AA, Airlie MA, Flenley DC, Douglas NJ: Dose of nebulized ipratropium bromide in acute severe asthma. *Respir Med* 85:517–520, 1991.

125. McFadden ER, elSanadi N, Strauss L, et al: The influence of parasympatholytics on the resolution of acute attacks of asthma. *Am J Med* 102(1):7–13, 1997.

126. Fitzgerald JM, Grunfeld A, Pare PD, et al: The clinical efficacy of combination nebulized anticholinergic and adrenergic bronchodilators vs nebulized adrenergic bronchodilator alone in acute asthma. Canadian Combivent Study Group. *Chest* 111(2):311–315, 1997.

127. Higenbottam T, Hay I: Has the treatment of asthma improved? *Chest* 98:706–712, 1990.

128. Darioli R, Perret C: Mechanical controlled hypoventilation in status asthmaticus. *Am Rev Respir Dis* 129:385–387, 1984.

129. Tuxen DV, Lane S: The effects of ventilatory pattern on hyperinflation, airway pressures, and circulation in mechanical ventilation of patients with severe air-flow obstruction. *Am Rev Respir Dis* 136:872–879, 1987.

130. Menitove SM, Goldring RM: Combined ventilator and bicarbonate strategy in the management of status asthmaticus. *Am J Med* 94:898–901, 1983.

131. Williams TJ, Tuxen DV, Scheinkenstel CD, Czarny D, Bowes G: Risk factors for morbidity in mechanically ventilated patients with acute severe asthma. *Am Rev Respir Dis* 146:607–615, 1992.

132. Beasley R, Cushley M, Holgate St: A self management plan in the treatment of adult asthma. *Thorax* 44:200–204, 1989.

133. Cross D, Nelson HS: The role of the peak flow meter in the diagnosis and management of asthma. *J Allergy Clin Immunol* 87:120–128, 1991.

134. Sherman JM, Capen CL: The Red Alert Program for life-threatening asthma. *Pediatrics* 100(2, pt 1):187–191, 1997.

135. Kolbe J, Vamos M, Fergusson W, Elkind G, Garret J: Differential influences on asthma self-

management knowledge and self-management behavior in acute severe asthma. *Chest* 110(6): 1463–1468, 1996.

136. Cowie RL, Revitt SG, Underwod MF, Field SK: The effect of a peak flow-based action plan in the prevention of exacerbations of asthma. *Chest* 112:1534–1538, 1997.

137. Levenson T, Grammer LC, Yarnold PR, Patterson R: Cost-effective management of malignant potentially fatal asthma. Allergy Asthma Proc 18(2):73–78, 1997.

138. McDermott MF, Murphy DG, Zalenski RJ, et al: A comparison between emergency diagnostic and treatment unit and inpatient care in the management of acute asthma. *Arch Intern Med* 157(18): 2055–2062, 1997.

139. Barger LW, Vollmer WM, Felt RW, Buist AS: Further investigation into the recent increase in asthma death rates: A review of 41 asthma deaths in Oregon in 1982. *Ann Allergy* 60:31–39, 1988.

140. Bates DV, Baker-Anderson M, Sizto R: Asthma attack periodicity: A study of hospital emergency visits in Vancouver. *Environ Res* 51(1):51–70, 1990.

141. Bates DV, Sizto R: The Ontario Air Pollution Study: Identification of the causative agent. *Environ Health Perspect* 79:69–72, 1989.

142. Bates DV, Sizto R: Relationship between air pollutant levels and hospital admissions in southern Ontario. *Can J Public Health* 74:117–12, 1983.

Chapter 4

PATHOLOGY OF ACUTE ASTHMA

Ritu Nayar
Anjana V. Yeldandi

INTRODUCTION

Since asthmatic patients are rarely biopsied for diagnostic purposes, morphologic descriptions of asthma are based primarily on autopsy findings from patients dying in status asthmaticus.[1–7] The findings described in *acute asthmatic* deaths have been supplemented by postmortem studies on lungs from asthmatic patients dying of unrelated causes,[1,8,9] as well as from lung biopsies,[10–12] and cytology specimens[13] in living patients. Recently, Sur and colleagues have raised the possibility that sudden-onset fatal asthma may be a distinct pathologic entity.[14]

GROSS FINDINGS

Lungs from asthmatic patients are often hyperinflated and do not retract when they are removed from the body at autopsy (Fig. 4-1). This is probably due in part to the presence of tenacious mucus plugs in small- and medium-sized bronchi. These gelatinous, gray-white mucus plugs are readily seen on the cut surface of the lung on autopsy. Distal to these plugs, areas of overdistention appear grossly pale, whereas dark areas represent atelectasis (Fig. 4-2). This mottled appearance has been attributed to varying degrees of airway obstruction. In partial airway obstruction, air enters the distal parenchyma through expanded airways during inspiration but cannot exit through narrowed airways during expiration, thus leading to air trapping by a ball-valve type effect. In complete obstruction, atelectasis occurs due to absorption of distal air.[15]

MICROSCOPIC FINDINGS

Basement Membrane Thickening

Thickening of the basement membrane seen on light microscopy is one of the pathologic hallmarks of asthma. It is pink, hyalinized, and approximately two-fold thicker in patients who die of status asthmaticus compared to nonasthmatic patients[16] (Fig. 4-3). Basement membrane thickening is believed to be caused largely by increased deposition of type III and type V collagen, along with fibronectin,[9,17] and perhaps is augmented by protein transudation.[8] Transmission electron microscopy has demonstrated that the basement membrane has at least two morphologically distinct layers: the basal lamina and a thicker reticular collagenous lamina. It is the latter that becomes thickened in atopic asthma, even in mild, stable disease.[17] The thickening appears to be most pronounced in areas of epithelial damage and submucosal inflammation.[15] Growth factors released as a result of epithelial damage and mucosal inflammation result in proliferation of myofibroblasts that are thought to secrete collagen types responsible for basement membrane thickening.[17] Thickening of the reticular lamina is a normal aging process and that may be hastened by chronic inflammation. Focal but variable thickening of the basement membrane also occurs in lung cancer,

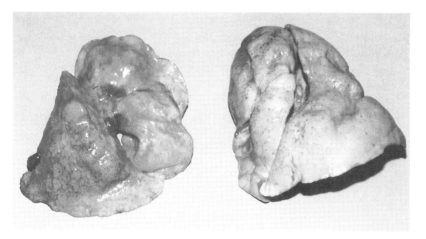

Figure 4-1
Hyperinflated lung specimens from a child who died of acute asthma. These have not been filled with formalin and represent failure to collapse upon removal from the body. H & E stain, medium magnification. (Courtesy of Monica Smiddy, MD, Office of Chief Medical Examiner, New York City.)

Figure 4-2
Hyperinflated adult lung at autopsy. Note the pale patchy areas representing overdistention with adjacent darker areas representing atelectasis. H & E stain, medium magnification. (Courtesy of Monica Smiddy, MD, Office of Chief Medical Examiner, New York City.)

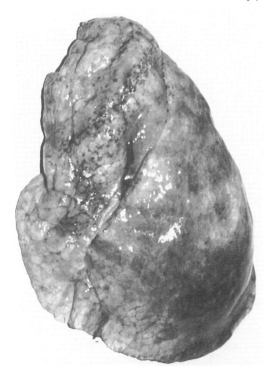

chronic obstructive airway disease, and chronic inflammatory conditions such as bronchiectasis and tuberculosis.

Bronchial Smooth Muscle

Smooth muscle hypertrophy (Fig. 4-4) of the airway is a well-recognized finding in asthmatics. While the etiology of muscular hypertrophy is not clearly understood, neural mediation is thought to play a role in both muscular hyperactivity and increased muscle thickness.[18,19] Sheils and colleagues postulated that vascular leakage in the airways in asthma is a primary event that leads to airway smooth muscle hyperplasia and hypertro-

Figure 4-3
Thickened basement membrane in a histologic section of an asthmatic. (H & E stain, medium magnification.)

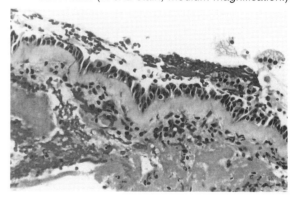

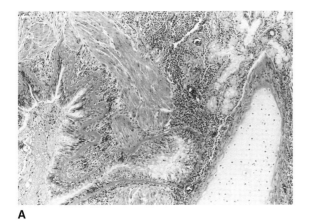

A

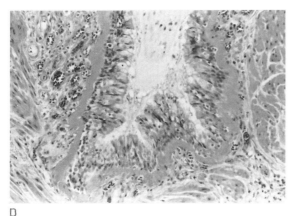

B

Figure 4-4

A and *B*: Bronchial submucosa with goblet cell hyperplasia, smooth muscle hypertrophy, submucosal edema, and mild inflammatory infiltrate. H & E stain, medium magnification. (*Courtesy of Monica Smiddy, MD, Office of Chief Medical Examiner, New York City.*)

phy.[20] Prolonged bronchoconstriction is also thought to contribute to the bronchial wall muscular hypertrophy seen in asthma patients.[21] Bronchial smooth muscle hypertrophy is not seen in chronic bronchitis and thus is helpful in separating it from asthma, pathologically.

Changes in the Respiratory Epithelial Lining

Major basic protein (MBP), a toxic protein released from eosinophilic granules, contributes to respiratory epithelial damage.[22] Airway edema may also indirectly contribute to epithelial sloughing.

Creola bodies are hyperplastic fragments of ciliated bronchial epithelium that can become detached from the basement membrane and form tight balls. They are named after the patient in whom they were first observed and described.[23] Creola bodies resemble bronchioloalveolar carcinoma on cytologic preparations; however, the presence of surface cilia on Creola bodies is a useful distinguishing feature. Creola bodies are seen in sputa, histologic sections, or within plugs/casts in the bronchial tree. The more proximal a Creola body travels in the bronchial tree, the more cellular degeneration occurs. Muscle spasm[2] or extreme transudation of fluid[8] have been proposed as possible mechanisms that result in this form of mucosal injury. The loss of ciliated mucosal surface cells further compromises bronchial tree clearance mechanisms. Atypical squamous metaplasia can also occur in the bronchial lining, secondary to injury and regeneration.

The bronchial mucosal lining and submucosal glands also demonstrate goblet cell hyperplasia: a concurrent decrease in ciliated bronchial cells occurs. Dail[15] has also pointed out that normally goblet cells line the proximal bronchi and are present up to the level of the cartilage in smaller bronchi measuring about 1 to 2 mm in diameter. In asthma patients, goblet cells are seen more peripherally, and in increased numbers.

Submucosal Changes

The bronchial submucosa shows varying degrees of vascular dilatation, edema, and inflammation (Figs. 4-4*A,B* and 4-5) that occur in response to local release of inflammatory mediators. The airway inflammatory response is present even at clinically early stages of the disease.[21] Eosinophils are often prominent among the inflammatory cells, and range between 5% to 50% of inflammatory cells. In some cases they can be minimal or absent, in which case lymphocytes and plasma cells predominate. The presence of an increased number of eosinophils in the mucosa in bronchial biopsies

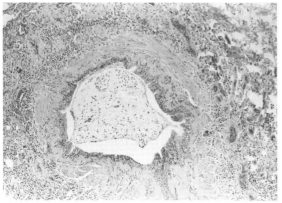

Figure 4-5
Section from a respiratory bronchiole showing luminal gelatinous contents with a few inflammatory cells. H & E stain, medium magnification. (Courtesy of Monica Smiddy, MD, Office of Chief Medical Examiner, New York City.)

has been correlated to deterioration of symptoms in asthma.[24] In asthmatic biopsy specimens, mast cells show various degrees of degranulation, suggesting that mast cell activation, with subsequent release of inflammatory mediators, may occur continuously within the airways.[25]

Olivieri and colleagues examined the relationship between bronchoalveolar lavage (BAL) fluid and lung histology in 13 asthmatics in remission.[26] The BAL content of inflammatory cells appeared to reflect the overall severity of the inflammatory process in the bronchial mucosa. An increased number of BAL eosinophils were found only in asthmatics with evidence of active disease.[27] Studies have also demonstrated that mast cells in BAL are increased in asthmatics compared to healthy controls, but are no higher than those in sarcoidosis or fibrosing alveolitis.[27] Sur and colleagues have demonstrated that interleukin-5 protein can be detected in BAL as asthma progresses from the asymptomatic to the clinically symptomatic state in patients with significant BAL eosinophilia.[28]

The volume and size of submucosal glands increases in asthma but not to the degree that is seen in chronic bronchitis.[11,15] The serous-to-mucus acinar ratio remains unaltered in asthma, but in bronchitis there is a relative reduction in serous acini, which contain antibacterial and antiproteolytic enzymes.

Outpouchings of the bronchial mucosa, which probably represent dilatation of the bronchial gland mouths,[8] apparently enlarge due to the forces of increased intraluminal pressure, muscle contraction, and mucus stasis in these areas. Monckeberg first described such a phenomenon in 1909 when he described a cryptlike protrusion of the epithelium.[29] Since then various other descriptors for this change have been coined including *diverticulosis*,[8] *bronchial gland duct ectasia*,[30] *bronchial sacculations*,[31] and *dilations of gland openings*.[32]

Airway Wall Nerves

In fatal asthma, immunohistologic studies have demonstrated an absence of vasoactive intestinal peptide (VIP) in mucosal nerve fibers and an increase in the number of P-containing fibers, which are stimulatory to bronchial smooth muscle.[33] Since the density of the β adrenoceptors and VIP receptors are normal, the degranulation seen in fatal asthma is thought to contribute to loss of intraaxonal VIP.[34]

Other Changes in the Airway Lumen

Mucus Plugs   Asthmatics often have gelatinous intraluminal material in their airways (Fig. 4-5). Formation of thick secretions is multifactorial in origin and includes increased mucus production from goblet cells and submucosal glands, increased fibrin formation,[8,35] and chemical changes in mucus that result in high levels of acidic glycoproteins and an alteration in the glycoprotein:proteoglycan ratio.[36] Leakage of albumin and other proteins from injured airways results in protein-mucus mixtures. The endothelium of bronchial postcapillary venules in asthmatics has wide gaps[37] that cause plasma exudation which might contribute to the development of inflammatory cell influx and increased epithelial shedding. Well-formed laminations are seen in older secretions. Studies performed on mucus plugs or casts of asthmatics have shown that eosinophils are usually well preserved as strands of cells and admixed with mucus in whorled patterns.[38] Treatment with corticosteroids is believed to decrease the cellular content in some cases of mucus plugs, but corticosteroids usually do not prevent the formation of these plugs.

Curschmann's Spirals Curschmann's spirals are formed from thick mucus plugs containing whorls of shed epithelium. They appear as small, linear, whorled strands of mucus that are twisted in a common direction and contain a central, highly refractile coil (Fig. 4-6). They were first described as originating in the distal bronchioles in asthma by Curschmann in 1883.[39] The tight coil produced implies that the mucus is secreted from gland necks, or flows in distal bronchioles in a common circumferential direction. Curschmann's spirals have subsequently been described in effusions and cervicovaginal smears. Their origin on serosal surfaces is believed to be secondary to rolling-up of a mucin-rich surface layer.[15]

Charcot-Leyden Crystals These are small hexagonal eosinophilic crystals formed by degranula-

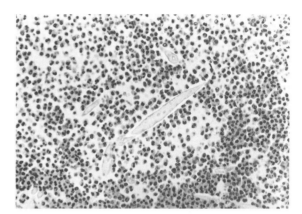

Figure 4-7
Charcot-Leyden crystals with numerous bilobed eosinophils. H & E stain, medium magnification.

tion of eosinophils (Fig. 4-7). In biochemical terms, they are pure phospholipases[40] derived from the cell membrane of degenerated eosinophils. Charcot-Leyden crystals form only in the presence of eosinophils. They have also been described in allergic sinusitis, and bloody/traumatic pleural effusions, which are other conditions characterized by the presence of eosinophils.

HISTOPATHOLOGIC CHANGES AND SEVERITY OF ASTHMA

In the last several decades, total asthma deaths have been increasing in the United States and worldwide.[41,42] In a study from the Office of the Chief Medical Examiner of the State of Maryland, at least two of the following gross or microscopic findings were seen in 62 asthmatic deaths: hyperinflation, mucus plugs, eosinophils, bronchial smooth muscle hypertrophy, thickening of bronchial epithelial basal lamina, prominent goblet cells, and bronchial epithelial sloughing.[43] In a comparative postmortem study by Cluroe and colleagues of 72 cases of asthmatic deaths and an equal number of matched control patients, asthma was defined by the presence of four out of five of the following criteria: mucus plugging, basement membrane thickening, submucosal eosinophilic infiltration, epithelial shedding, and submucosal

Figure 4-6
Curschmann's spiral in a background of mucus and inflammmatory cells in a cytologic preparation from the lung Papanicolaou stain, high magnification. (Courtesy of Denise VS DeFrias, MD, Professor, Northwestern University Medical School, Chicago, IL.)

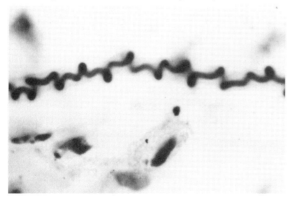

smooth muscle hypertrophy.[30] Using these criteria, the authors found histologic evidence of asthma in 74% of the asthma deaths compared to 7% in the control group. In the asthma cases, diverticulae were present in 54% of cases, of which 92% were in the histologically positive asthmatic group. Bronchial gland diverticulae were observed in seven patients in the control group, five of whom had histologic evidence of asthma, but in whom death had not been attributed to asthma. These authors also found interstitial emphysema in cases in which diverticulae ruptured. Interstitial emphysema was seen in 10 cases of fatal asthma, all of which had histologic evidence of asthma and gland ectasia, but this was not observed in the control group patients.

The immunopathologic features of asthmatic deaths suggest that the degree of inflammation increases from mild to severe disease, with parallel alterations in epithelial cell integrity, basement membrane changes, and increases in bronchial smooth muscle and mucous glands.[44] However, these similarities do not explain catastrophic acute asthmatic deaths characterized by the most common finding of occlusion of the bronchial lumen by tenacious inspissated mucus. The work of Sur and colleagues involving immunohistochemical quantitation of submucosal eosinophils, neutrophils, elastase, and major basic protein in autopsy lung tissue demonstrated that patients with sudden-onset fatal asthma had more neutrophils than eosinophils and less intraluminal mucus compared to the slow-onset fatal asthma group.[14] This observation led the authors to postulate that sudden-onset fatal asthma may be an immunohistologically distinct entity and to suggest the possibility of performing bronchial biopsies to determine which patients are at risk for sudden-onset fatal asthma.[45] However, autopsy findings indicate that asthma is associated with disease activity outside the airway, such as infiltration of lung parenchyma by eosinophils, suggesting that small mucosal and submucosal bronchial biopsies may not be sufficient to reflect the extent and severity of the disease process.[44] While bronchial biopsies may be illustrative in some cases, the current available data (at the time of this writing) do not suggest that biopsies should be used to risk-stratify or clinically manage patients and the need for a pathologic classification of asthma has been suggested.[46]

REFERENCES

1. Huber HL, Koessler KK: The pathology of asthma. *Arch Intern Med* 30:689–760, 1922.
2. Houston JC, de Nevasquez S, Trounce JR: A clinical and pathological study of fatal cases of status asthmaticus. *Thorax* 8:207–213, 1953.
3. Cardwell BS, Pearson RSB: Death in asthmatics. *Thorax* 14:341–352, 1959.
4. Messer JW, Peters GA: Causes of death and pathologic findings in 304 cases of bronchial asthma. *Dis Chest* 38:616–624, 1960.
5. Reid L: Pathological changes in asthma, in Clark TJK, Godfrey S (eds): *Asthma*. London, Chapman and Hall, 1977, pp 79–95.
6. Dunnill MS: Pathology of asthma, in Middleton E, Jr, Reed CE, Ellis EF (eds): *Allergy: Principles and Practice*. St Louis MO, Mosby, 1978, pp 678–686.
7. Dunnill MS: *Pulmonary Pathology*. Edinburgh, Churchill-Livingston, 1987, pp 61–79.
8. Dunnill MS: The pathology of asthma with special reference to changes in the bronchial mucosa. *J Clin Pathol* 13:27–33, 1960.
9. Sobonya RE: Concise clinical study. Quantitative structural alterations in long standing allergic asthma. *Am Rev Respir Dis* 130:289–292, 1984.
10. Glynn AA, Michaels L: Bronchial biopsy in chronic bronchitis and asthma. *Thorax* 23:142–153, 1960.
11. Salvato G: Some histologic changes in chronic bronchitis and asthma. *Thorax* 23:168–172, 1968.
12. Laitinen LA Heino M, Laitenen A, Haahtela T: Damage to the airway epithelium and bronchial reactivity in patients with asthma. *Am Rev Respir Dis* 131:599–606, 1985.
13. Sanerkin NG, Evans DMD: The sputum in bronchial asthma: Pathopneumonic patterns. *J Pathol* 89:535–541, 1965.
14. Sur S, Crotty TB, Kephart GM, et al: Sudden-onset fatal asthma. A distinct entity with few eosinophils and relatively more neutrophils in the airway mucosa? *Am Rev Respir Dis* 148 (3):550–552, 1993.
15. Dail DH: Eosinophilic infiltrates, in Dail DH, Hammar SP (eds): *Pulmonary Pathology*. New York, Springer-Verlag, 1993, pp 537–543.
16. McCarter JH, Vazquez JJ: The bronchial basement

membrane in asthma. *Arch Pathol Lab Med* 82:328–335, 1966.

17. Roche WR, Williams JH, Beasley R, Holgate ST: Subepithelial fibrosis in the bronchi of asthmatics. *Lancet* I:520–524, 1989.

18. Richardson JB: Airways smooth muscle. *J Allergy Clin Immunol* 80:409–411, 1987.

19. Hogg JC: Varieties of airway narrowing in severe and fatal asthma. *J Allergy Clin Immunol* 80:417–419, 1987.

20. Sheils IA, Bowler SD, Taylor SM: Airway smooth muscle proliferation in asthma: The potential of vascular leakage to contribute to pathogenesis. *Med Hypothesis* 45 (1):37–40, 1995.

21. Laitinen LA, Laitinen A, Haatela T: Airway mucosal inflammation even in patients with newly diagnosed asthma. *Am Rev Respir Dis* 147:697–704, 1993.

22. Gleich GJ, Frigas E, Loegering DA et al: Cytotoxic properties of eosinophil major basic protein. *J Immunol* 123:2925–2927, 1975.

23. Naylor B: The shedding of the mucosa of the bronchial tree in asthma. *Thorax* 17:69–72, 1962.

24. Laitinen LA, Laitinen A, Heino M, Haatela T: Eosinophilic airway inflammation during exacerbation of asthma and its treatment with inhaled corticosteroid. *Am Rev Resp Dis* 143:423–427, 1991.

25. Beasley R, Burgess C, Crane J, et al: Pathology of asthma and its clinical implications. *J Allergy Clin Immunol* 92:148–154, 1993.

26. Olivieri D, Foresi A: Correlation between cell content of bronchoalveolar lavage (BAL) fluid and histologic findings in asthma. *Respiration* 59(Suppl 1):3–5, 1992.

27. Wardlaw AJ, Dunnette S, Gleich GJ, et al: Eosinophils and mast cells in bronchoalveolar lavage in subjects with mild asthma. *Am Rev Respir Dis* 137:62–69, 1988.

28. Sur S, Gleich GJ, Swanson MC, et al: Eosinophilic inflammation is associated with elevation of IL-5 in the airways of patients with spontaneous symptomatic asthma. *J Allergy Clin Immunol* 96:661–668, 1995.

29. Monckeberg JG: Zur Pathologischen Anatomie des Bronchialasthmas. *Verh Dtsch Ges Pathol* 14:173–180, 1909.

30. Cluroe A, Holloway L, Thompson K, et al: Bronchial gland duct ectasia in fatal bronchial asthma:

association with interstitial emphysema. *J Clin Pathol* 42:1026–1031, 1989.

31. Macdonald IG: The local and constitutional pathology and bronchial asthma. *Ann Intern Med* 6:253–277, 1933.

32. Lamson RW, Butt EM: Fatal "asthma." A clinical and pathological correlation of 187 cases. *JAMA* 108:1843–1850, 1937.

33. Ollerenshaw S, Jarvis D, Woolcock A, et al: Absence of immunoreactive vasoactive intestinal polypeptide in tissue from lungs of patients with asthma. *N Engl J Med* 320:1244–1248, 1989.

34. Jeffery PK: Pathology of Asthma. *Br Med Bull* 48 (1):23–29, 1992.

35. Barton Ad, Lourenco RV: Bronchial secretions and mucociliary clearance. *Arch Intern Med* 131:140–144, 1973.

36. Reid LM: The presence or absence of bronchial mucus in fatal asthma. *J Allergy Clin Immunol* 80:415–416, 1987.

37. Laitinen LA, Laitinen A: Is asthma also a vascular disease? *Am Rev Respir Dis* 135:A474, 1987.

38. Jelihovsky T: The structure of bronchial plugs in mucoid impaction, bronchocentric granulomatosis and asthma. *Histopathology* 7:153–167, 1983.

39. Curschmann H: ber Bronchiolitis exsudativa und ihr verhaltnis zum. Asthma nervosum. *Dtsch Arch Klin Med (Liepzig)* 32:1–34, 1883.

40. Weller PF, Goetzl EJ, Austen AF: Human eosinophil lysophospholipase: The sole protein component of Charcot-Leyden crystals. *J Immunol* 128:1346–1349, 1982.

41. Sears MR: Increasing asthma mortality—fact or artifact? *J Allergy Clin Immunol* 82:957–960, 1988.

42. Asthma—United States, 1980–1990. *MMWR* 41:733–735, 1992.

43. Weitzman JB, Kanarek NF, Smialek JE: Medical examiner asthma death autopsies. A distinct subgroup of asthma deaths with implications for public health preventive strategies. *Arch Pathol Lab Med* 122:691–699, 1998.

44. Kay AB: Pathology of mild, severe and fatal asthma. *Am J Respir Crit Care Med* 154:S66–S69, 1996.

45. Sur S, Hunt LW, Crotty TB, Gleich GJ: Sudden-onset fatal asthma. *Mayo Clin Proc* 69:495–496, 1994. Editorial.

46. Holgate ST, Roche W, Djukanovic J, et al: The need for a pathologic classification of asthma. *Eur Respir J* 4(13):113S–122S, 1991.

Chapter 5

AIRFLOW OBSTRUCTION AND DYNAMIC PULMONARY HYPERINFLATION

Andrea Rossi
A. Ganassini
V. Brusasco

INTRODUCTION

Asthma is a chronic inflammatory disorder of the airways, probably due to genetic and environmental factors.[1,2] Typically, asthmatic airways narrow "too easily" and "too much" in response to stimuli that have little or no effect on normal airways.[3–5] This condition, known as airway hyperresponsiveness, has been widely recognized as a hallmark of asthma. Although the precise relationship between airway inflammation and airway hyperresponsiveness is still unknown, it is believed that bronchoconstrictor stimuli such as allergens, cold dry air, exercise, air pollutants, and respiratory infections enhance the inflammatory process through a complex network of humoral mediators, neurotransmitters, cytokines, and chemokines.[6] However, there is recent evidence suggesting that an abnormal mechanical response of the airways may be a prerequisite for airway hyperresponsiveness and severe asthma, and may not be closely associated with the magnitude of airway inflammation.[7]

The most clinically relevant mechanical consequences of airway hyperresponsiveness are an excessive airway narrowing and consequent changes in lung volumes. Generally, both acute and chronic bronchoconstriction are almost invariably accompanied by pulmonary hyperinflation.[8–14] Hyperventilation itself may represent an increased burden for the ventilatory pump, thus contributing to symptoms. Further complicating assessment is the likelihood that changes in lung volume affect the measurements of airway caliber and the assessment of airway responsiveness. This chapter explores the effects of hyperresponsiveness in asthma on airway resistance and, in turn, on lung volumes, lung mechanics, and respiratory muscle performance.

BRONCHIAL HYPERRESPONSIVENESS

In clinical settings, the degree of airway responsiveness is most frequently assessed by bronchial challenges with methacholine or histamine (i.e., pharmacologic stimuli acting directly on airway smooth muscle). The bronchoconstrictor substance is administered by inhalation until a targeted response (generally a 20% reduction of FEV_1) is achieved. The threshold dose (PD_{20}) or concentration (PC_{20}) causing the targeted response is commonly used to quantitate the degree of airway responsiveness. An abundant amount of literature has shown that PD_{20} or PC_{20} are remarkably lower in patients with asthma compared to atopic and normal patients without asthma.[3] Furthermore, the lowest PD_{20} and PC_{20} are generally found in the most severe asthmatics.

Some years ago, Orehek and colleagues demonstrated that the response to bronchoconstrictor stimuli is not completely described by the threshold dose or threshold concentration.[15] They observed that the airway response to methacholine and histamine can be characterized not only by a threshold level, but also by the slope of the dose-response curve and that these two parameters were poorly correlated. They observed that asthma patients with a low PD_{20} (referred to as hypersensitivity) exhibited two patterns of dose-response curve: flat and steep (referred to as hyperactivity). These researchers suggested both hypersensitivity and hyperactivity were useful concepts to understand the asthmatic airway response. Other researchers have also suggested that determination of PD_{20} or PC_{20} without a complete dose (or concentration)-response curve may be not only insufficient but also potentially misleading in the assessment of the severity of airway hyperresponsiveness.[4,5] If a bronchial challenge is stopped immediately after a 20% decrease of FEV_1 is attained, the maximum level of bronchoconstriction cannot be evaluated. It has been suggested that the dose (or concentration)-response curve to inhaled bronchoconstrictor agents may exhibit three basic shapes.[5]

1. In *healthy subjects*, high doses or concentrations of bronchoconstrictor agent may cause significant airway narrowing, but the magnitude of this response is limited, that is, there is a point at which no further constriction occurs when the dose or concentration of the agent is increased. In other words, a plateau appears in the dose (or concentration)—response curve before excessive bronchoconstriction (e.g., 40% decrease of FEV_1) is achieved.

2. In atopic individuals without asthma and those with *mild asthma*, the threshold dose or concentration may be low, revealing hypersensitivity, but the maximal response may be limited by a plateau similar to normal individuals.

3. In *moderate and severe asthma*, the threshold dose or concentration tends to be low (hypersensitivity) but, as important, the airways continue to narrow with increasing dose and with little plateau effect.[16–19] Although the occurrence of a plateau response does not necessarily indicate complete protection against excessive bronchoconstriction, it may indicate that some protective mechanisms are operative.[20] It has been suggested that bronchial hypersensitivity and excessive air-

way narrowing occur via different mechanisms[21] and have different consequences for lung function tests.[20]

How do these observations in patients receiving bronchial provocation relate to in vitro studies of smooth muscle function? More than 10 years ago, Macklem[5] addressed the importance of the in vitro studies conducted by Stephens which demonstrated that isolated airway smooth muscle can shorten isotonically to 20% to 30% of its resting length.[15,22] In vivo, this level of shortening would cause complete airway closure.[5,23] Since maximum bronchoconstriction is limited in normal subjects to a level much lower than predicted from the in vitro behavior of smooth muscle, it has been suggested that some mechanisms that limit airway smooth muscle shortening are operative in vivo and that the airway caliber in vivo is the result of a complex balance between forces favoring and opposing airway narrowing.[23] The former (favoring) is the force developed by the airway smooth muscle and the latter (opposing) is developed by the elastic load imposed on smooth muscle. In vitro, airway smooth muscle subjected to elastic load shortens much less compared to unloaded conditions and increases its tone.[24] The elastic load on airway smooth muscle is represented by parallel elastic elements lying within the airway wall and the elastic recoil force of the lung parenchyma surrounding the airways.[23]

The mechanisms leading to excessive airway narrowing in asthma are complex[4] and their detailed description goes beyond the purposes of this chapter. Whether the smooth muscle of asthmatic airways behaves differently from normal airways continues to be debated.[25] Recent experimental studies suggest that smooth muscle from sensitized airways may contract in response to stretching[25,26] and can shorten more and more rapidly[27] than smooth muscle from normal airways. Furthermore, the airway smooth muscle thickness may be increased in asthma as a consequence of hypertrophy and hyperplasia.[28] Although not proven, it is possible that an increased airway smooth muscle mass produces more contractile force and leads to excessive airway narrowing.[29–31] The thickening of airway walls as a result of inflammation may amplify the effect of airway smooth muscle shortening on airway caliber,[32] while peribronchial edema may unlink the airways from the surrounding parenchyma, thus reducing or even abolishing the stretching effect of lung elastic recoil on the airway.[5,21,33] Finally, the involvement of the lung periphery in an asthma attack may cause parenchymal hysteresis to exceed airway hysteresis, which results in a reduced bronchodilator force during expiration.[34] It has recently been suggested that the inability of lung inflation to dilate the constricted airways may be a major determinant of bronchial hyperresponsiveness in asthma.[35]

Clinically, the lack of limit to bronchoconstriction seems to be more relevant than simple hypersensitivity, since it implies the potential for an acute asthma attack to be very severe even in patients with chronically mild disease. The greater magnitude of airway narrowing may lead to status asthmaticus respiratory failure,[36–42] and fatal or near-fatal asthma.[43–45] Recognizing excessive airway narrowing may also have therapeutic implication since anti-inflammatory drugs, but not bronchodilators, seem to have the capability to limit the degree of bronchoconstriction.[21,46,47]

From a clinical viewpoint, the principal symptoms of acute severe asthma are dyspnea and wheezing. With progression to the extreme, breathlessness becomes unbearable, mental disturbances appear, and the "silent chest" replaces wheezing.[39] The term *acute* defines the brief interval through which clinically significant symptoms develop, which occasionally begins from a normal baseline. However, most often patients progress to an acute stage after a period of underestimated mild symptoms such as cough or dyspnea. The term *severe* not only refers to the level of symptoms but also to the fact that the attack is often refractory to treatment,[40,42] although even acute asthma with hypercapnia may reverse with appropriate therapy.[41] Life-threatening conditions stemming from mismanagement, and often the result of an underestimation of the severity of the disease, either by the patient or the care givers, are well recognized.[48] The key event in acute asthma is the rapidly increasing severity of bronchial obstruction, mainly due to bronchospasm,[4] the major cause of dyspnea. This increasing severity has ma-

jor consequences on lung mechanics and efficiency of breathing.

Understanding the pathophysiology of these processes is fundamental to the ability to appropriately treat patients with acute asthma.[49]

FUNCTIONAL CONSEQUENCES OF AIRWAY NARROWING

Progressive and unconstrained bronchoconstriction is the hallmark of an asthma attack and leads to 1) increased flow resistance, 2) pulmonary hyperinflation, and 3) ventilation to perfusion mismatching. The latter, which is regarded as the major mechanism of hypoxemia,[50,51] has been recently reviewed[52,53] and is discussed in detail elsewhere in this book (see Chapter 6). As an asthma attack progresses, hypercapnia and respiratory acidosis[36] may occur, requiring aggressive treatment, even with mechanical ventilation, to prevent asphyxia and respiratory arrest.[54]

Widespread airway narrowing in asthma causes a remarkable increase in airflow resistance, which can be as high as five times the baseline value.[55] Maximum expiratory flows are markedly reduced at all lung volumes and the peak expiratory flow (PEF) may be less than 150 to 100 L/min in acute asthma. Maximum inspiratory flow is reduced less than expiratory flow, yet the inspiratory work of breathing is increased.[56] Because of the inequality of time constants within the lungs, which is caused by a heterogeneous parallel distribution of airway narrowing,[55,57] dynamic lung compliance is reduced and becomes frequency-dependent.[57] The reduction of dynamic lung compliance increases the elastic work of breathing. Therefore airway narrowing per se has the potential for increasing both the elastic and resistive workload on the inspiratory muscles. Several studies have shown that the inspiratory muscle strength and endurance is normal or only slightly reduced in stable asthma patients,[58–61] suggesting that the ventilatory pump could easily tolerate this increase in workload. However, airway narrowing eventually causes an increase in end-expiratory lung volume, which may have a remarkable effect on the elastic work of breathing.[56] Even if breathing at higher lung volumes reduces the resistive work,[57] the overall pressure-generating capacity of the ventilatory pump may be impaired by operation at high lung volumes. This combination of increased workload and reduced ventilatory pump efficiency is common to acute asthma and exacerbations of chronic obstructive pulmonary disease (COPD), and may represent one of the major mechanisms leading to hypercapnic ventilatory failure.[37,62–66]

The changes in respiratory mechanics due to acute asthma and, in particular, the relationship between airflow obstruction and the changes in lung volumes commonly referred to as pulmonary hyperinflation are discussed below.

SUBDIVISION OF LUNG VOLUMES IN NORMAL INDIVIDUALS

In healthy subjects, the subdivision of lung volumes (Fig. 5-1) depends mainly on the elastic properties of the individual anatomic structures of the respiratory system.[67]

Residual Volume

The residual volume (RV) is the amount of gas remaining in the lungs and airways at the end of a maximum expiration (Fig. 5-1). It is determined in young healthy subjects by the balance between the expiratory muscle strength, which progressively decreases with decreasing volume, and the elastic recoil of the chest wall, which progressively increases at low lung volumes. In the elderly, small airways can become closed or near-closed at low lung volume, thus causing air trapping at the end of a maximum expiration.[68,69] It has been determined that peripheral airways close if the transpulmonary pressure (P_L) is reduced below -5 cm H_2O in the young and below $+4.5$ cm H_2O in the elderly.[69–73] This condition is not unusual, although the amount of trapped gas may be less than expected because some small airways in dependent lung regions remain patent,[72] allowing gas to escape slowly via collateral ventilation or diffusion from units with closed airways into units with open airways and

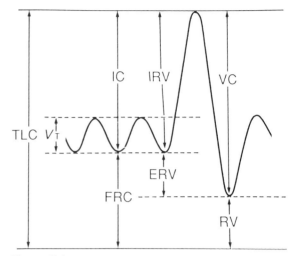

Figure 5-1

Spirometric division of lung volumes. TLC, total lung capacity; IC, inspiratory capacity; IRV, inspiratory reserve volume; FRC, functional residual capacity; ERV, expiratory reserve volume; VC, vital capacity; RV, residual volume; V_T, tidal volume.

hence, into upper lung regions. Aging is associated with a loss of lung elastic recoil, which reduces maximum flow, thus accounting for the increase in RV in the elderly.[73] In fact, when expiratory flows are very low near RV, the limited breath-holding ability of the subject may interrupt expiration before reaching the lung volume to which the expiratory muscles could have theoretically driven the system.

In summary, RV in normal subjects is mainly determined by the static balance between expiratory muscles strength and chest wall recoil; however, dynamic mechanisms (i.e., flow limitation and peripheral airway closure) may be determining factors in the elderly.

Total Lung Capacity

The total lung capacity (TLC) is the amount of gas present in the lungs and airways at the end of maximal inspiration (see Fig. 5-1). It is determined by the balance between the maximum strength of the inspiratory muscles, which progressively decreases with increasing lung volume, and the elastic recoil of the whole respiratory system (i.e., lung and chest wall), which progressively increases at high lung volume. In particular, the volume-pressure relationship of the lungs becomes essentially flat close to TLC.

Functional Residual Capacity

The functional residual capacity (FRC) is the amount of gas in the lungs and airways at the end of a tidal expiration (see Fig. 5-1). It is normally governed by the opposing elastic recoil forces of the lungs and the chest wall. In healthy subjects during quiet tidal breathing, the elastic energy stored in the respiratory system during inspiration is sufficient to exhale passively to a volume at which a static equilibrium is achieved (relaxation volume: Vr).[67] At this point, Vr is identical to FRC. Although electrical activity has been found to be present in some abdominal muscles during quiet tidal expiration, its mechanical consequences have not been fully elucidated.[74] The term *end-expiratory lung volume* (EELV) is also used. It is synonymous with FRC but is most often used in reference to an increased FRC resulting from dynamic hyperinflation.

The lung volume at which the FRC is positioned is of paramount importance in the dynamics of breathing as it sets the length at which the inspiratory muscles start their contraction. Due to their length-tension characteristics, the inspiratory ability of muscles to generate pressure decreases at high lung volumes.

Normal subjects spontaneously decrease FRC below Vr during exercise by activating the expiratory muscles in order to increase tidal volume. By contrast, there is no physiologic condition in which FRC is involuntarily increased above Vr, although as noted above it routinely occurs in instances of airflow obstruction.

SUBDIVISION OF LUNG VOLUMES IN ASTHMA

As previously mentioned, the excessive airway narrowing of acute asthma may cause a phenomenal increase in airflow resistance and a striking reduction in maximal expiratory flows. Both these events affect lung volumes, causing some of them to increase (namely RV, TLC, and FRC) and others to decrease (namely slow and forced vital capacity (VC and FVC, respectively), inspiratory capacity (IC), and expiratory reserve volume (ERV) (see Fig. 5-1). Several mechanisms are involved in these changes.[12]

Residual Volume

Acute asthma is associated with a reduction in lung elastic recoil similar in magnitude to that observed with aging, but less than that associated with pulmonary emphysema.[55,75,76] Thus, increased airway resistance in asthma can lead to flow limitation during passive expiration. Under conditions of flow limitation, the expiratory time may be inadequate for lung volume to decrease to a point at which the elastic recoil of the chest wall and the force of the expiratory muscles balance each other.[77] Thus, RV will increase, as described below.

It has also been shown that in patients with mild asthma and without clinical symptoms, the lung volume at which small airways close is higher than in normal individuals, probably as a consequence of the diffuse chronic inflammatory process in terminal bronchioles and inherent airway instability.[3,78] During an acute asthma attack, this phenomenon is enhanced by excessive airway narrowing, such that some airways close at TLC, with progressive closure of others in the course of expiration.[79] Closure or near-closure of small airways may also result from bronchial wall edema and mucus plugging. Alveolar gas is probably exhaled through a few severely narrowed airways until the capability to expire terminates, thus resulting in air trapping.[3,69] A consistent increase of RV has been observed during exacerbations of asthma,[80,81] after inhalation of allergens[82,83] or chemical agents, like methacholine or histamine,[12,84,85] after exposure to dust,[84,86,87] and after exercise.[10,11]

An interesting observation relevant to the understanding of the mechanism involved in the rise in RV in acute asthma has recently been reported by Pellegrino and colleagues.[87] They found that RV increased more in asthma patients than in normal individuals at similar levels of methacholine-induced bronchoconstriction. They hypothesized that the magnitude of increase in RV was determined by the site and mechanism of airway narrowing. In other studies, it was determined that methacholine caused a bronchoconstrictor response that was limited to conducting airways in healthy subjects but involved both conducting airways and lung parenchyma in asthma patients.[85,88–90] The involvement of the lung periphery in the bronchoconstrictor response was associated with a blunted bronchodilator effect of deep inhalation,[90] which has been attributed to an increase of parenchymal hysteresis.[34,88,90] A blunted bronchodilator effect of deep inhalation would result in lower forced expiratory flows at all lung volumes during a maximal expiration and a rise in RV due to airway closure or extreme flow limitation at low lung volumes.

Whatever the underlying mechanism, closure or near-closure of small airways early in expiration represents the major causative mechanism in the rise of RV during an acute asthma attack.[91] This is clinically relevant since it seems to be associated with excessive airway narrowing. Recently, Gibbons and colleagues[20] suggested that excessive bronchoconstriction could be detected during a bronchial challenge without the need for generation of a complete dose-response curve. They suggested that if a 20% reduction in FEV_1 is accompanied by a similar reduction of FVC (i.e., with little or no change in the FEV_1/FVC) during induced bronchoconstriction, excessive airway narrowing is likely to occur. Thus, measuring the changes in FVC, which reflect changes in RV, in addition to FEV_1, during a bronchial provocation challenge may be useful to detect the asthma patients at risk of serious airway obstruction. In fact, the decrease in FVC can be assumed to represent peripheral airway narrowing, probably linked to a diffuse inflammatory process in the small airways, whereas an isolated reduction of FEV_1 might reflect central bronchoconstriction and simple hypersensitivity.

Total Lung Capacity

Airway closure occurring at higher than normal lung volumes obviously reduces the VC.[4,5,92] However, the decrease in VC does not seem to be proportional to the rise in RV because TLC also augments in acute asthma,[93] probably as a consequence of loss of lung elastic recoil[80,94] or increased inspiratory muscle strength,[95,96] or both. There is evidence that lung elastic recoil is slightly reduced in acute asthma, especially at lung volumes close to TLC.[55] This change in TLC is reversible with resolution of the asthma.[75]

The mechanism of the change in lung elastic recoil during acute asthma[79,90,97–99] has not been well elucidated; changes in surface tension, elastic and connective fibers of the lungs, and stress relaxation have been suggested but not proven. An increase in TLC after inhalation of allergens,[83] histamine,[13] exercise,[10,11,79] or methacholine[97] was found by some, but not all, investigators.[100,101] It should be noted that measurements of TLC measured by body plethysmography[102] may overestimate thoracic gas volume because of the poor transmission of alveolar pressure changes to the mouth in the presence of abnormal peripheral airway resistance.[103–105] Nevertheless, TLC measured radiographically has also been shown to be increased during an acute asthma attack.[8,80,93,106] It is possible that these changes in TLC evolve over time, as suggested by animal experiments,[107] although a reversible remodelling of lung tissue due to sustained hyperinflation remains to be proven.

Functional Residual Capacity

From a clinical standpoint, the most important change in lung volumes during an asthma attack is the rise in FRC, which has substantial effects on respiratory muscle mechanics (see below) and hence on the capability of the ventilatory pump to sustain spontaneous breathing.

Pulmonary hyperinflation is defined as an increase in FRC above its predicted values. For example, in patients with COPD due to emphysema, FRC can increase above predicted TLC because of the loss of lung elastic recoil.[108] *Dynamic pulmo-*

nary hyperinflation (DPH) is defined as an increase in FRC above Vr due to the difference between the time needed to deflate the lungs to Vr and the time actually available between two consecutive inspirations.[109] Under these circumstances, end-expiration is determined by the ensuing inspiratory effort[110] and not the achievement of Vr.

DETERMINANTS OF DYNAMIC HYPERINFLATION

In acute severe asthma, the major determinants of the rise in FRC are the abnormal airflow resistance, expiratory flow limitation, and the post-inspiratory activity of the inspiratory muscles.

The Contribution of Airflow Resistance

The mechanism by which abnormal flow resistance may cause pulmonary hyperinflation is readily intuitive. In relaxed awake humans[111] and in anaesthetized cats with a linear tracheal cannula,[112] the time decay of expired volume can be described by the following monoexponential function:

$$V_{(t)} = V_0 \cdot e^{-t/\tau_{rs}} \tag{1}$$

where V is the exhaled volume at any time (t) during relaxed expiration, V_0 is the total exhaled volume, and τ_{rs} is the time constant of the respiratory system (rs):

$$\tau = R_{rs} \times C_{rs} \tag{2}$$

where R and C are resistance and compliance. It is clear from Eq. 2 that the time constant is increased any time R or C increase. In acute asthma, dynamic compliance (C_{dyn}) is reduced whereas static compliance (C_{st}) may increase because of a slight loss of lung elastic recoil. Hence, the changes in C_{rs} tend not to be large enough to significantly affect τ. However, τ is invariably increased because of the high R_{rs}. According to Equation 1, if τ is longer, the time necessary to expire a given volume of gas is also longer. In healthy individuals with a normal C_{rs} of 0.1 L/cm H_2O and R_{rs} of 2 cm H_2O/L per second, τ is approximately 0.2 seconds. A fivefold increase of R_{rs}, as may be

the case during acute severe asthma, would cause a fivefold increase of τ to a value of approximately 1 second. As an expiratory time (T_E) of 4 to 5 seconds is needed to drive the lungs to Vr, and, assuming a "duty cycle" [i.e., the ratio of inspiratory time (T_I) to total breathing cycle duration (T_{TOT})] of 0.4, a breathing frequency of about 8 breaths per minute would be necessary to allow a T_E of 4 to 5 seconds. By contrast, in normal individuals a T_E <1 second may be sufficient to exhale completely to Vr. Spontaneous breathing frequencies in the range of 8 breaths per minute have not been reported in patients with acute severe asthma. Indeed, these patients tend to increase breathing frequency and decrease tidal volume.[41] Therefore, under circumstances of long τ, the T_E available between two inspiratory efforts may be insufficient to achieve Vr, and FRC is increased.[110]

An additional increase in expiratory flow resistance during spontaneous breathing might be due to narrowing of the glottis, which has been shown to occur during induced bronchoconstriction in asthma patients. Analysis of upper airway activity[79,113,114] has shown that the oropharynx dilates during inspiration following bronchoprovocation, thus reducing inspiratory flow resistance. However, the upper airway narrows during expiration, which may contribute to the increase in expiratory flow resistance and, thereby, to pulmonary hyperinflation.

These effects may be particularly pronounced during mechanical ventilation of patients with acute severe asthma, since this subgroup of patients exhibits the most extreme increase in airflow resistance and the act of intubation adds an additional resistor in series with the patient's own airways. As shown in Figure 5-2, during ventilation this muscle-relaxed patient exhibited an FRC that was elevated to 1.4 L above Vr. As shown on the time axis of this plot of lung volume versus time, approximately 23 seconds of passive expiratory time is required for lung volume to fall to Vr. Since it is not possible to ventilate patients with respiratory rates so slow as to permit this protracted expiratory cycle, some degree of hyperinflation must usually be tolerated during mechani-

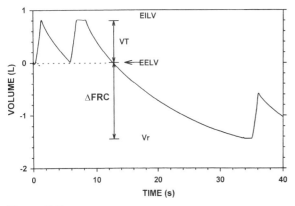

Figure 5-2

Volume/time relationship with a completely relaxed expiration following a brief end-inspiratory occlusion in a ventilator-dependent patient with asthma. EILV, end-inspiratory lung volume; V_T, tidal volume; EELV, end-expiratory lung volume; ΔFRC, difference in volume from EELV to the relaxed functional residual capacity (FRC) or relaxation volume (Vr). (From Rossi and Ganassini[130])

cal ventilatory support of patients with asthma (see Chapter 13). The impact of dynamic hyperinflation on a spontaneously breathing patient during mechanical ventilation is shown in Figure 5-3.

The Contribution of Expiratory Flow Limitation

Expiratory flow limitation can be defined as the inability to increase flow over the prevailing tidal volume (V_T) range by increasing transpulmonary pressure.[115] Under these circumstances, expiratory flow and, hence, ventilation cannot be increased by activation of the expiratory muscles unless the FRC is increased to allow breathing at higher lung volume where greater flows can be generated. The major consequence of expiratory flow limitation is that all compensatory mechanisms to defend alveolar ventilation must be inspiratory in nature and involve modifications in the intensity and pattern of inspiratory muscle activation.[116] In a recent study, it was shown that the prevalence of expiratory flow limitation detected by the negative pres-

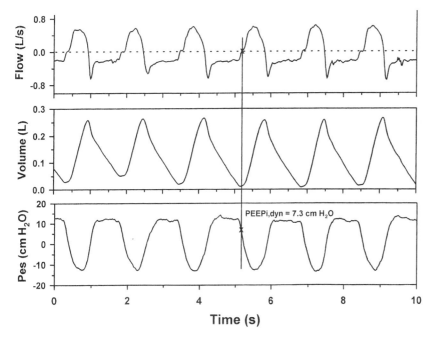

Figure 5-3

Representative record (flow, volume, and esophageal pressure, or Pes, from top to bottom) in an intubated, spontaneously breathing patient with an acute exacerbation of chronic airflow obstruction. The expiratory flow is abruptly cut at the end of expiration, while the Pes swing (namely the inspiration effort) has already begun. The difference between the point corresponding to the onset of the change in Pes and the point of zero flow on the Pes tracing represents PEEPi,dyn, which had to be counterbalanced by the contracting inspiratory muscles in order to start inspiration.

sure technique (NEP) in stable moderate asthma patients was much lower than in COPD patients for a comparable degree of reduction in FEV_1.[115] This difference was attributed to the lower lung elastic recoil in COPD as compared with asthma.

Pellegrino and Brusasco suggested the hypothesis that the attainment of tidal expiratory flow limitation during progressive bronchoconstriction could be the trigger for the initiation of inspiration[98] (Fig. 5-4). Indeed, when bronchoconstriction was induced by inhaled methacholine, individuals without asthma tended not to exhibit an increased FRC, despite a significant reduction of FEV_1, whereas most asthma patients consistently exhibited an increased FRC with decreasing forced expiratory flows. As illustrated in Figure 5-4, the increase in FRC was associated with a reduction of forced expiratory flow sufficient to equal tidal expiratory flow at FRC. This finding was interpreted as suggesting that, during progressive bronchoconstriction, expiration terminates only when flow limitation occurs, as revealed by the impingement of tidal flow on forced expiratory flow. It seems that asthma patients "choose" to increase their FRC when it would be impossible for them to keep tidal volume at the relaxation volume without expiring under conditions of flow limitation.

The Contribution of Post-inspiratory Activity of the Inspiratory Muscles

In normal individuals during tidal ventilation, inspiratory muscle action does not cease suddenly with the beginning of expiration but persists during the first portion of expiration, thus braking it.[117] In infants, post-inspiratory activity represents a mechanism, among others, to uphold FRC in the presence of stiff lungs and a floppy chest wall. In adults, the exact purpose of post-inspiratory activity is not clear, although it has been suggested that it results in an end-inspiratory hold optimizing distribution of inspired gas.

In stable COPD, the decay of the activity of the inspiratory muscles during expiration is faster than in normal individuals.[118] In both normal subjects and those with asthma, post-inspiratory activ-

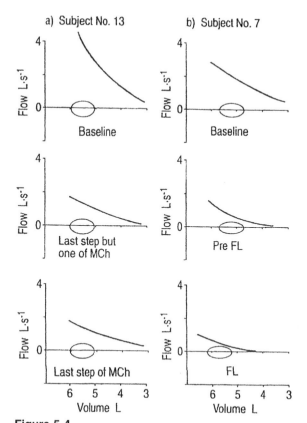

Figure 5-4

Tidal and partial (i.e., started from a lung volume below total lung capacity) forced expiratory flow-volume loops in two typical individuals in whom inhaling methacholine (MCh): a) did not increase FRC; and b) did increase FRC. Upper panels are baseline conditions. In subject b), FRC increased when the tidal flow–volume loop at a given dose of methacholine (middle panel) would have impinged on the partial loop of the next step (lower panel) (flow limitation conditions). In contrast, in subject a), FRC did not increase after methacholine, and the conditions of flow limitation never occurred, as inferred from the presence of expiratory flow reserve near end-expiration. FRC, functional residual capacity. (From Muller and Bryan[98])

ity of the inspiratory muscles was enhanced by external resistive loading and during induced bronchoconstriction.[95,119,120] In those with asthma, post-inspiratory activity was mainly present in intercostal and accessory muscles whereas the diaphragm relaxed early in expiration,[120] although

Table 5-1

Mechanisms of Pulmonary Hyperinflation in Asthma

- Abnormal airway resistance
- Expiratory flow limitation
- Glottis narrowing in expiration
- Post-inspiratory inspiratory muscle activity
- Airway closure and near-closure at higher lung volume
- Slight loss of lung elastic recoil

some post-inspiratory activity of the diaphragm has been found by other investigators.[95] Martin and co-workers suggested that this persistent post-inspiratory activity of the extradiaphragmatic inspiratory muscles is one of the mechanisms upholding FRC during bronchoconstriction, although the relative contributions of rib cage and abdominal displacement to the volume of hyperinflation are variable due to concomitant expiratory muscle activity.[121] This conclusion was based on the observation that pleural pressure remained negative during bronchoconstriction-induced pulmonary hyperinflation, indicating that the positive abdominal pressure generated by expiratory muscle contraction is not transmitted to the chest wall. A negative pleural pressure throughout expiration would prevent expiratory flow limitation, which would be consistent with the significant correlation between the changes in pulmonary resistance and the degree of pulmonary hyperinflation found by Martin and co-workers.[56] An alternative view has been advanced by Pellegrino and colleagues who hypothesized that expiratory flow limitation plays a key role in pulmonary hyperinflation during induced bronchoconstriction and the post-inspiratory activity of the inspiratory muscles is a consequence rather than a cause of hyperinflation.[18] However, Pellegrino and colleagues did not measure pleural pressure,[98] and Martin and colleagues did not analyze results relating tidal and maximum expiratory flows; these possibilities have not been fully sorted out.[120–122]

In summary, pulmonary hyperinflation invariably accompanies acute episodes of asthma. There are multiple causes (Table 5-1) including unconstrained airway narrowing, associated

changes in the mechanical properties of the lungs, and dynamic events such as long expiratory time constant and post-inspiratory activity of the inspiratory muscles. Both airway narrowing and pulmonary hyperinflation increase the work of breathing. Although some disagreement exists on the relative importance of each of the mechanisms underlying pulmonary hyperinflation, it is unanimously accepted that the increase in FRC has a negative impact on the pressure-generating capacity of the ventilatory pump.

CONSEQUENCES OF PULMONARY HYPERINFLATION

The most relevant consequences of pulmonary hyperinflation in bronchial asthma are summarized in Table 5-2.

Work of Breathing

Although there is controversy about the ultimate effects of combined bronchoconstriction and pulmonary hyperinflation on the overall work of breathing (WOB), mainly because very few measurements have been made during acute asthma,[56,57,120,122] it seems reasonable to assume that abnormal flow resistance increases the resistive WOB whereas pulmonary hyperinflation increases the elastic WOB.[123]

Because of the inverse relationship between airway resistance and lung volume,[124] an immediate consequence of the rise in lung volumes, particularly in FRC in asthma, is an increase of airway

Table 5-2

Consequences of Pulmonary Hyperinflation in Asthma

- Intrinsic PEEP (inspiratory threshold load)
- Reduced inspiratory muscle pressure generating capacity
- Increased elastic work of breathing
- Increased risk of barotrauma
- Decreased cardiac output
- Decreased "ohmic" resistive work of breathing

caliber. Therefore, during an asthma attack, pulmonary hyperinflation tends to limit airway narrowing.[57] Furthermore, a larger airway diameter can diminish the number of small airways that close during expiration, thus improving the intrapulmonary distribution of the inspired gas, while the lower flow resistance may reduce the WOB.

Martin and colleagues reported a substantial increase in WOB, both in its resistive and elastic components, during induced bronchoconstriction.[120] Patients with bronchoconstriction generated large swings in intrathoracic pressure to generate negative alveolar pressure, with a fivefold increase in magnitude of the inspiratory muscle effort. This occurred with recruitment of the intercostal-accessory and abdominal muscles to assist the diaphragm. Similar results were obtained by the same investigators in healthy subjects during external resistive loading.[119] They suggested that the increase in the elastic load as a result of pulmonary hyperinflation represents the major burden on the inspiratory muscles,[120] and that in patients with asthma this burden was borne primarily by the diaphragm and other inspiratory muscles.[120] They also suggested that continuous positive airway pressure (CPAP) applied during bronchoconstriction would augment the expiratory muscle activity (see below) to share the WOB between inspiratory and expiratory muscles.[122]

By contrast, Wheatley and colleagues reported that the increase in the elastic work during induced bronchoconstriction and hyperinflation was due not only to hyperinflation but to decreased dynamic lung compliance resulting from an increased time constant inequality, as well.[57] This latter mechanism may be less important during hyperinflation, which, by itself, tends to decrease heterogeneity. In addition, Wheatley and colleagues found a decrease in expiratory muscle load owing to a lower expiratory airway resistance, which they attributed to larger airway caliber at higher lung volume.[57] The reduction in work done by the expiratory muscles compensated for the increased inspiratory work and pulmonary hyperinflation owing to induced bronchoconstriction and did not result in a substantial increase in total

WOB. They concluded that the spontaneous increase of FRC in acute asthma is a mechanism minimizing the WOB and energy expenditure.[57] Unfortunately, no subsequent investigation was performed to clarify the changes in the WOB during acute asthma.

In assessing these studies, it should be mentioned that the relationships of respiratory system resistance and airway resistance to lung volume are different. By using the interrupter technique in both healthy anaesthetized subjects[125] and in ventilator-dependent patients with acute respiratory distress syndrome (ARDS)[126] or acute exacerbation of COPD,[127] it has been shown that, unlike the "ohmic" airway resistance which increases with increasing flow and decreases with increasing volume, the resistance of the respiratory system, which includes the "non-ohmic" component due to the viscoelasticity of lung and chest wall tissues, increases with increasing volume. The same technique (i.e., the interruption technique) was used by Sly and colleagues in anaesthetized cats during administration of methacholine and induced bronchoconstriction.[128] They found that both airway and pulmonary tissue resistance increased with use of methacholine. However, increasing lung volume decreased abnormal airway resistance but not pulmonary tissue resistance. In fact, airway caliber increased with increasing volume thereby reducing airway resistance, whereas lung tissue stress-adaptation phenomena increased with increasing lung volume, thus explaining the different behavior of tissue resistance. The modification of total respiratory system resistance with methacholine-induced bronchoconstriction and changes in lung volume depends upon the combined effects of airway and tissue resistance.

Intrinsic PEEP

If passive expiration is incomplete, the end-expiratory recoil pressure of the respiratory system (Pel,rs) results in a positive end-expiratory alveolar pressure.[129,130] The end-expiratory Pel,rs has been termed occult, auto- or intrinsic PEEP analogous to positive end-expiratory pressure (PEEP) set by the ventilator in ventilator-dependent patients.[131,132] In ventilator-dependent patients, intrinsic PEEP (PEEPi) may be promptly disclosed by end-expiratory airway occlusion as illustrated in Figure 5-5. Intrinsic PEEP has been also found in spontaneously breathing patients with chronic airflow obstruction, in whom it can be inferred from the change in pleural (esophageal) pressure preceding inspiratory flow, as illustrated in Figure 5-3. If FRC is above Vr, the end-expiratory Pel,rs must be counterbalanced by the contracting inspiratory muscles before creating a negative pressure in the central airway and hence inspiratory flow. Therefore, in terms of energetics of breathing, PEEPi constitutes an inspiratory threshold load.

Under those circumstances, the traditional, simplified, equation of motion:

$$P_{mus} = (E_{rs} \cdot V_T) + (V_T/T_I \cdot R_{tot}) \qquad (3)$$

becomes:

$$P_{mus} = PEEPi + (E_{rs} \cdot V_T) + (V_T/T_I \cdot R_{tot}) \qquad (4)$$

where P_{mus} is the pressure generated by the contracting inspiratory muscles, E_{rs} is the elastance of the total respiratory system, V_T is tidal volume, T_I is inspiratory time, V_T/T_I is mean inspiratory flow, and R_{tot} is total airflow resistance.

Figure 5-5
Representative record with measurement of PEEPi by single-breath end-expiratory airway occlusion (EEO) in a mechanically ventilated patient with acute exacerbation of chronic airflow obstruction during controlled ventilation. (From Rossi and Polese[129])

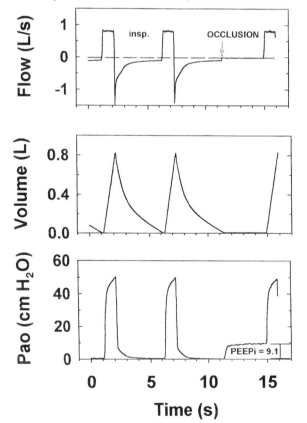

DYNAMIC INTRINSIC PEEP

Intrinsic PEEP measured from the decrease in pleural pressure (Ppl) preceding flow was named *dynamic intrinsic PEEP* (PEEPi,dyn) to distinguish it from PEEPi measured by end-expiratory occlusion under static condition (PEEPi,st) (i.e., after equilibration between lung regions with different time constants). PEEPi,dyn is lower than PEEPi,st because, under dynamic condition, the units with fast time constants start filling while those with slow time constants are still emptying. Hence PEEPi,dyn reflects mainly the end-expiratory Pel,rs of the fast units, whereas PEEPi,st reflects the average PEEPi,st after equilibration of alveolar pressure.[129] In general, PEEPi,dyn is 70% to 80% of PEEPi,st,[133] although greater differences have been reported during mechanical ventilation.[134] Clearly, PEEPi represents an extra burden upon the inspiratory muscles, which can contribute substantially to the ventilatory workload. In ventilator-dependent patients with advanced COPD, Appendini and colleagues[135] and Ranieri and colleagues[136] reported that PEEPi,dyn accounted for about 40% of the total ventilatory workload. If data collected in COPD patients can be extrapolated to patients with acute asthma, it appears obvious that the elastic load determined by pulmonary hyperinflation, which is provided in part by PEEPi and in part by the flatter volume-pressure relationship at high lung volume, can represent the greatest component of the workload, as

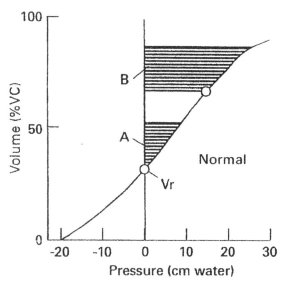

Figure 5-6

Static volume-pressure representation of dynamic hyperinflation. When inspiration starts from point B (increased end-expiratory lung volume, namely dynamic hyperinflation), the elastic work of breathing (shaded area) is higher than when inspiration starts from point A. Vr, relaxation volume of the respiratory system; VC, vital capacity. (From Pride and Milic-Emili[108])

illustrated in Figure 5-6. There are, however, two other considerations. First, both in COPD and asthma expiratory muscles may contribute to positive end-expiratory alveolar pressure. Second, the mechanisms of hyperinflation differ somewhat between asthma and COPD, with post-inspiratory activity of inspiratory muscles being almost negligible in COPD.[118]

EXPIRATORY MUSCLES AND PEEPi

Ninane and colleagues have shown that the expiratory muscles are active during spontaneous breathing in stable COPD patients,[137,138] while Lessard and colleagues,[139] Appendini and colleagues,[140,135] and Zakynthynos and colleagues,[141] found expiratory muscle activity in COPD patients with acute exacerbation and respiratory failure. Clearly, if the expiratory muscles are actively contracting during expiration, the decrease in pleural

pressure preceding flow might be due to expiratory muscle relaxation rather than to inspiratory muscle contraction (Fig. 5-7). Apart from the technical considerations related to the proper measurement of PEEPi, it is clear that the amount of positive end-expiratory alveolar pressure due to expiratory muscle activity has little to do with the magnitude of the inspiratory workload.[142] Gorini and colleagues have confirmed that expiratory muscle activity contributes significantly to the magnitude of PEEPi and this contribution increases with acute bronchoconstriction[143] (Figure 5-8). They hypothesized that abdominal muscle recruitment, which cannot increase expiratory flows because of expiratory flow limitation,[144] probably preserves diaphragmatic length at the beginning of inspiration under conditions of pulmonary hyperinflation. This explanation can be accepted, provided that inspiratory muscle contraction starts before expiratory muscle relaxation, which does not seem to always be the case[137] Therefore, the physiologic meaning of abdominal muscle activity in COPD patients with expiratory flow limitation needs to be further elucidated. Clearly, the condition might be different in asthma patients in whom expiratory flow limitation is less common than in COPD. However, the functional "barrier" provided by post-inspiratory activity can prevent the effects of abdominal muscle activity on expiratory flows. In fact, studies by Martin and colleagues,[56,120,122] Cormier and colleagues[145] and Wheatley and colleagues[57] determined that pleural pressure does not become positive during expiration in the course of induced bronchoconstriction, which indicates that the positive abdominal pressure determined by expiratory muscle contraction during expiration does not affect pleural pressure in the upper rib cage. This conclusion is supported also by some recent data by Gorini and colleagues who used a sophisticated technique to monitor changes in volume and shape of upper and lower rib cage and the abdomen, combined with measurement of pleural and gastric pressure.[146]

PEEPi and Post-inspiratory Muscle Activity

The second aspect of differing mechanisms underlying pulmonary hyperinflation in acute asthma

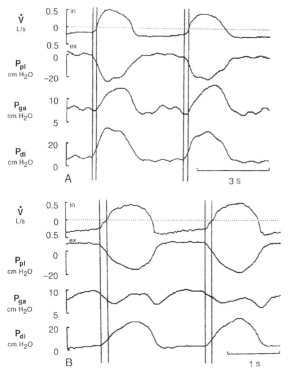

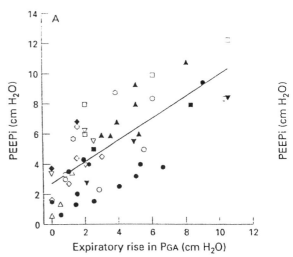

Figure 5-8

Relationship between dynamic PEEPi and the expiratory rise in gastric pressure (P_{ga}). The solid line is the regression lines and different symbols correspond to individual patients. (From Gorini and Misuri[143])

Figure 5-7

Experimental record illustrating the method used to determine the level of dynamic intrinsic PEEP (PEEP,dyn) during spontaneous unoccluded breathing efforts in two representative patients. From top to bottom, tracings represent flow ($\dot{V}$), pleural pressure (Ppl), gastric pressure (Pga), and transdiaphragmatic pressure (Pdi). The first vertical line indicates the point corresponding to the onset of the inspiratory effort (Pdi swing). The second vertical line indicates the point corresponding to the start of the inspiratory flow. The dotted horizontal line represents zero flow. A. The tidal volume is 0.46 L. Note that expiratory flow ends abruptly before inspiration, whereas the Pdi and Ppl swings have already begun and Pga has remained constant during that interval. In this case, PEEPi,dyn was measured as the negative deflection in Ppl between the point corresponding to the onset of the Pdi swing and the point of zero flow. B. The tidal volume is 0.33 L. Note that Pga increases throughout most of expiration. By contrast, Pga becomes less positive from the onset of the inspiratory effort indicated by the start of positive Pdi owing to the start of inspiratory flow. In this case PEEPi,dyn was measured as the negative Ppl deflection between the point corresponding to the onset of the Pdi swing and the point of zero flow subtracted by the amount of Pga

and COPD relates to the pattern of activation of the inspiratory muscles. As mentioned previously, the post-inspiratory activity of the inspiratory muscles, particularly the intercostals, is enhanced in acute asthma and may contribute to pulmonary hyperinflation. Such activity has never been found in COPD patients, in whom the post-inspiratory activity seems reduced, even when compared to normal individuals. In the Campbell diagram, PEEPi is given by the distance between the chest wall and lung static relaxation curves. Under those circumstances, PEEPi represents an inspiratory threshold load that becomes greater with increasing lung volume because of the increasing distance between the two lines. The post-inspiratory activity, which is illustrated graphically by the area between the actual expiration on the PV relationship and the chest wall relaxation line (Fig. 5-8), re-

negative deflection observed in the interval. In, inspiratory flow; Ex, expiratory flow. (From Appendini and Patessio[140])

Table 5-3

Respiratory Mechanics in Three Patients with Asthma During the First Day of Mechanical Ventilation in the Control Mode

Variable	A.F.(f, 36)	B.S.(f,17)	O.G.(f, 28)
V_E (L/min)	8.4	9.5	9.6
F (b/min)	12.0	13.0	12.0
V_T (L)	0.70	0.73	0.80
T_E (s)	3.1	2.9	3.7
PEEPi (cm H_2O)	12.9	13.6	8.0
δFRC (L)	0.81	0.30	0.48
Cst,rs (L/cm H_2O)	0.044	0.060	0.040
Rrs (cm H_2O/L/s)	36.5	17.8	33.1

ABBREVIATIONS: V_E, minute ventilation; f, ventilation frequency; V_T, inflation volume; T_E, expiratory time; PEEPi, intrinsic positive end-expiratory pressure; δFRC, difference between the static equilibrium volume of the respiratory system and the functional residual capacity during mechanical ventilation; Cst,rs, static respiratory compliance; Rrs, respiratory resistance after subtraction of endotracheal tube and measuring equipment.

duces PEEPi if the end-expiratory position does not lie on the chest wall relaxation line. In that condition, pleural pressure (Ppl) may be less positive or even negative at end-expiration due to the post-inspiratory activity rather than to the active isometric contraction of the inspiratory muscles to counterbalance PEEPi. It should be noted that the work done by the contracting inspiratory muscles during lengthening is less expensive in terms of energetics than the isometric work needed to offset PEEPi. Therefore, the post-inspiratory activity could represent a way to save energy during ventilation at high lung volume. In addition, the negative Ppl throughout expiration does not impair venous return or cardiac output and prevents expiratory flow limitation.

Table 5-3 shows data obtained in patients with status asthmaticus during controlled mechanical ventilation with the ventilatory pattern determined by the ventilator.[147] These data show that passive respiratory mechanics are similar in both asthma and COPD;[148] both are characterized by increased flow resistance and dynamic pulmonary hyperinflation with significant PEEPi (Fig. 5-9).

Hyperinflation and Mechanical Ventilation

Recent work has shown that measurement of total exhaled volume, as shown in Figure 5-2, may help to prevent barotrauma and asthma mortality during mechanical ventilation[149,150] by guiding adjustment of ventilator settings to reduce hyperinflation. Such a strategy, which usually requires controlled hypoventilation with permissive hypercapnia[151] (see Chapter 13), has been shown to reduce asthma mortality during mechanical ventilation substantially. However, reduction of dynamic hyperinflation might be more difficult in asthma than in COPD, because of some differences in the underlying pathophysiology. Most reports agree that a long expiratory time (e.g., more than 30 seconds),[152,153] results in full decompression of the lungs to Vr and hence, a substantial reduction of hyperinflation in mechanically ventilated patients with COPD. Thus, the use of long T_E during mechanical ventilation has been recommended to minimize PEEPi and its adverse effects.[129,130] Interestingly, it has been demonstrated that the use of smaller than conventional tidal volumes associ-

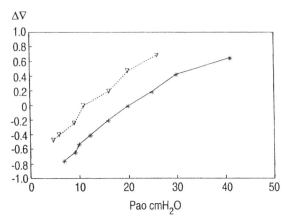

Figure 5-9

Static relationship between volume (V) and pressure at the airway opening (Pao) in a critically ill asthma patient (female, 32 yrs) on the first day of (controlled) mechanical ventilation, before (*) and after (∇) 0.1 mg of adrenaline i.v.. Experimental points have been obtained with the interrupter technique during relaxed expiration. ∆∇ = 0 represents the end-expiratory lung volume during regular mechanical ventilation. The value of Pao at ∆∇ = 0 provides the level of intrinsic positive end-expiratory pressure (PEEPi). Since the patient is dynamically hyperinflated, the relaxed expiration continues well below the end-expiratory lung volume during regular ventilation. However, although the expiratory time was about 30 seconds, the static equilibrium volume was not reached, because of the extremely high flow resistance. Adrenaline produced an important bronchodilatation as shown by the decrease of PEEPi from 20 to 10 cm H_2O, without changes in the slope of the ∆∇ = Pao relationship. (From Rossi and Appendini[147])

and Ravenscraft has suggested that PEEPi measured at the endotracheal tube may not reflect severe hyperinflation in patients with status asthmaticus who are undergoing mechanical ventilation.[155] These investigators reported a small number of asthma patients in ventilatory failure who exhibited all of the symptoms of extreme hyperinflation, including compromised cardiac output, radiographic hyperinflation, high-peak airway pressure, high-plateau airway pressure, and increased peak-plateau pressure gradient, and yet whose PEEPi was only minimally increased when assessed by an end-expiratory hold maneuver. These investigators then followed lung mechanics serially, and observed airway pressures that fell dramatically during treatment and resolution of the underlying status asthmaticus. They speculated that the disparity resulted from complete airway closure of many portions of the lung, with persistent gas trapping during an end-expiratory pause, and a failure of PEEPi to be measurable at the endotracheal tube. In an editorial to this report, it was suggested that patients undergoing mechanical ventilation may exhibit occult PEEP that is not readily assessed by the usual methods.[156] To the extent that this is true, significant portions of the hyperinflated lungs would not communicate with the airway opening, thus making the measurement of occlusion pressure at end-expiration insensitive to positive alveolar pressure distal to the point of small airways closure, as illustrated in Figure 5-10. The failure of postmortem asthmatic lungs to collapse supports this explanation[157,158] (see Chapter 4).

The fact that small airway closure occasionally plays a significant role in the determination of pulmonary hyperinflation has important implications for treatment of acute asthma, and particularly for mechanical ventilatory management.

First, volume trapped by completely occluded airways cannot be passively exhaled regardless of the duration of expiratory time.[159] Clearly, this does not mean that short T_E should be used in asthma, since much hyperinflation in most patients results from narrowed but still patent airways.[149,150,160] Rather, it means that a reduction in tidal volume may be also necessary in

ated with longer than usual T_E decreases PEEPi substantially, although this "controlled hypoventilation" type of ventilatory setting resulted in a deterioration in ventilation to perfusion matching, thus decreasing Pa_{O_2} and raising Pa_{CO_2}.[94,154] However, reduction in PEEPi caused a significant increase in cardiac output and in oxygen delivery such that tissue oxygenation improved.[94,154]

Unfortunately, there are no similar studies in status asthmaticus and data from ventilator-dependent COPD patients cannot be extrapolated to asthma. An interesting study by Leatherman

End-Expiratory Airway Occlusion

Measured A.P = 5 cm H_2O

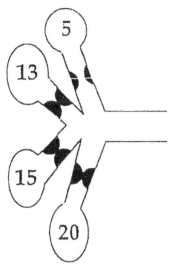

Figure 5-10
A hypothetical model to explain underestimation of end-expiratory alveolar pressure by measured auto-positive end-expiratory pressure (AP) in severe asthma. Alveolar pressure (cm H_2O) in four different lung units is shown. At end-expiration, only the upper lung unit is in communication with the central airway, causing the airway occlusion pressure (measured at positive end-expiration) to be much lower than end-expiratory alveolar pressure in the other hyperinflated, but noncommunicating, lung units. (From Leatherman and Ravenscraft[155])

some patients.[161] Second, this observation adds support to avoidance of external PEEP, which some investigators have suggested as a means to open closed airways.[162] Studies have shown that even small amounts of PEEP (e.g., 5 cm H_2O) can worsen hyperinflation and decrease cardiac output in asthma patients.[160] The distribution of airway closure is likely to be heterogeneous in patients with status asthmaticus, causing "recruiting" PEEP to cause regional hyperinflation,[163] as suggested in Figure 5-11. In a recent paper, Guerin and colleagues found that small airway closure

was common also in ventilator-dependent COPD during exacerbation and suggested that PEEP should be set to the level at which all airways were open[164] (Fig. 5-11). Borrowing the concept from the "open lung approach" applied to patients with ARDS,[165] Guerin and colleagues suggested that PEEP above closing pressure would prevent some

Figure 5-11
Relationships of inflation volume, relative to relaxation volume (Vr), to static pressure of total respiratory system (Pst,rs) obtained at four levels of PEEP in two representative patients. The static volume-pressure curves exhibit an inflexion point (Po) (white arrow). The broken lines below the inflexion point are extrapolated. EELV (black arrow): end-expiratory lung volume on ZEEP. In one patient, total PEEP on ZEEP was halfway between Vr and Po, whereas in another patient it was closer to Po. (From Guerin and LeMasson[164])

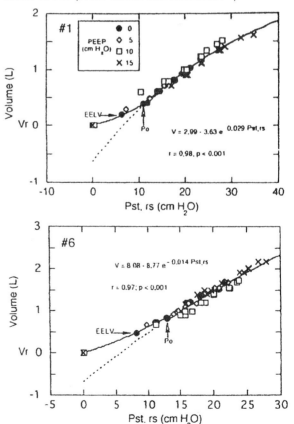

ventilator-induced injuries in COPD as well. However, in acute asthma small airways are likely to close at higher lung volume and throughout expiration, so that the approach suggested by Guerin and colleagues for COPD cannot be extrapolated to status asthmaticus without further research. Thus, application of PEEP in ventilator-dependent asthmatics is anecdotal and will remain controversial[166] until additional data are provided. While some studies have shown benefit from continuous positive airway pressure (CPAP) administered by mask to spontaneously breathing patients with acute asthma[167] (see Chapter 12), this benefit may result from reduction in load on the inspiratory muscles.[122] This mechanism seems to be completely different from the mechanism by which CPAP is thought to decrease the ventilatory workload in exacerbated COPD. In COPD, CPAP counterbalances PEEPi, thus reducing substantially the inspiratory threshold load, which may represent about 40% of the overall mechanics load in COPD.[135,136,140] However, Martin and colleagues did not evaluate PEEPi in their patients with asthma during induced bronchoconstriction so that a replacement of PEEPi by CPAP cannot be ruled out. This is an important issue, since application of low levels of PEEP or CPAP may improve the impact of non-invasive ventilation in acute asthma,[168] as has been shown in COPD.[140]

Respiratory Strength

Several studies have shown that the respiratory muscles of stable asthma patients have normal[58] or close to normal[59,169] maximum strength and endurance. In contrast, during an acute asthma attack, the maximum strength of the inspiratory muscles can be profoundly reduced. This likely results from length-tension and geometrical effects of hyperinflation. The reduced pressure-generating capacity during acute asthma can reduce the ability of the inspiratory muscles to bear a burden while both the resistive and elastic (including PEEPi) ventilatory workload can be significantly increased, as previously discussed. Although this association of decreased inspiratory muscle strength and increased load may theoreti-

cally expose muscle fibers to the risk of fatigue, there is no direct evidence of inspiratory muscle fatigue in patients with acute asthma.

A different condition may characterize patients with steroid-dependent asthma, in whom the inspiratory muscle strength may be severely reduced,[170,171] probably because of the effect of steroids on skeletal muscles.[172,173] Data by Weiner and colleagues suggest that patients with stable asthma, who have some degree of airway obstruction and pulmonary hyperinflation, exhibited reduced inspiratory muscle strength that increases after bronchodilation, in inverse relationship to the decrease in lung volume.[169] It is noteworthy that inspiratory muscle strength and efficiency were lower in healthy females than in males,[174] but in stable asthma patients, they were greater in females than in males; the reason(s) for this difference have not been elucidated.[169,174]

Inspiratory Muscle and Pulmonary Hyperinflation The remarkable increase in FRC occurring during acute asthma causes a reduction in the maximum inspiratory muscle strength because of a shorter than normal starting and operational length.[175] However, it has been suggested that the diaphragm and the rib cage inspiratory muscles are influenced differently by hyperinflation. It is unquestionable that, during hyperinflation, the ability of the diaphragm to lower intrathoracic pressure is reduced primarily because of shorter length.[93,175,176] Under normal mechanical conditions, the contraction of the diaphragm causes expansion of the lower rib cage not only because of "insertional" force but also because of "appositional" action.[176] The insertional force of the diaphragm is due to the insertion of its fibers on the upper margin of the lower ribs and the xiphoid process of the sternum, such that contraction lifts and rotates outward the lower ribs while the abdominal contents oppose the caudal movement of the central tendon. The appositional action of the diaphragm on the lower rib cage is due to the fact that, in standing humans, the diaphragmatic fibers separate approximately 30% of the rib cage surface from the abdominal content. Under these circumstances, when diaphragmatic contraction generates a positive abdominal pressure, it is transmitted to the lower rib cage with an expanding action. Pulmonary hyperinflation, by lowering the diaphragm, reduces significantly the area of apposition and increases the area of the rib cage exposed to negative pleural pressure. When FRC approaches TLC, the zone of apposition is virtually abolished and the increase in abdominal pressure cannot expand the lower rib cage. Therefore, although no direct measurement of inspiratory muscle strength and endurance has been reported in acute asthma, a reduction in the diaphragmatic pressure-generating capacity can be expected to occur on the basis of experimental data in animals and humans. In contrast, it appears that the diaphragmatic shape (i.e., the increase in radius) plays little or no role in determining the effect of hyperinflation on the pressure-generating capacity of the diaphragm.[176]

The progressive reduction in the pressure-generating ability of the diaphragm with increasing lung volume puts most of the ventilatory workload on the rib cage inspiratory muscles, in particular the parasternal intercostals, which represent the most important portion of the intercostal musculature.[177] Although intercostal muscles shorten less than the diaphragm with pulmonary hyperinflation (i.e., 7% to 10% versus 40%), the operating length of the parasternal intercostals is smaller than that of the diaphragm, such that even small changes in the length at which contraction starts may induce a severe mechanical disadvantage.[178] However, some experimental data suggested that the optimal length for the parasternal intercostals occurs close to TLC[178,179] rather than close to FRC, as is the case for the diaphragm. This conclusion, however, is not supported by all studies;[180] therefore, it cannot be stated that pulmonary hyperinflation, while detrimental for the diaphragm is beneficial for the parasternal intercostals, until further data are available. Data concerning the effects of hyperinflation on scalene and sternomastoid function are inconclusive.[177]

In summary, pulmonary hyperinflation is detrimental for diaphragmatic function and the inspiratory muscles of the rib cage must bear the ventilatory workload. This is not a result of changes in the pattern of the neural activation, but rather is the consequence of changes in the mechanical action of the inspiratory muscles. Theoretically, these mechanical changes may expose the diaphragm and the rib cage inspiratory muscles to the risk of fatigue, although this remains to be investigated in acute asthma.

Expiratory Muscles   Expiratory muscles are active in stable COPD patients[142] during tidal breathing. Recent data by Gorini and colleagues provided evidence of increasing expiratory muscle activation with progressive bronchoconstriction[143] (see Fig. 5-8). In asthma, expiratory muscles may be active at baseline conditions; their activity may increase with acute bronchospasm and pulmonary hyperinflation.[56,95,96,120–122] However, owing to the persistent post-inspiratory activity of the inspiratory intercostals, the positive expiratory abdominal pressure cannot be used to increase expiratory flows. Rather, it may prevent excessive diaphragmatic shortening by reducing the contribution of the lower rib cage and abdominal compartment to hyperinflation[121] with the purpose of optimizing the length of the diaphragmatic fibers for subsequent inspiration. The improvement in the efficiency of diaphragmatic function resulting from a more favorable position on its active length-tension curve might compensate for the added cost of breathing borne by the inspiratory intercostal and accessory muscles. Indeed, the observation that some distortion of the rib cage occurs during induced bronchoconstriction[181] supports the hypothesis that the rib cage accounts for most of the hyperinflation associated with airway narrowing.[146] In summary, activation of abdominal muscles during expiration occurs in asthma and seems to decrease the load on the inspiratory muscles and to optimize the length of the diaphragm.

CLINICAL CONSIDERATIONS

The prevalence and severity of bronchial asthma appears to be increasing worldwide, and all patients with asthma are at risk of developing an acute attack that may progress to status asthmaticus and to near-fatal or fatal asthma. As discussed in this chapter, airway narrowing and airway closure and near-closure determines pulmonary hyperinflation, with an increase in FRC that couples to an augmented workload with a reduced inspiratory muscle pressure-generating capacity. This may lead, in turn, to a profound load-capacity imbalance that can impair the capacity of an asthma patient to maintain ventilation during an acute attack. Although the mechanisms leading to life-threatening conditions are complex and may involve profound abnormalities in gas exchange, pulmonary mechanics, and control of breathing,[182] the major cause of respiratory failure and fatal asthma is an underestimation of the severity of the disease, particularly at the onset of acute attacks. Hypoxemia in acute severe asthma (see Chapter 6) may couple with hypercapnia and respiratory acidosis to further impair ventilatory pump function and a vicious cycle of deterioration.

REFERENCES

1. Manian P: Genetics of asthma: A review. *Chest* 112:1397–1408, 1997.
2. National Heart, Lung, and Blood Institute/World Health Organization: *Workshop Report, March 1993: Global initiative for asthma*. National Institutes of Health, Publ No. 95-3659, January 1995.
3. Woolcock AJ: Asthma, in Murray JF, Nadel JA (eds): *Textbook of Respiratory Medicine*, 2. Philadelphia, Saunders, 1994, pp 1288–1330.
4. Macklem PT: Mechanical factors determining maximum bronchoconstriction. *Eur Respir J* 2(Suppl):516s–519s, 1989.
5. Macklem PT: The clinical relevance of respiratory muscle research. *Am Rev Respir Dis* 134:812–815, 1986.
6. Haley KJ, Drazen JM: Editorial. Inflammation and airway function in asthma. What you see is not necessarily what you get. *Am J Respir Crit Care Med* 157:1–3, 1998.
7. Crimi E, Spanevello A, Neri M, et al: Dissociation between airway inflammation and airway hyperresponsiveness in allergic asthma. *Am J Respir Crit Care Med* 157:4–9, 1998.
8. Woolcock AJ, Read J: Lung volume in exacerbations of asthma. *Am J Med* 41:259–273, 1966.
9. Woolcock AJ, Rebuck AS, Cade JF, Read J: Lung volume changes in asthma measured concurrently by two methods. *Am Rev Respir Dis* 104:703–709, 1971.
10. Anderson SD, McEvoy JDS, Bianco S: Changes in lung volumes and airway resistance after exercise in asthmatic subjects. *Am Rev Respir Dis* 106:30–37, 1972.
11. Freedman S, Tattersfield AE, Price NB: Changes in lung mechanics during asthma induced by exercise. *J Appl Physiol* 38:974–982, 1975.
12. Cade JF, Woolcock AJ, Rebuck AS, Pain MCF: Lung mechanics during provocation of asthma. *Clin Sci* 40:381–391, 1971.
13. Stanescu DC, Frans A, Brasseur L: Acute increase of total lung capacity in asthma following histamine aerosols. *Bull Eur Physiopathol Respir (Nancy)* 9:523–530, 1973.
14. Mead J, Whittenberger JL: Physical properties of human lungs measured during spontaneous respiration. *J Appl Physiol* 5:770–796, 1953.
15. Orehek J, Gayrard P, Smith AP, et al: Airway response to carbachol in normal and asthmatic subjects. Distinction between bronchial sensitivity and reactivity. *Am Rev Respir Dis* 115:937, 1977.
16. Anthonisen NR: Tests of mechanical function, in Macklem PT, Mead J (eds): *Handbook of Physiology*, vol III, part 2: *The Respiratory System: Mechanics of Breathing*. Bethesda, American Physiological Society, 1986, pp 753–784.
17. Pride NB, Macklem PT: Lung mechanics in disease, in Macklem PT, Mead J (eds): *Handbook of Physiology*, vol III, part 2: *The Respiratory System: Mechanics of Breathing*. Bethesda, American Physiological Society, 1986, pp 659–692.
18. Pellegrino R, Violante B, Crimi E, Brusasco V: Effects of aerosol methacoline and histamine on airways and lung parenchyma in healthy humans. *J Appl Physiol* 74:2681–2686, 1993.
19. Pellegrino R, Violante B, Brusasco V: Maximal bronchoconstriction in humans. Relationship to deep inhalation and airway sensitivity. *Am J Respir Crit Care Med* 153:115–21, 1996.
20. Gibbons WJ, Sharma A, Lougheed D, Macklem PT: Detection of excessive bronchoconstriction in asthma. *Am J Respir Crit Care Med* 153:582–589, 1996.
21. Sterk PJ, Bel EH: Bronchial hyperresponsiveness: The need for a distinction between hypersensitivity and excessive airway narrowing. *Eur Respir J* 2: 267–274, 1989.

22. Stephens NL, Kroeget E, Mohta JA: Force-velocity characteristics of respiratory airway smooth muscle. *J Appl Physiol* 26:685–692, 1969.

23. Moreno RH, Hogg JC, Parè PD: Mechanics of airway narrowing. *Am Rev Respir Dis* 133:1171–1180, 1986.

24. Okazawa M, Ishida K, Road J, et al: In vivo and in vitro correlation of trachealis muscle contraction in dogs. *J Appl Physiol* 73:1486–1493, 1992.

25. Stephens NL, Hoppin FG: Mechanical properties of airway smooth muscle, in Macklem PT, Mead J (eds): *Handbook of Physiology,* vol III, part 2: *The Respiratory System: Mechanics of Breathing.* Bethesda, American Physiological Society, 1986, pp 263–276.

26. Mitchell RW, Rabe KF, Magnussen H, Leff AR: Passive sensitization of human airways induces myogenic contractile responses in vitro. *J Appl Physiol* 83:1276–1281, 1997.

27. Mitchell RW, Ruhlmann E, Magnussen H, et al: Passive sensitization of human bronchi augments smooth muscle shortening velocity and capacity. *Am J Physiol* 267:L218–L222, 1994.

28. Ebina M, Takahashi T, Tamihiko C, Motomiya M: Cellular hypertrophy and hyperplasia of airway smooth muscles underlying bronchial asthma. A 3-D morphometric study. *Am Rev Respir Dis* 148:720–726, 1993.

29. Lambert RK: Role of bronchial basement membrane in airway collapse. *J Appl Physiol* 71:666–673, 1991.

30. Lambert RK, Codd SL, Alley MR, Pack RJ: Physical determinant of bronchial mucosal folding. *J Appl Physiol* 77:1206–1216, 1994.

31. Lambert RK, Wiggs BR, Kuwano K, et al: Functional significance of increased airway smooth muscle in asthma and COPD. *J Appl Physiol* 74:2771–2781, 1993.

32. James AL, Parè PD, Hogg JC: The mechanics of airway narrowing in asthma. *Am Rev Respir Dis* 139:242–246, 1989.

33. Paré PD, Roberts CR, Bai TR, Wiggs BJ: The functional consequences of airway remodelling in asthma. *Monaldi Arch Chest Dis* 52:589–96, 1997.

34. Froeb HF, Mead J: Relative hysteresis of the dead space and lung in vivo. *J Appl Physiol* 25:244–248, 1968.

35. Skloot G, Permutt S, Togias AG: Airway hyperresponsiveness in asthma: a problem of limited smooth muscle relaxation with inspiration. *J Clin Invest* 96:2393–2403, 1995.

36. Wasserfallen JB, Schaller MD, Feihl F, Perret CH: Sudden asphyxic asthma: a distinct entity? *Am Rev Respir Dis* 142:108–111, 1990.

37. Soler M, Imhof E, Perruchoud AP: Severe acute asthma. Pathophysiology, clinical assessment, and treatment. *Respiration* 57:114–121, 1990.

38. Leatherman J: Life-threatening asthma. *Clin Chest Med* 15:453–479, 1994.

39. Corbridge TC, Hall JB: The assessment and management of adults with status asthmaticus. *Am J Respir Crit Care Med* 151:1296–1316, 1995.

40. Bone RC: Status asthmaticus, in Parrillo JE, Bone RC (eds): *Critical Care Medicine. Principles of Diagnosis and Management.* St. Louis, MO, Mosby, 1995, pp 627–638.

41. Mountain RD, Sahn SA: Clinical features and outcome in patients with acute asthma presenting with hypercapnia. *Am Rev Respir Dis* 138:535–539, 1988.

42. Levy BD, Kitch B, Fanta CH: Medical and ventilatory management of status asthmaticus. *Intensive Care Med* 24:105–117, 1998.

43. Strunk RC: Identification of the fatality-prone subject with asthma. *J Allergy Clin Immunol* 83:477–485, 1989.

44. Weiss KB, Wagener DK: Changing patterns of asthma mortality: identifying target populations at high risk. *JAMA* 264:1683–1687, 1990.

45. Molfino NA, Slutsky AS: Near-fatal asthma. *Eur Respir J* 7:981–990, 1994.

46. Rossi A, Ganassini A: Near-fatal asthma and mechanical ventilation. *Monaldi Arch Chest Dis* 51:2, 99–101, 1996.

47. Booms P, Cheung D, Timmers MC, et al: Respiratory pathophysiologic responses. Protective effect of inhaled budesonide against unlimited airway narrowing to methacholine in atopic patients with asthma. *J Allergy Clin Immunol* 99:330–337, 1997.

48. Guidelines on the management of asthma. *Thorax* 48:S1–S24, 1993.

49. Petty T: Treat status asthmaticus three days before it occurs. *J Intensive Care Med* 4:135–136, 1989.

50. McFadden ER, Lyons HA: Arterial-blood gas tension in asthma. *N Engl J Med* 278:1027–1032, 1968.

51. Giuntini C, Guerini C, Mariani M, et al: Il comportamento del rapporto ventilazione-perfusione e della circolazione polmonare nella sindrome asmatica. *Rass Pat App Respir* 1–15, 1968.

52. Rodriguez-Roisin R: Acute severe asthma: pathophysiology and pathobiology of gas exchange abnormalities. *Eur Respir J* 10:1359–1371, 1997.

53. Rodriguez-Roisin R, Roca J: Bronchial asthma. *Thorax* 49:1027–1033, 1994.

54. Sydow M, Burchardi H: Intensive care management of life-threatening status asthmaticus, in Vincent JL (ed): *Update in Intensive Care and Emergency Medicine,* 14. Berlin, Springer-Verlag, 1991, pp 313–323.

55. Ward ME, Roussos C, Macklem PT: Respiratory mechanics, in Murray JF, Nadel JA (eds): *Textbook of Respiratory Medicine,* 2d ed. Philadelphia, Saunders, 1994, pp 90–138.

56. Martin JG, Shore SA, Engel LA: Mechanical load and inspiratory muscle action during induced asthma. *Am Rev Respir Dis* 128:455–460, 1983.

57. Wheatley JR, West S, Cala SJ, Engel LA: The effect of hyperinflation on respiratory muscle work in acute induced asthma. *Eur Respir J* 3:625–632, 1990.

58. McKenzie DK, Gandevia SC: Strength and endurance of inspiratory, expiratory, and limb muscles in asthma. *Am Rev Respir Dis* 134:999–1004, 1986.

59. Sette L, Ganassini A, Boner AL, Rossi A: Maximal inspiratory pressure and inspiratory muscle endurance time in asthmatic children: reproducibility and relationship with pulmonary function tests. *Ped Pulmonol* 24(6):385–390, 1997.

60. Marks J, Pasterkamp H, Asher T, Leahy F: Relationship between respiratory muscle strength, nutritional status, and lung volume in cystic fibrosis and asthma. *Am Rev Respir Dis* 133:414–417, 1986.

61. Lands L, Desmond J, Demizio D, et al: The effect of nutritional status and hyperinflation on respiratory muscle strength in children and young adults. *Am Rev Respir Dis* 141:1506–1509, 1990.

62. Schmidt GA, Hall JB, Wood LDH: Management of ventilated patient, in Murray JF, Nadel JA (eds): *Textbook of Respiratory Medicine,* 2d ed. Philadelphia, Saunders, 1994, pp 2636–2657.

63. Tobin MJ, Mador MJ: Acute respiratory failure, in Calverley PMA, Pride NB (eds): *Chronic Obstructive Pulmonary Disease.* London, Chapman & Hall, 1995, pp 461–494.

64. Similowsky T, Milic-Emili J, Derenne JP: Respiratory mechanics during acute respiratory failure of chronic obstructive pulmonary disease, in Derenne JP, Whitelaw WA, Similowsky T (eds): *Acute Respiratory Failure in Chronic Obstructive Pulmonary Disease.* New York, Marcel Dekker, 1996, pp 23–46.

65. Rossi A, Polese G, De Sandre G: Respiratory failure in chronic airflow obstruction: recent advances and therapeutic implications in the critically ill patient. *Eur J Med* 1:349–357, 1992.

66. Perret C: Sudden asphyxia in asthma, in Vincent JL (ed): *Update in Intensive Care and Emergency Medicine,* 13. Berlin, Springer-Verlag, 1989, pp 86–90.

67. Agostoni E, Hyatt RE: Static behaviour of the respiratory system, in Macklem PT, Mead J (eds): *Handbook of Physiology,* vol III, part 2. *The Respiratory System: Mechanics of Breathing.* Bethesda, MD, American Physiological Society, 1986, pp 113–130.

68. Dollfuss RE, Milic-Emili J, Bates DV: Regional ventilation of the lung studied with boluses of 133 xenon. *Resp Physiol* 2:234–246, 1967.

69. Milic-Emili J: Ventilation, in West JB (ed): *Regional Differences in the Lung.* New York, Academic Press, 1977, pp 167–195.

70. Milic-Emili J: Topographical inequality of ventilation, in Crystal RG, West JB, Weibel ER, Barnes PJ (eds): *The Lung.* Philadelphia, Lippincott-Raven, 1997, pp 1415–1423.

71. Holland J, Milic-Emili J, Macklem PT, Bates DV: Regional distribution of pulmonary ventilation and perfusion in elderly subjects. *J Clin Invest* 47:81–92, 1968.

72. Engel LA, Grassino A, Anthonisen NR: Demonstration of airway closure in man. *J Appl Physiol* 38:1117–1125, 1975.

73. Rossi A, Ganassini A, Tantucci C, Grassi V: Aging and the respiratory system. *Aging Clin Exp Res* 8:143–161, 1996.

74. De Troyer A, Estenne M, Ninane V, et al: Transversus abdomis muscle function in humans. *J Appl Physiol* 68:1010–1016, 1990.

75. Gold WM, Kaufman HS, Nadel JA: Elastic recoil of the lungs in chronic asthmatic patients before and after therapy. *J Appl Physiol* 23:433–438, 1967.

76. Finucane KE, Colebatch HJH: Elastic behavior of the lung in patients with airway obstruction. *J Appl Physiol* 26:330–338, 1969.

77. Anthonisen NR: Closing volume, in West JB (ed): *Regional Differences in the Lung.* New York, Academic Press, 1977, pp 451–482.

78. McCarthy D, Milic-Emili J: Closing volume in asymptomatic asthma. *Am Rev Respir Dis* 107:559–570, 1973.

79. Peress L, Sybrecht G, Macklem PT: The mechanism of increase in total lung capacity during acute asthma. *Am J Med* 61:165–169, 1976.

80. Woolcock AJ, Read J: The static elastance proper-

ties of the lungs in asthma. *Am Rev Respir Dis* 98:788–794, 1968.

81. Engstrom I: Respiratory studies in children. XII. Serial studies of mechanics of breathing, lung volumes and ventilatory capacity in provoked asthmatic attacks. Acta Paediatr (Stockh) 53:345–355, 1964.

82. Fish JE, Ankin ML, Kelly JF, Peterman VI: Regulation of bronchomotor tone by lung inflation in asthmatic and non-asthmatic subjects. *J Appl Physiol* 50:1079–1086, 1980.

83. Olive JT, Hyatt RE: Maximal expiratory flow and total respiratory resistance during induced bronchoconstriction in asthmatic subjects. *Am Rev Respir Dis* 106:366–376, 1972.

84. Bouhuys A, Hunt VR, Kim BM, Zapletal A: Maximum expiratory flow rates in induced bronchoconstriction in man. *J Clin Invest* 48:1159–1168, 1969.

85. Fish JE, Rosenthal RR, Batra G, et al: Airway responses to methacholine in allergic and nonallergic subjects. *Am Rev Respir Dis* 113:579–586, 1976.

86. Bouhuys A, Van de Woestijne KP: Respiratory mechanics and dust exposure in byssinosis. *J Clin Invest* 49:106–118, 1970.

87. Pellegrino R, Violante B, Selleri R, Brusasco V: Changes in residual volume during induced bronchoconstriction in healthy and asthmatic subjects. *Am J Respir Crit Care Med* 150:363–368, 1994.

88. Burns CB, Taylor WR, Ingram RH: Effects of deep inhalation in asthma: relative airway and parenchymal hysteresis. *J Appl Physiol* 59:1590–1596, 1985.

89. Sekizawa K, Sasaki H, Shimizu Y, Takishima T: Dose-response effects of methacholine in normal and in asthmatic subjects. *Am Rev Respir Dis* 133:593–599, 1986.

90. Brusasco V, Pellegrino R, Violante B, Crimi E: Relationship between quasi-static pulmonary hysteresis and maximal airway narrowing in humans. *J Appl Physiol* 72:2075–2080, 1992.

91. Brusasco V, Pellegrino R, Rodarte JR: Vital capacities in acute and chronic airway obstruction: dependence on flow and volume histories. *Eur Respir J* 10:1316–1320, 1997.

92. Macklem PT: The importance of excessive bronchoconstriction in asthma. *Giorn It Allergol Immunol Clin* 2:275–281, 1992.

93. Blackie SP, Al-Majed S, Staples CA, et al: Changes in total lung capacity during acute spontaneous asthma. *Am Rev Respir Dis* 142:79–83, 1990.

94. Hillman DR, Finucane KE: The effect of hyperin-

flation on lung elasticity in healthy subjects. *Respir Physiol* 54:295–305, 1983.

95. Muller N, Bryan AC, Zamel N: Tonic inspiratory muscle activity as a cause of hyperinflation in histamine-induced asthma. *J Appl Physiol* 49:869–874, 1980.

96. Muller N, Bryan AC, Zamel N: Tonic inspiratory muscle activity as a cause of hyperinflation in asthma. *J Appl Physiol* 50:279–282, 1981.

97. Pellegrino R, Violante B, Nava S, et al: Relationship between expiratory airflow limitation and hyperinflation during methacholine induced bronchoconstriction. *J Appl Physiol* 75:1720–1727, 1993.

98. Pellegrino R, Brusasco V: On the causes of lung hyperinflation during bronchoconstriction. *Eur Respir J* 10:468–475, 1997.

99. Pellegrino R, Brusasco V: Lung hyperinflation and flow limitation in chronic airway obstruction. *Eur Respir J* 10:543–549, 1997.

100. Mansell A, Dubrawsky C, Levinson H, et al: Lung mechanics in antigen-induced asthma. *J Appl Physiol* 37:297–301, 1974.

101. Kirby JB, Juniper EF, Hargreave FE, Zamel N: Total lung capacity does not change during methacholine-stimulated airway narrowing. *J Appl Physiol* 61:2144–2147, 1986

102. DuBois AB, Botelho SY, Bedell GN, et al: A rapid plethysmographic method for measuring thoracic gas volume: a comparison with a nitrogen washout method for measuring functional residual capacity in normal subjects. *J Clin Invest* 35:322–326, 1956.

103. Rodenstein DO, Stanescu DC, Francis C: Demonstration of failure of body plethysmography in airway obstruction. *J Appl Physiol: Respirat Environ Exercise Physiol* 52:949–954, 1982.

104. Brown R, Ingram RH Jr, McFadden ER Jr: Problems in plethysmographic assessment of changes of total lung capacity in asthma. *Am Rev Respir Dis* 118:685–692, 1978.

105. Shore SA, Huk O, Mannix S, Martin JC: Effect of panting frequency on the plethysmographic determination of thoracic gas volume in chronic pulmonary obstructive disease. *Am Rev Respir Dis* 128:54–59, 1983.

106. Kinsella M, Muller NL, Staples C, et al: Hyperinflation in asthma and emphysema: assessment by pulmonary function testing and computed tomography. *Chest* 94:286–289, 1988.

107. Buhain WJ, Brody JS, Fisher AB: Effect of artifi-

cial airway obstruction on elastic properties of the lung. *J Appl Physiol* 33:589–594, 1972.

108. Pride NB, Milic-Emili J: Lung mechanics, in Calverley PMA, Pride NB (eds): *Chronic Obstructive Pulmonary Disease.* London, Chapman & Hall, 1995, pp 135–160.

109. Rossi A, Polese G, Brandi G: Dynamic hyperinflation, in Marini JJ, Roussos C (eds): V*entilatory Failure.* Berlin, Springer-Verlag, 1991, 15:199–218.

110. Vinegar A, Sinnett EE, Leith DE: Dynamic mechanisms determine functional residual capacity in mice, Mus musculus. *J Appl Physiol: Respirat Environ Exercise Physiol* 46:867–871, 1979.

111. McIlroy MB, Tierney DF, Nadel JA: A new method for measurement of compliance and resistance of lung and thorax. *J Appl Physiol* 17:424–427, 1963.

112. Zin WA, Pengelly LD, Milic-Emili J: Single-breath method for measurement of respiratory mechanics in anesthetized animals. *J Appl Physiol* 52:1266–1271, 1982.

113. Higgenbottam T: Narrowing of the glottis opening in humans associated with experimentally induced bronchoconstriction. *J Appl Physiol* 49:403–407, 1980.

114. Collett PW, Brancatisano T, Engel LA: Upper airway dimensions and movements in bronchial asthma. *Am Rev Respir Dis* 133:1143–1149, 1986.

115. Boczkowski J, Murciano D, Pichot MH, et al: Expiratory flow limitation in stable asthmatic patients during resting breathing. *Am J Respir Crit Care Med* 156:752–757, 1997.

116. Siafakas NM, Vermeire P, Pride NB, et al: Optimal assessment and management of chronic obstructive pulmonary disease (COPD). *Eur Respir J* 8:1398–1420, 1995.

117. Shee CD, Ploy-Song-Sang Y, Milic-Emili J: Decay of inspiratory muscle pressure during expiration in conscious humans. *J Appl Physiol* 58:1859–1865, 1985.

118. Citterio G, Agostoni E, Del Santo A, Marazzini L: Decay of inspiratory muscle activity in chronic airway obstruction. *J Appl Physiol* 51:1388–1397, 1981.

119. Martin JG, Habib M, Engel LA: Inspiratory muscle activity during induced hyperinflation. *Respir Physiol* 39:303–313, 1980.

120. Martin J, Powell E, Shore S, Emrich J, Engel A: The role of respiratory muscles in the hyperinflation of bronchial asthma. *Am Rev Respir Dis* 121:441–447, 1980.

121. Lennox S, Mengeot PM, Martin JG: The contributors of rib cage and abdominal displacements to the hyperinflation of acute bronchospasm. *Am Rev Respir Dis* 132:679–684, 1985.

122. Martin JG, Shore SA, Engel LA: Effect of continuous positive airway pressure on respiratory mechanics and pattern of breathing in induced asthma. *Am Rev Respir Dis* 126:812–817, 1982.

123. Agostoni E, Campbell EJM, Freedman S: The mechanical work of breathing, in Campbell EJM, Agostoni E, Newsom Davis J (eds): *The Respiratory Muscles. Mechanics and Neural Control.* London, Lloyd-Luke Ltd, 1970, pp 115–137.

124. DuBois AB, Botelho SY, Comroe JH Jr: A new method for measuring airway resistance in man using a body plethysmograph: values in normal subjects and in patients with respiratory disease. *J Clin Invest* 35:327–335, 1956.

125. D'Angelo E, Calderini E, Torri G, et al: Respiratory mechanics in anesthetized paralyzed humans: effects of flow, volume, and time. *J Appl Physiol* 67:2556–2564, 1989.

126. Eissa NT, Ranieri MV, Corbeil C, et al: Analysis of behaviour of the respiratory system in ARDS patients: effects of flow, volume, and time. *J Appl Physiol* 70:2719–2729, 1991.

127. Tantucci C, Corbeil C, Chassé M, et al: Flow resistance in patients with chronic obstructive pulmonary disease in acute respiratory failure. *Am Rev Respir Dis* 144:384–389, 1991.

128. Sly PD, Brown KA, Bates JHT, et al: Effect of lung volume on interrupter resistance in cats challenged with methacholine. *J Appl Physiol* 64:360–366, 1988.

129. Rossi A, Polese G, Brandi G, Conti G: The intrinsic positive end expiratory pressure (PEEPi). Physiology, implications, measurement, and treatment. *Intensive Care Med* 21:522–536, 1995.

130. Rossi A, Ganassini A, Polese G, Grassi V: Pulmonary hyperinflation and ventilator-dependent patients. *Eur Respir J* 10:1663–1674, 1997.

131. Pepe PE, Marini JJ: Occult positive end-expiratory pressure in mechanically ventilated patients with airflow obstruction. *Am Rev Respir Dis* 126:166–170, 1982.

132. Rossi A, Gottfried SB, Zocchi L, et al: Measurement of static compliance of the total respiratory system in patients with acute respiratory failure during mechanical ventilation: the effect of "intrinsic" PEEP. *Am Rev Respir Dis* 131:672–767, 1985.

133. Petroff BJ, Legare M, Goldberg P, et al: Continuous positive airway pressure reduces work of breathing and dyspnea during weaning from mechanical ventilation in severe chronic obstructive pulmonary disease. *Am Rev Respir Dis* 141:281–289, 1990.

134. Maltais F, Sovilj M, Goldberg P, Gottfried SB: Respiratory mechanics in status asthmaticus. Effect of inhalational anesthesia. *Chest* 106:1401–1406, 1994.

135. Appendini L, Purro A, Patessio A, et al: Partitioning of inspiratory muscle workload and pressure assistance in ventilator-dependent COPD patients. *Am J Respir Crit Care Med* 154:1301–1309, 1996.

136. Ranieri VM, Grasso S, Mascia L, et al: Effects of proportional assist ventilation on inspiratory muscle effort in patients with chronic obstructive pulmonary disease and acute respiratory failure. *Anesthesiology* 86:79–91, 1997.

137. Ninane V, Yernault JC, De Troyer A: Intrinsic PEEP in patients with chronic obstructive pulmonary disease. *Am Rev Respir Dis* 148:1037–1042, 1993.

138. Ninane V, Rypens F, Yernault JC, De Troyer A: The role of respiratory muscles in the hyperinflation of bronchial asthma. *Am Rev Respir Dis* 146:16–21, 1992.

139. Lessard MR, Lo Faso F, Brochard L: Expiratory muscle activity increases intrinsic positive end-expiratory pressure and mask pressure support during exacerbation of chronic obstructive pulmonary disease. *Am J Respir Crit Care Med* 151:562–569, 1995.

140. Appendini L , Patessio A, Zanaboni S et al: Physiologic effects of positive end-expiratory pressure during mask ventilatory assistance in patients with acute exacerbation of COPD. *Am J Respir Crit Care Med* 149:1069–1076, 1994.

141. Zakynthinos SG, Vassilakopoulos T, Zakynthinos E, Roussos C: Accurate measurement of intrinsic positive end-expiratory pressure: how to detect and correct for expiratory muscle activity. *Eur Respir J* 10:522–529, 1997.

142. Ninane V, Rypens F, Yernault JC, De Troyer A: Abdominal muscle use during breathing in patients with chronic airflow obstruction. *Am Rev Respir* 16–21, 1992.

143. Gorini M, Misuri G, Duranti R, et al: Abdominal muscle recruitment and PEEPi during broncho-constriction in chronic obstructive pulmonary disease. *Thorax* 52:355–361, 1997.

144. Valta P, Corbeil C, Lavoie A, et al: Detection of expiratory flow limitation during mechanical ventilation. *Am J Respir Crit Care Med* 150:1311–1317, 1994.

145. Cormier Y, Lecours R, Legris C: Mechanisms of hyperinflation in asthma. *Eur Respir J* 3:619–624, 1990.

146. Iandelli I, Gorini M, Bertoli F, et al: *Abdominal Muscle Recruitment Plays an Important Role in the Variability of Transdiaphragmatic Pressure during Sniff Maneuvers in Normal Subjects.* San Francisco, ALA/ATS International Conference, May 16–21, 1997.

147. Rossi A, Appendini L, Poggi R, et al: Acute bronchial asthma: indications for intensive care. *Eur Respir Rev* 3:400–403, 1993.

148. Rossi A, Polese G, Milic-Emili J: Mechanical ventilation in the passive patient, in Derenne JP, Whitelaw WA, Similowsky T (eds): *Acute Respiratory Failure in Chronic Obstructive Pulmonary Disease.* New York, Dekker, 1996, pp 709–746.

149. Tuxen DV, Williams TJ, Scheinkestel CD, et al: Use of a measurement of pulmonary hyperinflation to control the level of mechanical ventilation in patients with acute severe asthma. *Am Rev Respir Dis* 146:1136–1142, 1992.

150. Williams TJ, Tuxen DV, Scheinkestel CD, et al: Risk factors for morbidity in mechanically ventilated patients with acute severe asthma. *Am Rev Respir Dis* 146:607–615, 1992.

151. Feihl F, Perret C: Permissive hypercapnia. How permissive should we be? *Am J Respir Crit Care Med* 150:1722–1737, 1994.

152. Kimball WR, Leith DE, Robins AG: Dynamic hyperinflation and ventilator dependence in chronic obstructive pulmonary disease. *Am Rev Respir Dis* 126:991–995, 1982.

153. Broseghini C, Brandolese R, Poggi R, et al: Respiratory mechanics during the first day of mechanical ventilation in patients with pulmonary edema and chronic airway obstruction. *Am Rev Respir Dis* 138:355–361, 1988.

154. Rossi A, Santos C, Roca J, et al: Effects of PEEP on VA/Q mismatching in ventilated patients with chronic airflow obstruction. *Am J Respir Crit Care Med* 149:1077–1084, 1994.

155. Leatherman JW, Ravenscraft SA: Low measured auto-positive end-expiratory pressure during mechanical ventilation of patients with severe asthma:

Hidden auto-positive end-expiratory pressure. *Crit Care Med* 24:541–546, 1996.

156. Stewart TE, Slutsky AS: Occult, occult auto-PEEP in status asthmaticus. *Crit Care Med* 24:379–380, 1996.

157. Hogg JC: Pathology of asthma. *J Allergy Clin Immunol* 92:1–5, 1993.

158. Dunnill MS: The pathology of asthma, with special reference to changes in the bronchial mucosa. *J Clin Pathol* 13:27–33, 1960.

159. Tuxen DV, Lane S: The effects of ventilatory pattern on hyperinflation, airway pressures, and circulation in mechanical ventilation of patients with severe airflow obstruction. *Am Rev Respir Dis* 136:872–879, 1987.

160. Tuxen DV: Detrimental effects of positive end-expiratory pressure during controlled mechanical ventilation of patients with severe airflow obstruction. *Am Rev Respir Dis* 140:5–9, 1989.

161. Georgopoulos D, Mitrouska I, Markopoulou K, et al: Effects of breathing pattern on mechanically ventilated patients with chronic obstructive pulmonary disease and dynamic hyperinflation. *Intensive Care Med* 21:880–886, 1995.

162. Qvist J, Pemberton M, Bennike KA: High-level PEEP in severe asthma. *N Engl J Med* 307:1347–1348, 1982.

163. Suter PM, Fairley B, Isenberg MD: Optimum end-expiratory airway pressure in patients with acute pulmonary failure. *N Engl J Med* 292:284–289, 1975.

164. Guerin C, LeMasson S, De Varax R, et al: Small ariway closure and positive end-expiratory pressure in mechanically ventilated patients with chronic obstructive pulmonary disease. *Am J Respir Crit Care Med* 155:1949–1956, 1997.

165. Hudson LD: Protective ventilation for patients with acute respiratory distress syndrome. *N Engl J Med* 338:385–387, 1998.

166. Rossi A, Ranieri MV: Positive end-expiratory pressure. In: Tobin MJ, ed: *Principles and Practice of Mechanical Ventilation.* New York, McGraw-Hill, 1994, pp 259–303.

167. Schivaram U, Miro AM, Cash ME, et al: Cardiopulmonary responses to continuous positive airway pressure in acute asthma. *J Crit Care Med* 8:87–92, 1993.

168. Meduri GU: Noninvasive positive-pressure ventilation in patients with acute respiratory failure. *Clin Chest Med* 17:513–553, 1996.

169. Weiner P, Suo J, Fernandez E, Cherniack RM: The effect of hyperinflation on respiratory muscle strength and efficiency in healthy subjects and patients with asthma. *Am Rev Respir Dis* 14:1501–1505, 1990.

170. Bowyer SL, LaMothe MP, Hollister JR: Steroid myopathy: incidence and detection in a population with asthma. *J Allergy Clin Immunol* 76:234–42, 1985.

171. Melzer E, Souhrada JR: Decrease of respiratory muscle strength and static lung volumes in obese asthmatics. *Am Rev Respir Dis* 121:17–22, 1980.

172. Douglass JA, Tuxen DW, Horne M, et al: Myopathy in severe asthma. *Am Rev Respir Dis* 146:517–519, 1992.

173. Leatherman JW, Fluegel WL, David WS, et al: Muscle weakness in mechanically ventilated patients with severe asthma. *Am J Respir Crit Care Med* 153:1686–1690, 1996.

174. Weiner P, Suo J, Fernandez E, Cherniack RM: Efficiency of the respiratory muscles in healthy individuals. *Am Rev Respir Dis* 140:392–6, 1989.

175. Gibson GJ: Pulmonary hyperinflation a clinical overview. *Eur Respir J* 9:2640–2649, 1996.

176. De Troyer A: Effect of hyperinflation on the diaphragm. *Eur Respir J* 10:708–713.

177. Decramer M: Hyperinflation and respiratory muscle interaction. *Eur Respir J* 10:934–941, 1997.

178. Farkas G, Decramer M, Rochester DF, De Troyer A: Contractile properties of intercostal muscles and their functional significance. *J Appl Physiol* 59:528–535, 1985.

179. Jiang TX, Deschepper K, Demedts M, Decramer M: Effects of acute hyperinflation on the mechanical effectiveness of the parasternal intercostals. *Am Rev Respir Dis* 139:522–528, 1989.

180. Dimarco AF, Romaniuk JR, Supinski GS: Mechanical action of the interosseous intercostal muscles as a function of lung volume. *Am Rev Respir Dis* 142:1041–1046, 1990.

181. Ringe ER, Loring SH, McFadden ER Jr, Ingram RA Jr: Chest wall configurational changes before and during acute obstructive episodes in asthma. *Am Rev Respir Dis* 128:607–10, 1983.

182. Kikuchi Y, Okabe S, Tamura J, et al: Chemosensitivity and perception of dyspnea in patients with a history of near fatal asthma. *N Engl J Med* 330:1329–1334, 1994.

Chapter 6

GAS EXCHANGE IN ACUTE ASTHMA

R. Rodriguez-Roisin

INTRODUCTION

This chapter reviews evidence that demonstrates disturbances (with a wide range of magnitude) in gas exchange that are frequently associated with episodes of acute asthma (AA). It also addresses the most characteristic clinical hallmarks of abnormal gas exchange and evaluates the pathophysiology of gas exchange, focusing on ventilation-perfusion ($\dot{V}_A/\dot{Q}$) imbalance, which is the critical intrapulmonary determinant of arterial hypoxemia in bronchial asthma, particularly during severe attacks, and its relationship to more conventional lung function tests, such as the maximal airflow rate. Finally, the chapter compares and contrasts the effects of the most common pharmacologic agents used to treat attacks of AA and examines the pathophysiologic mechanisms in these critical conditions whereby gas exchange improves, worsens, or remains unchanged. This evaluation is based primarily on the information derived from the multiple inert gas elimination technique (MIGET) that is used to estimate, quantitively and qualitatively, the distributions of $\dot{V}_A/\dot{Q}$ ratios in the lung.[1] MIGET represents a major breakthrough in unraveling the complex interplay among the different intrapulmonary [$\dot{V}_A/\dot{Q}$ mismatching, intrapulmonary shunt, and alveolar to end-capillary diffusion limitation of oxygen (O_2)] and extrapulmonary (inspired O_2 fraction, overall ventilation, cardiac output, and O_2 consumption) factors that govern respiratory blood gases and in facilitating a more thorough interpretation of gas exchange in the clinical arena.

This chapter is designed to assist practicing clinicians in bridging the gap between basic principles and clinical application in the field of pulmonary gas exchange in AA. The reader is invited to review other sources for a more comprehensive description of the theoretical and practical principles of MIGET.[1]

CLINICAL PERSPECTIVE

Pulmonary gas exchange can be mildly to profoundly disturbed in patients with severe exacerbations of AA. Arterial blood gases, including Pa_{O_2}, Pa_{CO_2}, and the alveolar-arterial P_{O_2} difference (AaP_{O_2}), which are well-known conventional markers of abnormal pulmonary gas exchange, can fluctuate between slightly abnormal values and extremely altered levels during acute attacks that result in profound arterial hypoxemia with or without hypercapnia.[2-4] A review based on reports of arterial blood gases in more than 300 critically ill patients with severe AA in the 1970s revealed that only 2% of patients had Pa_{O_2} values less than 50 mm Hg, while 13% had values between 45 and 60 mm Hg.[5] In a study of a small series of patients with AA within the first hours after hospital admission, 5 of 10 patients (FEV_1 range, 12% to 57% of the predicted value; mean, 33% of the predicted value) had Pa_{O_2} values less than 50 mm Hg (only one patient required mechanical ventilation) and two patients had levels less than 45 mm Hg while breathing room air.[6] In a study of 18 patients with severe AA, Pa_{O_2} was less than 50 mm Hg in two patients, and Pa_{CO_2} was more than 45 mm Hg in two of nine patients admitted to the hospital (mean FEV_1, 31% of the predicted value) while they were breathing room air (Fig. 6-1).

Two of the most widely cited studies of arterial blood gas disturbances in patients with severe AA were published in the late 1960s. The first study included 12 patients with more severe AA, termed *status asthmaticus,* and 64 other patients with clinically less severe AA.[8] The second study investigated a more heterogeneous population composed of 101 patients with varying degrees of airflow obstruction (FEV_1 range, 18% to 59% of the predicted value).[9] Several conclusions were drawn from these studies. The first was that marked hypoxemia, hypercapnia, and respiratory acidosis were primary hallmarks of patients with the most serious conditions, occurring only at extreme degrees of bronchoconstriction, whereas hypoxemia by itself was the most outstanding finding in patients with less severe AA. Second, mild or no hypoxemia, along with hypocapnia and respiratory alkalosis constituted the most characteristic arterial blood gas pattern in patients with less severe acute airway narrowing. With progressive disease and lack of appropriate and effective therapy, further $\dot{V}_A/\dot{Q}$ worsening may develop and initial compensatory increases in alveolar ventilation can fail because of both increased airway resistance and increased work of breathing that progress to respiratory muscle weakness or fatigue,[10] with ensuing hypercapnia and respiratory or mixed acidosis resulting from lactic acid accumulation. Third, although there was a general linear correlation between the degree of reduction of FEV_1 and Pa_{O_2}, in particular, below an FEV_1 value of 1 L, the correlation was weak when the FEV_1 was above 1 L (Fig. 6-2). Equally important, a normal level of Pa_{CO_2} did not confirm that Pa_{O_2} was greater than 45 mm Hg. It was hypothesized that on the basis of the classic three-compartment model of gas exchange,[11] $\dot{V}_A/\dot{Q}$ imbalance was the most likely mechanism underlying arterial blood gas abnormalities in these patients. Overall, these patients had markedly increased AaP_{O_2}, abnormally large Bohr's physiologic dead space (V_D/V_T) and normal CO single-breath diffusing capacity (DL_{CO}) measurements; interestingly, the venous admixture ratio ($\dot{Q}_S/\dot{Q}_T$) was increased in only a few patients. These two historical studies[8,9] have been so influential that they continue to be quoted in the current medical literature.

Hypercapnia with respiratory acidosis in patients with severe exacerbations of AA is a serious event, but it does not always indicate the need for mechanical ventilatory support. However, the significance of the "crossover" phenomenon from the early hypocapnia associated with hyperventilation and respiratory alkalosis to normal ranges of both Pa_{CO_2} and pH as evidence of impending respiratory/mixed acidosis potentially leading to life-threatening acute respiratory failure, is a reliable sign of a deteriorating course of the disease[12] and should alert physicians to the need for more vigorous treatment, including mechanical support, if necessary.

Other studies from the late 1970s of patients with severe episodes of AA, mostly retrospective in design, have underlined both the clinical and the therapeutic relevance of an increased Pa_{CO_2}

Figure 6-1

Plots of individual Pa_{O_2} and Pa_{CO_2} values in AA patients while breathing room air obtained immediately after admission (<6 hours). Each data point represents a single individual. Closed symbols, hospitalized patients: open symbols, discharged patients. (With permission, from Ferrer, et al[7])

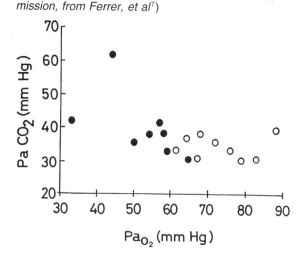

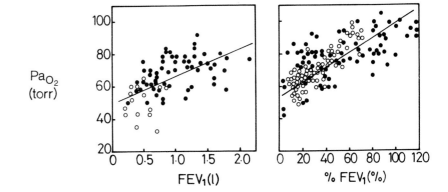

Figure 6-2
Schematic representation of the plots between FEV₁ expressed as both absolute values and percent of predicted and Pa_{O_2}.

value. Sheehy and colleagues emphasized the need for tracheal intubation and controlled mechanical ventilation along with aggressive drug therapy in a study in which 22 of 70 episodes of status asthmaticus were characterized by elevated Pa_{CO_2} levels.[13] In these patients, Pa_{CO_2} averaged 73 mm Hg. In a retrospective analysis of 811 patients admitted to the hospital for AA, Scoggin and colleagues recommended the implementation of mechanical ventilation as a life support strategy in 19 patients who became clinically obtunded and/or showed progressive hypercapnia, despite maximum vigorous medical therapy, including systemic glucocorticoids and systemic or inhaled bronchodilators.[14] Interestingly, in this subset of patients, mean arterial blood gas values were Pa_{O_2}, 62 mm Hg, Pa_{CO_2}, 61 mm Hg, and pH of 7.28. In another retrospective study, Westerman and colleagues reviewed 39 patients who required mechanical ventilation in whom Pa_{O_2} values averaged 66 mm Hg, Pa_{CO_2} values 77 mm Hg, and pH, 7.13.[15] Approximately 50% of these measurements were taken while administering oxygen-enriched mixtures. These investigators concluded that, in patients with gradually deteriorating airflow obstruction or markedly labile asthma, it was advisable to consider mechanical ventilatory support to minimize the risks of sudden near-fatal or fatal asthma. All three of these studies emphasized the clinical relevance of an elevated Pa_{CO_2} in AA patients and the necessity for physicians to treat these episodes more aggressively.

In a prospective study by Picado and col-

leagues, the features of 26 patients with severe AA who were admitted to an intensive care unit and who needed mechanical ventilation during a 6-year period, were analyzed.[16] Arterial blood gases were dramatically disturbed; arterial P_{O_2} ranged between 20 and 55 mm Hg, Pa_{CO_2} ranged between 105 and 23 mm Hg, and pH varied widely with frequent mixed respiratory and metabolic acidosis. Luksza and colleagues[17] and Higgins and colleagues[18] reported that patients with severe AA treated with mechanical ventilatory support showed results similar to the study of Picado and colleagues.[16]

However, Mountain and Sahn have challenged the concept that threshold levels of hypercapnia are an indication for the institution of mechanical ventilatory support.[19] They retrospectively compared 61 hypercapnic AA patients to 168 nonhypercapnic AA patients admitted to a hospital in Denver (altitude, 1600 m; normal Pa_{CO_2} values, <38 mm Hg). Compared with nonhypercapnic AA patients, patients with hypercapnia (Pa_{CO_2} values, >38 mm Hg) had a male gender predominance and a longer duration of severe persistent asthma, and were more likely to be treated regularly with glucocorticoids. Equally important, hypercapnic patients had more severe airflow obstruction, a greater respiratory rate, and a higher incidence of pulsus paradoxus than did those with normocapnia. Although only five patients ultimately needed mechanical ventilation, the presence of hypercapnia did not correlate closely with a need for ventilatory support. Furthermore, some patients with hypercapnia caused by asthma tended to reverse rapidly. Patients with normocapnia on hospital admission did not progress to hypercapnia after receiving appropriate therapy. In patients with hypercapnia who were readmissions, the values of Pa_{CO_2} in one episode correlated with those found during a subsequent hospitalization. This indicates that the premorbid status of ventilatory control may play a role in determining alveolar ventilation in response to the resistive load of acute airway narrowing.

A recently published clinical report of a middle-aged man admitted to an emergency department (ED) with an exacerbation of AA proposed that the combination of acute hypercapnia, cerebral hypoxemia, and elevated intrapulmonary pressures could have caused a dilated pupil due to intracranial hypertension, resulting in uncal herniation and third cranial nerve palsy.[20] Previously, Gaussorgues and colleagues had reported three severe AA patients with increased intracranial pressure (>21 mm Hg), all with fixed dilated pupils. A computed tomography (CT) scan of the head revealed generalized edema and effacement of the cerebral sulci in one of the patients.[21] It is known that high levels of Pa_{CO_2} (>200 mm Hg) produce maximal cerebral vasodilation that leads to increased intracranial blood volume.[22] In this context, the combination of severe hypoxemia and acidosis can be expected to facilitate substantial cellular swelling in the brain. Equally important, the enormous intrathoracic pressures generated during a severe asthma attack further aggravate increased intracranial pressure by increasing central venous pressure.

Hypercapnia-induced increased intracranial pressure that leads to reversible quadriparesis with hyperreflexia and abnormal plantar reflexes has been reported in a middle-aged female with severe AA who needed mechanical ventilation and was treated with halothane to minimize airflow resistance.[23] Halothane increases cerebral blood flow; thus, in the administration of inhalational anesthesia in extreme life-threatening AA, isoflurane is preferred to halothane.[23]

The development of striking subconjunctival hemorrhage in episodes of fulminant AA (see below) characterized by profound hypercapnic (mean Pa_{CO_2} 91 mm Hg) and respiratory/mixed acidotic (mean pH, 6.99) conditions has been observed and may be due to abrupt and intense congestion of blood in the territory of the superior vena cava induced by increased intrathoracic pressures.[24] This uncommon finding should be considered as a sign of severe AA.

Kikuchi and colleagues examined whether the sensation of dyspnea or hypoxia and hypercapnia chemosensitivity determine the fatal nature of many attacks of AA.[25] They demonstrated that patients with near-fatal asthma had a significantly lower hypoxic, but not hypercapnic, ventilatory drive and a lower airway occlusion pressure compared with normal individuals and asthma patients who were not at risk for near-fatal asthma. Similarly, the Borg scale, which is used to rate the sensation of difficulty in breathing during resistive loading, was lower in the patients at risk, and there was a significant positive correlation between hypoxic chemosensitivity and the perception of dyspnea. Altogether, these findings indicate that in addition to severe airway narrowing, dysfunction in the defense mechanisms protecting against profound hypoxemia and bronchoconstriction may play a pivotal role in predisposing patients to near-fatal exacerbations of AA. If chemosensitivity is blunted or minimized in patients with AA, severe respiratory insufficiency may ensue, ultimately leading to death.[26]

Molfino and colleagues studied 10 patients with AA who presented to the ED with respiratory arrest or overt respiratory insufficiency immediately after admission, despite aggressive medical treatment.[27] At the time of respiratory arrest, while oxygen was administered by a variety of approaches, these patients showed profound hypercapnia (Pa_{CO_2} values, 62 to 155 mm Hg) and mixed acidosis (pH, 7.19 to 6.87). It was assumed that the near-fatal nature of the exacerbations of AA was a consequence of intense asphyxia (i.e., unconsciousness or death resulting from lack of oxygen) rather than cardiac abnormalities related to the side effects of β_2 agonists. Asphyxia, or hypoxemia, pointed to undertreatment rather than overtreatment as one of the principal factors in the increased number of patients with fatal asthma.

Roca and colleagues, using MIGET analysis, were the first to characterize the underlying pathophysiologic mechanism of abnormal pulmonary gas exchange as $\dot{V}_A/\dot{Q}$ inequalities, in a series of 10 patients with severe AA on hospital admission and during subsequent recovery.[6] These patients manifested intense airflow obstruction and moderate to severe hypoxemia without CO_2 retention. The most novel finding was that there were no interindividual correlations between the severity of airflow obstruction and the deterioration of gas exchange on admission; this lack of correlation persisted throughout the period of hospitalization.

Wasserfallen and colleagues identified a subset of severe episodes of AA defined as a sudden, rapidly progressing attack of less than 3 hours duration. These asphyxic exacerbations of AA were characterized by their abrupt onset, the preponderance of male patients, and the striking levels of Pa_{CO_2} on admission. These fulminant exacerbations resolved quickly and required only a short duration of mechanical ventilatory support. Episodes were usually induced by massive exposure to allergens or a stressful circumstance.[28]

Similarly, thunderstorm activity[29] and heavy inhalation of airborne soybean dust in middle-aged or elderly patients[30] and *Alternaria alternata* in children and young adult patients[31] have been reported to cause acute asthmatic incidents. During the outbreaks in Barcelona caused by the inhalation of soybean dust that affected 687 patients and caused more than 1000 ED admissions,[32] epidemic patients were characteristically and significantly ventilated fewer hours (mean, 12 hours), admitted to intensive care for fewer days (<2 days), and hospitalized for fewer days (mean, 1 week) compared with nonepidemic asthma patients.[30] The term *sudden-onset fatal asthma* is useful to differentiate this form of asthma from the more common slow-onset form and to emphasize the different pathogenic mechanisms involved.[33]

CLINICAL OUTCOME

McFadden and colleagues demonstrated a correlation between lung mechanics and symptoms and physical findings in 22 patients with severe AA,

during exacerbations, and serially during recovery over a period of 5 hours.[34] In addition to the poor correlation between clinical signs and symptoms and functional abnormalities, one of the most outstanding findings was the manner in which these patients improved. When patients became asymptomatic, lung mechanics (i.e., specific airway conductance) and spirometry, including FEV_1 and maximal midexpiratory flow rates, along with static lung volumes (i.e., residual volume and functional residual capacity), ranged between 40% and 50% of those predicted; when the physical signs were no longer present, these lung function markers were still 60% to 70% of the predicted values. Since symptoms and signs of AA vanished earlier and with a far greater change in both airway resistance and FEV_1 compared with any of the other physiologic parameters, it was hypothesized that these clinical manifestations were largely related to improvement of large airway function, whereas a longer period of time was required for improvement of peripheral airflow obstruction.

In a serial study by Rudolf and colleagues, following patients over 1 week, the changes in arterial blood gases in 14 patients with severe AA were investigated.[35] All 14 patients received a standard therapeutic regime and had similar measurements at different time points. The investigators demonstrated that hypoxemia (Pa_{O_2} values, 43 to 71 mm Hg; mean, 57 mm Hg) reflected the severity of the acute attacks and constituted the most common arterial blood gas pattern on hospital admission; Pa_{O_2} often required a week or more to return to normal values. Equally important, there was no useful correlation between Pa_{O_2} and maximal airflow rates as assessed by peak expiratory flow rates (PEFR), thus supporting the very wide scatter of data in previous[8,9] and subsequent studies.[6,7] Age, duration of the acute episode, and severity of airway narrowing were all unrelated to changes in arterial blood gases, and pulse rate was found to be a poor predictor of hypoxemia in older patients. Since Pa_{O_2} is a surrogate marker of overall $\dot{V}_A/\dot{Q}$ imbalance and PEFR is a reliable descriptor of maximal airflow narrowing and airway resistance inpatients with AA, these investigators have speculated that these functional parameters assess two different pathophysiologic phenomena.

These findings, and the hypothesis of McFadden and colleagues[34] stimulated additional questions and suggested further directions for research, one of which was the significance of the intriguing dissociation between spirometric abnormalities and gas exchange disturbances within and between different clinical categories of asthma from severe AA to stable persistent or intermittent asthma.

The dissociation between spirometry and gas exchange abnormalities was confirmed subsequently by Roca and colleagues who used MIGET to characterize gas exchange on a daily basis during hospitalization and then weekly for 1 month after discharge, in a study of 8 patients with severe asthma.[6] The main finding of this study was the systematic lack of correlation between $\dot{V}_A/\dot{Q}$ inequality and spirometry, both on admission and throughout hospitalization. Nevertheless, significant negative correlations developed toward the end of the study, at weeks 3 and 4 after discharge from the hospital, when maximal recovery of both functional abnormalities associated with AA

was achieved (Fig. 6-3). Indeed, different time courses in the recovery of these two functional markers were demonstrated in all but one patient. Thus, while spirometric variables improved immediately after the onset of therapy, both Pa_{O_2} and $\dot{V}_A/\dot{Q}$ indices took longer to recover (Fig. 6-4). Since maximal expiratory airflow rates are related largely to clinical symptoms, it was hypothesized that $\dot{V}_A/\dot{Q}$ mismatching was a more silent and persistent manifestation of bronchial asthma. This may indicate that spirometric variables result from reversible bronchoconstriction and narrowing of large central airways, whereas $\dot{V}_A/\dot{Q}$ disturbances are more closely related to events that occur in the more peripheral small airways, where inflammation may play a significant role in luminal constriction. The authors of this study concluded that gas exchange abnormalities cannot be inferred from spirometric alterations. Moreover, the delay in the improvement of pulmonary gas exchange variables, specifically $\dot{V}_A/\dot{Q}$ mismatching, compared with symptoms and spirometric indices,

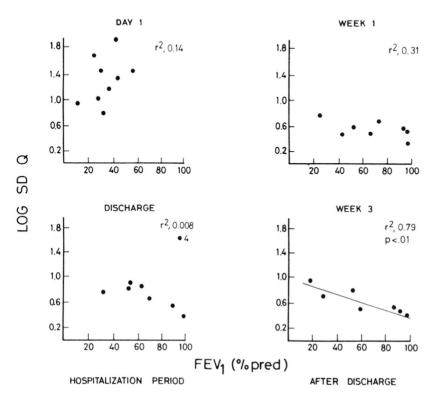

Figure 6-3
FEV_1 expressed as percent of predicted value and an index of $\dot{V}_A/\dot{Q}$ mismatching, expressed as the dispersion of blood flow (log SD Q) from day 1 through week 3, in AA patients who needed hospitalization. Each data point represents a single patient. All correlations, except for week 3, were very weak. Poor correlations also were observed between other indices of spirometry and gas exchange, suggesting a full dissociation between these two different functional outcomes. (With permission, from Roca, et al[6])

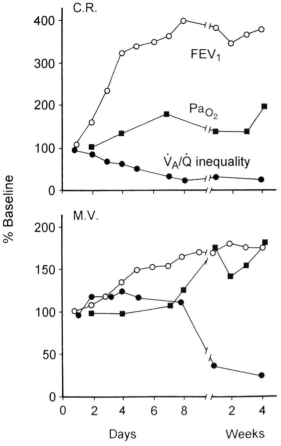

Figure 6-4

Time courses of spirometry and two indices of pulmonary gas exchange, expressed as percent of change from baseline, in two representative AA patients during hospitalization and after discharge. In patient CR (top), the three parameters improved sharply between hospitalization and discharge. By contrast, in patient MV (bottom), the correlation among the three variables was weak, with spirometry steadily improving by itself during hospital admission. After discharge, the recovery of the two gas exchange indices was evident but delayed in relation to the spirometric amelioration. The latter pattern was shown in seven of eight AA patients studied, whereas the former pattern was observed only in the remaining patient. (With permission, from Roca, et al[6])

supports the strategy of a more prolonged treatment of AA, including anti-inflammatory drugs.

The time course for recovery of arterial oxygen saturation (Sa_{O_2}) in children admitted to the hospital with AA was investigated by Mihatsch and colleagues[36] and the results of their study were similar to those of Roca's group.[6] Measurements of both PEFR and Sa_{O_2} that were assessed twice daily before and 30 minutes after the administration of nebulized salbutamol, for 4 days, demonstrated that PEFR plateaued in less than 48 hours after admission while Sa_{O_2} plateaued 12 hours later, when levels reached near-optimal values. In other words, as in adults,[6] arterial oxygenation in children, as assessed by pulse oximetry, took longer to recover than the PEFR, with a time lag of about 12 hours. The investigators suggested that, in children, Sa_{O_2} may be more accurate than PEFR in reflecting the events of uneven matching of alveolar ventilation and pulmonary perfusion owing to airflow obstruction caused by airway inflammation. Conceivably, this process resolves less rapidly than does the more widespread bronchospastic component of airway narrowing. Furthermore, PEFR may not be the most sensitive surrogate marker of lung function for detecting minor disturbances in the airway caliber of peripheral bronchi. A clinical inference of this study is that combining a measurement of airway function such as PEFR with Sa_{O_2} would allow a more comprehensive physiologic assessment and might lead to improvements in the management and assessment of AA in children, since PEFR reflects only a partial component of the relevant pathophysiologic hallmarks of AA. Thus, oximetry may prove to be a helpful tool in monitoring the severity of AA in children, particularly those too young to fully cooperate with PEFR assessments. When it is available, pulse oximetry should be performed in the ED for AA patients of all ages to assess both the severity and the outcome of arterial oxygen desaturation (below 90%) during the first hours of treatment.

Ferrer and colleagues, using MIGET, investigated whether patients with AA who were successfully discharged from the ED had a different time course of $\dot{V}_A/\dot{Q}$ inequalities and maximal expiratory airflow rates compared with those requiring hospitalization.[7] Their hypothesis was that a simultaneous recovery of both $\dot{V}_A/\dot{Q}$ disturbances and spirometry in patients discharged earlier from the ED would indicate fewer widespread inflammatory changes in the bronchial tree, specifically the most peripheral component. As expected, it was demonstrated that, in the ED, both airflow obstruction (decreased expiratory airflow rates) and gas exchange abnormalities were, on average,

more disturbed in hospitalized patients than in discharged patients (Fig. 6-5). However, the most novel finding was that while the rate of recovery of the spirometric alterations was similar in both subsets of patient, $\dot{V}_A/\dot{Q}$ disturbances recovered differently (Fig. 6-6). Thus, hospitalized patients showed a delay in the improvement of $\dot{V}_A/\dot{Q}$ inequalities in relation to airflow rates, similar to the study by Roca and colleagues.[6] In contrast, for discharged patients, the recovery of the two endpoint functional variables was identical. Together,

Figure 6-5

Time courses of FEV₁ expressed as percent of predicted value, and $\dot{V}_A/\dot{Q}$ inequalities, expressed as the dispersions of ventilation (log SD V) and blood flow (log SD Q) and an overall index of $\dot{V}_A/\dot{Q}$ heterogeneity (DISP R-E·) (all dimensionless) in hospitalized (closed symbols) and discharged (open symbols) patients, breathing room air. Shaded areas correspond to normal limits. Note that discharged patients always showed better lung function than did hospitalized patients (see text for further details). (With permission, from Ferrer, et al[7])

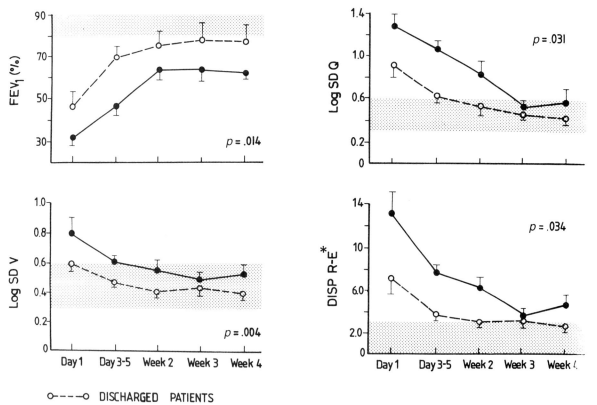

○----○ DISCHARGED PATIENTS
●——● HOSPITALIZED PATIENTS

Figure 6-6

Time courses of improvement of FEV_1 and $\dot{V}_A/\dot{Q}$ disturbances, expressed as the dispersion of blood flow (log SD Q) and an overall index of $\dot{V}_A/\dot{Q}$ heterogeneity (DISP R E') in AA patients, in the hospital or discharged, while breathing room air (variables are expressed in special arbitrary units: 100, the most normal value; 0, the most abnormal). When hospitalized patients approached their maximal improvement in FEV_1 at week 2, $\dot{V}_A/\dot{Q}$ imbalance was still at 60% of its best value; by contrast, in discharged patients both spirometric and gas exchange defects were similar and overlapped (see text for further details). (With permission, from Ferrer, et al[7])

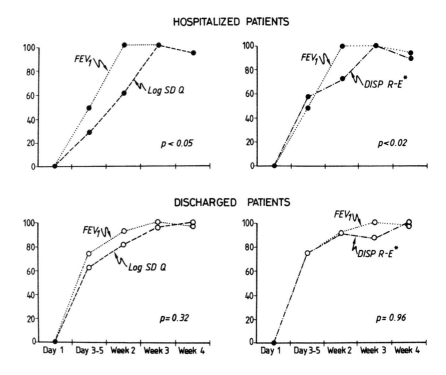

these findings indicate that patients who need hospitalization have more intense inflammation in the bronchial tree, which in turn takes longer to recover after initiation of adequate therapy. This is consistent with the hypothesis that pulmonary gas exchange reflects changes in peripheral airways whereas PEFR or FEV_1 reflect large airway function. Furthermore, it is likely that severe attacks of AA have more profound peripheral airway narrowing for any degree of proximal airway narrowing.

These findings have been reinforced by recent pathologic studies. Using both endobronchial and transbronchial biopsies, Kraft and colleagues demonstrated, in patients with stable persistent asthma, that the airway inflammatory response involves not only proximal but also distal airways, specifically the alveolar tissue.[37] Eosinophils and macrophages within alveoli may contribute more to lung function changes than does inflammation in more proximal airways. In a recent postmortem study, five cases of sudden asthma death were associated with inflammatory cellular infiltrates of proximal and distal lung tissues.[38] Furthermore, despite similar FEV_1 values peripheral airways resistance was significantly higher at night[39] while both peripheral tissue oxygen transport and cellular oxidation were jeopardized during the nadir of the nocturnal episode of airway narrowing.[40] Equally important, the finding of marked goblet cell hyperplasia in distal conducting airways, which are thought to be involved in the accumulation of large amounts of mucus in the lumen of distal airways (with associated impairment of mucociliary clearance and epithelial damage), led to the suggestion that this was a central structural hallmark in fatal AA.[41]

Although the prediction of outcome at admission of patients who require hospitalization for AA is not possible on an individual basis, Bolliger and colleagues identified several clinical and functional features that point to patients with incapacitating asthma and should alert clinicians to the need for hospital admission.[42] These factors are

1) a PEFR value less than 30% of predicted, 2) a Pa_{CO_2} value more than 45 mm Hg, 3) the presence of central cyanosis (and Pa_{O_2} less than 60 mm Hg), and 4) a history of poor long-term control of asthma (i.e., recurrent hospitalizations, maintenance glucocorticoid therapy, and regular use of β_2-agonist medications). By contrast, patients discharged successfully from the ED had an FEV_1 greater than 65% of predicted and PEFR values more than 75% of predicted values. These findings are of clinical interest in that different predictive indices in patients with severe AA at the time of hospital admission[43,44] have been found, prospectively, not to be of value.[45]

MECHANISMS OF HYPOXEMIA AND HYPERCAPNIA

It remains generally unquestioned that $\dot{V}_A/\dot{Q}$ mismatch in AA is the pivotal mechanism of abnormal arterial blood gases, since it is the primary factor that modulates the varying levels of arterial hypoxemia. Carbon dioxide retention during AA also can, in part, be associated with $\dot{V}_A/\dot{Q}$ inequality, although alveolar hypoventilation due to respiratory muscle weakness and/or fatigue also may play a central role.[2,3,10] By contrast, both increased intrapulmonary shunting and alveolar to end-capillary diffusion limitation of O_2—the two other major intrapulmonary factors that influence pulmonary gas exchange—are conspicuously negligible.

Although $\dot{V}_A/\dot{Q}$ inequality is the pivotal factor governing hypoxemia, the degree of imbalance between alveolar ventilation and pulmonary perfusion matching is a function of both the severity and the amplitude of an attack of AA (Fig. 6-7). Mild to moderate crises of AA may have nearly normal values that are close to the $\dot{V}_A/\dot{Q}$ distributions found in healthy individuals. In these

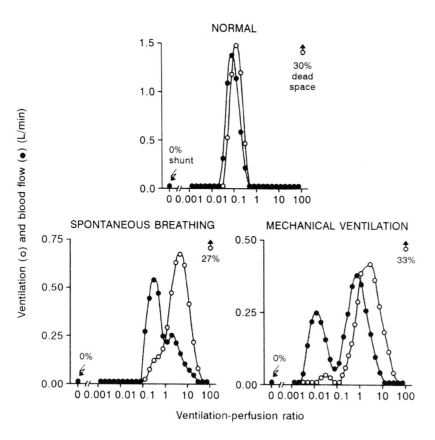

Figure 6-7

Three patterns of ventilation-perfusion distributions plotted against a $\dot{V}_A/\dot{Q}$ ratio on a log scale in patients breathing room air and during mechanical ventilation (Fi_{O_2}, 0.4). Note the narrow, unimodal, central, and symmetric distributions in a healthy subject (top) compared with the predominant bimodal blood flow pattern of the two AA patients (bottom). The dispersion of ventilation is discretely broadened, intrapulmonary shunting is conspicuously absent, and inert dead space is normal or slightly increased (during mechanical support by itself) in the uneven $\dot{V}_A/\dot{Q}$ relationships. Note also the lack of difference in the $\dot{V}_A/\dot{Q}$ patterns between the two AA patients (bottom). (With permission, from Rodriguez-Roisin, et al[55]; Ballester, et al[56]) cases, slightly broadened unimodal distributions of the pulmonary perfusion may induce only an increase in the dispersion of blood flow,[1] with normal or slightly decreased Pa_{O_2} and Pa_{CO_2} values, but increased AaP_{O_2} values.[2,3] This is due to the buffering effect that an inordinately high cardiac output (a distinctive feature of many AA patients) has on Pa_{O_2}.[46] The mechanism that causes the high cardiac output to help optimize Pa_{O_2} in the presence of the deleterious influence of underlying $\dot{V}_A/\dot{Q}$ inequality by itself remains uncertain, although it may be due to increased mixed venous P_{O_2}.[47] The anxiety caused by the severity of the AA attack, which probably increases the levels of circulating catecholamines, together with the use of bronchodilators, which have vasoactive effects, may, in part, explain increased cardiac output. Although AA patients show a more perturbed $\dot{V}_A/\dot{Q}$ status than do patients with chronic obstructive pulmonary disease (COPD) during severe acute exacerbations, Pa_{O_2} values are, in general, much lower in COPD patients. Conceivably, both a less elevated cardiac output and less efficient hypoxic pulmonary vasoconstriction (HPV) (see below) due to a more disrupted pulmonary vasculature are factors that explain the differences between the two patient groups.

Increased levels of exhaled nitric oxide (NO) are consistently found in patients with asthma, particularly in clinically unstable glucocorticoid-naïve patients.[48,49] Since endogenous NO is a potent vasodilating agent and may have a proinflammatory effect in the airways through upregulation of NO synthase, it may enhance plasma exudation in bronchial vasculature, thus facilitating narrowing of airway caliber. Similarly, increased NO may prevent an even matching of ventilation and blood flow in hypoxic alveolar units. However, a recent study with a randomized, double-blind, placebo-controlled design failed to show any correlation between basal levels of increased exhaled NO and the underlying abnormal $\dot{V}_A/\dot{Q}$ status in patients with mild asthma.[50] Moreover, inhibition of endogenous NO by N^G-nitro-L-arginine-methyl-esther (L-NAME) (a competitive antagonist of NO synthesis), did not influence $\dot{V}_A/\dot{Q}$ mismatching or

the basal conditions of pulmonary artery pressure.[50] By contrast, oral administration of nifedipine (20 mg, three times daily for 3 days), a systemic and pulmonary vasodilator, adversely affected pulmonary gas exchange in patients with mild asthma.[51] Nifedipine also resulted in a lowered Pa_{O_2} after methacholine challenge, possibly as a result of further $\dot{V}_A/\dot{Q}$ worsening.

Collectively, $\dot{V}_A/\dot{Q}$ abnormalities are commensurate with the underlying structural airway derangement commonly described in patients who die from severe AA attacks: obstruction, smooth muscle hypertrophy, peribronchial inflammatory infiltrates, and increased luminal mucus secretions. Narrowing and increased airway hyperresponsitivity in the bronchial tree with decreased ventilation in the dependent alveolar units are plausible explanations for the development of $\dot{V}_A/\dot{Q}$ defects. However, the precise mechanisms by which $\dot{V}_A/\dot{Q}$ imbalance develops in AA patients remain unclear. Several recent studies have suggested abnormal airway permeability, resulting from release of inflammatory mediators, may be important.[52–54] In a human model of asthma, using platelet-activating factor (PAF) as a bronchial challenge, the authors demonstrated the development of $\dot{V}_A/\dot{Q}$ inequalities that were qualitatively and quantitatively identical to those in patients with spontaneous forms of AA;[52] these data were replicated in healthy individuals.[53] Equally important, PAF-induced $\dot{V}_A/\dot{Q}$ abnormalities were diminished by pretreatment with inhaled salbutamol.[54] Conceivably, PAF and other mediators actively facilitate the development of $\dot{V}_A/\dot{Q}$ inequalities by enhancing airway plasma leakage.

Critically ill patients with life-threatening AA, with[55] or without[6,7,56] mechanical ventilatory support, exhibit extremely abnormal profiles of $\dot{V}_A/\dot{Q}$ imbalance (see Fig. 6-7). In these patients, a large percentage of pulmonary blood flow is distributed to alveolar units with poorly or very poorly ventilated lung units. All in all, the more severe the exacerbation of asthma, the worse the underlying $\dot{V}_A/\dot{Q}$ imbalance. Indeed, patients with extremely severe forms of AA[55] generate a profound bimodal profile of blood flow distribution as the most distinctive hallmark of the $\dot{V}_A/\dot{Q}$ spectrum (Fig. 6-8). It is conceivable that the high levels of inspired O_2 fractions that may, in part, minimize HPV, and the added pharmacologic effects of high doses of bronchodilators with potent vasodilating effects, may contribute to the enhancement of areas that are poorly ventilated and overperfused.

In AA patients with presumed narrowing of both proximal and distal airways there is a bimodal distribution of pulmonary blood flow. This contrasts with patients with persistent severe asthma who show minor $\dot{V}_A/\dot{Q}$ defects (with a mildly broadened distribution of blood flow) in spite of similar levels of airway obstruction (FEV_1 reductions on the order of 40% of predicted).[57] This mild $\dot{V}_A/\dot{Q}$ mismatch in severe persistent asthma may be modulated by airway remodeling along

with relatively well-preserved, effective pulmonary hypoxic vasoconstriction. In a dog model of artificial multiple airway occlusion,[58] it was demonstrated that when small airways were completely occluded, ventilation was preserved beyond these obstructed airways because of the efficiency of collateral ventilation to distal alveolar units. As experimental obstruction became more proximal, collateral ventilation was less efficacious so that the ventilation of distal units was meager, a status associated with a bimodal $\dot{V}_A/\dot{Q}$ profile. These experimental data may explain the range of $\dot{V}_A/\dot{Q}$ profiles seen in AA patients. No differences in the $\dot{V}_A/\dot{Q}$ patterns[55] have been shown between slow-onset and sudden-onset (fulminant) AA.[30,33]

Regardless of the amplitude and severity of

Figure 6-8

Ventilation-perfusion distributions recovered at maintenance Fi_{O_2} in eight AA patients who needed mechanical ventilation. These findings indicate that in all but two patients (patients 7 and 8), two different populations of gas exchange units (characterized by a bimodal blood flow pattern) were observed. Except in patient 4, intrapulmonary shunting was negligible; very small areas of high $\dot{V}_A/\dot{Q}$ units were shown in patients 2, 3, and 8; inert dead space (not shown) was slightly increased in patients 1 and 4, and moderately increased in patients 2, 3, and 5. (With permission, from Rodriguez-Roisin, et al[55])

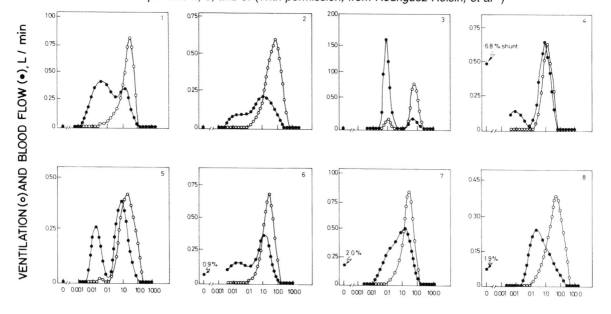

VENTILATION – PERFUSION RATIO

$\dot{V}_A/\dot{Q}$ inequalities, increased intrapulmonary shunting in patients with AA is remarkably trivial even in the most life-threatening conditions. This may reflect three underlying pathophysiologic events: 1) airway occlusion is rarely complete; 2) collateral ventilation may be very effective in preserving ventilation in distal alveolar units beyond more centrally located obstructed airways; and 3) HPV operates very actively in the pulmonary circulation, promoting an even match of ventilation and perfusion in alveolar units.

Two other pathophysiologic aspects of AA shown in MIGET studies are relevant in this context. The first is the minimal increase in lung units with high $\dot{V}_A/\dot{Q}$ ratios, that is, an augmented (altered) dispersion of alveolar ventilation; the second involves the presence of an increased dead space[55,56] (see Fig. 6-7). These phenomena, however, have little influence on ameliorating low Pa_{O_2} values. Regions of high $\dot{V}_A/\dot{Q}$ would be expected to exist in AA patients in whom gas trapping, along with increased intra-alveolar pressures, induced by check-valve mechanisms could exist. Hyperinflation would minimize blood flow in such lung areas, facilitating the development of areas, such as West's zone 1, where alveolar pressure exceeds pulmonary-capillary pressures.[59] In principle, inert dead space is always slightly lower than Bohr's dead space because it does not incorporate the dead space–like effects of alveolar units with a P_{CO_2} value less than arterial P_{CO_2}.[1] Alternatively, increased overall ventilation augments physiologic dead space, with all other factors being equal. Whatever the mechanism, the absence of high $\dot{V}_A/\dot{Q}$ and of a more substantially increased inert dead space observed in patients with AA is an intriguing feature that remains unsettled.

$\dot{V}_A/\dot{Q}$ defects in patients with AA are consistent with historical studies of gas exchange disturbance.[8,9] In the classic three-compartment lung model,[11] the effects of an increased $\dot{Q}_S/\dot{Q}_T$ and V_D/V_T are viewed as a rough estimate of the extent of the underlying $\dot{V}_A/\dot{Q}$ mismatch. The increased $\dot{Q}_S/\dot{Q}_T$ is similar to the presence of extensive areas of poorly ventilated $\dot{V}_A/\dot{Q}$ ratios, thereby producing an increment in the distribution or dispersion of pulmonary blood flow. Nonethe-

less, the absence of alveolar units with a high $\dot{V}_A/\dot{Q}$ ratio, even in patients who receive mechanical ventilation and in whom alveolar pressure is positive, is a consistent finding in all clinical forms of adult AA.

During severe exacerbations, patients with COPD also demonstrate a low $\dot{V}_A/\dot{Q}$ pattern. However, they exhibit two distinctive additional $\dot{V}_A/\dot{Q}$ findings. On the one hand, they always manifest mild to moderate increases in intrapulmonary shunting, usually at less than 10% of cardiac output, even at maintenance Fi_{O_2}, suggesting the complete occlusion of several airways and a less efficacious HPV. On the other hand, it is common to see areas of high $\dot{V}_A/\dot{Q}$ units and a markedly increased inert dead space, which probably is multifactorial from a pathophysiologic standpoint. Gas trapping, lung hyperinflation, intrinsic positive end-respiratory pressure ($PEEP_i$), and areas of pulmonary emphysema can underlie these high $\dot{V}_A/\dot{Q}$ areas.[60,61] Moreover, the dissociation between gas exchange and maximal airflow rates seen in patients with AA is less apparent in patients with COPD during acute exacerbations. In a sequential study of these patients, a parallel improvement in the spirometric and gas exchange indices during 6 weeks of recovery was demonstrated.[61]

While the mechanisms of arterial hypoxemia in AA have been thoroughly investigated, primarily through the use of MIGET, the causes of hypercapnia remain opaque. The coexistence of an excessive ventilatory load and an impaired ventilatory pump may lead to respiratory muscle fatigue and/or weakness and exhaustion, causing increased levels of Pa_{CO_2}.[10] This is a hypothesis that is often invoked, but has never been proven. Lung overinflation provoked by widespread airway narrowing can increase the work of breathing and cause respiratory muscle efficiency to deteriorate. This also is associated with high levels of intrinsic PEEP, representing an inspiratory threshold load that further increases the energy expenditure of breathing. However, whether hypercapnia in patients with AA represents impending or already established respiratory muscle fatigue and/or weakness has not been determined.[10]

PULMONARY CIRCULATION

Since arterial hypoxemia is governed primarily by $\dot{V}_A/\dot{Q}$ defects, it can be corrected promptly by the administration of relatively moderate doses of inspired O_2 (range, 0.4 to 0.6). However, from a pathophysiologic viewpoint, while a patient is breathing 100% O_2, there is further $\dot{V}_A/\dot{Q}$ deterioration. This results from increased dispersion of blood flow and suggests that HPV is attenuated even without accompanying pulmonary hemodynamic changes. Even in patients with the most abrupt forms of AA, pulmonary hypertension is usually not severe.[55] Through the mechanisms of vascular recruitment and dilatation, the pulmonary vascular bed may redistribute blood flow without influencing standard flow-pressure outcomes, but still provoke worsening in some of the indices of $\dot{V}_A/\dot{Q}$ mismatching. Teleologically, however, HPV is a mechanism that minimizes the extent of $\dot{V}_A/\dot{Q}$ mismatch and hence, hypoxemia. No correlation has been demonstrated between increased levels of exhaled NO and gas exchange disturbances in patients with mild asthma[50] (see "Mechanisms of Hypoxemia and Hypercapnia" section, above).

An intriguing finding demonstrated in AA patients who received mechanical ventilation[55] was that the administration of 100% O_2 facilitated the development of a moderate intrapulmonary shunt (usually less than 10% of cardiac output) that is not observed at maintenance Fi_{O_2}. This is not seen in AA patients who are breathing spontaneously[56] or have stable persistent asthma,[57] or in patients with other chronic lung disorders such as COPD or idiopathic lung fibrosis,[62] while breathing 100% O_2. Although the precise mechanism of this finding remains unexplained, it points to the development of areas with reabsorption atelectasis and/or to a substantial increment in regional blood flow in small preexisting intrapulmonary shunts.[55]

In clinical practice, nevertheless, the development of this mild to moderate increase in intrapulmonary shunting after the administration of 100% O_2 has little influence on Pa_{O_2} as it usually exceeds 450 to 500 mm Hg. Alternatively, a Pa_{O_2} value less than 300 mm Hg under hyperoxic

conditions in an AA patient should alert physicians to the urgent need to exclude the coexistence of consolidation (pneumonia), pulmonary collapse (pneumothorax or atelectasis), or generalized edema, which are easily visualized on a conventional chest radiograph. After high inspired-O_2 breathing fractions, in addition to the outstanding increases of Pa_{O_2} values, there are also increases in Pa_{CO_2} values, although smaller (3 to 5 mm Hg.)[55] Together, these arterial blood gas findings indicate further $\dot{V}_A/\dot{Q}$ deterioration, although the additional influence of a Haldane effect on Pa_{CO_2} values cannot be excluded.

McFadden and Hejal suggested that, in some patients with life-threatening AA, increases and falls in Pa_{CO_2} values with the administration and removal of 100% O_2, respectively, may point to a depressant effect on ventilation similar to that observed in patients with unstable COPD who receive high inspired-O_2 fractions.[5] This point of view is not supported by the existing studies of gas exchange abnormalities in AA disease, as reviewed above.

Experimentally, in normal lungs, hypocapnia can cause $\dot{V}_A/\dot{Q}$ matching to deteriorate, suggesting that HPV is abrogated; by contrast, hypercapnia does not result in significant changes in $\dot{V}_A/\dot{Q}$ heterogeneity.[63] In patients with severe acute respiratory failure who need mechanical ventilation, metabolic alkalosis disturbs $\dot{V}_A/\dot{Q}$ imbalance; conversely, reversing this effect with hydrochloric acid (HCl) results in an improvement in Pa_{O_2},[64] possibly due to blood pH. The acidosis-induced improvement in gas exchange has been related to a dual mechanism: a shift of the oxyhemoglobin dissociation curve caused by Bohr's effect, and more importantly, an improvement in $\dot{V}_A/\dot{Q}$ mismatch, possibly by enhancing HPV through redistribution of pulmonary blood flow away from hypoxic areas. Taken together, these findings are consistent with the notion that acidosis and alkalosis enhance and mitigate, respectively, the hypoxic vascular response of the lungs.[65] Similarly, it has been demonstrated that hypocapnia-induced $\dot{V}_A/\dot{Q}$ imbalance in hyperventilated normal canine lungs is pH-mediated and is not a function of Pa_{CO_2}, per se.[66] In another study with intact dogs, metabolic acidosis and alkalosis, respectively, magnified and palliated HPV; respiratory acidosis did not alter HPV, whereas respiratory alkalosis decreased HPV, suggesting a pH-independent vasodilating effect of CO_2.[67]

RESPONSE TO BRONCHODILATORS

Several guidelines,[68,69] are available to guide drug treatment of AA.[68,69] Different classes of β agonists, including adrenaline or epinephrine, short-acting β_2 adrenergics such as albuterol (salbutamol) and terbutaline; along with parenteral glucocorticoids and oxygen are viewed as standard first-line therapies.[4]

The levels of P_{O_2} and P_{CO_2} in any alveolar unit depend on three key factors: 1) the $\dot{V}_A/\dot{Q}$ relationship per se, 2) the composition of O_2 in the inspired air, and 3) the composition of O_2 in the mixed venous blood of the pulmonary artery.[70] Since both β_2 agonists and oxygen (see "Pulmonary Circulation" section, above) are associated with vasoactive effects, it may be useful to review their pathophysiologic influence on pulmonary gas exchange in the clinical setting of the AA patient.

One of the most commonly used bronchodilators is salbutamol (albuterol), which is known to be very effective in patients with asthma, by any method of administration. Ballester and colleagues demonstrated that 600 μg administered by inhalation using a conventional metered-dose inhaler (MDI) without spacer, for more than 30 minutes, was a very effective bronchodilator, with FEV_1 increasing 50% from baseline (from 1.0 to 1.5 L), an effect not associated with changes in Pa_{O_2}, cardiac output, or $\dot{V}_A/\dot{Q}$ imbalance.[56] In the same study, in another subset of AA patients, intravenous salbutamol, at a dose rate of 4 μg per minute through a 90-minute period, had a bronchodilator efficacy similar to that of a MDI; however, cardiac output increased approximately 50% from baseline (from 6 to 9 L per minute). This was paralleled by a simultaneous further deterioration of $\dot{V}_A/\dot{Q}$ heterogeneity, while the Pa_{O_2} values remained essentially unchanged. Similarly, there was a significant increase in O_2 uptake (con-

sumption). Thus, in spite of an identical beneficial bronchodilator effect on maximal airflow rates, with either method of administration, $\dot{V}_A/\dot{Q}$ inequalities deteriorated only during intravenous infusion by itself.

In another population of patients with AA, both the efficacy and the safety of nebulized salbutamol (2.5 mg) and epinephrine (1 mg) were compared in a randomized, parallel study. No significant differences in bronchodilator effects as assessed by PEFR measurements were detected.[71] Nevertheless, there was a mild but significant increase in Pa_{O_2} after epinephrine, compared with salbutamol; effects on Pa_{CO_2} were similar. Earlier, in their first MIGET study, Wagner and colleagues demonstrated that in patients with moderate asthma the administration of nebulized isoproterenol produced a transient worsening in $\dot{V}_A/\dot{Q}$ defects along with a substantial increase in cardiac output.[72] Similarly, in a canine model of bronchoconstriction, nebulization of epinephrine, isoproterenol, and salbutamol provoked distinct pulmonary gas exchange responses despite similar airflow improvement, indicating that salbutamol and epinephrine were less deleterious to gas exchange than isoproterenol.[73]

The question arises as to why similar patients respond differently to the use of salbutamol and epinephrine. Conceivably, this can be related to the α- and β-adrenergic properties of these pharmacologic agents.[73] Although these drugs are effective bronchodilators that improve Pa_{O_2} values very slightly through local improvement of regional ventilation, they may also increase cardiac output, thereby inducing some vasodilation in the pulmonary circulation. This bronchodilator-induced hyperdynamic response has a dual cardiovascular effect (Fig. 6-9). On one hand, it is beneficial to pulmonary gas exchange by increasing the levels of O_2 content in the mixed venous blood, thus optimizing Pa_{O_2} values, other factors being equal; but on the other hand, it is deleterious to gas exchange because it causes further deterioration in the $\dot{V}_A/\dot{Q}$ mismatch through passive redistribution of pulmonary blood flow and/or active pulmonary vasodilation, thus minimizing baseline levels of Pa_{O_2}.[47] Ultimately, the end-point Pa_{O_2} value results

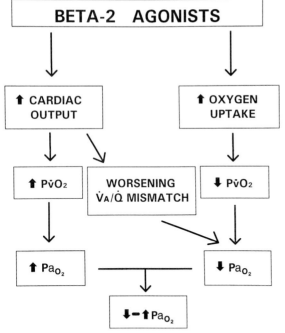

Figure 6-9
Pathophysiologic algorithm for interactions among bronchodilation, increased cardiac output, and increased O_2 consumption (uptake) and $\dot{V}_A/\dot{Q}$ inequalities in AA patients after the administration of β-adrenergics at high doses. As a result of the most influential effects of each of these factors governing gas exchange, Pa_{O_2} may decrease, remain unchanged, or even decrease (see text for further details).

from a balance between these two opposing pathophysiologic mechanisms. In clinical practice, therefore, Pa_{O_2} can decrease, a finding traditionally known as *paradoxical* hypoxemia,[74] or remain unaltered, according to the dose given and the method of administration of the β_2-adrenergic agent. Obviously, epinephrine with its associated α-adrenergic effects induces pulmonary vasoconstriction, enhancing pulmonary gas exchange; therefore, it is more beneficial because it minimizes the underlying $\dot{V}_A/\dot{Q}$ imbalance and tends to improve Pa_{O_2}, other factors being equal.[47] From a clinical point of view, however, these effects have a minor impact on both the daily management and the clinical outcome of AA patients, since all the Pa_{O_2} changes are rapidly and easily reversed with

supplemental oxygen (Fi_{O_2} range, 0.4 to 0.6). Similarly, these findings indicate that salbutamol can be administered more safely by inhalation than by vein. They also remind clinicians that the bronchodilator potency of epinephrine is similar to that of salbutamol. It is of note that the massive administration of β_2-adrenergic agonists also can increase O_2 consumption,[56,75] thereby having an additional detrimental effect on gas exchange by inducing a trend toward decreased Pa_{O_2} through a reduction of mixed venous P_{O_2}, other factors being equal[47] (Fig. 6-9).

Furthermore, the results of these relatively simple studies may have implications for bronchodilator therapy that is administered during mechanical ventilation.[76] Recent studies have established the efficacy of MDIs for delivering bronchodilators in AA patients who need mechanical support, assuming use of a spacing device and proper technique. Currently, it is generally accepted that in mechanically ventilated patients, largely those with COPD, MDIs routinely offer several advantages over nebulizers for achieving effective bronchodilation.

Salbutamol may be given either by inhalation or by vein. The efficacy and safety of these two routes of administration were compared in a parallel, randomized study by Salmeron and colleagues in 47 patients with hypercapnia who were spontaneously breathing.[77] After both therapeutic regimes, PEFR and a specific clinical index score that included dyspnea, wheezing, accessory muscle use, respiratory rate, and pulsus paradoxus, improved significantly. However, Pa_{CO_2} levels decreased after administration of nebulized salbutamol; moreover, nebulized salbutamol induced fewer side effects (both hypokalemia and tachycardia) than salbutamol administered intravenously. These data suggest that nebulized salbutamol is more effective and safer than the systemic administration method, despite similar plasma concentrations, in spontaneously breathing AA patients. In addition, nebulization likely improves the underlying $\dot{V}_A/\dot{Q}$ imbalance more effectively. Thus, local deposition plays a major role even in severe bronchial narrowing.

Interestingly, acute hyperoxia (Fi_{O_2}, 1.0) in

patients with stable bronchial asthma did not potentiate the effect of nebulized salbutamol at three incremental concentrations (from 0.05 mg/mL through 5 mg/mL) at 15-minute intervals, in a randomized double-blind study;[78] similarly, no significant change in FEV_1 was observed after hyperoxic breathing.

Recent experimental findings have suggested a role for combining oxygen therapy with salbutamol in asthma patients who are already in a hypoxic state.[79] In this study, it was shown that in bovine isolated bronchial rings, salbutamol was the only bronchodilator that was more effective in normoxia than in hypoxia.[79] The same group observed, using the same experimental model, that changes in oxygen tension substantially altered the ability of bronchodilators, including salbutamol, to protect against methacholine-induced bronchoconstriction.[80] This suggests that the responses evoked by bronchodilators under hyperoxic conditions may not necessarily predict those in the physiologic range of Pa_{O_2}; it also indicates that the relative efficacy of bronchodilators may vary between normoxia and hypoxia.

In a randomized double-blind study in stable asthma patients, the pulmonary and extrapulmonary effects of three different β agonists, administered by nebulizer, were compared.[81] Two doses of either fenoterol (5 mg), salbutamol (5 mg), or ipratropium bromide (5 mg) were nebulized at 60-minute intervals. It was clearly demonstrated that both fenoterol and salbutamol were more effective than ipratropium bromide as bronchodilators. However, fenoterol induced more harmful metabolic (hypokalemia) and cardiac (tachycardia) effects than did salbutamol or ipratropium bromide. These two side effects were repeatedly invoked to explain epidemics of fatal or near-fatal asthma in New Zealand in the 1980s.[82] In recent years, there has been increased interest in the undesirable effects of fenoterol because, with the high doses used in clinical practice, this β agonist can cause more harmful cardiac inotropic and systemic effects than do other bronchodilators of the same family.[82,83] In addition to its use at a higher dosage, the most likely explanation is that fenoterol may be less selective for β receptors.[83] It has been demon-

strated in patients with asthma, on a microgram equivalent basis, that inhaled fenoterol exhibited greater systemic potency than did salbutamol, while there was no difference in bronchodilator effectiveness.[84]

Alternatively, these data indicate that anticholinergics such as ipratropium bromide can be considered as a second-line bronchodilator treatment to strengthen the use of selective β agonists when patients respond poorly or insufficiently to the administration of more standard adrenergic compounds and parenteral glucocorticoids. Furthermore, the magnitude of the undesirable effects after a high dose of fenoterol suggests avoiding its use in all clinical categories of asthma, including AA. In a laboratory-induced human model of asthma, pretreatment with salbutamol successfully blocked PAF-induced increases in airway resistance and gas exchange abnormalities, whereas ipratropium bromide pretreatment only blocked PAF effects on airway resistance.[54] The efficacy of salbutamol was attributed to enhanced relaxation of endothelial cells in the bronchial postcapillary venules, vasodilation of the bronchial vessels, or both.[3,54]

The use of theophylline in the treatment of AA has been the subject of controversy for many years.[85] Nevertheless, several guidelines have recommended the use of methylxanthines in patients with asthma who need hospital admission because of AA.[68,69] Furthermore, in view of the potential anti-inflammatory effect of this drug,[86] a reappraisal of its role in asthma management has recently begun. A study to evaluate the effects of intravenous aminophylline on pulmonary gas exchange in patients hospitalized with AA was designed by the author.[87] In addition to a standard treatment with both inhaled salbutamol and intravenous glucocorticoids, one subset of patients received intravenous aminophylline, while the other subset received placebo. In the theophylline-treated group, a discrete but significant bronchodilator effect (17% from baseline) was demonstrated compared with the placebo-treated group. Importantly, however, aminophylline administered at therapeutic plasma levels (mean, 15 μg/mL) did not improve Pa_{O_2} values compared to placebo; yet in the placebo-treated group, $\dot{V}_A/\dot{Q}$ mismatch deteriorated slightly, probably due to the constraints of the time course of the study and the lack of sufficient bronchodilator therapy imposed by the limitations of the experimental design. Accordingly, these data indicated that the combination of theophylline with β agonists resulted in optimal bronchodilation without disturbing pulmonary gas exchange and appeared to be a reasonable second-line bronchodilator therapeutic approach, as was proposed in consensus guidelines.[68,69]

Most of these clinical trials have provided evidence for the appealing hypothesis that there is dissociation between spirometry and pulmonary gas exchange in AA patients.[6,7,46] From these data, it can be clinically helpful, in AA patients, to reinforce the monitoring of arterial oxygen saturation by pulse oximetry.

ACKNOWLEDGEMENT

This work is supported by grants from the Commisionat per a Universitats i Recerca (1997 SGR 00086) de la Generalitat de Catalunya and the Fondo de Investigación Sanitaria (FIS) 97/0126.

REFERENCES

1. Roca J, Wagner PD: Contributions of multiple inert gas elimination technique to pulmonary medicine: 1. Principles and information content of the multiple inert gas elimination technique. *Thorax* 49:815–824, 1994.
2. Rodriguez-Roisin R, Roca J: Contributions of multiple inert gas elimination technique to pulmonary medicine: 3-Bronchial asthma. *Thorax* 49:1027–1033, 1994.
3. Rodriguez-Roisin R: Acute severe asthma: pathophysiology and pathobiology of gas exchange abnormalities. *Eur Respir J* 10:1359–1371, 1997.
4. Corbridge TC, Hall J: The assessment and management of adults with status asthmaticus. *Am J Respir Crit Care Med* 151:1296–1316, 1995.
5. McFadden ER Jr. Hejal R: Asthma. *Lancet* 345:1215–1220, 1995.
6. Roca J, Ramis LI, Rodriguez-Roisin R, et al: Serial relationships between ventilation-perfusion inequality and spirometry in acute severe asthma requiring hospitalization. *Am Rev Respir Dis* 137:1055–1061, 1988.
7. Ferrer A, Roca J, Wagner P, et al: Airway obstruction and ventilation-perfusion relationships in acute severe asthma. *Am Rev Respir Dis* 147:579–584, 1993.
8. Tai E, Read J: Arterial-blood gas tension in asthma. *Lancet* 1:644–646, 1967.
9. McFadden ER Jr, Lyons H: Arterial blood gas tension in asthma. *N Engl J Med* 278:1027–1032, 1968.
10. Rossi A, Appendini L, Poggi R, et al: Acute bronchial asthma: indications for intensive care. *Eur Respir Rev* 14(Suppl 3):400–403, 1993.
11. Riley RL, Cournand A: "Ideal" alveolar air and the analysis of ventilation-perfusion relationships in the lung. *J Appl Physiol* 1:825–847, 1949.
12. Weiss AB, Faling U: Clinical significance of Pa_{CO_2} during status asthma: the cross-over point. *Ann Allergy* 26:545–551, 1968.
13. Sheehy AF, DiBenedetto R, Lefrak S, Lyons HA: Treatment of status asthmaticus. *Arch Intern Med* 130:37–42, 1972.
14. Scoggin CH, Sahn SA, Petty TL: Status asthmaticus. A nine-year experience. *JAMA* 238:1158–1162, 1977.
15. Westerman DE, Benatar SR, Potgieter PD, Ferguson AD: Identification of high-risk asthmatic patients. Experience with 39 patients undergoing ventilation for status asthmaticus. *Am J Med* 66:565–572, 1979.
16. Picado C, Montserrat JM, Roca J, et al: Mechanical ventilation in severe exacerbation of asthma. Study of 26 cases with six deaths. *Eur J Respir Dis* 64:102–107, 1983.
17. Luksza AR, Smith P, Coakley J, et al: Acute severe asthma treated by mechanical ventilation: 10 years' experience from a district general hospital. *Thorax* 41:459–463, 1986.
18. Higgins B, Greening AP, Crompton AK: Assisted ventilation in severe acute asthma. *Thorax* 41:464–467, 1986.
19. Mountain RD, Sahn SA: Clinical features and outcome in patients with acute asthma presenting with hypercapnia. *Am Rev Respir Dis* 138:535–539, 1988.
20. Dimond J P, Palazzo MG: An unconscious man with asthma and a fixed dilated pupil. *Lancet* 349:98, 1997.
21. Gaussorgues P, Piperno D, Fouqué P, et al: Hypertension intracranienne au cours de l'état asthmatique. *Ann Fr Anesth Réanim* 6:38–41, 1987.

22. Nunn JF. *Applied Respiratory Physiology,* 3d ed. London, Butterworths, 1987, p 462.

23. Zender HO, Eggimann, Bulpa P, et al: Quadriparesia following permissive hypercapnia and inhalational anesthesia in a patient with severe status asthmaticus (letter). *Intensive Care Med* 22:1001, 1996.

24. Rodriguez-Roisin R, Torres A, Agustí AGN, et al: Subconjunctival haemorrhage: a feature of acute severe asthma. *Postgrad Med J* 61:579–581, 1985.

25. Kikuchi Y, Okabe S, Tamura G, et al: Chemosensitivity and perception of dyspnea in patients with a history of near-fatal asthma. *N Engl J Med* 330: 1329–1334, 1994.

26. McFadden ER Jr: Fatal and near-fatal asthma. *N Engl J Med* 324:409–411, 1991.

27. Molfino N, Nannini U, Martelli AN, Slutsky A: Respiratory arrest in near fatal asthma. *N Engl J Med* 324:285–288, 1991.

28. Wasserfallen JB, Schaller MD, Feihl F, Perret C: Sudden asphyxic asthma: A distinct entity? *Am Rev Respir Dis* 142:108–111, 1990.

29. Murray V, Venables K, Laing-Morton T, et al: Epidemic of asthma possibly related to thunderstorms. *Br Med J* 309:131–132, 1994.

30. Ferrer A, Torres A, Roca J, et al: Characteristics of patients with soybean dust-induced acute severe asthma requiring mechanical ventilation. *Eur Respir J* 3:429–433, 1990.

31. O'Hallaren MT, Yunginger JW, Offord KP, et al: Exposure to an aeroallergen as a possible precipitating factor in respiratory arrest in young patients with asthma. *N Engl J Med* 324:359–363, 1991.

32. Antó JM, Sunyer J, Rodriguez-Roisin R, et al: Community outbreaks of asthma associated with inhalation of soybean dust. *N Engl J Med* 320:1097–1102, 1989.

33. Sur S, Crotty TB, Kephart GM, et al: Sudden-onset fatal asthma. A distinct entity with few eosinophils and relatively more neutrophils in the airway submucosa. *Am Rev Respir Dis* 148:713–719, 1993.

34. McFadden ER Jr, Kiser R, DeGroot WJ: Acute bronchial asthma. Relations between clinical and physiologic manifestations. *N Engl J Med* 288:221–225, 1973.

35. Rudolf M, Riordan JF, Grant BJB, et al: Arterial blood gases in acute severe asthma. *Eur J Clin Invest* 10:55–62, 1980.

36. Mihatsch W, Geelhoed GC, Landau LI, LeSouëf PN: Time course of change in oxygen saturation and peak expiratory flow in children admitted to hospital with acute asthma. *Thorax* 45:438–441, 1990.

37. Kraft M, Djukanovic R, Wilson S, et al: Alveolar tissue inflammation in asthma. *Am J Respir Crit Care Med* 154:1505–1510, 1996.

38. Fauls JL, Tormey VJ, Leonard C, et al: Lung immunopathology in cases of sudden asthma death. *Eur Respir J* 10:301–307, 1997.

39. Kraft M, Pak J, Martin RJ, Irvin CG: Peripheral airway resistance increases at night in nocturnal asthma (abstract). *Am J Respir Crit Care Med* 155(Part 2):A679, 1997.

40. Kraft M, Williams BT, Walther JM, Martin RJ, Cairns CB: Impairment of peripheral tissue oxygenation and cellular oxidation in patients with nocturnal asthma (abstract). *Am J Respir Crit Care Med* 155(Part 2):A895, 1997.

41. Aikawa T, Shimura S, Sasaki H, et al: Marked goblet cell hyperplasia with mucus accumulation in the airways of patients who died of acute severe asthma attack. *Chest* 101:916–921, 1992.

42. Bolliger CT, Fourie PR, Kotze D, Joubert JR: Relation of measures of asthma severity and response to treatment to outcome in acute severe asthma. *Thorax* 47:943–947, 1992.

43. Fischl MA, Pitchenick A, Gardner LB: An index predicting relapse and need for hospitalization in patients with acute severe asthma. *N Engl J Med* 305:783–789, 1981.

44. Rose CC, Murphy JG, Schwartz J: Performance of an index predicting the response of patients with acute bronchial asthma to intensive emergency department treatment. *N Engl J Med* 310:573–577, 1984.

45. Centor RM, Yarbrough B, Wood JP: Inability to predict relapse in acute asthma. *N Engl J Med* 310:577–579, 1984.

46. Wagner PD, Hedenstierna G, Rodriguez-Roisin R: Gas exchange, expiratory flow obstruction and the clinical spectrum of asthma. *Eur Respir J* 9:1278–1282, 1996.

47. Rodriguez-Roisin R, Wagner PD: Clinical relevance of ventilation-perfusion inequality determined by inert gas elimination. *Eur Respir J* 3:469–482, 1990.

48. Kharitonov SA, Yates D, Robbins RA, et al: Increased nitric oxide in exhaled air of asthmatic patients. *Lancet* 343:133–135, 1994.

49. Massaro AF, Gaston B, Kita D, et al: Expired nitric oxide levels during treatment of acute asthma. *Am J Respir Crit Care Med* 152:800–802, 1995.

50. Gómez FP, Barberà JA, Roca J, et al: Effect of

nitric oxide synthesis inhibition with nebulized L-NAME on ventilation-perfusion distributions in bronchial asthma. *Eur Respir* 12:865–871, 1998.

51. Ballester E, Roca J, Rodriguez-Rosin R, Agustí-Vidal A: Effect of nifedipine on arterial hypoxaemia occurring after methacholine challenge in asthma. *Thorax* 41:468–472, 1986.

52. Félez MA, Roca J, Barberà JA, et al: Inhaled platelet-activating factor worsens gas exchange in mild asthma. *Am J Respir Crit Care Med* 150:369–373, 1994.

53. Rodriguez-Roisin R, Félez MA, Fan Chung K, et al: Platelet-activating factor causes ventilation-perfusion mismatch in humans. *J Clin Invest* 93:188–194, 1994.

54. Díaz O, Barberà JA, Marrades R, et al: Inhibition of PAF-induced gas exchange defects by beta-adrenergic agonists in mild asthma is not due to bronchodilation. *Am J Respir Crit Care Med* 156:17–22, 1997.

55. Rodriguez-Roisin R, Ballester E, Torres A, et al: Mechanisms of abnormal gas exchange in patients with status asthmaticus needing mechanical ventilation. *Am Rev Respir Dis* 139:732–739, 1989.

56. Ballester E, Reyes A, Roca J, et al: Ventilation-perfusion mismatching in acute severe asthma: effects of salbutamol and 100% oxygen. *Thorax* 44:258–267, 1989.

57. Ballester E, Roca J, Ramis LI, et al:. Pulmonary gas exchange in severe chronic asthma. Response to 100% oxygen and salbutamol. *Am Rev Respir Dis* 141:558–562, 1990.

58. Lee LN, Ueno O, Wagner PD, West JB: Pulmonary gas exchange after multiple airway occlusion by beads in the dog. *Am Rev Respir Dis* 140:1216–1221, 1989.

59. West JB, Dollery CT, Naimark A: Distribution of bloodflow in isolated lung: relation to vascular and alveolar pressures. *J Appl Physiol* 19:713–724, 1964.

60. Rodriguez-Roisin R, Roca J: Gas exchange in COPD, in Calverley PMA, Pride NB (eds): *Chronic Obstructive Pulmonary Disease*. London: Chapman & Hall, 1994, pp 161–184.

61. Barberà JA, Roca J, Ferrer A, et al: Mechanisms of worsening gas exchange during acute exacerbations of chronic obstructive pulmonary disease. *Eur Respir J* 10:1285–1291, 1997.

62. Agustí AGN, Barberà JA: Contributions of multiple inert gas elimination technique to pulmonary medicine: 2. Chronic pulmonary disease: chronic obstruc-

tive pulmonary disease and idiopathic pulmonary fibrosis. *Thorax* 49:924–932, 1994.

63. Domino KB, Swenson ER, Polissar NL, et al: Effect of inspired CO_2 on ventilation and perfusion heterogeneity in hyperventilated dogs. *J Appl Physiol* 75:1306–1314, 1993.

64. Brimioulle S, Kahn RJ: Effects of metabolic acidosis on pulmonary gas exchange. *Am Rev Respir Dis* 141:1185–1189, 1990.

65. Nattie EE: Gas exchange in acid-base disturbances, in Fahri LE, Tenney SM (eds): *Handbook of Physiology*, vol 4: *The Respiratory System. Gas Exchange.* Bethesda, American Physiological Society, 1987, pp 421–438.

66. Domino KB, Swenson ER, Hlastala MP: Hypocapnia-induced ventilation/perfusion mismatch: A direct CO_2 or pH-mediated effect? *Am J Respir Crit Care Med* 152:1534–1539, 1995.

67. Brimioulle S, Lejeune P, Vachiery JL, et al: Effect of acidosis and alkalosis on hypoxic pulmonary vasoconstriction in dogs. *Am J Physiol* 258:H347–353, 1990.

68. National Heart, Lung and Blood Institute: International consensus report on diagnosis and treatment of asthma. *Eur Respir J* 5:601–641, 1991.

69. British Thoracic Society et al: Guidelines on the management of asthma. *Thorax* 48(Suppl):S1–S24, 1993.

70. West JB: Ventilation-perfusion relationships. *Am Rev Respir Dis* 116:919–943, 1977.

71. Coupe MO, Guly U, Brown E, Barnes PJ: Nebulized adrenaline in acute severe asthma: Comparison with salbutamol. *Eur J Respir Dis* 71:227–232, 1987.

72. Wagner PD, Dantzker DR, Iacovoni VE, et al: Ventilation-perfusion inequality in asymptomatic asthma. *Am Rev Respir Dis* 118:511–524,1978.

73. Rodriguez-Roisin R, Bencowitz HZ, Wagner PD: Gas exchange responses to bronchodilators following methacholine challenge. *Am Rev Respir Dis* 130:617–626, 1983.

74. Halmagyi DF, Cotes JE: Reduction of systemic blood oxygen as a result of procedures affecting the pulmonary circulation in patients with chronic pulmonary disease. *Clin Sci* 18:475–489, 1959.

75. Amoroso P, Wilson SR, Moxham J, Ponte J: Acute effects of inhaled salbutamol on the metabolic rate of normal subjects. *Thorax* 48:882–885, 1993.

76. Dhand R, Tobin MJ: Inhaled bronchodilator therapy in mechanically ventilated patients. *Am J Respir Crit Care Med* 156:3–10, 1997.

77. Salmeron S, Brochard L, Mal H, et al: Nebulized

versus intravenous albuterol in hypercapnic acute asthma. *Am J Respir Crit Care Med* 149:1466–1470, 1994.

78. Dagg KD, Thomson LJ, Ramsay SG, Thomson NC: Effect of hyperoxia on the bronchodilator response to salbutamol in stable asthmatic patients. *Thorax* 51:853–854, 1996.

79. Clayton RA, Nally JE, Thomson NC, McGrath JC: The effect of oxygen tension on responses evoked by methacholine and bronchodilators in isolated bovine bronchial rings. *Pulm Pharmacol* 9:123–128, 1996.

80. Clayton RA, Nally JE, Thomson NC, McGrath JC: Changing the oxygen tension alters the ability of bronchodilators to protect against methacholine-induced challenge in bovine isolated bronchial rings. *Pulm Pharmacol Ther* 10:51–60, 1997.

81. Bremner P, Burgess C, Beasley R, et al: Nebulized fenoterol causes greater cardiovascular and hypokalemic effects than equivalent bronchodilator doses of salbutamol in asthmatics. *Respir Med* 86:419–423, 1992.

82. Blaw GJ, Westendorp RGJ: Asthma deaths in New Zealand: Whodunnit? *Lancet* 345:2–3, 1995.

83. Wong CS, Pavord ID, Withams J, et al: Bronchodilator, cardiovascular and hypokalaemic effects of fenoterol, salbutamol and terbutaline in asthma. *Lancet* 336:1396–1399, 1990.

84. Lipworth BJ, Newnham DM, Clark RA, et al: Comparison of the relative airways and systemic potencies of inhaled fenoterol and salbutamol in asthmatic patients. *Thorax* 50:54–61, 1995.

85. McFadden ER: Methylxanthines in the treatment of asthma: the rise, the fall and the possible rise again. *Ann Intern Med* 115:323–324, 1991.

86. Evans DJ, Taylor DA, Zetterstrom O, et al: A comparison of low-dose inhaled budesonide plus teophylline and high dose inhaled budesonide for moderate asthma. *N Engl J Med* 337:1412–1418, 1997.

87. Montserrat JM, Barberà JA, Viegas C, et al: Gas exchange response to intravenous aminophylline in patients with a severe exacerbation of asthma. *Eur Respir J* 8:28–33, 1995.

Chapter 7

CARDIOPULMONARY INTERACTIONS ASSOCIATED WITH AIRFLOW OBSTRUCTION

Michael R. Pinsky

INTRODUCTION

The heart and lungs are intimately coupled by their anatomical proximity within the thorax and, more importantly, by their responsibility to deliver the oxygen requirements of individual cells and organs. During critical illness, if these two organ systems fail by themselves or in combination, the end result is an inadequate oxygen delivery to the body, with inevitable tissue ischemia, progressive organ dysfunction, and if untreated, death. Severe acute asthma may result in not only ventilatory failure but, because of heart-lung interactions, cardiovascular collapse as well, despite otherwise normal cardiovascular reserve. Thus, restoration and maintenance of normalized cardiopulmonary function is an essential and primary goal in the management of the critically ill asthma patient.

However, severe bouts of bronchospasm may still carry an appreciable mortality. Studies have demonstrated mortality rates as high as 22%[1] for all patients requiring mechanical ventilation and 16% for all hospitalized patients with severe asthma.[2] Although many deaths are attributed to anoxic brain injury, barotrauma and hypotension represent the two primary complications of mechanical ventilation.[3] These and other studies underscore the importance of preventing lung over-distention in the management of patients with severe asthma. An understanding of how cardiovascular dysfunction can occur in severe asthma is therefore of prime importance in the management of these patients.

CARDIOPULMONARY PHYSIOLOGY

Respiration can affect global cardiovascular performance through its effects on the determinants of cardiovascular function. To simplify this analysis, heart-lung interactions can be separated into three primary concepts. First, ventilation is exercise, since it consumes O_2, produces CO_2, and the respiratory muscles can be fatigued.[4] Thus, if either the work of breathing is too excessive or the ability of the cardiovascular system to deliver O_2 to the exercising muscles is too limited, the patient will either not be able to sustain spontaneous ventilation or not be able to be weaned from mechanical ventilation. Second, both spontaneous and positive-pressure ventilation increase lung volume above some end-expiratory baseline level. Severe bronchospasm with air trapping can increase lung volumes above normal resting levels. This increase in lung volume may exist even at end-expiration and increase further with each inspiratory cycle. Increases in lung volume alter pulmonary vascular resistance, cardiac filling, and autonomic tone. Third, spontaneous inspiratory efforts and positive-pressure ventilation cause opposite swings in intrathoracic pressure (ITP). Thus, during spontaneous inspiration ITP decreases as the respiratory muscles contract expanding the lungs. In contrast, during positive pressure ventilation, ITP increases during inspiration as the expanding lungs push against the heart and chest wall. Accordingly, one needs to understand the separate effects of changes in lung volume and ITP on cardiovascular performance in order to comprehend the similar and different aspects of each type of ventilation on cardiovascular function. The hemodynamic differences between spontaneous and positive-pressure ventilation reflect primarily these differences in ITP swings and the energy necessary to produce them.

To assess cardiac function in a simplified fashion, the determinants can be grouped into four interrelated processes: those forces or processes that affect heart rate, preload, contractility, and afterload.[5] Our current understanding of cardiovascular function also emphasizes both the independence and dependence of right ventricular (RV) and left ventricular (LV) performance on each other and to external stresses. Phasic changes in lung volume and ITP can simultaneously change all four of these hemodynamic determinants for both the RV and LV. Complicating these matters further, the direction of these changes in lung volume and ITP can be in similar or opposite directions. It is clear, therefore, that a comprehensive understanding of cardiopulmonary interactions is a nearly impossible goal to achieve in most patients. However, by understanding the components of this process, it is possible to come to a better realization of their determinants, and, to a greater or lesser degree for any individual patient, predict the limits of these interactions and how the patient may respond to stresses imposed by either adding or removing artificial ventilatory support. Finally, by defining these interactions, the logic of pressure-limited ventilation with its associated permissive hypercapnia becomes obvious (see Chapter 12).

Ventilation Is Exercise

Spontaneous ventilatory efforts are induced by contraction of the respiratory muscles, of which the diaphragm and intercostal muscles comprise the bulk of the tissue. However, with marked hyperpnea, abdominal wall muscles and muscles of the shoulder girdle also function as accessory respiratory muscles. Blood flow to these muscles is derived from several arterial circuits whose abso-

lute flow is believed to exceed the highest metabolic demand of maximally exercising skeletal muscle under normal conditions.[4] Thus, under conditions of normal cardiovascular function, blood flow is not the limiting factor that determines maximal ventilatory effort. Although ventilation normally requires less than 5% of total O_2 delivery to meet its demand,[4] in lung disease states, where the work of breathing is increased such as in pulmonary edema or bronchospasm, the requirements for O_2 may increase to 25% or 30% of total O_2 delivery.[4,6-8] Furthermore, if cardiac output is limited, blood flow to vital organs, including the respiratory muscles, may be compromised, inducing both tissue hypoperfusion and lactic acidosis.[9-11] The institution of mechanical ventilation for ventilatory and hypoxemic respiratory failure may reduce metabolic demand on the stressed cardiovascular system by increasing Sv_{O_2} for a constant cardiac output and Ca_{O_2};[10] this may, in turn, have a salutary effect on arterial P_{O_2}. Intubation and mechanical ventilation, when adjusted to the metabolic demands of the patient, may dramatically decrease the work of breathing, resulting in increased O_2 delivery to other vital organs and decreased serum lactic acid levels.[11] Finally, as the metabolic demands of the various muscle groups are varied by changes in ventilatory support to and from spontaneous to mechanical ventilation,[12-15] blood flow distribution as well tends to be redirected toward the more active muscle groups and away from the visceral organs.[16]

Hemodynamic Effects of Lung Volume Changes

Respiratory-induced changes in lung volume may profoundly affect cardiovascular performance. These interactions are mediated by several different mechanisms through changes in autonomic tone, pulmonary vascular resistance, direct mechanical compression of the cardiac fossa, ventricular interdependence, and increases in intraabdominal pressure. These heart-lung interactions are common to both spontaneously breathing patients and those on positive-pressure mechanical ventilation. In addition to the cyclic increase in lung volume during inspiration, a more sustained increase in end-expiratory lung volume can be accomplished with positive end-expiratory pressure (PEEP) or continuous positive airway pressure (CPAP) by mask on patients who are mechanically ventilated or spontaneously breathing, respectively, and by hyperinflation in patients with airflow obstruction.[17]

Autonomic Tone Lung inflation, both phasically and tonically, alters autonomic tone by varying both sympathetic and parasympathetic tone. Normal spontaneous inspiration with increases in lung volume of less than 15 mL/kg increases heart rate owing to withdrawal of vagal tone.[18,19] This inspiration-associated heart rate increase and expiration-associated heart rate decrease is referred to as *respiratory sinus arrhythmia*. Respiratory sinus arrhythmia reflects the relative sensitivity of the coupling of the autonomic nervous system and the cardiovascular system.[20] In diseases associated with dysautonomia, respiratory sinus arrhythmia is either markedly diminished or absent. As lung inflation increases with higher tidal volumes (>15 ml/kg) heart-rate decreases.[21] Reflex arterial vasodilation can also occur in association with this decrease in heart rate.[22-24] Although not proven, this inflation-vasodilation response may contribute to the initial hypotension seen with the hyperinflation of bronchospasm or when such patients are placed on mechanical ventilation. This cardiodepressive reflex appears to be mediated at least partially by afferent vagal fibers, since it is abolished by selective vagotomy. However, hexamethonium, guanethidine, and beryllium also block this reflex.[24-27] These data suggest that lung inflation mediates its reflex cardiovascular effects by modulating central autonomic tone. However, except as a diagnostic tool to assess autonomic dysfunction, inflation-associated cardiovascular responses do not appear to be significant clinically except, perhaps, in the extreme.[25,26]

Lung inflation also can cause release of humeral factors from the pulmonary endothelial cells, which can also induce a depressor response,[28-30] presumably by stretch-induced release of prostacyclin, because this response can be inhibited by blocking prostaglandin synthesis.[31,32] No specific role for nitric oxide metabolism has been found in inflation-induced vasodilation, although nitric oxide production is stimulated by vascular wall shear stress.

Pulmonary Vascular Resistance Pulmonary vascular resistance (PVR) can be markedly altered by changes in lung volume. Indeed, a major determinant of pulmonary blood flow other than right ventricular pump function, is lung volume. To better understand the effects of respiration on PVR, it is necessary to review some aspects of the anatomical relations of the normal pulmonary circulation.[33-36] The pulmonary vasculature can be divided into two categories of blood vessels, based on the effects of the pressure that surrounds them. One population of blood vessels is termed the *alveolar vessels*. These vessels are located within the alveolar walls and are surrounded by alveolar pressure. Anatomically, these vessels comprise the small arterioles, venules, and most of the pulmonary capillaries. As alveoli distend during inspiration, alveolar vessels are compressed by the expanding alveoli as the result of the obligatory increase in transpulmonary pressure.[37] These points are summarized in Figure 7-1. This inspiratory compression causes the resistance in these vessels to increase and their capacitance to decrease. This alveolar vessel compression is similar whether lung volume increases due to spontaneous inspiration or to positive-pressure ventilation. The other population of pulmonary blood vessels is termed *extra-alveolar vessels*; these vessels sense interstitial pressure as their surrounding pressure. The normal radial interstitial forces that act upon the airways act upon these vessels. Interstitial pressure is similar to ITP and changes in proportion to ITP during breathing.[38] As lung volume increases, the radial forces stretching the extra-alveolar vessels also increase, which increases their capacitance and decreases their resistance to blood flow.[39] However, as lung volume decreases these extra-alveolar vessels decrease their diameter. Although this process decreases vascular capacitance, its effect on pulmonary vascular resistance per se is small.[36]

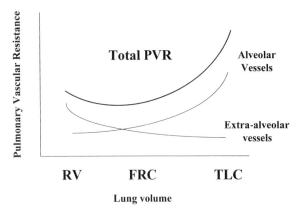

Figure 7-1

Schematic representation of the effects of changes in lung volume on total pulmonary vascular resistance (PVR). Changes in lung volume that deviate from normal functional residual capacity (FRC) cause total PVR to increase. Thus at both extremes of lung volume, residual volume (RV) and total lung capacity (TLC), PVR is maximal. Relation between lung volume and alveolar or extra-alveolar pulmonary vascular resistance are quite different from each other.

Interestingly, in neonates, the increased PVR induced by hyperinflation may persist following removal of the increased airway pressure and the return of lung volume to its preinflation state.[40] This suggests that when pulmonary vasomotor tone is high and pulmonary vasculature is hypertrophied, as in the neonate, reflex vasoconstriction can also occur during lung inflation.[41,42] This increased vasomotor tone does not appear to exist in adults with normal pulmonary vasculature, although it is not clear if it is an operative mechanism in patients with cor pulmonale or vasoreactive pulmonary hypertension, as may exist in patients with asthma.

Severe acute asthma is almost universally associated with significant increases in lung volume (see Chapter 5). These lung volume increases directly increase PVR. The causes of this increase are multiple and include a disproportionate increase in expiratory resistance over inspiratory resistance, better respiratory muscle strength during inspiration than expiration, and expiratory braking such that end-expiratory lung volume is held

above that volume to which it would otherwise decrease. However, in patients with severe status asthmaticus who are sedated and paralyzed on mechanical ventilation, hyperinflation also commonly occurs.[43,44] The contribution of voluntary expiratory braking to the state of hyperinflation in these circumstances is nil. Fortunately, maximal increases in lung volume only occur at end-inspiration. Accordingly, the maximal lung volume–induced increase in PVR is usually small, even in patients with hyperinflation. The increase in PVR, however, will increase RV afterload, which in itself may precipitate acute cor pulmonale.[45] Similarly, diseases associated with acute-on-chronic hyperinflation such as chronic asthmatic bronchitis and emphysema can overload the right ventricle and decrease cardiac output (cor pulmonale) during bouts of further hyperinflation.

Regional lung volumes may decrease during acute asthma, as when segmental lung collapse results from peribronchial edema and mucus plugging. This causes terminal airways to close, decreasing downstream alveolar ventilation with its resultant alveolar hypoxia. Pulmonary vasomotor tone increases when alveolar P_{O_2} decreases below 60 mm Hg.[46] Similarly, decreases in mixed venous P_{O_2} and blood pH can both induce increased pulmonary vasomotor tone through this mechanism.[47] This local pulmonary vasoconstrictive process is referred to as *hypoxic pulmonary vasoconstriction* and is the result of both loss of active vasodilation and active increase in pulmonary vasomotor tone.[48–50] This acidemia- and hypoxia-induced increase in pulmonary vasomotor tone is mediated through local inhibition of a constitutively expressed nitric oxide synthase on the vascular endothelium. Although a useful reflex to minimize ventilation-perfusion mismatching when alveolar collapse occurs in only one region of the lung, it induces a global increase in pulmonary vasomotor tone when the entire lung volume is nonspecifically reduced. Fortunately, even in severe status asthmaticus requiring intubation, alveolar hypoxia is readily reversed by modest amounts of supplemental oxygen (see Chapter 6).

One major goal of patient management during acute asthma is to minimize these effects of increased lung volumes. Thus, incorrect ventilatory parameter settings during mechanical ventilation can cause deterioration of cardiovascular performance. Excessively large tidal volumes or inadequate expiratory time resulting in dynamic hyperinflation (auto-PEEP) can further increase PVR.[43,51,52] Approaches to these difficult patient management issues are presented in Chapter 13.

Mechanical Heart-Lung Interactions The heart within the thorax is surrounded by the sternum anteriorly, the spinal column posteriorly, the lungs laterally, and the diaphragm inferiorly. This space is referred to as the *cardiac fossa.* As the lungs expand within the thorax, they push against the heart, chest wall, and diaphragm. The chest wall can expand outwardly and the diaphragm can descend. However, the heart is trapped within the cardiac fossa.[17,53] Thus, juxtacardiac pleural pressure increases more than lateral chest wall pleural pressure as lung volume increases.[54–61] Normally, this compressive effect is small and transient. However, with large tidal breaths and with hyperinflation, significant mechanical compression of the heart can occur, resembling cardiac tamponade in every fashion. Indeed, under these circumstances, both pericardial and juxtacardiac pleural pressures are increased equally.[17,62] The hemodynamic consequence of this form of mechanical cardiopulmonary interaction is usually a decrease in RV and LV preload.[63–65] If it occurs only during inspiration, this process primarily reflects a transient decrease in LV end-diastolic volume due to increasing pericardial pressure. However, if it is due to sustained increases in lung volume, the decrease in preload may be due to both a decrease in venous return, as described below, and a decrease in the distending pressure of the two ventricles. If the surrounding pressure of the heart continues to rise with progressive hyperinflation, there can also be mechanical compression of the coronary vessels that can lead to myocardial ischemia and a deterioration in cardiac function.[66–68]

Mechanical compression of the heart within the cardiac fossa does not alter LV diastolic compliance, since the relation between intraluminal pressure and pericardial pressure is unchanged.[52]

However, "effective" LV diastolic compliance, measured as intraluminal pressure by itself, does decrease. Thus, if measures of LV pressure were used without reference to pericardial pressure, such as pulmonary artery occlusion pressure (Ppao), it would then appear that LV diastolic compliance decreased. At significantly increased lung volume, for the same end-diastolic volume, Ppao would have to be greater. However, these interrelations are complicated by another factor termed *ventricular interdependence,* discussed below.

Recently Takata and colleagues proposed a novel approach to understanding mechanical heart-lung interactions.[69] Although these researchers use their model to describe the differences between the effect of tamponade and constrictive pericarditis on pericardial pressure using the terms *coupled* and *uncoupled* pericardial restraint, their analysis may be useful in examining the effects of hyperinflation and inspiration, respectively, on cardiac fossal pressure. They proposed that pericardial stiffness (or elastance) over the right and left ventricles is different in constrictive pericarditis but similar in tamponade. Accordingly, in constrictive pericarditis, changes in venous return should selectively alter RV filling, whereas in tamponade they should alter both RV and LV filling. If this is extrapolated to ventilation, it appears that tidal increases in lung volume represent uncoupled pericardial restraint because they selectively limit RV filling and not LV diastolic compliance. Previous researchers have suggested that positive-pressure inspiration selectively decreases RV filling because the pressure gradient for systemic venous return, rather than pulmonary blood flow, is reduced by the increase in ITP. Although this argument is valid, as will be discussed in greater detail in the following section, the magnitude of the reduction in RV filling is often excessive when compared to either the increase in ITP or the decrease in the pressure gradient for systemic venous return. The model proposed by Takata and colleagues demonstrates that when mechanical compression of the heart occurs during inspiration, the local surface pressure over the RA and RV may increase more than it does over the left atrium and left ventricle.[70] Thus, RV filling could be selectively impaired independent of any change in the pressure gradient for systemic venous return. This would be a non-steady-state effect and would only occur during inspiration. In contrast, if hyperinflation were to occur, inducing a sustained increase in lung volume, then the uncoupled cardiac fossal restraint would become coupled cardiac fossal restraint. Thus, hyperinflation, as occurs in severe asthma, would produce a clinical picture indistinguishable from tamponade. Indeed, more than 25 years ago Rebuck and Read made this identical observation in their analysis of the hemodynamic effects of severe asthma, although they did not postulate a specific mechanism to explain this phenomenon.[71]

Ventricular Interdependence Ventricular interdependence refers to the interaction of one ventricle on the other.[72] Any process that causes RV end-diastolic volume to increase will decrease LV diastolic compliance by both intraventricular septal shift and pericardial limitations of absolute biventricular volumes.[73,74] Usually described during diastole, diastolic ventricular interdependence is primarily an RV to LV effect.[75,76] This RV to LV interaction is a parallel interaction, in that it occurs in phase between the two ventricles. The reason for the parallel interaction is that absolute biventricular volume is remarkably constant throughout the cardiac cycle due to cardiac limitation.[77,78]

Increases in pericardial pressure can occur as lung volume increases due to one of several mechanisms. Compression of the heart within the cardiac fossa will increase pericardial pressure more than lateral chest wall pleural pressure.[79] However, increases in ITP, as seen during positive pressure inspiration and during the strain phase of a Valsalva maneuver, primarily increase all ITP pressure equally.[79–81] Since under normal conditions, RV diastolic compliance is greater than LV diastolic compliance, similar increases in pericardial pressure will have a greater effect on reducing RV end-diastolic volume than on LV end-diastolic volume. Once RV filling pressure approximates LV filling pressure, however, further increases in pericardial pressure will decrease both ventricular

end-diastolic volumes. This pericardial pressure-dependent decrease in ventricular filling is analogous to tamponade wherein differential effects of tamponade on RV and LV filling were first described.

Ventricular interdependence can also occur through shifts of the intraventricular septum.[73] If RV end-diastolic volume were to increase sufficiently to shift the intraventricular septum leftward, LV diastolic compliance would be reduced. If RV end-diastolic volume were to increase, as it often does during spontaneous inspiration or with fluid loading, then LV diastolic compliance would decrease.[74] With spontaneous respiratory efforts, this scenario would give rise to an inspiration-associated fall in LV stroke volume and aortic pulse pressure.[82] This phenomenon is referred to as *pulsus paradoxus* and can explain most of the observed arterial pulse pressure variations seen during ventilation,[83,84] especially during the increased inspiratory effort frequently seen in asthma.[71,73]

Ventricular interdependence can also occur in a series fashion as RV blood flows through the lungs into the left ventricle. Thus, changes in RV output must eventually affect steady-state LV output. If RV output were to increase, for example, the LV output must also increase after a few heartbeats.

Diaphragmatic Descent Increasing lung volume not only causes the chest wall to expand outwardly, but also causes the diaphragm to descend. This occurs passively during positive-pressure ventilation and actively during spontaneous ventilation. In both cases, however, diaphragmatic descent compresses the liver and increases intra-abdominal pressure. This causes many hemodynamic effects. The combined hepatic compression and increased abdominal pressure increases intrahepatic vascular resistance, decreasing portal blood flow through the liver and accelerating nonsplanchinic inferior venal blood flow.[85] Diaphragmatic descent also pulls down on the diaphragmatic pericardial attachments, decreasing pericardial volume and increasing pericardial pressure.[86]

The effect of increasing abdominal pressure and hepatic outflow resistance on venous return to the heart is complex. By increasing abdominal pressure, the vascular pressures in the abdomen are also increased by a similar amount.[87] This should increase the upstream pressure for venous return, as described below. Since positive-pressure ventilation tends to decrease venous return by increasing right atrial pressure (the downstream pressure for venous return), this matched increase in upstream pressure tends to preserve venous blood flow despite positive-pressure breaths. However, since hepatic outflow resistance increases, the resistance to venous return is also increased. Thus, under conditions of low cardiac outputs (e.g., hypovolemia in an asthma patient), the increased outflow resistance effect predominates, decreasing venous return.[88–90] Diaphragmatic compression also alters hepatic metabolic function by changing the blood flow distribution through the liver and by altering the relation between hepatic blood flow and the space of Diessé.[91]

Hemodynamic Effects of Changes in Intrathoracic Pressure

Much confusion exists in both the literature and in the practical understanding of heart-lung interactions because of the problems encountered in conceptualizing ITP, pleural pressure, alveolar pressure and how they change during ventilation and ventilatory maneuvers, and how they relate to changes in lung volume and cardiovascular pressures. The relation between ITP and pleural pressure and the effects of ITP on cardiovascular performance are discussed below.

Relation between Intrathoracic Pressure and Pleural Pressure   Pleural pressure is the surface pressure between the opposing surfaces of the thorax separated by the visceral and parietal pleura. Ventilation alters pleural pressure. Local differences in mean pleural pressure exist from base to apex and anterior to posterior due to local differences in surface forces and hydrostatic pressure gradients.[79] Pleural pressure is higher in de-

pendent regions owing to hydrostatic forces. This gravity-dependent difference in regional pleural pressure explains the greater degree of distention of the lungs in the nondependent portions of the chest as compared to the dependent portions, since alveolar pressure at end-expiration is similar throughout the lungs. The change in pleural pressure with breathing is also different in different portions of the lung. These differences, however, are due neither to hydrostatic forces nor to regional differences in lung distention, but to local differences in surface forces. As the lung expands, the chest wall and diaphragm move away, but the heart is trapped within the cardiac fossa and cannot move. Accordingly, juxtacardiac pleural pressure increases more than lateral chest wall pleural pressure as lung volume increases, but it increases by a similar amount if lung volume remains constant (as during a Valsalva maneuver).[61,92] This pleural pressure difference accounts for some of the hemodynamic sensitivity observed during both hyperinflation and positive-pressure ventilation. In general, the "generic" pleural pressure is referred to as ITP. Within this context, it will be assumed to reflect the relevant pleural pressure under the specific condition addressed. Clinically, esophageal pressure is often used to estimate changes in ITP.[93]

Transthoracic Pressure Gradients for Blood Flow   Spontaneous and positive-pressure inspiration will induce opposite changes in ITP. ITP decreases with spontaneous inspiration as the respiratory muscles contract, whereas ITP increases during positive-pressure inspiration as the expanding lungs push on the chest wall and diaphragm. If inspiratory airway resistance is increased (as occurs during acute asthma), lung compliance is decreased (as occurs during pulmonary edema and interstitial fibrosis states), or when the inspiratory efforts are exaggerated (as occurs during dyspneic hyperventilation), then the inspiration-associated decrease in ITP seen during spontaneous ventilation will be greater. None of these factors would be expected to influence the change in ITP seen with positive-pressure inspiration, since the only determinant of the increase in ITP during positive-pressure inspiration would be the increase in lung volume.[55] Using this same construct, the inspiration-associated increase in ITP seen during positive-pressure ventilation will be greater if chest wall compliance is reduced (as occurs with ankylosing spondylitis or tense ascities)[63] or large tidal volume ventilation is administered. Neither of these factors would be expected to influence the change in ITP that is seen with spontaneous ventilation.

Changes in airway resistance and lung compliance, per se, do not directly alter the change in ITP seen during positive-pressure ventilation[55] if no spontaneous ventilatory efforts are being made. They do affect the associated increase in airway pressure and they can easily lead to a secondary increase in ITP if dynamic hyperinflation develops, such that the positive-pressure breath occurs from an increased end-expiratory lung volume. This is typical of the asthma patient undergoing positive-pressure ventilation (see Chapter 13). Accordingly, changes in airway pressure cannot be used to estimate the probable changes in ITP produced by positive-pressure ventilation, because the determinants of these two pressures (airway pressure and intrathoracic pressure) are different. However, changes in airway pressure can be used to identify the development of hyperinflation in an otherwise stable ventilatory condition.

Mean ITP over the ventilatory cycle and changes in ITP during ventilation are major determinants of cardiovascular function.[51,94] Changes in ITP reflect the primary differences in the hemodynamic effects of ventilation between spontaneous and positive-pressure ventilation. Changes in ITP alter cardiovascular function primarily by altering the pressure gradients for both systemic venous return and LV ejection.[95,96] Conceptually, the circulation can be represented by two compartments, one within the thorax that senses ITP as its surrounding pressure and another outside the thorax that senses atmospheric pressure as its surrounding pressure. Since volume changes and ventilatory efforts alter ITP but not atmospheric pressure, a variable pressure gradient will be induced between these two compartments by ventilation. Increasing ITP will increase all the vascular

pressures within the thorax more than in the nonthoracic compartment, whereas decreasing ITP will have the opposite effect. The interface of this two-compartment model is at the junction of the large systemic veins as they enter the chest to drain into the right atrium, and at the aortic valve as the left ventricle ejects its blood into an aorta with free extrathoracic drainage. Thus, changes in ITP primarily affect cardiac function by altering the pressure gradients between the vasculature within the thorax and the rest of the body. Since the heart resides within the chest, it can be viewed as a pressure chamber within a pressure chamber (the thorax). Accordingly, changes in ITP will affect the pressure gradients for systemic venous return to the heart (RV) and LV ejection pressure, independent of the heart itself.

Accordingly, negative swings in ITP will increase these pressure gradients, whereas positive swings in ITP will decrease them. Spontaneous inspiration is associated with an acceleration of venous blood flow back to the right heart (increasing RV end-diastolic volume), as well as an increase in transmural LV ejection pressure (impeding LV ejection and increasing LV end-systolic volume). These effects combine to increase both biventricular blood volume and intrathoracic blood volume. By contrast, positive-pressure inspiration is associated with a deceleration of blood flow back to the right heart (decreasing RV end-diastolic volume), as well as a decrease in transmural LV ejection pressure (augmenting LV ejection and decreasing LV end-systolic volume). The combined effects of these interactions is to decrease both biventricular blood volume and intrathoracic blood volume. Importantly, diaphragmatic descent, by altering both the resistance to venous return and the upstream pressure to venous return, tends to minimize the venous return differences but not the hemodynamic effects of changes in ITP on LV ejection.

The effects of changes in ITP on cardiac output can also be examined from the perspective of venous return to the right ventricle. As described by Guyton and colleagues, venous return is a function of the pressure gradient for venous return and resistance to venous return.[95] As we discussed above, inspiration alters venous outflow resistance across the liver, in particular, and the diaphragm, in general. The relation between right atrial pressure and venous return as right atrial pressure is varied is called the *venous return curve.* Since the right atrium resides in the thorax, changes in ITP directly alter right atrial pressure.[97] Increasing ITP increases right atrial pressure, decreasing RV output, whereas decreasing ITP has the opposite effect.[98] Interestingly, right atrial pressure relative to atmosphere usually decreases during spontaneous inspiration if the RV is filling, presumably because the right ventricle is not presenting a significant distending resistance pressure.[81] In fact, Magder and colleagues suggested using the presence of an inspiratory decrease in right atrial pressure to identify patients who retained preload responsiveness.[99] However, LV filling occurs relative to an intrathoracic pressure background; therefore changes in ITP do not independently alter LV filling pressure. The effects of changes in ITP on the relation between venous return and LV output can be described by plotting both on a venous return curve diagram. As can be seen from this diagram, depicted in Figure 7-2, decreases in ITP cannot increase venous return greatly because of flow limitation to maximal venous blood flow. However, increases in ITP can progressively reduce blood flow to a standstill.[100]

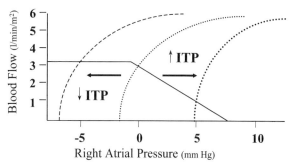

Figure 7-2

Schematic representation of the effects of changes in intrathoracic pressure (ITP) on steady-state cardiac output (blood flow) as determined by the interaction between venous return (solid line) and left ventricular ejection (dotted line) as right atrial pressure varies. Changes in right atrial pressure alter venous return. Increasing right atrial pressure decreases venous return. When venous return decreases to zero, right atrial pressure equals mean systemic pressure. When right atrial pressure decreases to subatmospheric values, as during spontaneous inspiration, venous return reaches a maximal flow limitation, such that further reductions in right atrial pressure do not increase venous return more. Left ventricular output varies in proportion with right atrial pressure (Starling's law of the heart). However changes in ITP shift the left ventricle function curve to the left equal to the amount of decrease in ITP or to the right with increases in ITP. Thus, decreases in ITP increase cardiac output, but only marginally, whereas increases progressively decrease cardiac output toward zero.

Changes in Intrathoracic Pressure and Right Ventricle Function Right ventricular end-diastolic volume is determined by the systemic venous return to the RA, RV diastolic compliance, and the volume of blood remaining in the RV after the prior heartbeat (RV end-systolic volume). During a spontaneous inspiration, venous blood flow back to the right side of the heart increases the RV end-diastolic volume. Functionally, how does this occur? Since right atrial pressure (Pra) reflects the back-pressure against which venous return must flow, if Pra decreases, the pressure gradient for venous return will increase as well.[97,101,102]

Since diaphragmatic descent compresses the abdomen (increasing intraabdominal pressure),

the increase in the driving pressure for venous return can be even greater than that presumed to occur from the decrease in Pra alone.[87] Furthermore, this upstream pressure for venous return is also determined by vascular tone, blood volume in the venous reservoirs of the systemic circulation, and blood flow distribution within these venous reservoirs.[102] The average pressure of all these vascular reservoirs is termed the *mean systemic pressure* (Pms). Pms is a concept rather than an actual vascular pressure because different vascular beds, if measured simultaneously, would have different venous pressures. Still, the conceptual use of a Pms to represent the upstream pressure that drives blood flow from the systemic circulation towards the RA has merit. Although diaphragmatic descent induced by inspiration-associated increases in lung volume can increase Pms, this effect is probably only operative during periods of sustained hyperinflation and with the application of high levels of PEEP. Importantly, if diaphragmatic descent due to hyperinflation is enough to significantly increase Pms by increasing intraabdominal pressure, then pulmonary vascular resistance should also be markedly increased by the same lung overdistention. Thus, RV systolic function is often compromised by hyperinflation due to the combined effects of increased venous return (increasing RV end-diastolic volume) and increased pulmonary vascular resistance (increasing RV end-systolic volume).[103]

Acute attacks of bronchospasm are associated with profound negative swings in ITP.[104] During such vigorous spontaneous inspiratory efforts Pra can decrease to values much less than zero relative to atmospheric pressure. Since the great veins of the thorax do not have the structural integrity to sustain a negative wall pressure, they will collapse when their transmural pressure falls below zero, limiting maximal venous flow at some defined level. This vascular collapse occurs at the junction of the thoracic and extrathoracic vessels. Further decreases in Pra below this collapse point are associated with matched increases in venous resistance such that maximal flow remains constant.[95,100,105] This phenomenon has been referred to as a *Starling resistor mechanism* that induces a flow-limitation of venous return at some maximal plateau value. Since inspiratory muscles can induce reductions in ITP well below 100 mm Hg, such a flow limitation mechanism is important in limiting RV filling and in preventing massive RV dilation. However, the left ventricle is not spared this pressure limitation. As ITP decreases, the pressure gradient for LV ejection progressively increases until it exceeds the pressure limit of ejection pressures capable for that left ventricle for that defined end-diastolic volume. Thus, profoundly negative swings in ITP as occur with spontaneous inspiratory efforts during bouts of severe bronchospasm should selectively increase LV afterload, placing a very large metabolic load on the ejecting left ventricle. Although logical, this hypothesis that profoundly negative swings in ITP selectively increase LV afterload has never been rigorously tested.

During a positive-pressure breath, ITP increases during inspiration. The increases in ITP cause Pra to also increase limiting venous return. Hyperinflation, if associated with an increase in end-expiratory ITP, will decrease venous return. In patients with normal cardiovascular function, cardiac output is primarily preload-dependent and relatively afterload insensitive. Thus, ventilator-induced increases in ITP decreasing RV end-diastolic volume can profoundly reduce cardiac output.[6,51,94,106] Diminished venous return limiting cardiac output is one of the most common deleterious heart-lung interactions encountered during mechanical ventilation of patients with acute asthma.[51,94] Conversely, patients with congestive heart failure are relatively insensitive to LV end-diastolic volume and are primarily affected by changes in LV afterload.[107,108] Under these circumstances, the institution of positive-pressure ventilation can improve cardiovascular performance through its effects on decreasing afterload, despite the obligatory associated decrease in venous return.[57,107,108]

Expiratory Muscles and Intrathoracic Pressure   Expiration is normally a passive phenomenon. It usually relies on the elastic recoil properties of the respiratory system to return lung volume to its original functional residual capacity. However, active expiratory muscle recruitment assists in sustaining an elevated minute ventilation or in maintaining a normal minute ventilation in the setting of increased expiratory flow resistance.[109,110] There are several potential mechanisms through which expiratory muscle contraction may assist in inspiration. First, contraction of the abdominal musculature can cause cephalad displacement of the diaphragm during hyperinflation, which results in a more favorable diaphragmatic length-tension relationship. This reduces the work cost of diaphragmatic contraction on the subsequent inspiration.

Second, an increased intraabdominal pressure provides a fulcrum for the diaphragm to help it lift the rib cage. Furthermore, by increasing intraabdominal pressure, as described above, that portion of the venous system within the abdomen is also pressurized, increasing mean systemic pressure.

The hemodynamic consequences of expiratory muscle recruitment have not been defined. Presumably, active expiratory efforts share similar effects to those seen in a Valsalva maneuver. During a Valsalva maneuver the initial increase in ITP is directly transmitted to the intrathoracic aorta, and arterial blood pressure rises by the same amount as the ITP. Eventually, if the strain maneuver is sustained, venous return usually begins to fall and arterial pulse pressure, as a manifestation of LV stroke volume, decreases below pre-Valsalva maneuver values. Finally, upon release of the Valsalva strain, the depleted thoracic aorta loses its externally sustained mean pressure and falls to very low levels.[92] In patients with a normal cardiovascular system, reflex sympathetic responses result in a mean and pulse pressure overshoot. However, in the presence of impaired cardiac performance and adequate intravascular volume, a Valsalva maneuver results in completely different hemodynamic responses that can be described as a "square wave" profile. Arterial blood pressure increases at the start of the Valsalva maneuver, and both mean arterial pressure and pulse pressure remain constant until its release, without any detectable pressure fall on release or overshoot of systolic arterial pressure.

Therefore, during active abdominal musculature contraction, as exemplified by the Valsalva maneuver, the hemodynamic consequences of expiratory muscle recruitment during increased respiratory loads are probably dependent on many factors, including the duration of expiratory time, intravascular volume status, level of sympathetic tone, and baseline cardiac contractile function. Accordingly, patients with different initial cardiovascular states may manifest different responses during breathing with active expiration. In a volume overload state with heart failure, cardiac aug-

mentation may be seen, whereas in a hypovolemic patient, marked arterial pressure swings may occur with hemodynamic instability. This latter state may be more representative of the patient with acute asthma.

Changes in Intrathoracic Pressure and Left Ventricle Ejection   Left ventricular afterload is also significantly affected by negative ITP changes that occur during a spontaneous breath.[104,108,111,112] During LV systole, the intraluminal pressure of the LV and the aorta are nearly identical. However, the LV and the intrathoracic aorta are surrounded by ITP, which is more negative (subatmospheric) relative to the extrathoracic aorta. Thus, the inward direction of contraction of the LV during systole is impeded by the directionally opposite forces of the ITP, which tends to pull outward on the LV while it is ejecting.[75,113,114] Therefore, negative inspiratory ITP changes during spontaneous breathing increase LV afterload. Normally, this small increase in afterload does not interfere with steady-state hemodynamics. However, during conditions of extremely negative swings in ITP, such as during marked inspiratory efforts in the setting of acute airway obstruction, the combination of increases in preload and afterload may precipitate LV dysfunction and even, rarely, pulmonary edema.[104,115–120] Cardiovascular decompensation from increases in LV afterload can also be observed when weaning patients from positive-pressure ventilation to resumption of spontaneous breathing.[121,122] Although not quantitated, this decompensation is believed to be a frequent cause of weaning failure in the ICU.[123,124] Profound LV systolic[111,125] and diastolic[126] dysfunction can occur during episodes of negative swings in ITP, whereas increasing ITP, as may occur with expiratory grunting,[127–129] or the institution of positive-pressure ventilation can augment LV ejection[125,130–135] by decreasing LV ejection pressure as well as LV filling.[76] The combined effects of decreased LV volumes and ejection pressure reduce myocardial O_2 demands. However, these effects are not unlimited. Ejection can only proceed until end-systolic volume approaches the minimal ventricular volume possible, which in normal individuals is near its resting end-systolic volume.[136] Furthermore, coronary perfusion pressure is reduced if the increases in ITP are associated with baroreceptor-induced vasodilation. Thus, decreases in coronary blood flow may occur if the increases in ITP are high enough, or initial coronary perfusion pressure is low enough.[137–139]

Another mechanism through which increased respiratory workload may have a detrimental effect on cardiovascular function is through metabolic increase of the respiratory muscles and the work cost of breathing. Normally, the oxygen cost of breathing under resting conditions accounts for approximately 5% of the total oxygen consumption.[4] However, when either the oxygen demand of the respiratory muscles increases excessively or the compensatory ability of the cardiovascular system to meet it is limited, respiratory pump failure and death may ensue because of inadequate blood flow to the respiratory muscles.[9,11,12,140]

With pulmonary disease, oxygen cost of breathing may account for values over 50% of the total O_2 consumption. This is especially well documented in patients during failed ventilator weaning attempts.[4] As the work of breathing increases, blood flow to the respiratory muscles will also increase and may, in blood flow-limited states, compromise blood flow to other vital organs.[8] In normal individuals, increases in total oxygen demand, including increased demand by the respiratory muscles (e.g., occurring during exercise), is easily compensated by the cardiovascular reserve. However, critically ill patients often have limited cardiovascular reserve secondary to ischemia, sepsis, or other organ failure, and are unable to generate the necessary increase in cardiac output. In these conditions, mechanical ventilation may reduce or eliminate the oxygen cost of breathing and restore an adequate oxygen supply/demand relationship.[9] Furthermore, merely instituting positive-pressure ventilation may not abolish the work cost of breathing in a dyspneic patient because of the continued inspiratory ventilatory efforts that may occur and because of poor patient-ventilator synchrony.[141–143]

CLINICAL CONDITIONS

Bronchospasm and Obstructed Breathing

In conditions associated with large negative swings in ITP (spontaneous inspiratory efforts in the presence of increased resistive or elastic loads), including restrictive lung disease, acute asthma, obstructive sleep apnea, upper airway obstruction, and vocal cord paralysis, venous return may be markedly increased, and predispose the patient to pulmonary edema formation.[104,117,118] The incidence of pulmonary edema associated with acute upper airway obstruction in both the pediatric and adult patient population is reported to be between 9% and 12%.[115,119,120] In children, the most common causes of acute upper airway obstruction leading to pulmonary edema are croup and epiglottitis. Postextubation laryngospasm is also frequently reported in association with pulmonary edema, in both children and adults.[115,119] Several concurrent mechanisms have been proposed to explain the pathogenesis of pulmonary edema associated with acute upper airway obstruction.

Fortunately, a plateau of maximal venous return is reached as Pra becomes negative where further decreases in Pra will no longer increase blood flow to the heart.[95,144,145] This venous flow limitation is caused by the collapse of thoracic veins leading into the RA, as ITP becomes more subatmospheric as described above. This naturally occurring flow limitation prevents massive volume overloading of the right heart and central circulation during large swings in ITP. Thus, the exaggerated negative ITP changes that lead to increases in venous return are only one of several factors that can result in pulmonary edema during loaded inspiration. Clearly, the more negative the swings in ITP during loaded inspiration, the greater will be the increase in LV afterload.[111]

Cardiopulmonary management is directed towards reducing ITP swings by resolution of airflow obstruction. Intubation and controlled mechanical ventilation may be clinically useful in removing these negative swings in ITP and correcting gas exchange abnormalities;[117,118] pulmonary artery catheters, diuretics, and inotropic agents are not usually required since this is readily reversible within hours following appropriate ventilatory supportive care and therapy towards the underlying process.

During acute exacerbations of asthma, mean ITP during tidal breathing becomes progressively more negative in order to generate the larger transpulmonary pressures necessary for lung inflation.[104] Furthermore, to prevent airway collapse during expiration, there is persistent inspiratory muscle activity during exhalation that may result in a negative ITP throughout much of the respiratory cycle. This persistently subatmospheric ITP can cause a predisposition to pulmonary edema formation via the associated increases in intrathoracic blood volume.

Furthermore, when loaded spontaneous respirations are associated with highly negative ITP and hyperinflation, as in acute asthma, RV afterload may be increased to an extent that it adversely affects RV performance. Jardin and colleagues demonstrated by two-dimensional echocardiography that highly negative ITP swings in acute asthma patients reduced RV ejection by restraining its systolic inward motion.[103] Excessive manually delivered tidal breaths in patients with airflow obstruction also induced profound cardiovascular compromise and ultimately led to electromechanical dissociation similar to that seen with acute tamponade.[146] Benefits observed while employing continuous positive-airway pressure, with or without endotracheal intubation, in airflow-limited diseases may be due in part to either abolishing negative swings in ITP and/or to decreasing hyperinflation.[147,148]

Ventricular interdependence reductions in LV preload appear to be the primary mechanism producing a pulsus paradoxus in patients with pericardial tamponade. However, the paradoxical pulse that is seen with exaggerated negative swings in ITP, such as an acute exacerbation of asthma or obstructive lung disease, is a combination of both decreased LV preload from ventricular interdependence and also an increase in LV afterload.[148] The presence and magnitude of a pulsus paradoxus has been shown to be directly pro-

portional to the inspiratory-expiratory changes in ITP and inversely related with forced expiratory flow in 1 second (FEV_1) during acute bronchospasm.[71] In contrast, with tamponade the arterial diastolic pressure is constant and systolic pressure decreases with inspiration; in hyperinflation the pulse pressure remains constant as the mean pressure decreases with inspiration.[71]

Hemodynamic Effects of Initiating Positive-Pressure Ventilation

Positive pressure-induced reduction in systemic venous return is the most commonly observed heart-lung interaction in the intensive care unit. This is most likely responsible for the acute cardiovascular collapse frequently observed in patients immediately following endotracheal intubation and "bagging" for acute respiratory failure.[146,149] Furthermore, a similar mechanism can explain the hypotension associated with significant hyperinflation or auto-PEEP in patients with airflow limitation (inadequate expiratory time).[43,146] Under these circumstances, management should be directed to interventions that will either decrease Pra (decrease ITP) or increase venous driving pressure (increase mean systemic pressure). During bagging after intubation of the asthma patient, slow rates (e.g., 4 per minute) are often necessary until additional volume resuscitation has occurred. During mechanical ventilation, mean ITP can be reduced through ventilator manipulations such as decreasing respiratory rate, increasing inspiratory flow rates, and decreasing tidal volume.[51] Another option to lower mean ITP, if status of the patient permits, is to select a mode of mechanical ventilation associated with spontaneous breathing, such as intermittent mandatory ventilation, pressure support ventilation, or continuous positive airway pressure.[108,141,142]

Recently, increased attention has been placed on the use of noninvasive ventilatory techniques to manage patients with acute respiratory failure. Importantly, although these techniques may benefit patients with chronic airflow obstruction by reducing the work-cost of breathing and improving LV performance,[150–152] their use in asthma has been recommended but has not been validated (see Chapters 12 and 13). Since hyperinflation and the resultant cardiovascular collapse represent very real concerns in asthma patients, extreme care and vigilance need to be applied if these methodologies are to be used in the management of acute asthma. Alternatively, mean systemic venous pressure can be increased by fluid resuscitation, leg elevation, or vasopressors.[102]

Alveolar dead space (high V/Q) is increased during mechanical ventilation when the lungs are over-distended or Ppa is decreased.[153] During low cardiac-output states caused, for instance, by hypovolemia in an asthma patient, there is pulmonary vascular hypovolemia. Mechanical ventilation even with normal tidal volume results in over-distended lungs relative to their perfusion pressure, increasing zone 1 and 2 conditions in the lungs. Thus, the dead space to tidal volume ratio (V_D/V_T) will increase. Often alveolar ventilation and Pa_{CO_2} can be improved in the patient with severe asthma undergoing mechanical ventilation by decreasing minute volume and volume loading,[154] and thus reducing V_D/V_T.

SUMMARY

In summary, the predominant adverse effects of acute asthma on the circulation arise from changes in lung volume (largely hyperinflation) and swings in intrathoracic pressure. These events relate directly to airflow obstruction and impair cardiac output in a variety of ways. The most significant mechanisms of cardiovascular compromise are diminished venous return, cardiac tamponade by direct compression, and increased RV afterload. During spontaneous breathing in severe airflow obstruction, a variety of mechanisms contribute to the existence of increased pulsus paradoxus, which can be used to gauge the severity of the obstruction. If positive-pressure ventilation is undertaken, cardiovascular compromise is exceedingly common. It can be minimized by volume administration to sustain venous return and ventilator strategies to minimize hyperinflation.

REFERENCES

1. Mansel JK, Stogner SW, Petrini MF, Norman JR: Mechanical ventilation in patients with acute severe asthma. *Am J Med* 89:42–8, 1990.
2. Marquette CH, Saulnier F, Leroy O, et al: Long-term prognosis of near-fatal asthma. A 6-year follow-up study of 145 asthmatic patients who underwent mechanical ventilation for a near-fatal attack of asthma. *Am Rev Respir Dis* 146:76–81, 1992.
3. Williams TJ, Tuxen DV, Scheinkestel CD, et al: Risk factors for morbidity in mechanically ventilated patients with acute severe asthma. *Am Rev Respir Dis* 146:607–15, 1992.
4. Roussos C, Macklem PT: The respiratory muscles. *N Engl J Med* 307:786–797, 1982.
5. Patterson SW, Piper H, Starling EH: The regulation of the heartbeat. *J Physiol* 48:465, 1914.
6. Grenvik A: Respiratory, circulatory and metabolic effects of respiratory treatment. *Acta Anaesth Scand* (Suppl) 1966.
7. Shuey CB, Pierce AK, Johnson RL: An evaluation of exercise tests in chronic obstructive lung disease. *J Appl Physiol* 27:256–261, 1969.
8. Viires N, Sillye G, Rassidakis A, et al: Effect of mechanical ventilation on respiratory muscle blood flow during shock. *Physiologist* 23:1, 1980.
9. Aubier M, Trippenbach T, Roussos C: Respiratory muscle fatigue during cardiogenic shock. *J Appl Physiol* 51:499–508, 1981.
10. Stock MC, David DW, Manning JW, Ryan ML: Lung mechanics and oxygen consumption during spontaneous ventilation and severe heart failure. *Chest* 102:279–283, 1992.
11. Aubier M, Vires N, Sillye G, et al: Respiratory muscle contribution to lactic acidosis in low cardiac output. *Am Rev Respir Dis* 126:648–652, 1982.
12. Aubier M, Murciano D, Menu D, et al: Dopamine effects diaphragmatic strength during acute respiratory failure in chronic obstructive pulmonary disease. *Ann Intern Med* 110:17, 1989.
13. Aubier M, Murciano D, Viires N, et al: Effects of digoxin on diaphragmatic strength generation in patients with chronic obstructive pulmonary disease during acute respiratory failure. *Am Rev Respir Dis* 135:544–548, 1987.
14. Aubier M, De Troyer A, Sampson M, et al: Aminophylline improves diaphragmatic contractility. *N Engl J Med* 305:249–252, 1981.
15. Beach T, Millen E, Grenvik A: Hemodynamic re-

sponse to discontinuance of mechanical ventilation. *Crit Care Med* 1:85–90, 1973.

16. Dorinsky PM, Hamlin RL, Gadek JE: Alterations in regional blood flow during positive end-expiratory pressure ventilation. *Crit Care Med* 15:106–115, 1987.

17. Butler J: The heart is in good hands. *Circulation* 67:1163–1168, 1983.

18. Anrep GV, Pascual W, Rossler R: Respiratory variations in the heart rate. I. The reflex mechanism of the respiratory arrhythmia. *Proc R Soc Lond [Biol]* 119:191–217, 1936.

19. Coon RL, Zuperku EJ, Kampine JP: Respiratory arrhythmias and the airway CO_2 lung receptors, and central inspiratory activity. *J Appl Physiol* 60:1713–1721, 1986.

20. Bernardi L, Calciati A, Gratarola A, et al: Heart rate-respiration relationship: computerized method for early assessment of cardiac autonomic damage in diabetic patients. *Acta Cardiol* 41:197–206, 1986.

21. Glick G, Wechsler A, Epstein S: Reflex cardiovascular depression produced by stimulation of pulmonary stretch receptors in the dog. *J Clin Invest* 48:467–472, 1969.

22. Taha BH, Simon PM, Dempsey JA, Skatrud JB, Iber C: Respiratory sinus arrhythmia in humans: an obligatory role for Vagal feedback from the lungs. *J Appl Physiol* 78:638–645, 1995.

23. Cassidy SS, Eschenbacher WI, Johnson RL Jr: Reflex cardiovascular depression during unilateral lung hyperinflation in the dog. *J Clin Invest* 64:620–626, 1979.

24. Daly MB, Hazzledine JL, Ungar A: The reflex effects of alterations in lung volume on systemic vascular resistance in the dog. *J Physiol* (London) 188:331–51, 1967.

25. Shepherd JT: The lungs as receptor sites for cardiovascular regulation. *Circulation* 63:1–10, 1981.

26. Vatner SF, Rutherford JD: Control of the myocardial contractile state by carotid chemo- and baroreceptor and pulmonary inflation reflexes in conscious dogs. *J Clin Invest* 63:1593–1601, 1978.

27. Ashton JH, SS Cassidy: Reflex depression of cardiovascular function during lung inflation. *J Appl Physiol* 58:137–145, 1985.

28. Said SI, Kitamura S, Vreim C: Prostaglandins: Release from the lung during mechanical ventilation at large tidal ventilation. *J Clin Invest* 51:83a, 1972.

29. Fuhrman BP, Everitt J, Lock JE: Cardiopulmonary effects of unilateral airway pressure changes in intact lambs. *J Appl Physiol* 56:1439–1448, 1984.

30. Grindlinger G, Manny J, Justice R, et al: Presence of negative inotropic agents in canine plasma during positive end-expiratory pressure. *Circ Res* 45:460–467, 1979.

31. Dunham B, Grindlinger G, Utsonomiya T, et al: Role of prostaglandins in positive end-expiratory pressure-induced negative inotropism. *Am J Physiol* 241:H783–H788, 1981.

32. Said SI, Foda HD: Humoral aspects of pulmonary-cardiovascular interactions, in Cassidy SS and Scharf SM (eds.): *Heart-Lung Interactions in Health and Disease.* New York, Mercel Dekker, 1989, pp 407–422.

33. Whittenberger JL, McGregor M, Berglund E, et al: Influence of state of inflation of the lung on pulmonary vascular resistance. *J Appl Physiol* 15:878–882, 1960.

34. Howell JBL, Permutt S, Proctor DF, et al: Effect of inflation of the lung on different parts of the pulmonary vascular bed. *J Appl Physiol* 16:71–76, 1961.

35. West JB, Dollery CT, Naimark A: Distribution of blood flow in isolated lung; relation to vascular and alveolar pressures. *J Appl Physiol* 19:713–724, 1964.

36. Permutt S, Howell JBL, Proctor DF, et al: Effect of lung inflation on static pressure-volume characteristics of pulmonary vessels. *J Appl Physiol* 16:64–70, 1961.

37. Lopez-Muniz R, Stephens NL, Bromberger-Barnea B, et al; Critical closure of pulmonary vessels analyzed in terms of Starling resistor model. *J Appl Physiol* 24:625–635, 1968.

38. West JB, Wagner PD: Pulmonary gas exchange, in West JB, Wagner PD (eds): *Bioengineering Aspects of the Lung.* New York, Marcel Dekker, 1977, p 361.

39. Hakim TS, Michel RP, Chang HK: Effect of lung inflation on pulmonary vascular resistance by arterial and venous occlusion. *J Appl Physiol* 53:1110–1115, 1982.

40. Fuhrman BP, Smith-Wright DL, Venkataraman S, et al: Pulmonary vascular resistance after cessation of positive end-expiratory pressure. *J Appl Physiol* 66:660–668, 1989.

41. Fuhrman BP, Everitt J, Lock JE: Cardiopulmonary effects of unilateral airway pressure changes in intact infant lambs. *J Appl Physiol* 56:1439–1448, 1984.

42. Fuhrman BP, Smith-Wright DL, Kulik TJ, Lock JE: Effects of static and fluctuating airway pressure on the intact, immature pulmonary circulation. *J Appl Physiol* 60:114–122, 1986.

43. Rossi A, Gottfried SB, Milic-Emili J: Dynamic hyperinflation, intrinsic PEEP and the mechanically ventilated patient. *Intensive Crit Care Digest* 5:30–33, 1986.

44. Pinsky MR: Through the past darkly: Ventilatory management of patients with chronic obstructive pulmonary disease. *Crit Care Med* 22:1714–1717, 1994.

45. Piene H, Sund T: Does pulmonary impedance constitute the optimal load for the right ventricle? *Am J Physiol* 242:H154–H160, 1982.

46. Marshall BE, Marshall C: Continuity of response to hypoxic pulmonary vasoconstriction. *J Appl Physiol* 49:189–196, 1980.

47. Marshall BE, Marshall C: A model for hypoxic constriction of the pulmonary circulation. *J Appl Physiol* 64:68–77, 1988.

48. Brower RG, Gottlieb J, Wise RA, Permutt W, Sylvester JT: Locus of hypoxic vasoconstriction in isolated ferret lungs. *J Appl Physiol* 63:58–65, 1987.

49. Hakim TS, Michel RP, Minami H, Chang K: Site of pulmonary hypoxic vasoconstriction studied with arterial and venous occlusion. *J Appl Physiol* 54:1298–1302, 1983.

50. Dawson CA, Grimm DJ, Linehan JH: Lung inflation and longitudinal distribution of pulmonary vascular resistance during hypoxia. *J Appl Physiol* 47:532–536, 1979.

51. Cournand A, Motley HL, Werko L, et al: Physiological studies of the effect intermittent positive pressure breathing on cardiac output in man. *Am J Physiol* 152:162–174, 1948.

52. Marini JJ, Culver BN, Butler J: Mechanical effects of lung distention with positive pressure in cardiac function. *Am Rev Respir Dis* 124:382–386, 1981.

53. Cabrera MR, Nakamura GE, Montague DA, et al: Effect of airway pressure on pericardial pressure. *Am Rev Respir Dis* 140:659–667, 1989.

54. Ellman H, Denbin H: Lack of diverse hemodynamic effect of PEEP in patients with acute respiratory failure. *Crit Care Med* 10:706–711, 1982.

55. Romand JA, Shi W, Pinsky MR: Cardiopulmonary effects of positive pressure ventilation during acute lung injury. *Chest* 108:1041–1048, 1995.

56. Canada E, Benumof JL, Tousdale FR: Pulmonary vascular resistance correlated in intact normal and abnormal canine lungs. *Crit Care Med* 10:719–723, 1982.

57. Grace MP, Greenbaum DM: Cardiac performance in response to PEEP in patients with cardiac dysfunction. *Crit Care Med* 20:358–360, 1982.

58. Pinsky MR, Vincent JL, DeSmet JM. Effect of positive end-expiratory pressure on right ventricular function in man. *Am Rev Respir Dis* 146:681–687, 1992.

59. Schulman DS, Biondi JW, Matthay RA, et al: Effect of positive end-expiratory pressure on right ventricular performance: importance of baseline right ventricular function. *Am J Med* 84:57–67, 1988.

60. Dhainaut JF, Bricard C, Monsallier JF, et al: Left ventricular contractility using isovolumic phase indices during PEEP in ARDS patients. *Crit Care Med* 10:631–635, 1982.

61. Brookhart JM, Boyd TE: Local differences in intrathoracic pressure and their relationship to cardiac filling pressures in the dog. *Am J Physiol* 148:434–444, 1947.

62. Wallis TW, Robotham JL, Compean R, et al: Mechanical heart-lung interaction with positive end-expiratory pressure. *J Appl Physiol* 54:1039–1047, 1983.

63. O'Quinn RJ, Marini JJ, Culver BH, et al: Transmission of airway pressure to pleural pressure during lung edema and chest wall restriction. *J Appl Physiol* 59:1171–1177, 1985.

64. Kingma I, Smiseth OA, Frais MA, et al: Left ventricular external constraint: relationship between pericardial, pleural and esophageal pressures during positive end-expiratory pressure and volume loading in dogs. *Ann Biomed Eng* 15:331–346, 1987.

65. Jardin FF, Farcot JC, Gueret P, et al: Echocardiographic evaluation of ventricles during continuous positive pressure breathing. *J Appl Physiol* 56:619–627, 1984.

66. Brooks H, Kirk E, Volonas P, et al: Performance of the right ventricle under stress: relation to right coronary flow. *J Clin Invest* 50:2176–2183, 1971.

67. Fessler HE, Brower RG, Wise R, et al: Positive pleural pressure decrease coronary perfusion. *Am J Physiol* 258:H814–H820, 1990.

68. Schulman DS, Biondi JW, Zohgbi S, et al: Coronary flow limits right ventricular performance during positive end-expiratory pressure. *Am Rev Respir Dis* 141:1531–1537, 1990.

69. M. Takata, Harasawa Y, Beloucif S, Robotham

JL: Coupled vs. Uncoupled pericardial restraint: effects on cardiac chamber interactions. *J Appl Physiol* 83:1799–1813, 1997.

71. Rebuck AS, Read J: Assessment and management of severe asthma. *Am J Med* 81:788–798, 1971.

72. Janicki JS, Weber KT: The pericardium and ventricular interaction, distensibility and function. *Am J Physiol* 238:H494–H503, 1980.

73. Brinker JA Weiss I, Lappe DL, et al: Leftward septal displacement during right ventricular loading in man. *Circulation* 61:626–633, 1980.

74. Taylor RR, Corell JW, Sonnenblick EH, Ross J Jr: Dependence of ventricular distensibility on filling the opposite ventricle. *Am J Physiol* 213:711–718, 1967.

75. Cassidy SS, Wead WB, Seibert GB, Ramanathan M: Changes in left ventricular geometry during spontaneous breathing. *J Appl Physiol* 63:803–811, 1987.

76. Olsen CO, Tyson GS, Maier GW, et al: Dynamic ventricular interaction in the conscious dog. *Circ Res* 52:85–104, 1983.

77. Hoffman EA, Ritman EL: Heart-lung interaction: effect on regional lung air content and total heart volume. *Ann Biomed Eng* 15:241–257, 1987.

78. Olson LE, Hoffman EA: Heart-lung interactions determined by electron beam X-ray CT in laterally recumbent rabbits. *J Appl Physiol* 78:417–427, 1995.

79. Novak RA, Matuschak GM, Pinsky MR: Effect of ventilatory frequency on regional pleural pressure. *J Appl Physiol* 65:1314–1323, 1988.

80. Jardin F, Farcot JC, Boisante L: Influence of positive end-expiratory pressure on left ventricular performance. *N Engl J Med* 304:387–392, 1981.

81. Tyberg JV, Taichman GC, Smith ER, et al: The relationship between pericardial pressure and right atrial pressure: An intraoperative study. *Circulation* 73:428–432, 1986.

82. Bromberger-Barnea B: Mechanical effects of inspiration on heart functions: A review. *Fed Proc* 40:2172–2177, 1981.

83. Guntheroth WG, Morgan BC, Mullins GL: Effect of respiration on venous return and stroke volume in cardiac tamponade. Mechanism of pulsus paradoxus. *Circ Res* 20:381–390, 1967.

84. Viola AR, Puy RJM, Goldman E: Mechanisms of pulsus paradoxus in airway obstruction. *J Appl Physiol* 68:1927–1931, 1990.

85. Takata M, Wise RA, Robotham JL: Effects of abdominal pressure on venous return: abdominal

86. Wise RA, Robotham JL, Summer WR: Effects of spontaneous ventilation on the circulation. *Lung* 159:175–192, 1981.

87. Fessler HE, Brower RG, Wise RA, et al: Effects of positive end-expiratory pressure on the gradient for venous return. *Am Rev Respir Dis* 143:19–24, 1991.

88. Fessler HE, Brower RG, Wise RA, Permutt S: Effects of positive end-expiratory pressure on the canine venous return curve. *Am Rev Respir Dis* 146:4–10, 1992.

89. Takata M, Robotham JL: Effects of inspiratory diaphragmatic descent on inferior vena caval venous return. *J Appl Physiol* 72:597–607, 1992.

90. Chihara E, Hasimoto S, Kinoshita T, et al: Elevated mean systemic filling pressure due to intermittent positive-pressure ventilation. *Am J Physiol* 262:H1116–H1121, 1992.

91. Matuschak GM, Pinsky MR, Rogers RM: Effects of positive end-expiratory pressure on hepatic blood flow and hepatic performance. *J Appl Physiol* 62:1377–1383, 1987.

92. Sharpey-Schaffer EP: Effects of Valsalva maneuver on the normal and failing circulation. *Br Med J* 1:693–699, 1955.

93. Milic-Emili J, Mead J, Turner JM: Improved method for assessing the validity of the esophageal balloon technique. *J Appl Physiol* 19:207–211, 1964.

94. Braunwald E, Binion JT, Morgan WL, Sarnoff SJ: Alterations in central blood volume and cardiac output induced by positive pressure breathing and counteracted by metraminol (Aramine). *Circ Res* 5:670–675, 1957.

95. Guyton AC, Lindsey AW, Abernathy B, et al: Venous Return at various right atrial pressures at the normal venous return curve. *Am J Physiol* 189:609–615, 1957.

96. Pinsky, MR, Guimond JG: The effects of positive end-expiratory pressure on heart-lung interactions. *J Crit Care* 6:1–11, 1991.

97. Pinsky MR: Instantaneous venous return curves in an intact canine preparation. *J Appl Physiol* 56:765–771, 1984.

98. Pinsky MR: Determinants of pulmonary artery flow variation during respiration. *J Appl Physiol* 56:1237–1245, 1984.

99. Magder S, Georgiadis G, Cheong T: Respiratory

vascular zone conditions. *J Appl Physiol* 69:1961–1972, 1990.

variation in right atrial pressure predict the response to fluid challenge. *J Crit Care* 7:76–85, 1992.

100. Morgan BC, Abel FL, Mullins GL, et al: Flow patterns in cavae, pulmonary artery, pulmonary vein and aorta in intact dogs. *Am J Physiol* 210:903–909, 1966.

101. Morgan BC, Martin WE, Hornbein TF, et al: Hemodynamic effects of intermittent positive pressure respiration. *Anesthesiology* 27:584–590, 1960.

102. Rothe C: Physiology of venous return: an unappreciated boost to the heart. *Arch Intern Med* 146:977–982, 1986.

103. Jardin F, Dubourg O, Margairaz A, et al: Inspiratory impairment in right ventricular performance during acute asthma. *Chest* 92:789–795, 1987.

104. Stalcup SA, Mellins RB: Mechanical forces producing pulmonary edema in acute asthma. *N Engl J Med* 297:592–596, 1977.

105. Holt JP: The effect of positive and negative intrathoracic pressure on cardiac output and venous return in the dog. *Am J Physiol* 142:594–603, 1944.

106. Johnston WE, Vinten-Johansen J, Santamore WP, et al: Mechanism of reduced cardiac output during positive end-expiratory pressure in the dog. *Am Rev Respir Dis* 140:1257–1264, 1989.

107. Calvin JE, Driedger AA, Sibbald WJ: Positive end-expiratory pressure (PEEP) does not depress left ventricular function in patients with pulmonary edema. *Am Rev Respir Dis* 124:121–128, 1981.

108. Vuori A, Jalonen J, Laaksonen V: Continuous positive airway pressure during mechanical ventilation and spontaneous ventilation: effect on central hemodynamics and oxygen transport. *Acta Anaesthesiol Scand* 23:453–461, 1979.

109. Jayaweera AR, Ehrlich W: Changes of phasic pleural pressure in awake dogs during exercise: potential effects on cardiac output. *Ann Biomed Eng* 15:311–318, 1987.

110. Strohl KP, Scharf SM, Brown R, Ingram RH Jr: Cardiovascular performance during bronchospasm in dogs. *Respiration* 51:39–48, 1987.

111. Buda AS, Pinsky MR, Ingles NB, et al: Effect of intrathoracic pressure on left ventricular performance. *N Engl J Med* 301:453–459, 1979.

112. Scharf SM, Brown R, Saunders N, et al: Effects of normal and loaded spontaneous inspiration on cardiovascular function. *J Appl Physiol* 47:582–590, 1979.

113. Robotham JL, Rabson J, Permutt S, Bromberger-Barnea B: Left ventricular hemodynamics during respiration. *J Appl Physiol* 47:1295–1303, 1979.

114. Scharf SM, Brown R, Warner KG, Khuri S: Intrathoracic pressure and left ventricular configuration with respiratory maneuvers. *J Appl Physiol* 66:481–491, 1989.

115. Kanter RK, Watchko JF: Pulmonary edema associated with upper airway obstruction. *Am J Dis Child* 138:356–358, 1984.

116. Luke MJ, Mehrizi A, Folger GM, et al: Chronic nasopharyngeal obstruction as a cause of cardiomegaly, cor pulmonale, and pulmonary edema. *Pediatrics* 37:762–768, 1966.

117. Miro AM, Shivaram U, Finch PJP: Noncardiogenic pulmonary edema following laser treatment of a tracheal neoplasm. *Chest* 96:1430–1431, 1989.

118. Oswalt CE, Gates GA, Holstrom FMG: Pulmonary edema as a complication of acute airway obstruction. *JAMA* 238:1833–1835, 1977.

119. Soliman MG, Richer P: Epiglottitis and pulmonary oedema in children. *Can Anaesth Soc J* 26:145–146, 1979.

120. Tami TA, Chu F, Wildes TO, et al: Pulmonary edema and acute upper airway obstruction. *Laryngoscope* 96:506–509, 1986.

121. Richard C, Teboul J-L, Archambaud F, et al: Left ventricular function during weaning of patients with chronic obstructive pulmonary disease. *Intensive Care Med* 20:181–186, 1994.

122. Mohsenifar Z, Hay A, Hay J, et al: Gastric intramural pH as a predictor of success or failure in weaning patients from mechanical ventilation. *Ann Intern Med* 119:794–798, 1993.

123. Rasanen J, Nikki P, Heikkila J: Acute myocardial infarction complicated by respiratory failure. The effects of mechanical ventilation. *Chest* 85:21–28, 1984.

124. Scharf SM, Graver LM, Khilnani S, Balaban K: Respiratory phasic effects of inspiratory loading on left ventricular hemodynamics in vagotomized dogs. *J Appl Physiol* 73:995–1003, 1992.

125. Pinsky MR, Marquez J, Martin D, et al: Ventricular assist by cardiac cycle-specific increases in intrathoracic pressure. *Chest* 91:709–715, 1987.

126. Sibbald WH, Calvin J, Driedge AA: Right and left ventricular preload and diastolic ventricular compliance: Implications for therapy in critically ill patients. *Critical Care State of the Art*, Vol 3. Fullerton, CA, Society of Critical Care Medicine, 1982 pp 188–201.

127. Harrison VC, Heese HV, Klein M: The significance of grunting in hyaline membrane disease. *Pediatrics* 41:549–559, 196

128. Pinsky MR, Matuschak GM. Itzkoff JM: Respiratory augmentation of left ventricular function during spontaneous ventilation in severe left ventricular failure by grunting: an auto-EPAP effect. *Chest* 86:267–269, 1984.

129. Prec KJ, Cassels DE: Oximeter studies in newborn infants during crying. *Pediatrics* 9:756–761, 1952.

130. Killian A, Stein K, Guthrie RD, et al: Cardiac augmentation by cardiac cycle specific increases in intrathoracic pressure in a model of neonatal heart failure. *Am Rev Respir Dis* 139:A21, 1989. Abstract.

131. Pinsky MR, Matuschak GM, Klain M: Determinants of cardiac augmentation by increase in intrathoracic pressure. *J Appl Physiol* 58:1189–1198, 1985.

132. Pinsky MR, Matuschak GM, Bernardi L, Klain M: Hemodynamic effects of cardiac cycle-specific increases in intrathoracic pressure. *J Appl Physiol* 60:604–612, 1986.

133. Prewitt RM, Wood LDH: Effect of positive end-expiratory pressure on ventricular function in dogs. *Am J Physiol* 236:H534–H544, 1979.

134. Stein K, Kramer DJ, Killian A, et al: Hemodynamic effects of synchronous high-frequency jet ventilation in mitral regurgitation. *J Appl Physiol* 69:2120–2125, 1990.

135. Ruskin J, Bache RJ, Rembert JC, Greenfield Jr: Pressure-flow studies in man: Effect of respiration on left ventricular stroke volume. *Circulation* 48:79–85, 1973.

136. Rankin JS, Olsen CO, Arentzen CE, et al: The effects of airway pressure on cardiac function in intact dogs and man. *Circulation* 66:108–120, 1982.

137. Abel FL, Mihailescu LS, Lader AS, Starr RG: Effects of pericardial pressure on systemic and coronary hemodynamics in dogs. *Am J Physiol* 268:H1583–H1605, 1995.

138. Khilnani S, Graver LM, Balaban K, Scharf SM: Effects of inspiratory loading on left ventricular myocardial blood flow and metabolism. *J Appl Physiol* 72:1488–1492, 1992.

139. Satoh S, Watanabe J, Keitoku M, et al: Influences of pressure surrounding the heart and intracardiac pressure on the diastolic coronary pressure-flow relation in excised canine heart. *Circ Res* 63:788–797, 1988.

140. Yanos J, Keamy MF, Leisk L, et al: The mechanism of respiratory arrest in inspiratory loading and hypoxemia. *Am Rev Respir Dis* 141:933–937, 1990.

141. Marini JJ, Capps JS, Culver BH: The inspiratory work of breathing during assisted mechanical ventilation. *Chest* 87:612–618, 1985.

142. Marini JJ, Smith TC, Lamb VJ: External work output during synchronized intermittent mechanical ventilation. *Am Rev Resp Dis* 138:1169–1179, 1988.

143. Marini JJ, Rodriguez RM, Lamb V: The inspiratory workload of patient-initiated mechanical ventilation. *Am Rev Respir Dis* 134:902–909, 1986.

144. Brecher GA, Hubay CA: Pulmonary blood flow and venous return during spontaneous respiration. *Circ Res* 3:40–214, 1955.

145. Guyton AC: Effect of cardiac output by respiration, opening the chest, and cardiac tamponade, in *Circulatory Physiology: Cardiac Output and Its Regulation.* Philadelphia, WB Saunders, 1963, pp 378-386.

146. Roger PL, Schlichtig R, Miro AM, et al: Auto-PEEP during CPR: an 'occult' cause of electromechanical dissociation. *Chest* 99:492–493, 1991.

147. Granton JT, Naughton MT, Benard DC, et al: CPAP improves inspiratory muscle strength in patients with heart failure and central sleep apnea. *Am J Respir Crit Care Med* 153:277–282, 1996.

148. Blaustein AS, Risser TA, Weiss JW, et al: Mechanisms of pulsus paradoxus during resistive loading and asthma. *J Am Coll Cardiol* 8:529–536, 1986.

149. Harken AH, Brennan MF, Smith B, et al: The hemodynamic response to positive and end-expiratory ventilation in hypovolemic patients. *Surgery* 76:786–793, 1974.

150. Ambrosino N, Nava S, Torbicki A, et al: Hemodynamic effects of pressure support and PEEP ventilation by nasal route in patients with stable chronic obstructive pulmonary disease. *Thorax* 48:523–528, 1993.

151. Ambrosino N, Cobelli F, Torbicki A, et al: Hemodynamic effects of negative-pressure ventilation in patients with COPD. *Chest* 97:850–856, 1990.

152. Brochard L, Isabey D, Piquet J, et al: Reversal of acute exacerbations of chronic obstructive lung disease by inspiratory assistance with a face mask. *N Engl J Med* 323:1523–1530, 1990.

153. Murray JF: *The Normal Lung.* 2d ed. Philadelphia, WB Saunders, 1986.

154. Manthous CA, Goulding P: The effect of volume infusion on dead space in mechanically ventilated patients with severe asthma. *Chest* 112:843–846, 1997.

Chapter 8

EMERGENCY DEPARTMENT ASSESSMENT: SEVERITY AND OUTCOME PREDICTION

Gustavo J. Rodrigo
Carlos Rodrigo

INTRODUCTION

The fatality rate from asthma has been increasing over the last decade.[1–4] The prevention of asthma-related deaths begins with the use of appropriate medications and depends on the ability of care givers and patients to recognize the danger signs of more severe disease. A useful practice is to assume that every exacerbation is potentially fatal and act accordingly.[5] Most deaths from asthma occur in patients with severe, poorly controlled disease whose condition gradually deteriorates over a period of days, and in patients who have a history of unstable illness, are partially responsive to treatment, and in whom a major attack occurs.[6–8] Rarely, death can be rapid and unexpected, termed *sudden-onset fatal asthma.*[9–11] Almost one half of these deaths occurred in a hospital[1,2,6,8,12]; in nearly 85% of asthma deaths, the final episode lasted at least 12 hours, which would have allowed sufficient time for treatment.[6,12–14] Surveys have documented inadequate or incomplete assessments in both outpatient[6] and inpatient settings.[12] Consequently, close monitoring of a patient's condition and response to treatment, including serial measurements of lung function, is an essential part of care.[15]

This chapter reviews acute asthma assessment in the emergency department (ED) setting. It emphasizes three key areas: 1) acute asthma as a multidimensional entity, 2) clinical assessment, including response to therapy and outcome measures, and 3) indications for hospitalization.

ACUTE ASTHMA AS A MULTIDIMENSIONAL ENTITY

Asthma exacerbations are characterized by acute or subacute episodes of progressively worsening shortness of breath, cough, wheezing, chest tightness, or a combination of these symptoms.[15] They involve decreases in expiratory airflow that can be documented and quantified by measurement of lung function. A variety of measures are used to assess the severity of this condition; most are logical and seem reasonably effective but have not been scientifically tested in a comprehensive manner.[16] Data from adults receiving outpatient treatment have shown that asthma appears to be multidimensional, with varying severity across this domain of symptoms and physiologic measurements.[17] However, only one study has examined the most common clinical and objective measures used in ED assessment of acute asthma. In that study, Rodrigo and Rodrigo used multivariate factor analysis to determine whether variables constitute separate or distinct dimensions.[18] This technique was used to examine the underlying relationships of a large number of variables and to determine whether information can be condensed into a smaller set of factors or components. The results from this analysis indicate that a description of acute adult asthma includes several independent factors or dimensions. This research presented a four-factor solution as most clinically and statistically appropriate. The first factor extracted from the data set contained the three lung function measures [peak expiratory flow rate (PEFR), forced expiratory volume in the first second (FEV_1), and forced vital capacity (FVC)] and early response to treatment (as a percent variation of FEV_1 at 30 minutes over the baseline value). The second factor contained three clinical measures (respiratory rate, accessory muscle use, and dyspnea) and the third factor included heart rate and wheezing. The fourth factor contained three demographic variables (age, duration of attack, and steroid use).

The results from this study indicated that a description of acute asthma severity should include these independent factors or dimensions. This factor analysis supported the hypothesis that most of the subjective and objective measures used in the assessment of these asthma patients represent separate and nonoverlapping dimensions and provide a useful summary for clinical application. In addition, these dimensions should be considered and included in research protocols to stratify study populations. Furthermore, the results of this study provide justification for the use of a small number of measures in the assessment of airflow obstruction and the prediction of the outcome of acute asthma episodes.

CLINICAL ASSESSMENT

The mean age of acute asthma patients seen in the ED is between 30 to 35 years, and two thirds of these patients are women.[19–20] Despite the considerable variability in the diagnostic evaluation of acute severe asthma patients in the ED,[21–23] their assessment should always include a medical history, measures of airflow obstruction, response to initial therapy, and monitoring of oxygen saturation. However, in a retrospective study, Reed

and colleagues found that the observations and measures used to assess the severity of asthma were recorded with variable frequency (e.g., heart rate in 84% of examinations, pulsus paradoxus in 13%, and PEFR in 11%).[21] This failure to record more objective measurements of the severity of asthma, and in particular, the extent of airflow obstruction, gives cause for concern. Although there was a significant increase in the percentage of patients who had objective measures of airflow obstruction recorded in the ED over the course of a longitudinal study,[24] there was still a substantial percentage of patients in whom flow rates were not monitored in the ED.

Medical History

A brief history pertinent to any exacerbation should be obtained. The objectives of this history are to determine time of onset of symptoms and cause of current exacerbation; severity of symptoms, especially compared with previous exacerbations; all current medications and time of last dose; prior hospitalizations and ED visits for asthma, particularly within the past year; prior episodes of respiratory insufficiency caused by asthma (intubation, mechanical ventilation, barotrauma); and underlying psychiatric illness. Patients with severe disease are thought to be at the greatest risk, but those with mild illness also may die if the therapy they receive is inappropriate.[25,26] Marked circadian variation in lung function, a large bronchodilation response, psychosocial instability, the use of three or more medications, frequent visits to the ED, recurrent hospitalizations, and previous life-threatening asthma attacks have been associated with poor outcomes.[25,27–32] The existence of such events is extremely important in an individual patient, but their absence does not assure low risk. Additionally, poorly controlled asthma is especially likely to occur in a setting of poverty. Many components of poverty may contribute to increased risk, including poor access to appropriate health care, lack of continuity of care, decreased likelihood of treatment with anti-inflammatory drugs, poor systems of social support, and low levels of education.[33–35] Finally, it is important to know that sudden-onset asthma attacks have a rapid deterioration followed by a more rapid response to treatment than slow-onset asthma attacks.[36]

Physical Examination

Particular attention should be paid to the general appearance of the patient. Brenner and colleagues observed that adults with acute asthma who assumed an upright position had a significantly higher pulse rate, respiratory rate, and rate of pulsus paradoxus (PP) and a significantly lower Pa_{O_2} value and PEFR than did patients who were able to remain supine.[37] All the patients in this study demonstrated sternocleidomastoid retraction, a finding that commonly indicates severe airflow obstruction.

A respiratory rate greater than 30 breaths per minute, tachycardia greater than 120 beats per minute, and PP greater than 12 mm Hg have been described as vital signs of acute severe asthma. The PP of acute severe asthma is an exaggeration of the normal fall in systolic blood pressure during inspiration. Its magnitude is thought to be related to the severity of the attack.[38] In severe airflow obstruction, PP is greater than the normal value of 4 to 10 mm Hg and typically greater than 15 mm Hg. However, disagreement exists about how often it is present and the level that should be considered abnormal. Rebuck and Read[39] found that PP greater than 10 mm Hg always indicated an FEV_1 of 1.25 L or less, usually below 0.9 L. Pulsus paradoxus can indicate asthma severity,[40] but PP also falls in a fatiguing asthmatic who is unable to generate significant changes in pleural pressure and the absence of an increased PP does not always indicate a mild attack.[41] More recently, Pearson and colleagues minimized the importance of PP in the assessment of acute severe asthma.[42] They found a weak association between airflow obstruction and PP; this sign was not found in one third of patients with the most severe obstruction and was found in one third of those with PEFR above 200 L per minute. Only severe PP ($\geq$25 mm Hg) was a reliable indicator of severe asthma. In summary, *a single PP determination* is a poor guide to the severity of acute asthma in individual patients. Some authors have recommend that PP should be abandoned as an indicator of severity of attack (see the revised British Thoracic Society guidelines on asthma management[43]), but there may be a role for serial measurements in selected patients.

Wheeze and dyspnea are present in virtually all acute asthma patients. Nevertheless, they correlate poorly with the degree of airflow limitation.[44] A patient who reports a marked increase in the severity of dyspnea should be assumed to have potentially severe airflow obstruction until this possibility is disproved. The converse is not true, however. Two groups of patients have abnormal responses to airway narrowing that put them at risk for respiratory failure. One group is unable to sense the presence of even marked airway obstruction and does not develop symptoms until the respiratory reserve is almost exhausted.[45,46] The other group has a blunted hypoxic ventilatory drive and does not develop the hyperpnea characteristic of acute asthma attacks.[47,48] In this group, alveolar hypoventilation can develop rapidly, even in the presence of moderate degrees of obstruction. In addition, severely obstructed patients may have a silent chest, if there is insufficient alveolar ventilation and airflow for wheezes to occur.[49] In these patients, the development of wheezes generally indicates improved airflow.

Composite data from two large clinical trials[50,51] have demonstrated that 67% of acute severe asthma patients have heart rates ranging between 90 and 120 beats per minute, with only 15% exceeding this value. Overall, successful treatment of airflow obstruction usually is associated with a decrease in heart rate, although some improving patients remain tachycardic because of the chronotropic effects of bronchodilators. Specifically, older patients (>35 years of age) tend toward treatment-related tachycardia, but at presentation they have a mean heart rate significantly lower than that of younger patients.[52] Data from these trials also showed that respiratory rates range between 20 and 30 breaths per minute in 60% of patients and are 30 or more in 16%.

The use of accessory muscles has received attention as an indicator of severe airflow obstruction. However, Kelsen and colleagues.[53] showed that 52% of patients with an FEV_1 less than 1 L did not demonstrate retractions. By contrast, in a review of 268 patients who presented to an ED for acute exacerbation of asthma (age between 18 and 50 years, FEV_1 below 50% of the predicted value), Rodrigo and Rodrigo (personal communication) found that only 5.2% of these patients did not show accessory muscle use. Only three patients with an FEV_1 less than 1 L did not present with suprasternal retraction. Thus, accessory muscle use can be considered a useful sign of severe airflow obstruction.

Arterial Blood Gases

Arterial blood gas determination is rarely necessary before the initiation of treatment. Only patients with an FEV_1 or PEFR less than 20% of the predicted value and with other signs of severe airflow obstruction are at risk for significant hypercapnia or acidosis.[54–59] Repeat blood gas sampling usually is not needed to determine whether a patient is deteriorating or improving. In most cases, valid judgments can be based on serial physical examinations with attention to patient posture, use of accessory muscles, diaphoresis, estimates of air movement during chest auscultation, and PEFR determinations. An exception might be a patient in extremis who cannot perform pulmonary function tests or for whom intubation and mechanical ventilation are being considered; in this situation, arterial blood should be sampled while the initial treatment is being given. Patients in the early stages of acute asthma exhibit mild hypoxemia and respiratory alkalosis as result of low ventilation-perfusion ratios.[60–62] As the severity of airflow obstruction increases, carbon dioxide tension (Pa_{CO_2}) generally increases because of patient exhaustion and inadequate alveolar ventilation and/or an increase in physiologic dead space. Analysis of blood gases in over 350 acutely ill asthma patients in published reports[54–57] showed that only 13% had a Pa_{CO_2} between 45 and 60 mm Hg, and 4% had an oxygen tension (Pa_{O_2}) below 50 mm Hg.

Oxygen saturation measured by pulse oximetry (on air) can indicate which patients who pres-

ent with acute severe asthma are likely to be in respiratory failure and therefore require more intensive management.[63] When oxygen saturation is 92% or greater, respiratory failure is unlikely.[64] Thus, blood gas tension should be measured in patients with acute severe asthma whose Sa_{O_2} is below 92% on admission, regardless of their inspired oxygen concentration. Arterial sampling is not required in patients with an Sa_{O_2} of 92% or higher unless their condition does not improve objectively, or deteriorates.

Radiographic Studies

Chest radiography plays only a small role in the assessment and management of patients with acute asthma. Many studies have demonstrated that the incidence of specific abnormalities on chest radiography in adults with uncomplicated acute asthma is low and have suggested that the information obtained is rarely helpful in ED management.[65–70] Findley and Sahn reviewed chest radiographs in 90 episodes of acute asthma among 60 patients.[65] Fifty-five percent of these films were interpreted as normal, 37% as demonstrating hyperinflation, and 7% as showing minimal interstitial markings that were unchanged from previous radiographs. There was no significant correlation between chest radiograph interpretation and hospitalization. Lavechia and colleagues evaluated initial chest radiographs in 48 asthmatic adult patients seen in the ED setting.[70] Forty-two percent of these films were interpreted as normal, whereas the remaining 58% showed hyperinflation, an enlarged cardiac silhouette, increased interstitial markings, focal parenchymal opacity, or pulmonary vascular congestion. These investigators concluded that their findings support the policy of not routinely performing chest radiography in the assessment of acute asthma patients. On the basis of these data, chest radiographs are indicated only in patients who present with signs or symptoms of barotrauma (e.g., chest pain, mediastinal crunch, subcutaneous emphysema, cardiovascular instability, or asymmetric breath sounds), in patients with clinical findings suggestive of pneumonia, or in an asthmatic patient who, after 6 to 12 hours, does not respond to therapy.

Monitoring of Cardiac Rhythm

Electrocardiograms (EKG) need not be routinely obtained, but continual monitoring of cardiac rhythm is appropriate in patients older than 50 years of age[49] and in those with coexisting heart disease.[15] When EKG monitoring is conducted, abnormalities are common, even in younger patients without known cardiac disease. The usual rhythm is sinus tachycardia, although supraventricular arrhythmias are not uncommon. Acute asthma can cause examination and EKG findings of right heart strain that can resolve after successful treatment. Common transient electrocardiographic findings include right axis deviation, clockwise rotation, and evidence of right ventricular strain. If due to asthma alone, reversal within hours of response to therapy is to be expected.

Measurement of Airflow Obstruction

The severity of airflow obstruction cannot be accurately judged by means of symptoms and physical examination by themselves. Acute asthma exacerbations are characterized by decreases in expiratory flow that can be documented and quantified through the measurement of lung function. This objective measure indicates the severity of an exacerbation more reliably than does the severity of symptoms. In fact, one of the most significant factors contributing to avoidable deaths is failure by the physician to appreciate the severity of the attack.[9,12,49] On presentation, after the initial treatment, and at ensuing frequent intervals, this measure constitutes an integral part of the assessment of disease severity and the response to therapy in any patient over 5 years of age.[15]

Measurement of airflow obstruction should be made using one of following techniques: 1) PEFR measured with a peak flow meter or 2) FEV_1 determined by spirometry. Many studies have found satisfactory correlations between PEFR and FEV_1 among healthy and asthmatic subjects.[71–83] However, in spite of the significance of this fact, few studies have analyzed the relationship between these two measures in the ED setting. Nowak and colleagues[84] compared PEFR and FEV_1 after bronchodilator therapy in patients treated in the ED and found that both measures correlated well at all stages of treatment (correlations ranged between 0.73 and 0.86). More recently, Rodrigo and Rodrigo compared measures of FEV_1 and PEFR in 114 patients who presented for treatment of acute asthma.[85] High correlations were observed with a value of 0.90 for all measures (Table 8-1). PEFR values tended to have more variability when pulmonary function was more impaired. Peak expiratory flow rate as a percent of predicted value was consistently higher than FEV_1. This phenomenon confirmed the tendency of % of predicted PEFR to underestimate the degree of pulmonary impairment.[86–88] Nonetheless, both PEFR and FEV_1 provide objective measures of airflow obstruction.

Importantly, the intensive and prolonged use of peak expiratory flow meters did not yield unreliable mean peak expiratory flow values in long-term studies. Douma and colleagues tested the reliability of PEFR values measured with mini-Wright PEFR meters that had been used fre-

Table 8-1
Correlations between PEFR and FEV_1

Comparison	r^a
PEFR (L/min) vs. FEV_1 (L) (pretreatment)	0.73
PEFR (% of predicted) vs. FEV_1 (% of predicted) (pretreatment)	0.61
PEFR (L/min) vs. FEV_1 (L) (30 minutes)	0.88
PEFR (% of predicted) vs. FEV_1 (% of predicted) (30 minutes)	0.83
PEFR (L/min) vs. FEV_1 (L) (end of treatment)	0.88
PEFR (% of predicted) vs. FEV_1 (% of predicted) (end of treatment)	0.81
PEFR (L/min) vs. FEV_1 (L) (all measures)	0.90
PEFR (% of predicted) vs. FEV_1 (% of predicted) (all measures)	0.84

^{a} NOTE: All values $p < .001$.
SOURCE: From Rodrigo and Rodrigo.[85]

quently for 5 years and concluded that mean peak expiratory flow values are still reliable after this interval.[89]

Even though spirometry is the gold standard for the measurement of airflow obstruction, in most asthma patients it is easier to measure PEFR than FEV_1; nevertheless, this maneuver is still difficult for severely dyspneic patients to perform. In these patients, deep inhalation may worsen bronchospasm[90] and, in rare cases, precipitate respiratory arrest.[91] Still, PEFR measurement is safe in most acute asthma patients.

On average, the mean level of lung function (FEV_1 or PEFR) in asthmatic patients who present for care to a hospital-based ED is 25% to 35% of the predicted value.[19,21,50,51,53,92–95] In its guidelines, the Expert Panel Report 2 (EPR-2)[15] recommended that any FEV_1 or PEFR less than 50% of the predicted value should be considered to represent a serious and severe asthma attack. Decision making that is based on the measured obstruction of airflow presumes that when asymptomatic, an asthma patient has normal or nearly normal lung function. However, some asthma patients may have significant fixed airflow obstruction even when they are asymptomatic. Knowledge of this fixed airflow obstruction during asymptomatic periods is useful in interpreting lung function measurements made during the acute exacerbation. Finally, both measurements require 1) patient cooperation in making a maximal expiratory effort and 2) coaching by a person trained in making these measurements. Measurements obtained without meeting these requirements will be erroneous and may lead to errors in assessment and measurement.

Differential Diagnosis

A number of conditions may mimic or complicate the diagnosis of acute asthma (Table 8-2). Usually, they can be identified by history and physical examination. The absence of a prior history of asthma, particularly in an adult, should alert the clinician to an alternative diagnosis.[96]

Congestive heart failure, particularly predominant left ventricular failure or mitral stenosis,

Table 8-2
Differential diagnosis of wheezing

Myocardial ischemia and/or congestive heart failure
COPD
Upper airway obstruction and/or foreign body
Pulmonary embolism
Hyperventilation syndrome
Vocal cord dysfunction

occasionally may present with episodic shortness of breath accompanied by wheezing. This symptom complex is sufficiently widely recognized to have been labeled *cardiac asthma.*[97] Clinical signs of heart failure will lead to the appropriate diagnosis.

Perhaps the most common and most difficult diagnostic problem in asthma is its differentiation from *chronic obstructive pulmonary disease* (COPD). In subjects more than 40 years of age, a distinction between COPD and asthma is often difficult, if not impossible. However, patients with COPD can be identified by prolonged tobacco use, chronic ventilatory failure, signs of pulmonary hypertension or cor pulmonae, and failure to reverse airflow obstruction significantly between acute exacerbations.[98]

Laryngeal/tracheal/bronchial obstruction resulting from any of a number of causes may produce shortness of breath, localized wheezing, inspiratory stridor localized over the trachea, or unilateral hyperinflation noted on chest radiography.[99] Often, unstable patients in the ED must be stabilized and definitive diagnostic tests must be performed at a later time.

Vocal cord dysfunction (VCD) often mimics asthma. Patients with VCD can present with recurrent severe shortness of breath and wheezing. VCD may even cause alveolar hypoventilation with increases in Pa_{CO_2} that prompt urgent intubation and mechanical ventilation. VCD that mimics asthma occurs more commonly in young adults with psychological disorders. It should be suspected when physical examination reveals a monophonic wheeze that is heard loudest over the glottis. Definitive diagnosis and exclusion of organic causes of vocal cord narrowing require direct visualization of the vocal cords.[100–102]

Recurrent small pulmonary emboli may be manifested by attacks of shortness of breath and, very rarely, wheezing heard on careful auscultation. However, in large series of angiographically proven pulmonary embolus, wheezing was not a reported sign,[103] but, if dyspnea is greatly disproportionate to the degree of obstruction and sudden in onset, pulmonary embolism should be considered as a possible diagnosis.[96]

Finally, recurrent attacks of shortness of breath at rest may be due to the *hyperventilation syndrome*. It usually is possible to base this diagnosis on the history alone. Hyperventilation attacks often occur under specific circumstances, for instance, in enclosed spaces or on public transport, and often are worse during the evening or occasionally at night. Attacks usually are associated with paraesthesias of the hands and feet, carpopedal spasm, dryness of the mouth, dizziness, and chest pain. Hyperventilation attacks occur commonly in patients with organic chest pain disease, and thus a diagnosis of hyperventilation syndrome does not exclude the possibility that the patient is also an asthmatic.[104]

Response to Therapy

Previous studies have demonstrated that the failure of initial therapy to improve expiratory flow predicts a more severe course and the need for hospitalization.[19,105–107] Therefore, measurement of the change in PEFR or FEV_1 over time may be one of the best ways to assess asthma patients acutely and predict the need for hospital admission. The response to initial treatment in the ED is a better predictor of the need for hospitalization than is the severity of an exacerbation at presentation.[19,108]

In 1982, Fanta and colleagues showed that a major variable that influenced the duration of the therapy needed to produce a remission was the severity of the obstruction at presentation.[106] Subjects whose initial FEV_1 was less than 30% of predicted value and who did not improve significantly at the end of 60 minutes of intense treatment ulti-

mately required prolonged ED therapy and/or hospital admission. Similarly, Nowak and colleagues found that an initial PEFR less than 100 L per minute and an improvement less than 60 L per minute after initial β agonist therapy are early indicators of severe resistant disease requiring aggressive therapy.[84] In another trial, Nowak and colleagues demonstrated a relatively poor correlation between FEV_1 and Pa_{O_2} or Pa_{CO_2}.[59] Similarly, they found that the mean Pa_{O_2}, Pa_{CO_2}, and pH in each of three clinical outcome groups (hospitalized, discharged, and relapsed patients) were not statistically different. The PEFR and the FEV_1, however, consistently differentiated these clinical groups. In contrast to these findings Martin and colleagues found that a change in PEFR that occurred 20 minutes after subcutaneous epinephrine did not predict the clinical outcome in patients with asthma.[58]

More recently, Stein and Cole found that a change in PEFR after 2 hours of bronchodilator treatment predicted the need for hospital admission.[107] Peak flow rate on entry did not predict the need for admission. After 2 hours of treatment, patients who ultimately were discharged from the ED had a significantly higher PEFR than did patients who required admission (in whom PEFR did not change significantly from that at entry). In the same way, Rodrigo and Rodrigo showed that the response of PEFR after 30 minutes of bronchodilator treatment was the most important predictor of time required before leaving the ED (Figure 8-1).[108]

Finally, in a trial that included 194 acute asthma patients, Rodrigo and Rodrigo demonstrated that early response to treatment (measured by the percent increase in FEV_1 at 30 minutes over the baseline value) was the most important predictor of outcome.[18] The patients who were discharged earliest from the ED were those with the greatest improvement in FEV_1 after 30 minutes of treatment. The use FEV_1 or PEFR response at 30 minutes of treatment has now been incorporated in recent asthma guidelines.[15]

Attempts have been made to create multifactorial scoring systems that would allow early identification of patients who are likely to require hos-

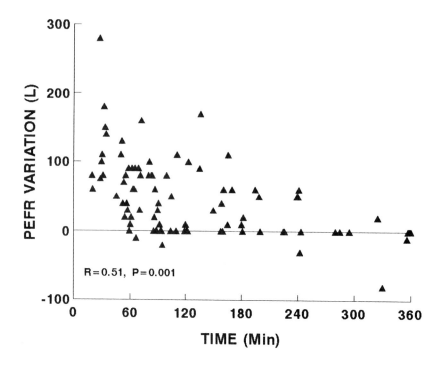

R = 0.51, P = 0.001

Figure 8-1
Correlation between variation of PEFR at 30 minutes from baseline value and duration of treatment. (Modified from Rodrigo and Rodrigo[108]).

pitalization for asthma. Various scoring systems have been elaborated for this purpose. Fischl and colleagues developed a predictive index using a combination of presenting factors: pulse rate, ≥ 120 per minute; respiratory rate, ≥ 30 per minute; pulsus paradoxus, ≥ 18 mm Hg; PEFR, ≤ 120 L per minute; moderate to severe dyspnea; accessory muscle use; and wheezing.[109] A score of 4 or higher (range, 0 to 7) was 95 % accurate in predicting the risk of relapse and 96% accurate in predicting the need for hospitalization. However, subsequent prospective studies failed to confirm the predictive accuracy of this index. For example, Rose and colleagues did not corroborate the precision of Fischl's index for evaluating patients with asthma who presented to an ED.[110] With index scores ≥ 4, the index exhibited a sensitivity of 0.40 and a specificity of 0.71. In the same way, Centor and colleagues failed to confirm the predictive accuracy of the index.[111] With a score of 4 or higher considered a positive test, the sensitivity for predicting hospital admission was 50%, whereas the specificity was 84.2%. When the test was used for predicting a relapse, the sensitivity was only 18.1%

with a specificity of 82.4%. Conflicting results also were obtained when scoring systems were applied to children with asthma in acute care settings. Kerem and colleagues studied prospectively 200 children with acute asthma.[112] A clinical score based on standard physical examination (i.e., heart and respiratory rates, pulsus paradoxus, dyspnea, accessory muscle use, and wheezing) was found to be the most effective in predicting outcome (hospitalized versus discharged patients). When each individual component of the clinical score on presentation was analyzed as an independent variable, the dyspnea score was the most predictive, with higher sensitivity but lower specificity than the overall clinical score. Neither the initial pulmonary function nor the absolute change in its value with treatment was helpful in predicting outcomes in this study.

Contrary to the Kerem study, Schuh and colleagues, in a retrospective review of data from a randomized, double-blind, placebo-controlled trial of 120 asthma patients 5 to 17 years of age, concluded that an $FEV_1 \leq 30\%$ of the predicted value and an asthma score ≥ 6 (i.e., accessory muscle use, wheezing, and dyspnea), both at 2 hours after the initiation of therapy, predicted the need for hospitalization.[113] By contrast, patients with an $FEV_1 \geq 60\%$ and an asthma score <3 had a high probability of being discharged. The system they employed was based on and modified from the score used by Fischl and colleagues and Kerem and co-workers.

Recently, in an effort to identify variables that can predict the outcome of patients with acute asthma, Rodrigo and Rodrigo retrospectively studied 163 adults with asthma (analysis sample) who presented to an ED.[114] All patients with persistent wheezing, dyspnea, and accessory muscle use at rest despite 6 hours of ED treatment were hospitalized. A multivariate analysis (discriminant analysis) identified three independent variables that made the greatest contribution in differentiating the two groups studied (discharged and hospitalized patients): PEFR variation over baseline, PEFR as percentage of the predicted value, and accessory muscle use, all measured at 30 minute after the beginning of treatment. A multifactorial index (range, 0 to 6) was developed using these variables (Table 8-3).

With a score of 4 or higher considered a positive test, a sensitivity of 0.86, a specificity of 0.96, a positive predictive value of 0.75, and a negative predictive value of 0.97 were obtained. To test the validity, the index was applied prospectively to a second sample (validation sample) of 91 acute asthma patients. The sensitivity, specificity, and predictive positive and negative values were 0.83, 0.97, 0.83, and 0.97, respectively.

Table 8-3
Predictive index scoring system

Variable	Score 0	Score 1	Score 2
Change in PEFR at 30 minutes (L/min)	>50	50-20	<20
PEFR at 30 minutes (% of predicted)	>45	45-35	<35
Accessory muscle use at 30 minutes	0-1	2	3

SOURCE: From Rodrigo and Rodrigo.[114]

Therefore, this simple index composed of three variables can facilitate an early decision (at 30 minutes of treatment) to hospitalize patients with severe asthma.

The EPR-2[15] stated that patients with a poor response are those who, despite a few hours of treatment in the ED, still have significant wheezing, shortness of breath, and persistent reduction of lung function ($FEV_1 \leq 40\%$ of predicted value). To elaborate, an acute asthma index for utilization in the early differentiation between patients with poor and good therapeutic respones in the ED setting, Rodrigo and Rodrigo studied 145 consecutive adult patients who presented to an ED (analysis sample).[115] The outcome was defined as the FEV_1 value after 3 hours of treatment in a dichotomized form: ≤45% of predicted value or poor response and >45% of predicted value or good response. Again, PEFR % of predicted value and PEFR increase from baseline, both measured at 30 minutes, were the most important predictors of the outcome after 3 hours of treatment.

INDICATIONS FOR HOSPITALIZATION

It usually takes days to weeks for a patient to return to normal lung function after a severe asthma exacerbation. McFadden and colleagues assessed changes in lung function before and after therapy in acute asthma patients.[116] When patients report that their symptoms have resolved, their FEV_1 may continue to be significantly low. The critical question facing the physician in the ED is whether outpatient therapy can safely and effectively achieve this return to normal lung function, or whether hospitalization is required. The decision to hospitalize a patient should be based on duration and severity of symptoms, severity of airflow obstruction, course and severity of prior exacerbations, medication use at the time of the exacerbation, access to medical care and medication, adequacy of support and home conditions, and presence of psychiatric illness. At either end of the severity spectrum, the decision whether to hospitalize patients with asthma is easy. As such, if despite 1 to 2 hours of treatment in the ED a patient still has significant wheezing, accessory muscle use, exercise limitation, and a persistent reduction in lung function (FEV_1 or PEFR $\leq 40\%$ of normal), the patient should be hospitalized. On the other hand, if a patient is free of symptoms, does not wheeze on auscultation and has normal or nearly normal lung function (FEV_1 or PEFR 60% of normal,[113]) the patient can be discharged from the ED. Observation for a minimum of 30 minutes after the last dose of a β agonist is recommended to ensure stability before discharge.

The greatest risk lies in determining whether to hospitalize asthmatic patients who fall between these two extremes (i.e., have an incomplete response to therapy). Patients in this group require continued treatment, but keeping patients for many hours in the ED while awaiting sufficient improvement constitutes inappropriate use of ED resources. We believe that a decision should be reached within 2 hours of the initiation of treatment. We recommend measurement of lung function before disposition and the use of the results of PEFR or FEV_1 at 30 minutes in the decision-making process.[18,108,114,115] Almost two thirds of patients have a quick response to high doses of inhaled β agonists (67% obtain the discharge threshold within 1 hour of treatment).[117,118] In the remaining one third of patients, β agonists have little effect. It is clear that there is little to be gained by prolonging treatment in the ED. If an attack does not resolve within a brief period (i.e., 1 to 2 hours), it is unlikely to do so. Patients with a poor response also have a greater number of recent ED visits and should be targeted for more aggressive management of their asthma.[119] This approach typically is associated with a low rate of relapses within 24 hours.[48,114,120]

Finally, patients with findings of severe airflow obstruction (i.e., use of accessory muscles of respiration, hypercapnia, or PEFR $\leq 40\%$ of predicted value) who deteriorate despite therapy should be admitted to an ICU. Other indications for ICU admission include respiratory arrest and altered mental status. We also recommend ICU admission for patients who present initially with mild or moderate obstruction but who deteriorate in the ED, despite therapy.

CONCLUSIONS

The death rate from asthma has increased in the last decade. Surveys have shown inadequate or incomplete assessment in outpatient and inpatient settings. Consequently, close monitoring of an asthma patient's condition and response to treatment, including serial measurements of lung function, is an essential part of care. The severity of airflow obstruction may not be accurately judged on the basis of symptoms and physical examination. Accordingly, it is very important to use an objective measure of airway obstruction (spirometry or peak flow meter) in the ED. Failure of initial therapy to improve expiratory flow predicts a more severe course and need for hospitalization. Thus, FEV_1 or PEFR measures at 30 minutes of treatment are the variables most predictive of outcome. The presence of accessory muscle use also can be considered a sign of severity. Arterial blood gas determination is rarely necessary. However, oxygen saturation, measured by pulse oximetry, can give an indication of which patients with acute severe asthma are likely to be in respiratory failure and therefore in need of more intensive management. Keeping patients for many hours in the ED, while awaiting sufficient improvement so that they can be sent home, constitutes inappropriate use of ED resources. A decision should be reached within 2 hours of the initiation of treatment.

REFERENCES

 1. Sly RM: Mortality from asthma. 1979–1984. *J Allergy Clin Immunol* 82:705–717, 1988.
 2. Sly RM: Mortality from asthma in children. 1979–1984. *Ann Allergy* 60:433–443, 1988.
 3. Sears MR: Worldwide trends in asthma mortality. *Bull Int Tuberc Lung Dis* 66:79–83, 1991.
 4. Strunk RC: Deaths due to asthma. *Am Rev Respir Dis* 148:550–555, 1993.
 5. McFadden ER, Warren EL: Observations on asthma mortality. *Ann Intern Med* 127:142–147, 1997.
 6. MacDonald JB, MacDonald ET, Seaton A, Williams DA: Asthma deaths in Cardiff 1963–74: 53 deaths in hospital. *Br Med J* 2:721–723, 1976.
 7. British Thoracic Association: Death from asthma

in two regions of England. *Br Med Jr* 285:1251–1255, 1982.

8. Robertson CF, Rubinfeld AR, Bowes G: Deaths from asthma in Victoria: A 12-month study. *Med J Aust* 152:511–517, 1990.

9. Roe PF: Sudden death in asthma. *Br J Dis Chest* 59:158–163, 1965.

10. Crompton G: The catastrophic asthmatic. *Br J Dis Chest* 81:321–325, 1987.

11. Wasserfallen JB, Schaller MD, Feihl F, Perret CH: Sudden asphyxic asthma: A distinct entity? *Am Rev Respir Dis* 142:108–111, 1990.

12. Rothwell RP, Rea HH, Sears MR, et al: Lessons from the national asthma mortality study: Deaths in hospital. *N Z Med J* 100:199–202, 1987.

13. Burney PG: Asthma mortality in England and Wales: evidence for a further increase, 1974–84. *Lancet* 2:323–326, 1986.

14. Barger LW, Vollmer WM, Felt RW, Buist AS: Further investigation into the recent increase in asthma death rates: A review of 41 deaths in Oregon in 1982. *Ann Allergy* 60:31–39, 1988.

15. National Blood, Lung, and Heart Institute: *National Asthma Education and Prevention Program Expert Panel Report 2: Guidelines for the diagnosis and management of asthma.* Bethesda, National Institutes of Health, Publ No. 55-4051, 1997.

16. FitzGerald JM, Hargreave FE: The assessment and management of acute life-threatening asthma. *Chest* 95:888–894, 1989.

17. Bailey WC, Higgins DM, Richards BM, Richards JM: Asthma severity: A factor analytic investigation. *Am J Med* 93:263–269, 1992.

18. Rodrigo G, Rodrigo C: Assessment of the patient with acute asthma in the emergency department. A factor analytic study. *Chest* 104:1325–1328, 1993.

19. Fanta CH, Israel E, Sheffer Al: Managing and preventing severe asthma attacks. *J Respir Dis* 13:94–108, 1993.

20. Dales RE, Schweitzer I, Kerr P, et al: Risk factors for the recurrent emergency department visits for asthma. *Thorax* 50:520–24, 1995.

21. Reed S, Diggle S, Cushley MJ, Sleet RA, Tattersfield AE: Assessment and management of asthma in an accident and emergency department. *Thorax* 40:897–902, 1985.

22. Daley JD, Kopelman RI, Comeau E, et al: Practice patterns in the treatment of acutely ill hospitalized asthmatic patients at three teaching hospitals. *Chest* 100:51–56, 1991.

23. Spevetz A, Bartter T, Dubois J, Pratter MR: Inpa-tient management of status asthmaticus. *Chest* 102:1392–1396, 1992.

24. Kuo E, Kesten S: A retrospective comparative study of in-hospital management of acute severe asthma: 1984 vs 1989. *Chest* 103:1655–1661, 1993.

25. Robertson CF, Rubinfeld AR, Bowes G: Pediatric asthma deaths in Victoria: The mild are of risk. *Pediatr Pulmonol* 13:95–100, 1992.

26. Foucard T, Graff-Lonnevig V: Asthma mortality rate in Swedish children and young adults 1973–88. *Allergy* 49:616–619, 1994.

27. Rea HH, Scragg R, Jackson R, Beaglehole R, et al: A case-controlled study of deaths from asthma. *Thorax* 41:833–839, 1986.

28. Sears MR, Rea HH, Rothwell RP, et al: Asthma mortality: Comparison between New Zealand and England. *Br Med J* 293:1342–1345, 1986.

29. Ryan G, Musk AW, Perera DM, et al: Risk factors for death in patients admitted to hospital with asthma: A follow up study. *Aust N Z Med* 21:681–685, 1991.

30. Greenberger PA, Miller TP, Lifschultz B: Circumstances surrounding deaths from asthma in Cook County (Chicago) Illinois. *Allergy Proc* 14:321—236, 1993.

31. Kallembach JM, Frankel AH, Lapinsky SE, et al: Determinants of near fatality in acute severe asthma. *Am J Med* 95:265–272, 1993.

32. Suissa S, Ernst P, Bolvin JF et al: A cohort analysis of excess mortality in asthma and the use of inhaled β-agonists. *Am J Respir Crit Care Med* 49:604–610, 1994.

33. Buist AS. Vollmer WM: Preventing deaths from asthma. *N Engl J Med* 331:1584–1585, 1994.

34. Gottlieb DJ. Beiser A, O'Conoor GT: Poverty, race and medication use are correlates of asthma hospitalization rates. A small are analysis in Boston. *Chest* 108:28–35, 1995.

35. Hanania NA, Wang AD, Kesten S. Chapman KR: Factors associated with emergency department dependence of patients with asthma. *Chest* 111:290–295, 1997.

36. Woodruff PG, Edmond SD, Singh AK, Camargo CA. Sudden-onset acute asthma: clinical features and response to therapy. *Acad Emerg Med* 5:695–701, 1998.

37. Brenner BE, Abraham E, Simon RR: Position and diaphoresis in acute asthma. *Am J Med* 74:1005–1009, 1983.

38. Edelson JD, Rebuck AS: The clinical assessment of severe asthma. *Arch Intern Med* 145:321–323, 1985.

39. Rebuck AS, Read J: Assessment and management of severe asthma. *AM J Med* 51:788, 1971.

40. Knowles G, Clark TJH: Pulsus paradoxus as a valuable sign indicating severity of asthma. *Lancet* 2:1356–1359, 1973.

41. Permutt S, Wise RA: Mechanichal interactions of respiration and circulation, in Fishman A (ed): *Handbook of Physiology,* vol 3. Baltimore, Williams and Wilkins, 1986, pp 647–662.

42. Pearson MG, Spence DP, Ryland I, Harrison BDW: Value of pulsus paradoxus in assessing acute severe asthma. British Thoracic Society Standards of Care Committee. *Br Med J* 307:659, 1993.

43. British Asthma Guidelines Coordinating Committee: British guidelines on asthma management: 1995 review and position statement. *Thorax* 52: S1–21, 1997.

44. Shim CS, Williams MH: Relationship of wheezing to the severity of obstruction in asthma. *Arch Intern Med* 143:890–892, 1983.

45. Rubinfeld AR, Pain MCF: Relationship between bronchial reactivity, airway caliber, and the severity of asthma. *Am Rev Respir Dis* 115:381–387, 1977.

46. Kendrick AH, Higss CMB, Whitfield MJ, Laszlo G: Accuracy of perception of severity of asthma: Patients treated in general practice. *Br Med J* 307:422–424, 1993.

47. Hudgel DW, Weil JV: Asthma associated with decreased hypoxic ventilatory drive. A family study. *Ann Intern Med* 80:623–625, 1974.

48. Kikuchi Y, Okabe S, Tamura G, et al: Chemosensitivity and perception of dyspnea in patients with a history of near-fatal asthma. *N Engl J Med* 330:1329–1334, 1994.

49. Shim CS, Williams MH: Evaluation of the severity of asthma: Patients versus physicians. *Am J Med* 68:11–13, 1980.

50. Rodrigo C, Rodrigo G: Early administration of hydrocortisone in the emergency room treatment of acute asthma: A controlled clinical trial. *Resp Med* 88:755–761, 1994.

51. Rodrigo C, Rodrigo G: Treatment of acute asthma. Lack of therapeutic benefit and increase of the toxicity from aminophylline given in addition to high doses of salbutamol delivered by metered-dose inhaler with spacer. *Chest* 106:1071–1076, 1994.

52. Rodrigo G, Rodrigo C: Effect of age on bronchodilator response in the acute asthma treatment. *Chest* 112:19–23, 1997.

53. Kelsen SG, Kelsen DP, Fleegler BF, et al: Emergency room assessment and treatment of patients with acute asthma. *Am J Med* 64:622–628, 1978.

54. Tai R, Read J: Blood-gas tensions in bronchial asthma. *Lancet* 1:644–646, 1967.

55. McFadden ER Jr, Lyons HA: Arterial-blood tensions in asthma. *N Engl J Med* 278:1027–1032, 1968.

56. Miyamoto T, Mizuno K, Furuya K: Arterial blood gases in bronchial asthma. *J Allergy.* 45:248–254, 1970.

57. Weng TR, Langer HM, Featherby EA, Levison H: Arterial blood gas tensions and acid-base balance in symptomatic and asymptomatic asthma in childhood. *Am Rev Respir Dis* 101:274–282, 1970.

58. Martin TG, Elenbaas RM, Pingleton SH: Use of peak expiratory flow rates to eliminate unnecessary arterial blood gases in the acute asthma. *Ann Emerg Med* 11:70–73, 1982.

59. Nowak RM, Tomlanovich MC, Sarkar DD, et al: Arterial blood gases and pulmonary function testing in acute bronchial asthma. *JAMA* 249:2043–2046, 1983.

60. Roca J, Ramis LI, Rodriguez-Roisin R, et al: Serial relationships between ventilation-perfusion inequality and spirometry in acute severe asthma requiring hospitalization. *Am Rev Respir Dis* 137:1055–1061, 1988.

61. Ballester E, Reyes A, Roca J, et al: Ventilation-perfusion mismatching in acute severe asthma: Effects of salbutamol and 100% oxygen. *Thorax* 44:258–267, 1989.

62. Rodriguez-Roisin R: Acute severe asthma: Pathophysiology and pathobiology of gas exchange abnormalities. *Eur Respir J* 10:1359–1371, 1997.

63. Geelhoed GC, Landau LI, Le Souef PN: Evaluation of SaO_2 as a predictor of outcome in 280 children presenting with acute asthma. *Ann Emerg Med* 23:1236–1241, 1994.

64. Carruthers DM, Harrison BDW: Arterial blood gas analysis or oxygen saturation in the assessment of acute asthma? *Thorax* 50:186–188, 1995.

65. Findley LJ, Sahn SA: The value of chest roentgenograms in acute asthma in adults. *Chest* 5:535–536, 1980.

66. Zieverink SE, Harper AP, Holden RW, et al: Emergency room radiography of asthma: An efficacy study. *Radiology* 145:27–29, 1982.

67. Blair DN, Coppage L, Shaw C: Medical imaging in asthma. *J Thorac Imaging* 1:23–25, 1986.

68. Sherman S, Skoney JA, Ravikrishnan KP: Routine

chest radiographs in exacerbations of acute obstructive pulmonary disease. *Arch Intern Med* 149:2493–2496, 1989.

69. White CS, Cole P, Lubetsky HW, Austin JHM: Acute asthma: Admission chest radiography in hospitalized adult patients. *Chest* 100:14–16, 1991.

70. Lavechia V, Rodrigo C, Maraffi L, Rodrigo G: Valor de la radiografía de tórax en pacientes asmáticos agudos que consultan en un servicio de emergencia. *Pac Critico* 5:128–132, 1992.

71. Friedman M, Walker S: Assessment of lung function using an airflow meter. *Lancet* 1:310–311, 1975.

72. Haydu SP, Chapman TT, Hughes DD: Pulmonary monitor for assessment of airways obstruction. *Lancet* 2:1225–1226, 1976.

73. Katz DN: The mini-Wright peak flow meter for evaluating airway obstruction in a family practice. *J Fam Pract* 17:51–57, 1983.

74. Daman HR: Pulmonary function testing: Use of the peak expiratory flow rate in an out-patient or office setting. *J Asthma* 21:331–337, 1984.

75. Litvan H, Canet J, Balañá LI, Sanchis J: Medidores simples de flujo espiratorio en la valoración preoperatoria de la función pulmonar. *Revista Española de Anestesiología y Reanimación* 31:131–143, 1984.

76. Cherniack RM: Use of pulmonary function tests in the assessment and treatment of patients with airway hyperreactivity. *Clin Rev Allergy* 3:395–409, 1985.

77. Williams AI, Church SE: Availability of mini peak flow meters for the management of severe asthma. *Lancet* 1:1341, 1985.

78. Connolly CK, Chan NS: Relationship between different measurements of respiratory function in asthma *Respiration* 52:22–33, 1987.

79. Kelly CA, Gibson GJ: Relation between FEV_1 and peak expiratory flow in patients with chronic airflow obstruction. *Thorax* 43:335–336, 1988.

80. Meltzer AA, Smolensky MH, D'Alonzo GE, et al: An assessment of peak expiratory flow as a surrogate measurement of FEV_1 in stable asthmatic children. *Chest* 96:329–333, 1989.

81. Vaughan MTR, Weber CRW, Tipton WR, Nelson HS: Comparison of PEFR and FEV_1 in patients with varying degrees of airway obstruction. Effect of modest altitude. *Chest* 95:558–562, 1989.

82. Bérubé D, Cartier A, L'Archeveque J, et al: Comparison of peak expiratory flow rate and FEV_1 in assessing bronchomotor tone after challenges with occupational sensitizers. *Chest* 99:831–836, 1991.

83. Paggiaro PL, Moscato G, Gianninni D, et al: Relationship between peak expiratory flow (PEF) and FEV_1 *Eur Respir J* 10(Suppl):39–41, 1997.

84. Nowak RM, Pensler MI, Sarkar DD, et al: Comparison of peak expiratory flow and FEV_1 admission criteria for acute bronchial asthma. *Ann Emerg Med* 11:64–69, 1982.

85. Rodrigo C, Rodrigo G: Comparación entre el pico de flujo espiratorio y el volumen espiratorio forzado en el primer segundo en pacientes en crisis asmática. *Rev Med Uruguay* 10:15–19, 1994.

86. Shapiro SM, Hendler JM, Ogirala RG, et al: An evaluation of the accuracy of assess and mini-Wright peak flowmeters. *Chest* 99:358–62, 1991.

87. Miller MR, Dickinson SA, Hitchings DJ: The accuracy of portable peak flow meters. *Thorax* 47:904–909, 1992.

88. Gardner RM, Crapo RO, Jackson BR, Jensen RL: Evaluation of accuracy and reproducibility of peak flow meters at 1400 m. *Chest* 101:948–952, 1992.

89. Douma WR, van der Mark ThW, Folgering HThM. Kort E, et al: Mini-Wright peak flow meters are reliable after 5 years use. *Eur Respir J* 10:457–459, 1997.

90. Lim TK, Ang SM, Rossing TH, et al: The effects of deep inhalation on maximal expiratory flow during intensive treatment of spontaneous asthmatic episodes. *Am Rev Respir Dis* 140:1168–1169, 1989.

91. Lemarchand PS, Herer LB, Huchon GJ: Cardiorespiratory arrest following peak expiratory flow measurement during attack of asthma. *Chest* 100:1168–1169, 1991.

92. Miller TP, Greenberg PA: The diagnosis of potentially fatal asthma in hospitalized adults. Patients characteristics and increased severity of asthma. *Chest* 102:515–518, 1992.

93. Rodrigo G, Rodrigo C: Comparison of salbutamol delivered by nebulizer or metered dose inhaler with a pear-shaped spacer in acute asthma. *Curr Ther Res* 54:797–808, 1993.

94. Rodrigo C, Rodrigo G: High-dose MDI salbutamol treatment of asthma in the ED. *Am J Emerg Med* 13:21–26, 1995.

95. Rodrigo G, Rodrigo C: Metered dose inhaler salbutamol treatment of asthma in the ED: Comparison of two doses with plasma levels. *Am J Emerg Med* 144–150, 1996.

96. Hall JB, Wood LDH: Management of the critically ill asthmatic patient. *Med Clin N Am* 74:779–796, 1990.

97. Fishman AP: Cardiac asthma. A fresh look at an old wheeze. *N Engl J Med* 320:1346–1348, 1989.

98. Schmidt GA, Hall JB: Acute on chronic respiratory failure. Assessment and management of patients with COPD in the emergent setting. *JAMA* 251:2688–2689, 1984.

99. Baughman RP, Loudon RC: Stridor: Differentiation from wheezing or upper airway noise. *Am Rev Respir Dis* 139:1407–1409, 1989.

100. Christopher KL, Wood RP, Eckert RC, et al: Vocal cord dysfunction presenting as asthma. *N Engl J Med* 308:1566–1570, 1983.

101. Bucca C, Rolla G, Brussino L, De Rose V, Bugiani M: Are asthma-like symptoms due to the bronchial or extrathoracic airway dysfunction? *Lancet* 346:791–795, 1995.

102. Newman KB, Mason UG, Schmaling KB: Clinical features of vocal cord dysfunction. *Am J Respir Crit Care Med* 152:1382–1386, 1995.

103. Stein PD, Willis PW, DeMets DL: History and physical examination in acute pulmonary embolism in patients without preexisting cardiac or pulmonary disease. *Am J Cardiol* 47:218–223, 1981.

104. Pauwels R, Snashall PD: *A Practical Approach to Asthma.* London, CBA Publishing Services, 1986, pp 67–69.

105. Banner AS, Shah RS, Addington WW: Rapid prediction of need for hospitalization in acute asthma. *JAMA* 235:1337–1338, 1976.

106. Fanta CH, Rossing TH, McFadden Jr ED: Emergency room treatment of asthma: Relationships among therapeutic combinations, severity of obstruction and time course of response. *Am J Med* 72:416–422, 1982.

107. Stein LM, Cole RP: Early administration of corticosteroids in emergency room treatment of acute asthma. *Ann Intern Med* 112:822–827, 1990.

108. Rodrigo G, Rodrigo C: Tratamiento de la crisis asmática: comparación entre fenoterol y salbutamol en altas dosis administradas con inhalador de dosis medida con inhalocámara (Volumatic) y aminofilina intravenosa. *Pac Crítico* 4:194–209, 1991.

109. Fischl MA, Pitchenik A, Gardner LB: An index predicting relapse and need for hospitalization in patients with acute bronchial asthma. *N Engl J Med* 305:783–789, 1981.

110. Rose CC, Murphy JG, Schwartz JS: Performance of an index predicting the response of patients with acute bronchial asthma to intensive emergency department treatment. *N Engl J Med* 310:573–577, 1984.

111. Centor RM, Yarbrough B, Wood JP: Inability to predict relapse in acute asthma. *N Engl J Med* 310:577–580, 1984.

112. Kerem E, Tibshirani R, Canny G, et al: Predicting the need for hospitalization in children with acute asthma. *Chest* 98:1355–1361, 1990.

113. Schuh S, Johnson D, Stephens D, et al: Hospitalization patterns in severe acute asthma in children. *Pediatr Pulmonol* 23:184–192, 1997.

114. Rodrigo G, Rodrigo C: A new index for early prediction of hospitalization in patients with acute asthma. *Am J Emerg Med* 15:8–13, 1997.

115. Rodrigo G, Rodrigo C: Early prediction of poor response acute asthma patients in the emergency department. *Chest.* 114:1016–1021, 1999.

116. McFadden ER, Kiser R, DeGroot W: Acute bronchial asthma: Relationship between clinical and physiological manifestations. *N Engl J Med* 288:221–225, 1973.

117. Strauss L, Hejal R, Galan G, et al: Observations on the effects of aerosolized albuterol in acute asthma. *Am J Respir Crit Care Med* 155:454–458, 1997.

118. Rodrigo C, Rodrigo G. Therapeutic response patterns to high and cumulative doses of salbutamol in acute severe asthma. *Chest.* 113:593–598, 1998.

119. Emerman CL, Cydulka RK: Factors associated with relapse after emergency department treatment for acute asthma. *Ann Emerg Med* 26:6–11, 1995.

120. McFadden ER, Elsandi N, Dixon L, et al: Protocol therapy for acute asthma: Therapeutic benefits and cost savings. *Am J Med* 99:651–661, 1995.

CHAPTER 9

PHARMACOTHERAPY OF ACUTE ASTHMA

Patrick T. Murray
Thomas Corbridge

INTRODUCTION

Asthma is a disease characterized by wheezing, dyspnea, and cough resulting from airway wall inflammation, airway hyperreactivity, and variable degrees of reversible airflow obstruction. Current paradigms emphasize the role of airway wall inflammation, smooth-muscle mediated bronchoconstriction, airway wall remodeling, and intraluminal mucus in the pathogenesis of this disease.[1-3] All asthmatics are at risk of developing a severe attack that places them at risk of developing respiratory failure. This disorder is referred to as *status asthmaticus* (SA).[4] Asthma attacks can occur at any time and at any place. A sudden and unexpected increase in airflow obstruction results primarily from bronchial smooth muscle-mediated bronchospasm and is termed *sudden asphyxic asthma*. Such acute deterioration may be triggered by allergens, medications including aspirin or β blockers, and inhalation of illicit drugs such as heroin[4a] or cocaine. Often, a trigger is never identified. More commonly, asthma worsens over several hours (>3 hours) or days. In this situation, airway wall inflammation, edema, and intraluminal mucus also contribute to airflow obstruction. Despite the relatively slow evolution of this form of SA, many patients miss the opportunity to treat worsening airway inflammation, choosing instead to increase their use of β agonists as a sole treatment strategy.[5]

No matter the time course, patients with SA have a life-threatening illness that can result in respiratory failure and death. Aggressive pharmacotherapy is crucial to improve airflow obstruction and help avert the progression to respiratory failure requiring assisted ventilation. The purpose of this chapter is to provide a basis for rational pharmacotherapy of acute asthma by reviewing common and novel drugs with attention to pertinent studies, drug dosing, the potential for adverse drug reactions, drug deposition, pharmacodynamic features, and outcome data for each drug administered. Additional information regarding inhaled therapy in nonintubated and intubated patients can be found in chapters 10 and 11, respectively.

β AGONISTS

Inhaled β agonists are the drugs of choice to treat smooth muscle-mediated bronchoconstriction in acute asthma (Table 9-1). Their onset of action is rapid and their side effects are generally well tolerated. Albuterol is the most frequently used drug in adults. Many experienced clinicians choose albuterol because it has a slightly longer duration of action and greater β_2-adrenoreceptor selectivity than metaproterenol, and results in less cardiac stimulation.[6-8] Some clinicians prefer metaproterenol or isoetharine for initial therapy because of their faster onset of action, despite their tendency to increase side effects.[9] Long-acting β agonists, such as salmeterol, have not been studied adequately in acute asthma. They are generally not recommended because of their slow onset of action and also because their effects, in conjunction with short-acting drugs in acute illness, are un-

Table 9-1
Drugs Used in the Treatment of Acute Asthma

Agents	Regimens
Albuterol	0.5 ml of 5% solution (2.5 mg; 5 mg/mL) in 2.5 mL normal saline by nebulization for 3 doses, then 2.5–10 mg every 1–4 h as needed, ⟨or⟩ 10–15 mg/h continuously ⟨or⟩ 4–8 puffs (90 μg/puff) by MDI with spacer every 20 min up to 4 h, then every 1–4 h as needed
Epinephrine	0.3–0.5 mL of a 1:1,000 solution (1 mg/mL) subcutaneously every 20 min for 3 doses; terbutaline (0.25 mg/dose) is favored in pregnant patients when parenteral therapy is indicated. Use with caution in patients older than 40 yr of age and in patients with coronay artery disease
Corticosteroids	Methylprednisolone 60–125 mg given intravenously every 6 h ⟨or⟩ prednisone 30–40 mg orally every 6 h
Oxygen	1–3 L/min by nasal cannula; titrate using pulse oximeter
Anticholinergics	Ipratropium bromide 0.5 mg by nebulization every 30 min for 3 doses, then every 2–4 h as needed; may be mixed with albuterol, and should be added to β_2 agonist rather than used as 1st-line therapy ⟨or⟩ 4–8 puffs by MDI (18 μg/puff) with spacer every 20 min × 3 ⟨or⟩ Glycopyrrolate 2 mg by nebulization every hour × 3
Theophylline	5 mg/kg intravenously over 30 min loading dose (in patients not previously receiving theophylline), followed by 0.4 mg/kg/h intravenous maintenance infusion. Check serum level within 6 h of loading dose. Watch for adverse drug reactions due to drug-drug and drug-disease interactions (see text).
Alternate Therapies Magnesium sulfate	2 g intravenously over 20 min; if hypomagnesemic, dose adequately to normalize serum concentration
Heliox	80:20, 70:30, or 60:40 helium:oxygen mix (%) by tight-fitting, nonrebreathing face mask. Higher helium concentrations are required for maximal effect

SOURCE: From National Institutes of Health[3]; Corbridge and Hall.[4]

known. An interesting new development in the arena of inhaled β agonist therapy is the availability of levalbuterol. Racemic albuterol is an equal mixture of the active enantiomer, (R) albuterol or levalbuterol, and inactive, or possibly even detrimental, (S) albuterol. In a recent study of stable asthma patients, levalbuterol appeared to provide a better therapeutic index than the standard dose of racemic albuterol.[10] In a subgroup of patients with pretreatment FEV_1 of 60% of predicted normal or less, 1.25 mg levalbuterol by nebulization increased FEV_1 to a greater extent than 2.5 mg racemic albuterol. Levalbuterol may prove to be more efficacious and less toxic than racemic albuterol, but further studies in SA are clearly needed before strong conclusions can be drawn.

Although overreliance on inhaled β agonists is unwise in the outpatient setting, underuse of these agents is a mistake in acute asthma management. These drugs should be used in a repetitive or continuous manner until there is a convincing clinical response or toxic side effects limit further drug administration.[11–13] Recent intensified use of β agonists should not preclude high-dose β agonist administration in the emergency department (ED) unless serious β agonist side effects are identified.[14] Many patients improve after additional therapy, which suggests poor outpatient drug delivery technique and/or the need for even greater drug doses. Larger and more frequent doses may be needed in acute asthma because the dose-response curve and duration of activity of these drugs are affected adversely by the degree of bronchoconstriction.[15]

The optimal dose of albuterol has yet to be established in acute asthma. McFadden and colleagues have compared two 5 mg treatments of albuterol by nebulization over 40 minutes to the standard dose of three 2.5 mg albuterol every 20 minutes, in 160 patients with acute asthma.[16] Peak expiratory flow rates (PEFR) improved in a dose-response fashion as the cumulative quantity of albuterol increased. That is, a single treatment of 5 mg albuterol achieved the same effect as two doses of 2.5 mg each, and 10 mg albuterol increased bronchodilation more than did 7.5 mg. Overall, the 5 mg regimen increased peak flows more rapidly and to a greater extent than the standard 2.5 mg approach. Patients receiving 5 mg doses also reached predetermined discharge criteria more rapidly and left the ED with their peak flow rates closer to normal. There was a trend toward fewer hospitalizations in the high-dose group (25 of 80 patients, 31%) than in the lower dose group (37 of 80 patients, 46%) ($P = .06$). Not surprisingly, patients admitted to the hospital had a blunted cumulative dose-response relationship to albuterol.

Emerman and colleagues compared the effects of 2.5 mg to 7.5 mg albuterol every 20 minutes for a total of 3 doses in 160 patients with acute asthma in an ED.[17] There was no difference in improvement in FEV_1 or admission rates between groups. McDermott and colleagues conducted a randomized, double-blind trial of two regimens of nebulized metaproterenol in 71 acute asthmatics presenting to an ED.[17a] The experimental group received 3 treatments in the first hour and hourly thereafter to hour 7. The control group was treated at time 0 and at hours 1, 3, 5 and 7. There were no differences in PEFR, time to discharge, or admission rates, but the experimental group had more tachycardia and ECG changes (atrial fibrillation in 1 patient and ischemia in another). Rodrigo and Rodrigo gave 4 puffs of albuterol (400 μg) at 10 minute intervals to 116 acute asthma patients in an ED.[18] After administration of 2.4 mg albuterol, 67% of patients obtained discharge criteria within 1 hour, one half of whom met discharge criteria after receiving only 12 puffs. Similarly, Strauss and colleagues found that two thirds of patients with acute asthma could be discharged from an ED after three 2.5 mg doses of albuterol by nebulization every 20 minutes.[19] These data demonstrate that about two thirds of acutely ill asthma patients seen in an ED can be successfully treated with albuterol alone and discharged home (with either inhaled or oral corticosteroids), and that the early response to albuterol is a good predictor of the need for hospitalization.[20]

β agonists should be given continuously to severely obstructed patients until there is a clinical response or adverse effects limit further drug administration (e.g., excessive tachycardia, arrhythmias, or tremor). High-dose inhaled β agonists are generally well tolerated. Tremor and tachycardia are common, but significant cardiovascular morbidity is not.[21] Since β-adrenoreceptor stimulation increases cellular Na-K-ATPase activity, hypokalemia requiring replacement therapy is routine in acutely ill patients receiving high-dose β agonists. This is particularly true when other agents that cause hypokalemia are added, such as corticosteroids and theophylline. High-dose β-adrenoreceptor stimulation also seems to contribute to the pathogenesis of lactic acidosis during SA, which more commonly develops in patients receiving injected β agonists (terbutaline, epinephrine).[22] The relative contribution of β agonists to the development of lactic acidosis is unknown given the other possible mechanisms for lactic acid accumulation (namely, increased work of breathing, tissue hypoxia, intracellular alkalosis, and changes in hepatic blood flow caused by hyperinflation).

Inhaled β agonists may be delivered equally well by metered dose inhaler (MDI) with spacer or by hand-held nebulizer, in patients able to use each effectively. Anywhere from 4 to 12 puffs by MDI with spacer achieves the same degree of bronchodilation as does one nebulized treatment.[23–27] Even in patients with severe disease, Idris and colleagues demonstrated that four puffs of albuterol (0.36 mg) delivered by MDI with spacer was as effective as 2.5 mg of albuterol by nebulization.[23] Turner and colleagues demonstrated equal efficacy between three puffs of metaproterenol delivered by MDI with spacer and 15 mg of metaproterenol by nebulization in the treatment of acute airflow obstruction.[26] Similarly, Rodrigo and Rodrigo recently demonstrated that inhaled bronchodilators can be delivered effectively by either MDI with spacer or hand-held nebulizer in acute asthma.[27] In recently extubated patients, MDIs can be used successfully in most cases. Tenholder and colleagues demonstrated a 70% success rate for conversion from nebulized therapy to MDI.[28] Failed conversions were seen mainly in patients unable to follow instructions and in patients with neuromuscular disease. Despite these data supporting the use of MDIs in the acute setting, many clinicians still prefer hand-held nebulizers because fewer instructions are needed, less coordination is required, and less supervision is necessary.

There is no advantage to the delivery of β agonists by the subcutaneous route in the initial treatment of SA unless the patient is unable to comply with inhaled therapy (such as those in cardiopulmonary arrest or those with an impaired sensorium).[29–31] In such dire circumstances, epinephrine may be delivered by the subcutaneous route, by vein, or by the endotracheal tube, when there is no intravenous access. Interestingly, subcutaneous epinephrine may benefit patients not responding adequately to several hours of inhaled

β agonists. Appel and colleagues found expiratory flow increased after administration of subcutaneous epinephrine in 60% of patients not responding to 2 hours of inhaled metaproterenol.[32] Caution is advised when administering parenteral therapy to older patients and to patients with coronary artery disease. Patients who are more than 40 years old have more sinus tachycardia, premature ventricular contractions, and atrial arrhythmias during epinephrine therapy.[33] In the absence of recent myocardial infarction or angina, however, older patients tolerate subcutaneous epinephrine reasonably well. Thus, inactive cardiac disease and age (>40 years) are only relative contraindications to parenteral therapy. With the possible exception of the pregnant patient, there is no advantage to giving the more β_2-specific agent, terbutaline sulfate, which may, in fact, result in greater tachycardia for the same degree of bronchodilation than does epinephrine.[34] In pregnancy, terbutaline may be the preferred parenteral β agonist because epinephrine has been associated with congenital malformations and decreased uterine blood flow in sheep.[35] In addition, there is extensive experience with the use of terbutaline as a tocolytic agent in pregnancy.

The available data do not support the routine use of IV infusion of β agonists in the treatment of patients with SA. Several studies have demonstrated inhaled therapy to be equal to or better than IV therapy in treating airflow obstruction, and less likely to cause cardiac toxicity,[36–39] including rare fatal myocardial necrosis.[40] Bloomfield and colleagues compared salbutamol given as a 0.5 mg IV injection over 3 minutes with a 0.5% solution of salbutamol by intermittent positive-pressure breathing for 3 minutes in a double-blind crossover trial during 22 episodes of asthma.[38] Both treatments significantly improved PEFR, but use of the inhaled route resulted in greater improvement in pulsus paradoxus and less tachycardia than did the IV route. Salermon and colleagues compared the effects of nebulized albuterol (5 mg administered twice during the first hour of treatment) with IV albuterol (0.5 mg over 60 minutes) in 47 patients with severe acute asthma defined by a PEFR of less than 150 L per minute.[39] The mean increase in PEFR at 1 hour was greater in the group treated with inhaled albuterol (107 L/min versus 42 L/min in the IV group). Inhaled therapy also resulted in a greater fall in Pa_{CO_2} and less β agonist-induced hypokalemia.

On the other hand, Cheong and colleagues found that 4 hours of continuous intravenous salbutamol (0.72 mg/h) resulted in a greater PEFR than did 5 mg salbutamol nebulized at 30 and 120 minutes.[41] However, the difference was modest (25% increase in PEFR in the IV group vs 14% in the inhaled group) and at the cost of more tachycardia. Also, it can be argued that had higher doses of inhaled salbutamol been given (as is common in clinical practice), there may have been no difference in PEFR response between groups. In the authors' practice, use of intravenous β agonists in the treatment of SA is rare. On an individual basis, however, we consider their use in patients (preferably those <40 years old) who have not responded to inhaled or subcutaneous therapy, and in whom respiratory arrest is imminent or in whom persistent severe airflow obstruction is associated with alarming levels of lung hyperinflation during mechanical ventilation. If parenteral β agonists are used, extreme care must be taken to avoid hypokalemia, lactic acidosis, and cardiac arrhythmias.

A number of studies have established a correlation between the long-term use of inhaled β agonists and asthma morbidity and mortality.[42–44] Patients who use β agonists most frequently are also those who are at the greatest risk of asthma death, but whether β agonists are the cause of death or a marker of disease severity is yet to be established.[45] In a 1994 report, Suissa and colleagues demonstrated that the risk of asthma death increased significantly at about 1.4 canisters of β agonist medication per month, and that the association between β agonist use and asthma mortality was confined primarily to the overuse of these drugs.[46] In the 1997 NIH Expert Panel Practical Guide for the Diagnosis and Management of Asthma, the importance of minimizing inhaled β agonist use through the use of inhaled corticoste-

roids or other anti-inflammatory medications was stressed.[3] It is important to note, however, that in acute asthma β agonists should not be withheld or underdosed because of concerns regarding the safety of regular use.

ANTICHOLINERGICS

The available data generally demonstrate a modest benefit to the addition of anticholinergics to β agonists in the treatment of acute asthma.[47–58b] However, these drugs produce less bronchodilation at peak effect than β agonists, and achieve a somewhat more variable clinical response, indicating the variable role of cholinergic mechanisms in acute asthma. Anticholinergics may be particularly useful in patients with bronchospasm induced by β blockade[59] or in patients with severe airflow obstruction (FEV_1 <25% predicted).[60]

There are three anticholinergic drugs available (atropine sulfate, ipratropium bromide, and glycopyrrolate). Atropine sulfate is the least desirable and is not recommended in the treatment of acute asthma. It is inferior to metaproterenol as a sole drug and does not produce further improvement in airflow in patients already treated with metaproterenol.[61] Its tertiary amine structure allows for absorption from the airway and unwanted systemic effects. Atropine may also impair mucociliary clearance.

Ipratropium bromide and glycopyrrolate, on the other hand, can both be marginally recommended in the treatment of acute asthma, mainly because of their good safety profile. Their quaternary amine structures limit absorption from the airway (minimizing systemic effects) and they are not thought to impair mucociliary clearance. Of the two drugs, ipratropium bromide is preferred because it is readily available for use by MDI or as a pre-mixed solution for nebulization, and it has been studied extensively in acute asthma. In contrast, nebulized glycopyrrolate has not been studied extensively in acute asthma, although it has been shown to be as effective as metaproterenol with fewer side effects.[62] The addition of a single aerosolized dose of glycopyrrolate to albuterol does not appear to be better than albuterol alone in patients with acute asthma.[62a]

Ipratropium bromide marginally augments the bronchodilating effect of β agonists in acute asthma, an effect that is not explained by inadequate dosing of β agonists.[48] Bryant and colleagues demonstrated that ipratropium bromide, 0.25 mg by nebulizer, combined with 5 mg of nebulized albuterol resulted in greater improvement in FEV_1 than did albuterol by itself.[47] In this study, a significant response to ipratropium bromide was detected within 1 minute of administration, and the mean time to highest FEV_1 was only 19 minutes. One in twenty-five patients in this study had a paradoxical bronchoconstrictive response to ipratropium, which contrasts to prior reports that as many as 20% of patients with acute asthma may have a bronchoconstrictive response.[63] In the single patient with bronchoconstrictive response, administration of a preservative-free solution subsequently prevented the paradoxical response.

Several other studies have demonstrated possible benefit to combination therapy. Karpel and colleagues randomized 384 ED patients to receive nebulized albuterol (2.5 mg) or albuterol (2.5 mg) combined with ipratropium, (0.5 mg) at entry and at 45 minutes.[52] At 45 minutes, there were significantly more responders in the ipratropium group; however, the median change of FEV_1 from baseline did not differ between groups and by 90 minutes, there was no difference in the percentage of responders or median change in FEV_1 between groups. Additionally, there were no significant differences in the number of patients requiring additional ED or hospital treatment. Garrett and colleagues randomized 338 asthma patients in the ED to receive a single dose of nebulized ipratropium bromide (0.5 mg) combined with salbutamol (3 mg) or salbutamol (3 mg) by itself.[53] Mean FEV_1 at 45 and 90 minutes was significantly higher with combined therapy. Of note, the observed gain in bronchodilation with combination therapy was greatest in those using the least amount of inhaled β agonists. More recently, Lin and colleagues demonstrated that ipratropium bromide added to albuterol resulted in greater improvement in PEFR than did albuterol by itself, in their study of 55 adult asthma patients.[54] Results of 2 separate meta-analyses published in 1999 also suggest that combination therapy is superior to β_2 agonists alone in adults.[55,58a] Similarly, a pooled analysis of three studies demonstrated that adding ipratropium bromide to albuterol produced a small improvement in lung function and reduced the risk of hospitalization and subsequent exacerbations.[56] In children, combination therapy decreased ED treatment time, albuterol dose requirements prior to discharge,[57] and hospitalization rates.[58]

To the contrary, Weber and colleagues reported the results of their prospective, randomized, double-blind, placebo-controlled trial of 67 patients receiving either a combination of albuterol (10 mg per hour) plus ipratropium bromide (1 mg per hour) or albuterol by itself via continuous nebulization for a maximum of 3 hours.[64] Primary outcome measures were improvement in PEFR and reduced hospital admission rates and length of stay in the ED. The direction of all three outcome measures favored combination therapy; however, differences did not reach statistical significance. Fitzgerald and colleagues randomized 342 asthma patients in the ED to receive nebulized ipratropium bromide (0.5 mg) combined with salbutamol (3 mg) or salbutamol (3 mg) by itself, in addition to oxygen and methylprednisolone (125 mg) intravenously.[65] Mean FEV_1 at 45 and 90 minutes trended higher with combined therapy, but values did not reach statistical significance. There was a trend toward fewer admissions in the group receiving combination therapy (5.9% vs 11.2%), but again, this difference was not statistically significant. Additionally, Ducharme and Davis did not demonstrate benefit from combination therapy in their study of nearly 300 children with mild to moderate acute asthma.[66] Other small studies examining the addition of ipratropium bromide to β agonist therapy in acute asthma have yielded mixed results.[67,68]

The optimal dose of ipratropium bromide is not known. Most investigators have used doses between 0.25 mg and 0.5 mg by nebulization in non-intubated patients, which would require over

10 puffs by MDI (0.018 mg per puff) if delivery to the airways were equivalent. The authors' approach in patients not responding to initial treatment with β agonists is to give 4 to 10 puffs of ipratropium bromide by MDI with spacer every 20 to 60 minutes. Alternatively, ipratropium bromide inhalation solution unit-dose vial (0.5 mg in 2.5 ml) may be added to albuterol concentrate (2.5 mg in 0.5 mL).

OXYGEN

Obstruction of peripheral airways causes ventilation/perfusion mismatch (low V/Q) and hypoxemia. True shunt averages only 1.5% of the pulmonary blood flow,[69] so correction of hypoxemia requires only modest enrichment of inspired oxygen (1 to 3 L per minute by nasal cannula). Hypoxemia in acute asthma may occur sooner and/or resolve later than do airflow rates, likely because gas exchange reflects peripheral airways disease and airflow rates reflect large airway function.[70] There is a rough correlation between the degree of airflow obstruction as measured by the FEV_1 or PEFR and hypoxemia;[71] however, there is no cut-off value for either measurement that accurately predicts significant hypoxemia mandating assessment of oxygenation by pulsed oximetry or arterial blood gas measurement in acutely ill patients with asthma. Supplemental oxygen by nasal cannula is recommended to maintain arterial oxygen saturation at greater than 90% (>95% in pregnant women and in patients with coronary artery disease). Routine administration of supplemental oxygen may not be required in all patients. McFadden and colleagues found that only 5% of acute asthma patients who were younger than 45 years old had an initial Pa_{O_2} of 55 mm Hg or less at low altitude.[72] However, supplemental oxygen does protect against hypoxemia resulting from β-agonist induced pulmonary vasodilation and minimizes hypoxemia-induced vasoconstriction.[73,74] Normoxia may also improve oxygen delivery to peripheral tissues (including respiratory muscles) and may protect against cardiac arrhythmias. Refractory hypoxemia is rare and suggests other pa-

thology, such as pneumonia, aspiration, acute lobar atelectasis, or barotrauma.

CORTICOSTEROIDS

Airway wall inflammation invariably contributes to airway wall narrowing and acute airflow obstruction in patients with SA. Systemic corticosteroids are the most potent and effective treatment of this inflammatory process and should be used in most patients. One exception may be the patient in mild exacerbation who responds completely to initial β-agonist therapy;[3] this patient may be treated effectively by continuing β agonists and inhaled corticosteroid therapy.

Corticosteroids suppress the generation of cytokines, recruitment of airway eosinophils, and release of inflammatory mediators.[3] They potentiate the effects of β agonists on smooth muscle relaxation, decrease β-agonist tachyphylaxis, and decrease mucus production.[75,76] Clinically, they improve the speed of resolution of SA, the number of relapses in the first week or two after treatment,[77–81] and decrease risk of asthma death.[82] In the study by Littenberg and Gluck, acute asthma patients were enrolled in a double-blind, randomized placebo-controlled trial of methylprednisolone, 125 mg IV given on presentation to the ED, in addition to other standard treatments.[83] Only 9 of 48 (19%) of patients treated with methylprednisolone were hospitalized, as compared with 23 of 49 patients (47%) in the control group.

Ideally, intensification of an anti-inflammatory regimen should begin at the first indication of worsening asthma control. Unfortunately, many patients (or their clinicians) fail to intervene early or aggressively in the course of worsening asthma, and airway wall inflammation is allowed to proceed unchecked. Indeed, in McFadden's study of albuterol use in the emergency department, only 44 of 160 of patients (28%) were using inhaled steroids and 20 of 160 patients (13%) were using oral steroids at baseline.[15] It is likely that inadequately treated inflammation results in progressive architectural distortion of the airway, accumulation of edema fluid within airway walls, and formation of thick intraluminal mucus plugs, which then limits the efficacy of corticosteroids and β agonists.

Whether there is a dose-response relationship to systemic steroids in SA is not clear. In the meta-analysis by Rowe and colleagues, doses lower than 30 mg of prednisone (or its equivalent) every six hours were less effective, but higher doses were no more effective.[81] Haskell and colleagues demonstrated that patients who received 125 mg IV of solumedrol every 6 hours improved more rapidly than patients who received 40 mg, although there was no difference in peak improvement.[84] In this study, both 125 mg and 40 mg doses of solumedrol were superior to 15 mg every 6 hours, in terms of rate and absolute level of improvement. Emerman and Cydulka compared 500 mg and 100 mg doses of methylprednisolone in ED treatment of asthma and found no benefit to higher-dose therapy.[85]

Further studies are needed to establish the best dose and dosing frequency of corticosteroids in SA. The recommendation by the Expert Panel from the NIH is to deliver 120 to 180 mg per day of either prednisone, methylprednisolone, or prednisolone in 3 or 4 divided doses for 48 hours, then 60 to 80 mg per day until the PEFR reaches 70% of predicted or the patient's personal best.[3] The authors recommend 40 to 60 mg of solumedrol (or its equivalent) every 6 hours intravenously during initial management. Dose equivalence should be selected based upon glucocorticoid/anti-inflammatory activity[65,86] (see Table 9-2). The first dose is administered immediately in the ED, since anti-inflammatory effects are not seen clinically for hours.[75] Indeed this delayed benefit may not reduce the need for hospitalization.[86a,86b] Still, clinical benefit may occur sooner as demonstrated in a recent study by Lin and colleagues.[87] They studied 56 patients with acute asthma, randomly assigned to either 125 mg methylprednisolone IV or placebo in addition to bronchodilators. There was a greater increase in PEFR at 60 and 120 minutes and a trend toward fewer admissions in the steroid group.

Once improvement is evident, the authors change patient medication to prednisone, in doses ranging from 60 to 80 mg daily (in single or divided doses). This dose is continued until the PEFR returns to baseline after which prednisone dose is tapered at various rates depending on a number of patient factors including PEFR readings, the duration of high-dose therapy required to treat the acute exacerbation, and whether oral corticosteroids have been used as maintenance therapy. Although automatic tapering schedules may result in patients decreasing their corticosteroid dose prematurely, recent data suggested that in patients discharged from the ED, an 8-day tapering schedule is as efficacious as an 8-day course of 40 mg per day of prednisone.[88] A single dose of triamcinolone diacetate (40 mg IM) has also

Table 9-2
Systemic Corticosteroids: Dose Equivalents, Pharmacokinetic and Pharmacodynamic Profiles

Corticosteroid	Equivalent dose, mg	Glucocorticoid potency	Mineralocorticoid potency	Plasma $T_{\frac{1}{2}}$, minutes	Biologic $T_{\frac{1}{2}}$, hours
Hydrocortisone	20	1	2	80–118	8–12
Prednisone	5	4	1	6	12–36
Prednisolone	5	4	1	115–212	12–36
Methylprednisolone	4	5	0	78–110	12–36
Dexamethasone	0.75	20–30	0	110–210	36–54

SOURCE: Adapted from Lacy et al[86]; Schimmer and Parker.[95]

been shown to be as effective as prednisone, 40 mg per day for 5 days, after ED treatment for asthma, and may be attractive in noncompliant patients.[89]

There does not appear to be an advantage to intravenous compared with oral administration of corticosteroids in terms of efficacy.[81] However, most clinicians prefer intravenous administration in patients at risk for intubation (thereby minimizing stomach contents), patients with dyspepsia (as may occur in the setting of theophylline intoxication or acute viral illness), and in patients who are hypovolemic from inadequate volume intake and high insensible volume losses.

Several recent trials have addressed the effects of inhaled corticosteroids in acute asthma. Rodrigo and Rodrigo conducted a randomized, double-blind trial of the addition of 1 mg of flunisolide versus placebo to 400 μg of salbutamol (both given by MDI with spacer, every 10 minutes for 3 hours) in 94 ED subjects.[90] They found that PEFR and FEV_1 were approximately 20% higher in the flunisolide group, beginning at 90 minutes. In an accompanying editorial, McFadden suggested that this early benefit may stem from high-dose inhaled steroid-induced vasoconstriction, decreasing airway wall edema, vascular congestion, and plasma exudation and their contributions to airway narrowing.[91] In another study in children discharged from the ED, a short-term dose schedule of inhaled budesonide, starting at a high dose and then tapered over 1 week was shown to be as effective as a tapering course of oral prednisolone.[92] However, Guttman and colleagues found no benefit from the addition of beclomethasone (7 mg every 8 hours by MDI with spacer) to nebulized salbutamol and systemic corticosteroid therapy (methylprednisolone 80 mg IV, followed by 40 mg six hours later).[93] Similarly, these researchers have also demonstrated that beclomethasone (5 mg delivered by MDI) during the initial 4 hours of ED treatment did not confer added benefit to albuterol in adults with mild to moderately severe asthma.[94]

Our own view is that there is little benefit to the addition of inhaled steroids to high-dose β agonists and systemic corticosteroids in the management of acute asthma. However, it is intriguing to consider the use of high-dose inhaled corticosteroids in refractory patients. Further studies addressing the mechanism of this benefit, including the possible role for topical vasoconstrictor therapy, should be done.

Care must be taken during administration of systemic corticosteroids to identify and treat steroid-induced side effects. Problems that may be encountered include hyperglycemia, hypertension, hypokalemia, alterations in mood (including anxiety, insomnia and frank psychosis), metabolic alkalosis, and peripheral hand or leg edema.[95] Systemic corticosteroids also appear to play a causative role in the development of myopathy in acute severe asthma[96,97] (see Chapter 14). It must also be remembered that corticosteroids induce metabolism of numerous drugs through induction of hepatic cytochrome p450 subfamily 3A enzymes, which may result in subtherapeutic levels of some narrow therapeutic index agents (e.g., augmented clearance of the p450 CYP 3A4-metabolized immunosuppressive agents cyclosporine and tacrolimus).[98]

THEOPHYLLINE

As monotherapy, theophylline is inferior to β agonists in the ED treatment of asthma. Rossing and colleagues[99] randomized 48 patients with acute asthma to treatment with nebulized isoproterenol, subcutaneous epinephrine or IV theophylline (each delivered as monotherapy). The mean improvement in FEV_1 after 60 minutes of treatment was greater in patients treated with isoproterenol or epinephrine than in patients given theophylline. Additionally, the mean duration of therapy required prior to discharge was significantly longer in the theophylline group. Several convincing studies have demonstrated that the addition of theophylline to β agonists in the first few hours of treatment did not confer additional benefit, and the use of theophylline increased the incidence of tremor, nausea, anxiety, palpitations, and tachycardia/tachyarrhythmia.[100–104] In a prospective, double-blind, randomized placebo-controlled trial of 44 patients (18 to 45 years old), Murphy and colleagues found that theophylline added to other standard medications did not improve PEFR during 5 hours of therapy, but that theophylline did cause more tremor, nausea or vomiting, and palpitations.[101] Similarly, recent data from Nuhoglu and colleagues did not demonstrate a benefit to aminophylline in 38 children admitted for asthma.[105]

Fewer studies are available demonstrating a benefit to theophylline in the early management of SA. Pierson and colleagues demonstrated that, in children treated with theophylline, ventilatory function improved after 1 and 24 hours of treatment without adverse effects.[106] Huang and colleagues conducted a double-blind, randomized placebo-controlled study of 21 adults treated with IV theophylline added to frequent nebulizations of albuterol and IV steroids.[107] The rate of improvement in FEV_1 during the first 3 hours was more rapid in patients receiving theophylline than in patients receiving placebo, a difference which persisted over the 48 hours of study. Recently, Yung and colleagues studied 163 children admitted for asthma unresponsive to albuterol.[108] Children receiving aminophylline had a greater improvement in spirometry at 6 hours and higher oxygen saturation in the first 30 hours, compared to controls.

Wrenn and colleagues demonstrated that ED administration of theophylline resulted in fewer hospitalizations, even though airflow rates were no different from patients receiving placebo.[109] This finding raises the possibility that theophylline benefits patients in ways distinct from bronchodilation,[110] including effects on inflammation,[111,112] respiratory muscle function, or mucus clearance. Finally, Kelly and Murphy have pointed out that even when benefit is not detected in the first few hours of therapy, theophylline may improve lung function after 8 to 24 hours of therapy.[113] They believe that it is inappropriate to extrapolate data from short-term studies performed in the ED to hospitalized patients with SA in whom administration of theophylline has been demonstrated to be beneficial at 24 hours.[106,114]

Review of the available data does not allow for strong conclusions to be made regarding the use of theophylline in acute asthma. In 1988, Littenberg analyzed 13 trials of theophylline use in

the ED treatment of asthma and concluded that there was inadequate evidence to support or reject the use of theophylline in this setting[115]; little has changed to refute this statement 10 years later. While debate continues,[116,117] and until more data are available, our approach is to administer theophylline to patients with a poor or incomplete response to β agonists and corticosteroids. This approach is safe if attention is paid to serum drug levels and to factors that increase serum levels.[118–120] We prefer IV dosing to limit oral intake in patients who may require intubation, although IV administration does not confer additional therapeutic benefit compared to orally administered drug. The loading dose of theophylline is 5 mg/kg (aminophylline, 6 mg/kg) by peripheral vein over 30 minutes in patients not taking theophylline, followed by a continuous infusion of 0.4 mg/kg per hour (aminophylline, 0.5 mg/kg per hour). In patients receiving theophylline, serum levels should be checked on arrival to the ED before additional theophylline is given. If the level is within the therapeutic range, a continuous infusion may be started, or the oral preparation may be continued. Serum levels should be checked within 6 hours of IV loading to avoid toxicity and to guide further dosing. The authors suggest levels between 8 and 12 μg/ml, although 20 μg/ml is commonly stated to be the upper limit of the target therapeutic concentration range (10 to 20 μg/ml). In some patients, the therapeutic index is lower than expected, resulting in development of significant side effects within the 15 to 20 μg/ml range. Appropriate drug monitoring procedures should be followed, including attention to serial serum drug levels and to drug-disease and drug-drug interactions that impair theophylline clearance (thus increasing serum levels), such as congestive heart failure, cirrhosis, and medications (quinolones, macrolide antibiotics, cimetidine) that competitively inhibit cytochrome p450 CYP 1A2.[98] Conversely, theophylline metabolism is enhanced by cigarette smoking (but not nicotine replacement) and several medications (oral contraceptives, fluvoxamine, omeprazole, rifabutin, rifampin), and is also much higher in pediatric patients than in adults; maintenance dosing requirements are accordingly increased under these conditions. Finally, pharmacodynamic monitoring for side effects must be emphasized for safe use of theophylline, with discontinuation in the presence of significant tachyarrhythmias, even when serum levels are within the target therapeutic range.

MAGNESIUM SULFATE

Intravenous magnesium sulfate has been reported to be a useful adjunctive therapy in patients with acute asthma refractory to treatment with inhaled β agonists.[121-131] Inhaled preparations of magnesium sulfate have also been reported to have a bronchodilator effect.[132-134] Benefits to IV magnesium have been described in patients with normal serum magnesium levels, although hypomagnesemia has been reported in up to 50% of patients with acute asthma.[135] The mechanisms of action are unknown. One possibility is that magnesium inhibits calcium channels of airway smooth muscle, thus interfering in calcium-mediated smooth muscle contraction.[136] Magnesium also decreases acetylcholine release at the neuromuscular junction, which may interfere with bronchoconstriction from parasympathetic stimulation. Magnesium reduces histamine-induced[137] and methacholine-induced[138] bronchoconstriction in asthma patients and increases respiratory muscle force generation.[139]

In the late 1980s and early 1990s, magnesium sulfate was used extensively in the ED treatment of SA. This practice was based on several reports demonstrating benefit; however, these studies suffered from small patient numbers, and many were anecdotal. One patient in acute hypercapnic respiratory failure in whom magnesium sulfate (1 g IV) delivered over 15 minutes was associated with dramatic improvement midway into infusion, thereby preventing intubation and mechanical ventilation, has been described.[127] Additional evidence supporting benefit in severe disease has been reported by Sydow and colleagues.[128] In their study of five mechanically ventilated asthma patients, high-dose magnesium sulfate (range, 10 to 20 g) over 1 hour caused a fall in peak airway

pressure (43 cm H_2O to 32 cm H_2O) with minimal side effects (moderate systemic hypotension was reported in 2 of 5 patients). Additional data supporting the use of magnesium sulfate was reported in a recent small, randomized placebo-controlled trial in children with moderate to severe acute asthma, in whom intravenous magnesium therapy improved FEV_1 at 50 and 110 minutes and increased ED discharge rates, compared to placebo.[129]

In the study by Bloch and colleagues, 135 patients with mild to severe asthma were randomized to a dose of 2 g magnesium sulfate IV or placebo after 30 minutes in the ED and followed for 4 hours.[130] For the group as a whole, hospital admission rates and FEV_1 were no different between magnesium-treated patients and controls. However, subgroup analysis of patients with the most severe asthma (FEV_1 <25% of predicted normal), showed that magnesium sulfate significantly decreased admission rates and improved FEV_1. Subsequently, an abstract of a prospective, randomized placebo-controlled trial of magnesium in patients with FEV_1 less than 25% demonstrated similar findings.[131]

Other studies have failed to confirm a benefit to magnesium sulfate use in the ED treatment of SA. Green and colleagues studied 120 consecutive ED patients with acute asthma unresponsive to inhaled albuterol.[140] Patients received magnesium sulfate (2 g IV) if they presented on odd days and no magnesium if they were seen on even days. Physicians were not blinded, but respiratory therapists and patients were unaware of the study. There were no differences in hospitalization rates, duration of ED treatment or changes in PEFR between treated and untreated groups. Similarly, Tiffany and colleagues conducted a randomized, double-blind placebo-controlled trial of 48 patients given magnesium or placebo if their initial PEFR was less than 200 L per minute and failed to double after two albuterol treatments.[141] Patients were randomized to three groups receiving a dose of: 2 g magnesium sulfate IV over 20 minutes followed by an infusion of 2 g per hour for 4 hours; 2 g magnesium sulfate IV followed by placebo infusion; or placebo-loading dose and infusion.

There was no benefit to either of the two magnesium dosing regimens in this study. The authors stated, however, that their conclusions may not apply to less severely ill patients who are not receiving high-dose β agonists or to more severely ill (i.e., mechanically ventilated) patients. They also raised the possibility that premenopausal women may be more responsive to magnesium therapy since estrogen has been reported to augment bronchodilator effect of magnesium.[142] Indeed there was a trend toward female responsiveness in the study by Tiffany and colleagues and in a study by Skobellof and colleagues that demonstrated a magnesium benefit, 25 of 34 (74%) patients were women.[121]

In general, magnesium sulfate is a safe and inexpensive drug, particularly in the usual clinical dose of 2 g IV over 20 minutes, a dose which increases serum levels to about twice the original level,[125] and most studies have not reported major complications from magnesium administration. However, care must be taken to avoid magnesium intoxication, particularly in patients with impaired renal function. Minor side effects of magnesium therapy include flushing and mild sedation. Intoxication may result in loss of deep tendon reflexes and hypotension.

Further data are needed to establish the role of magnesium in SA. Currently, routine use of this agent is not justified, with the possible exceptions of patients with severe disease and premenopausal women. Further studies should help clarify efficacy and subgroups of patients most likely to respond. In our practice, we consider magnesium sulfate in patients who have failed treatment with standard agents, prescribing a dose of 2 g magnesium sulfate IV over 20 minutes (unless the patient is hypomagnesemic, in which case we normalize serum levels).

HELIOX

Heliox is a blend of gas consisting of 80% helium and 20% oxygen. Other mixtures (such as 70:30% and 60:40%) are available for inhalation, but as the percentage of helium decreases, so does the benefit of breathing this gas blend (>60% helium is required for benefit), thereby precluding its use in patients requiring significant enrichment of inspired oxygen. Heliox is slightly more viscous than air, but significantly less dense, resulting in a more than three-fold increase in kinematic viscosity (the ratio of gas viscosity to gas density) compared to air. Theoretically, this property decreases the driving pressure required for gas flow by two mechanisms. First, for any level of turbulent flow, breathing low-density gas decreases the pressure gradient required for flow. Second, heliox decreases the Reynold's number (Re = pdV/u, where p is gas density, d is airway diameter, V is the mean linear velocity, and u is gas viscosity), favoring conversion of turbulent flow to laminar flow.[143] Heliox does not treat bronchospasm or airway wall inflammation.

Heliox improves distal airway delivery of inhaled radiolabeled aerosolized particles compared to air, in normal subjects[144] and in asthmatics.[145] Whether heliox augments the bronchodilator effect (as assessed by peak flows) of inhaled β agonists in acute severe asthma, compared to delivery in air, is unclear; results of the study by Melmed and colleagues suggest that it does.[146] However, results of the study by Henderson and colleagues suggest that it does not.[147]

Heliox can be delivered through a tight-fitting non-rebreathing face mask in nonintubated patients (Fig. 1) or through the inspiratory limb of the ventilator circuit in mechanically ventilated patients. The reader is directed to a comprehensive critical review of heliox use in the treatment of airflow obstruction that discusses the logistics of administering heliox to nonintubated and intubated patients.[148] In nonintubated patients with upper airway obstruction, heliox promptly improves dyspnea, work of breathing, and arterial blood gas abnormalities.[149] Effects in asthma are less clear. Manthous and colleagues treated adults with asthma for 15 minutes in the ED with 80:20% heliox delivered by tight-fitting face mask and demonstrated a significant decrease in pulsus paradoxus and an increase in peak flow.[150] A more recent randomized controlled trial of 23 adults with acute severe asthma similarly demonstrated

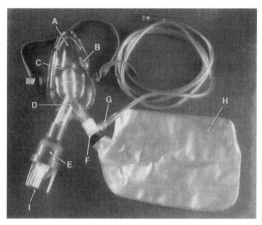

Figure 9-1
A face-mask delivery system for concurrent administration of heliox and bronchodilator medications in a spontaneously breathing patient with acute asthma. A = partial nonrebreather mask; B = exhalation valve; C = 22 mm ID adapter; D = ventilator Y; E = Mini-Heart™ Nebulizer or Uni Nebulizer™; F = one-way valve; G = connection for tubing to heliox tank; H = reservoir bag; I = port for nebulizing medication. A nonrebreather face mask is used to reduce the amount of external air entrained on inspiration so as not to dilute the concentration of helium. Flows of 5–10 L/min are generally sufficient to ensure that the reservoir bag has enough gas for tidal breathing. If supplemental oxygen is required to maintain adequate arterial oxygen saturation, a nasal cannula is placed beneath the mask and supplemental oxygen is titrated as required. The goal is to dilute helium as little as possible to maximize its effects. (With permission, from Manthous et al[148])

improved dyspnea and PEFR in heliox-treated patients.[150a] Eighty-two percent of patients receiving 70:30% heliox had greater than 25% improvement in PEFR at 20 minutes compared to 17% in the placebo group. However, Verbeek and colleagues were unable to demonstrate an improvement in FEV_1 with 70:30% heliox in their study of 13 acutely ill asthma patients.[151] Moreover, Rodrigo and colleagues recently reviewed the results of 4 randomized controlled trials of heliox use, concluding it does not im-

prove spirometry or alter outcome in acute asthma.[151a]

Additional data from uncontrolled studies suggest that heliox given to spontaneously breathing patients with acute severe asthma ameliorates respiratory acidosis.[152,153] The mechanism involves some combination of decreased CO_2 production from decreased work of breathing and increased alveolar ventilation, possibly resulting from less lung hyperinflation and dead space ventilation. Similar results have also been published in children.[154]

If favorable results are confirmed, heliox may prove to be a useful bridge to effective bronchodilator/anti-inflammatory therapy, thereby averting the need for intubation, in some cases. Of theoretical concern is the potential for heliox to mask increasing airflow obstruction. If this occurs during heliox breathing, there may be less time (and no margin for error) to control the airway and institute mechanical ventilation.

Heliox may also be useful in patients with SA requiring mechanical ventilation. Gluck and colleagues administered a 60:40% blend of heliox to seven intubated asthma patients[155]; within minutes, heliox decreased peak airway pressure by a mean of 33 cm H_2O and Pa_{CO_2} by a mean of 35.7 mm Hg. Data also suggest that heliox use in mechanically ventilated asthmatics improves the alveolar-to-arterial oxygen gradient [(A-a) gradient], allowing reduction in concentration of inspired oxygen to levels that maximize helium concentration and the benefits of heliox.[155a] Although these data are interesting, it is important to note that heliox is rarely needed in the routine management of ventilated patients, particularly if attention is paid to minimizing lung hyperinflation during mechanical ventilation (see Chapter 13). It is also important to be cognizant that recalibration of gas blenders and flow meters to this low-density gas is required to obtain accurate measures of oxygen concentration or tidal volume.[155b] Careful planning, including a trial of heliox in a lung model is mandatory prior to patient use; during patient use, a spirometer should be placed on the expiratory limb of the ventilator to confirm tidal volume changes.

ANTIBIOTICS

In the study of Teichtahl and colleagues, 37% of hospitalized asthma patients had evidence for an infectious trigger and 79% of the identified pathogens were viral.[156] Thus, in the majority of cases, including those triggered by respiratory infection, antibiotics are not indicated. This statement is supported by Graham and colleagues, who conducted a randomized double-blind study of amoxicillin and placebo in 60 adult patients admitted to hospital with acute asthma exacerbations.[157] There was no difference in improvement between groups for length of hospitalization, patient's self-assessment, or spirometry measurements.

Still, antibiotics are often prescribed in acute asthma because of an increase in sputum volume or purulence. However, sputum that looks purulent in this setting may contain an abundance of eosinophils, and not polymorphonuclear leukocytes, a distinction that can be made under the microscope. Indeed, transtracheal aspirates obtained from adults thought to have acute "infective" asthma often have culture results similar to those from normal controls.[158]

Antibiotics are indicated for patients with fever and sputum containing polymorphonuclear leukocytes, clinical findings of pneumonia, or signs and symptoms of acute sinusitis. The authors also favor the use of antibiotics in patients who have clinical findings suggestive of mycoplasmal or chlamydial infection.

INHALED ANESTHETIC AGENTS

In the rare instances where the above pharmacologic therapies in combination with expert ventilator strategies fail to stabilize a patient with SA, inhaled general anesthetics may be used to provide additional bronchodilation (although the basis for this recommendation comes primarily from anecdotal reports). Halothane and enflurane are most frequently used for this purpose.[159,160] Side effects include hypotension (due to myocardial depression and vasorelaxation) and arrhythmias. Prolonged therapy may be required pending resolu-

tion of airway wall edema and inflammation because the bronchodilator effect reverses soon after drug administration is discontinued. A relatively novel inhaled anesthetic agent, sevoflurane, has also been safely used in two subjects for this purpose, despite the potential for nephrotoxicity during prolonged administration of this drug.[161]

NOVEL THERAPIES

Numerous other agents have been suggested to be of benefit for acute asthma therapy, including some that have yet to be tested clinically in acute asthma patients; among these are leukotriene modifiers, inhaled nitric oxide therapy, lidocaine, surfactant, and diuretics. Inhibitors of leukotriene synthesis (5-lipoxygenase inhibitors) or effect (leukotriene receptor antagonists) are now available for clinical use, but there are no data to support the utility of these agents in acute asthma.[162] Inhaled nitric oxide (NO) is theoretically attractive in this setting, not only to optimize ventilation-perfusion matching in patients with mucus plugs and atelectasis, but also potentially to achieve a direct bronchodilator effect by stimulation of guanylyl cyclase activity in bronchial smooth muscle, analogous to the vasodilator effect of NO on vascular smooth muscle.[163,164] To date, however, the main focus of NO research in asthma has involved the diagnostic utility of exhaled NO measurements in following asthma disease activity, since airway inflammation presumably results in presence of the inducible NOS (iNOS) isoform, thus increasing exhaled NO concentrations.[165] However, this correlation may be absent in the setting of significant airflow obstruction.[166] Although data from some animal models suggest that NO may be beneficial for acute asthma therapy,[167] inhaled NO (80 ppm) worsened hypoxemia in methacholine-challenged human subjects.[168] Conversely, pharmacological inhibition of NO synthesis exacerbated bradykinin-induced bronchoconstriction in asthmatic human subjects, suggesting that NO could have a bronchoprotective role in asthma.[169] There is currently insufficient knowledge to define the complex interplay between the constitutive role of NO as a mediator of nonadrenergic noncholinergic airway neurotransmission, and the potential beneficial (bronchodilation) versus toxic (peroxynitrite-induced tissue injury) effects of iNOS-derived NO from inflamed airway epithelial and smooth muscle cells during asthma exacerbation.[170] Until further data become available, inhaled NO is not recommended for acute asthma therapy. Effects of inhaled furosemide added to conventional therapy were recently reported by Pendino and colleagues.[171] In their double-blind, randomized placebo-controlled trial of 42 patients in the ED, the authors found no significant differences in PEFR or clinical variables 15 and 30 minutes after therapy, except when they examined, as a subgroup, patients whose exacerbations were of relatively short duration (<8 hours). In this subgroup, PEFR improved more in the furosemide group. In another study by Karpel and colleagues, the combination of inhaled furosemide and metaproterenol was no better than metaproterenol alone in the ED treatment of acute asthma.[172] For now, there are insufficient data to recommend diuretics in the management of acute asthma.

Inhaled lidocaine has been reported to be beneficial in patients with severe steroid-dependent asthma.[173,174] Insufficient data are available in acute asthma to recommend this drug, although there are two interesting cases of epidural lidocaine improving airflow obstruction.[175,176] It should be noted that inhaled lidocaine has the potential to cause bronchoconstriction in asthmatics.[177]

Similarly limited data are available regarding surfactant inhalation in acute asthma.[178,179] In one small study of 11 acute asthmatics (who were stable for at least 6 hours), inhaled surfactant improved FEV_1 and Pa_{O_2} in all patients.[179] Additional data are needed before strong conclusions can be drawn; for now, surfactant cannot be recommended outside study protocol.

CONCLUSION

In conclusion, frequently dosed inhaled β agonist therapy, systemic corticosteroids, and supplemental oxygen remain the mainstays of pharmacotherapy of acute asthma (Table 9-1). Asthma patients may gain further benefit from addition of inhaled anticholinergic agents, theophylline, magnesium sulfate, or heliox inhalation. Whatever regimen is chosen, care must be taken to minimize the occurrence of adverse drug reactions and to maximize the therapeutic benefit gained from each agent administered.

REFERENCES

1. Busse WW, Calhoun WF, Sedgewick JD: Mechanism of airway inflammation in asthma. *Am Rev Respir Dis* 147:S20–S24, 1993.
2. Reed CE: New therapeutic approaches to asthma. *J Allergy Clin Immunol* 77:537–543, 1986.
3. *Guidelines for the Diagnosis and Management of Asthma: Expert Panel Report II.* Bethesda, National Institutes of Health, publ No. 97–405, 1997.
4. Corbridge T, Hall JB: The assessment and management of adults with status asthmaticus. *Am J Respir Crit Care Med* 151:1296–1316, 1995.
4a. Cygan J, Trunsky M, Corbridge T: Inhaled heroin-induced status asthmaticus: five cases and a review of the literature. *Chest* 117:272–275, 2000.
5. Petty TL: Treat status asthmaticus three days before it occurs. *J Intensive Care Med* 4:135–136, 1989.
6. Gern JE, Lemanske RF: Beta-adrenergic agonist therapy. *Immunol Allergy Clin North Am* 13(4):839–860, 1993.
7. Kennedy MCS, Simpson WT: Human pharmacological and clinical studies on salbutamol: a specific beta-adrenergic bronchodilator. *Br J Dis Chest* 63:165–174, 1969.
8. Paterson JW, Evans RJC, Prime FJ: Selectivity of bronchodilator action of salbutamol in asthmatic patients. *Br J Dis Chest* 65:21–38, 1971.
9. Shreshta M, Gourlay S, Robertson S, et al: Isoetharine versus albuterol for acute asthma: greater immediate effect, but more side effects. *Am J Med* 100:323, 1996.
10. Nelson H, Bensch G, Pleskow WW, et al: Improved bronchodilation with levalbuterol compared with racemic albuterol in patients with asthma. *J Allergy Clin Immunol* 102:943, 1998.
11. Rudnitsky GS, Eberlein RS, Schoffstall JM, et al.: Comparison of intermittent and continuously nebulized albuterol for treatment of asthma in an ur-

ban emergency department. *Ann Emerg Med* 22:1842–1846, 1993.

12. Lin RY, Sauter D, Newman T, et al: Continuous versus intermittent albuterol nebulization in the treatment of acute asthma. *Ann Emerg Med* 22:1847–1853, 1993.

13. Lipworth BJ, Clark RA, Dhillon DP, et al.: Beta-adrenoceptor responses to high doses of inhaled salbutamol in patients with bronchial asthma. *Br J Clin Pharmacol* 26:527–533, 1988.

14. Rossing TH, Fanta CH, McFadden ER: Effect of outpatient treatment of asthma with beta-agonists on the response to sympathomimetics in the ED. *Am J Med* 75:781–784, 1983.

15. Kelly HW. New beta2-agonist aerosols. Clin Pharm 4:393–403, 1985.

16. McFadden ER Jr, Strauss L, Hejal R, et al: Comparison of two dosage regimens of albuterol in acute asthma. *Am J Med* 105:12, 1998.

17. Emerman CL, Cydulka RK, McFadden ER Jr: Comparison of 2.5 mg vs 7.5 mg of inhaled albuterol in the treatment of acute asthma. *Chest* 115:92, 1999.

17a. McDermott MF, Nasr I, Rydman RJ, et al: Comparison of two regimens of beta-adrenergics in acute asthma. *J Med Syst* 23:269–272, 1999.

18. Rodrigo C, Rodrigo G: Therapeutic response patterns to high and cumulative doses of salbutamol in acute severe asthma. *Chest* 113:593, 1998.

19. Strauss L, Hejal R, Galan G, et al: Observations of the effects of aerosolized albuterol in acute asthma. *Am J Resp Crit Care Med* 155:454, 1997.

20. Rodrigo G, Rodrigo C. Early prediction of poor response in acute asthma patients in the emergency department. *Chest* 114:1016, 1998.

21. Newhouse MT, Chapman KR, McCallum AL, et al: Cardiovascular safety of high doses of inhaled fenoterol and albuterol in acute severe asthma. *Chest* 110:595, 1996.

22. O'Connell MB, Iber C: Continuous intravenous terbutaline infusions for adult patients with status asthmaticus. *Ann Allergy* 64:213–218, 1990.

23. Idris AH, McDermott MF, Raucci JC, et al: Emergency department treatment of severe asthma: metered-dose inhaler plus holding chamber is equivalent in effectiveness to nebulizer. *Chest* 103:665–672, 1993.

24. Jasper AC, Mohsenifar Z, Kahan S, et al: Cost-benefit comparison of aerosol bronchodilator delivery methods in hospitalized patients. *Chest* 91:614–618, 1987.

25. Newhouse MT: Emergency department management of life-threatening asthma: are nebulizers obsolete? *Chest* 103:661–663, 1993.

26. Turner JR, Corkery KJ, Eckman D, et al: Equivalence of continuous flow nebulizer and metered-dose inhaler with reservoir bag for treatment of acute airflow obstruction. *Chest* 93:476–481, 1988.

27. Rodrigo C, Rodrigo G: Salbutamol treatment of acute severe asthma in the ED: MDI vs hand-held nebulizer. *Am J Med* 16:637, 1998.

28. Tenholder MF, Bryson MJ, Waller RF, Faircloth TT: Can MDIs be used effectively by extubated ICU patients? *J Crit Illness* 7(1):111–117, 1992.

29. Fanta CH, Rossing TH, McFadden ER: Treatment of acute asthma: is combination therapy with sympathomimetics and methylxanthines indicated? *Am J Med* 80:5–10, 1986.

30. Uden DL, Goetz, DR, Kohen DP, Fifield GC: Comparison of nebulized terbutaline and subcutaneous epinephrine in the treatment of acute asthma. *Ann Emerg Med* 14:229–232, 1985.

31. Becker AB, Nelson NA, Simons FER: Inhaled salbutamol (albuterol) vs injected epinephrine in the treatment of acute asthma in children. *J Pediatrics* 102:465–469, 1983.

32. Appel D, Karpel JP, Sherman M: Epinephrine improves expiratory airflow rates in patients with asthma who do not respond to inhaled metaproterenol sulfate. *J Allergy Clin Immunol* 84:90–98, 1989.

33. Cydulka R, Davison R, Grammer L, et al: The use of epinephrine in the treatment of older adult asthmatics. *Ann Emerg Med* 17:322–326, 1990.

34. Amory DW, Burnham SC, Cheney FW Jr: Comparison of the cardiopulmonary effects of subcutaneously administered epinephrine and terbutaline in patients with reversible airway obstruction. *Chest* 67:279–286, 1975.

35. Rosenfeld CR, Barton MD, Meschia G: Effects of epinephrine on distribution of blood flow in the pregnant ewe. *Am J Obstet Gynecol* 124:156–163, 1976.

36. Lawford P, Jones BMJ, Milledge JS: Comparison of intravenous and nebulised salbutamol in initial treatment of severe asthma. *Br Med J* 1:84, 1978.

37. Williams SJ, Winner SJ, Clark TJH: Comparison of inhaled and intravenous terbutaline in acute severe asthma. *Thorax* 36:629–631, 1981.

38. Bloomfield P, Carmichael J, Petrie GR, et al: Comparison of salbutamol given intravenously and by

intermittent positive-pressure breathing in life-threatening asthma. *Br Med J* 1:848–850, 1979.

39. Salmeron S, Brochard L, Mal H, et al: Nebulized versus intravenous albuterol in hypercapnic acute asthma: a multicenter, double-blind, randomized study. *Am J Respir Crit Care Med* 149:1466–1470, 1994.

40. Kurland G, Williams J, Lewiston NJ: Fatal myocardial infarction during continuous infusion of intravenous isoproterenol during therapy of asthma. *J Allergy Clin Immunol* 63:407–11, 1979.

41. Cheong B, Reynolds SR, Rajan G, Ward MJ: Intravenous beta-agonist in severe acute asthma. *Br Med J* 297:448–450, 1988.

42. Sears MR, Taylor DR, Print CG, et al: Regular inhaled beta-agonist treatment in bronchial asthma. *Lancet* 336:1391–1396, 1990.

43. Spitzer WO, Suissa S, Ernst P, et al: The use of beta-agonists and the risk of death and near death from asthma. *N Engl J Med* 326:501–506, 1992.

44. Taylor DR, Sears MR, Herbison GP, et al: Regular inhaled beta-agonists in asthma: effects on exacerbations and lung function. *Thorax* 48:134–138, 1993.

45. Taylor DR, Sears MR, Cockroft DW: The beta-agonist controversy. *Med Clin N Am* 80:719–748, 1996.

46. Suissa S, Ernst P, Boivin JF, et al: A cohort analysis of excess mortality in asthma and the use of inhaled beta-agonists. *Am J Respir Crit Care Med* 149:604–610, 1994.

47. Bryant DH, Rogers P: Effects of ipratropium bromide nebulizer solution with and without preservatives in the treatment of acute and stable asthma. *Chest* 102:742–47, 1992.

48. Bryant DH: Nebulised ipratropium bromide in the treatment of acute asthma. *Chest* 88:24–29, 1985.

49. Shuh S, Johnson DW, Callahan S, et al: Efficacy of frequent nebulized ipratropium bromide added to frequent high-dose albuterol in severe childhood asthma. *J Pediatr* 126:639–645, 1995.

50. Rebuck AS, Chapman KR, Abboud R, et al: Nebulized anticholinergic and sympathomimetic treatment of asthma and chronic airways disease in the ED. *Am J Med* 82:59–64, 1987.

51. Kelly HW, Murphy S: Should anticholinergics be used in acute severe asthma? DICP *Ann Pharmacother* 24:409–414, 1990.

52. Karpel JP, Schacter EN, Fanta C, et al: A comparison of ipratropium and albuterol vs albuterol alone for treatment of acute asthma. *Chest* 110:611, 1996.

53. Garrett JE, Town GI, Rodwell P, Kelly AM: nebulized salbutamol with and without ipratropium bromide in the treatment of acute asthma. *J Allerg Clin Immunol* 100:165–170, 1997.

54. Lin RY, Pesola GR, Bakalchuk L, et al: Superiority of ipratropium bromide plus albuterol over albuterol alone in the emergency department management of adult asthma: a randomized clinical trial. *Ann Emerg Med* 31:208, 1998.

55. Stoodley RG, Aaron SD, Dales RE: The role of ipratropium bromide in the emergency management of acute asthma exacerbation: a meta-analysis of randomized clinical trials. *Ann Emerg Med* 34:8, 1999.

56. Lanes SF, Garrett JE, Wentworth CE, et al: The effect of adding ipratropium bromide to salbutamol in the treatment of acute asthma: a pooled analysis of three trials. *Chest* 114:365, 1998.

57. Zorc JJ, Pusic MV, Ogborn CJ, et al: Ipratropium bromide added to asthma treatment in the pediatric emergency department. *Pediatrics* 103:748, 1999.

58. Qureshi F, Pestian J, Davis P, Zaritsky A: Effect of nebulized ipratropium on hospitalization rates of children with asthma. *N Engl J Med* 339:1030–1035, 1998.

58a. Rodrigo G, Rodrigo C, Burschtin O: A meta-analysis of the effects of ipratropium bromide in adults with acute asthma. *Am J Med* 107:363–370, 1999.

58b. Calvo GM, Calvo AM, Marin HF, Moya GJ: Is it useful to add an anticholinergic treatment to beta 2-adrenergic medication in acute asthma attack? *J Invest All Clin Immunol* 8:30–34, 1998.

59. Gross N: The use of anticholinergic agents in the treatment of airways disease. *Clin Chest Med* 9:591–598, 1988.

60. Ward MJ, Fentem PH, Smith WHR, Davies D: Ipratropium bromide in acute asthma. *Br Med J* 282:598–600, 1981.

61. Karpel JP, Appel D, Breidbart D, Fusco MJ: A comparison of atropine sulfate and metaproterenol sulfate in the ED treatment of asthma. *Am Rev Respir Dis* 133:727–729, 1986.

62. Gilman MJ, Meyer L, Carter J, Slovis C: Comparison of aerosolized glycopyrrolate and metaproterenol in acute asthma. *Chest* 98:1095–1098, 1990.

62a. Cydulka RK, Emerman CL: Effects of combined treatment with glycopyrrolate and albuterol in acute exacerbation of asthma, *Ann Emerg Med* 23:270–274, 1994.

63. Rafferty P, Beasley R, Howarth PH: Bronchoconstriction induced by ipratropium bromide in asthma: relation to bromide ion. *Br Med J* 293:1538–1539, 1986.

64. Weber EJ, Levitt A, Covington JK, Gambrioli E: Effect of continuously nebulized ipratropium bromide plus albuterol on emergency department length of stay and hospital admission rates in patients with acute bronchospasm. *Chest* 115:937–944, 1999.

65. Fitzgerald JM, Grunfeld A, Pare PD, et al: The clinical efficacy of combination nebulized anticholinergic and adrenergic bronchodilators vs nebulized adrenergic bronchodilator alone in acute asthma. *Chest* 111:311–315, 1997.

66. Ducharme FM, Davis GM: Randomized controlled trial of ipratropium bromide and frequent low doses of salbutamol in the management of mild and moderate acute pediatric asthma. *J Pediatr* 133:479, 1998.

67. O'Driscoll BR, Taylor RJ, Horsley MG, et al: Nebulised salbutamol with and without ipratropium in acute airflow obstruction. *Lancet* 1:1418–1420, 1989.

68. McFadden ER, El Sanadi N, Strauss L, et al: The influence of parasympatholytics on the resolution of acute attacks of asthma. *Am J Med* 102:7–13, 1997.

69. Rodriguez-Roisin R, Ballester E, Roca J, Torres A, Wagner PD: Mechanisms of hypoxemia in patients with status asthmaticus requiring mechanical ventilation. *Am Rev Respir Dis* 139:732–39, 1989.

70. Ferrer A, Roca J, Wagner PD, et al: Airway obstruction and ventilation-perfusion relationships in acute severe asthma. *Am Rev Respir Dis* 147:579–584, 1993.

71. Nowak RM, Tomlanovich MC, Sarker DD, et al: Arterial blood gases and pulmonary function testing in acute bronchial asthma: predicting patient outcomes. *JAMA* 249:2043, 1993.

72. McFadden ER, Lyons HA: Arterial blood gas tension in asthma. *N Engl J Med* 278:1017–1032, 1968.

73. West JB. State of the art: Ventilation-perfusion relationships. *Am Rev Respir Dis* 116:919–943, 1977.

74. Ballester E, Reyes A, Roca J, et al: Ventilation-perfusion mismatching in acute severe asthma: effects of salbutamol and 100% oxygen. *Thorax* 44:258–267, 1989.

75. Barnes PJ, Pedersen S, Busse WW: Efficacy and safety of inhaled corticosteroids. New developments. *Am J Respir Crit Care Med* 157:S1–S53, 1998.

76. Schimmer BP, Parker KL: Adrenocorticotropic hormone; adrenocortical steroids and their synthetic analogs; inhibitors of the synthesis and actions of adrenocortical hormones, in Hardman JG, Limbird LE, Molinoff PB, et al (eds): *The Pharmacological Basis of Therapeutics,* 9th ed. New York, McGraw-Hill, 1996, p 1459.

77. Connett GJ, Warde C, Wooler E, et al: Prednisolone and salbutamol in the hospital treatment of acute asthma. *Arch Dis Child* 70:170–3, 1994.

78. Fanta CH, Rossing TH, McFadden ER Jr: Glucocorticoids in acute asthma. A critical controlled trial. *Am J Med* 74:845–51, 1983.

79. Scarfone RJ, Fuchs SM, Nager AL, et al: Controlled trial of oral prednisone in the ED treatment of children with acute asthma. *Pediatrics* 2:513–8, 1993.

80. Chapman KR, Verbeek PR, White JG, et al: Effect of a short course of prednisone in the prevention of early relapse after the ED treatment of acute asthma. *N Engl J Med* 324:788–94, 1991.

81. Rowe BH, Keller JL, Oxman AD: Effectiveness of steroid therapy in acute exacerbations of asthma: a meta-analysis. *Am J Emerg Med* 10(4):301–10, 1992.

82. Benatar SR: Fatal asthma. *N Engl J Med* 314:423–29, 1986.

83. Littenberg B, Gluck EH: A controlled trial of methylprednisolone in the emergency treatment of acute asthma. *N Engl J Med* 314:150–152, 1986.

84. Haskell RJ, Wong BM, Hansen JE. A double-blind, randomized clinical trial of methylprednisolone in status asthmaticus. *Arch Intern Med* 143:1324–27, 1983.

85. Emerman CL, Cydulka RK: A randomized comparison of 100-mg vs 500-mg dose of methylprednisolone in the treatment of acute asthma. *Chest* 107:1559–63, 1995.

86. Lacy CF, Armstrong LL, Ingrim NB, Lance LL (eds): *Drug Information Handbook 1998–1999,* 6th ed. Hudson (Cleveland), OH, Lexi-Comp, Inc, 1998.

86a. Rodrigo G, Rodrigo C: Corticosteroids in the emergency department therapy of acute adult asthma: an evidence-based evaluation. *Chest* 116:285–95, 1999.

86b. Rodrigo C, Rodrigo G: Early administration of hydrocortisone in the emergency room treatment of acute asthma: a controlled clinical trial. *Respir Med* 88:755–761, 1994.

87. Lin RY, Pesola GR, Bakalchuk L, et al: Rapid improvement of peak flow in asthmatic patients treated with parenteral methylprednisolone in the emergency department: a randomized controlled study. *Ann Emerg Med* 33:487–494, 1999.

88. Cydulka RK, Emerman CL. A pilot study of steroid therapy after emergency department treatment of acute asthma: is a taper needed? *J Emerg Med* 16:15, 1998.

89. Schuckman H, DeJulius DP, Blanda M, et al: Comparison of intramuscular triamcinolone and oral prednisone in the outpatient treatment of acute asthma: a randomized controlled trial. *Ann Emerg Med* 31:333, 1998.

90. Rodrigo G, Rodrigo C: Inhaled flunisolide for acute severe asthma. *Am J Respir Crit Care Med* 157:698–703, 1998.

91. McFadden Jr, ER: Inhaled glucocorticoids in acute asthma. Therapeutic breakthrough or nonspecfic effect. *Am J Respir Crit Care Med* 157:677–678, 1998.

92. Volovitz B, Bentur L, Finkelstein Y, et al: Effectiveness and safety of inhaled corticosteroids in controlling acute asthma attacks in children who were treated in the emergency department: a controlled comparative study with oral prednisone. *J Allergy Clin Immunol* 102:605, 1998.

93. Guttman A, Afilalo M, Colacone A, et al: The effects of combined intravenous and inhaled steroids (beclomethasone dipropionate) for the emergency treatment of acute asthma. The Asthma ED Study Group. *Acad Emerg Med* 4(2):100–106, 1997.

94. Afilalo M, Guttman A, Colacone A, et al: Efficacy of inhaled steroids (beclomethasone dipropionate) for treatment of mild to moderately severe asthma in the emergency department: a randomized clinical trial. *Ann Emerg Med* 33:304–309, 1999.

95. Schimmer BP, Parker KL: Adrenocorticotropic hormone; adrenocortical steroids and their synthetic analogs; inhibitors of the synthesis and actions of adrenocortical hormones, in Hardman JG, Limbird, LE, Molinoff, PB, et al (eds): *The Pharmacological Basis of Therapeutics,* 9th ed. New York, McGraw-Hill, 1996, p 1459.

96. Leatherman JW, Fluegel WL, David WS, et al: Muscle weakness in mechanically ventilated patients with severe asthma. *Am J Respir Crit Care Med* 153:1686–1690, 1996.

97. Behbehani NA, Al-Mane F, D'yachkova Y, et al: Myopathy following mechanical ventilation for acute severe asthma: the role of muscle relaxants and corticosteroids. *Chest* 115:1627, 1999.

98. Murray PT, Corbridge TC: Critical care pharmacology, in Hall JB, Schmidt GA, Wood LDH (eds): *The Principles of Critical Care,* 2d ed. New York, McGraw-Hill, 1997.

99. Rossing TH, Fanta CH, Goldstein DH, et al: Emergency therapy of asthma: comparison of the acute effects of parenteral and inhaled sympathomimetics and infused aminophylline. *Am Rev Respir Dis* 122:365–371, 1980.

100. Siegel D, Sheppard D, Gelb A, Weinberg PF: Aminophylline increases the toxicity but not the efficacy of an inhaled beta-adrenergic agonist in the treatment of acute exacerbations of asthma. *Am Rev Respir Dis* 132:283–286, 1985.

101. Murphy DG, McDermott MF, Rydman RJ, et al: Aminophylline in the treatment of acute asthma when $\beta2$-agonists and steroids are provided. *Arch Intern Med* 153:1784–1788, 1993.

102. Josephson GW, Kennedy HL, MacKenzie EJ, Gibson G: Cardiac dysrhythmias during the treatment of acute asthma: A comparison of two treatment regimens by double blind protocol. *Chest* 78:429–435, 1980.

103. Coleridge J, Cameron P, Epstein J, et al: Intravenous aminophylline confers no benefit in acute asthma treated with intravenous steroids and inhaled bronchodilators. *Aust N Z J Med* 23:348–54, 1993.

104. Rodrigo C, Rodrigo G: Treatment of acute asthma: lack of therapeutic benefit and increase of toxicity from aminophylline given in addition to high doses of salbutamol delivered by metered-dose inhaler with a spacer. *Chest* 106:1071–1076, 1994.

105. Nuhoglu Y, Dai A, Barlan IB, Basaran MM: Efficacy of aminophylline in the treatment of acute asthma exacerbation in children. *Ann Allergy Asthma Immunol* 80:395, 1998.

106. Pierson WE, Bierman CW, Stamm SJ, VanArsdel Jr PP: Double-blind trial of aminophylline in status asthmaticus. *Pediatrics* 48:642–646, 1971.

107. Huang D, O'Brien RG, Harman E, et al: Does aminophylline benefit adults admitted to the hospital for an acute exacerbation of asthma? *Ann Intern Med* 119:1155–1160, 1993.

108. Yung M, South M: Randomised controlled trial of aminophylline for severe acute asthma. *Arch Dis Child,* 79:405, 1998.

109. Wrenn K, Slovis CM, Murphy F, Greenberg RS: Aminophylline therapy for acute bronchospastic disease in the ED. *Ann Intern Med* 115:241–247, 1991.

110. Milgrom H, Bender B: Current issues in the use of theophylline. *Am Rev Respir Dis* 147:S33–S39, 1993.

111. Persson CGA: Xanthines as airway anti-inflammatory drugs. *J Allergy Clin Immunol* 81:615–617, 1988.

112. Pauwels RA: New aspects of the therapeutic potential of theophylline in asthma. *J Allergy Clin Immunol* 83:548–553, 1989.

113. Kelly HW, Murphy S: Should we stop using theophylline for the treatment of the hospitalized patient with status asthmaticus? *DICP* 23:995–998, 1989.

114. Evans WV, Monie RDH, Crimmins J, Seaton A: Aminophylline, salbutamol and combined intravenous infusions in acute severe asthma. *Br J Dis Chest* 74:385–389, 1980.

115. Littenberg B: Aminophylline in severe, acute asthma: a meta-analysis. *JAMA* 259:1678–1084, 1988.

116. Newhouse MT: Is theophylline obsolete? *Chest* 98:1–2, 1990.

117. McFadden ER: Methylxanthines in the treatment of asthma: the rise, the fall, and the possible rise again. *Ann Intern Med* 115:323–324, 1991.

118. Weinberger M, Hendeles L: Slow-release theophylline: rationale and basis for product selection. *N Engl J Med* 308:760–764, 1983.

119. Reynolds RJ, Buford JG, George RB: Treating asthma and COPD in patients with heart disease. *J Respir Dis* 3(10):41–51, 1982.

120. George RB: Preventing arrhythmias in acute asthma. *J Respir Dis* 12(6):545–561, 1991.

121. Skobeloff EM, Spivey WH, McNamara RM, Greenspon L: Intravenous magnesium sulfate for the treatment of acute asthma in the emergency department. *JAMA* 262:1210–1213, 1989.

122. Noppen M, Vanmaele L, Impens N, Schandevyl W: Bronchodilating effect of intravenous magnesium sulfate in acute severe asthma. *Chest* 97:373–376, 1990.

123. Rolla G, Bucca C, Caria E, et al: Acute effect of intravenous magnesium sulfate on airway obstruction of asthmatic patients. *Ann Allergy* 61:388–391, 1988.

124. Okayama H, Okayama M, Aikawa T, et al: Treatment of status asthmaticus with intravenous magnesium sulfate. *J Asthma* 28:11–17, 1991.

125. Okayama H, Aikawa T, Okayama M, et al: Bronchodilating effect of intravenous magnesium sulfate in bronchial asthma. *JAMA* 257:1076–1078, 1987.

126. Bloch H, Silverman R, Mancherje N, et al: Magnesium sulfate is a useful adjunct to standard therapy for acute severe asthma. *Chest* 102 (Suppl):83S, 1992.

127. McNamara RM, Spivey WH, Skobeloff EM, Jacubowitz S: Intravenous magnesium sulfate in the management of acute respiratory failure complicating asthma. *Ann Emerg Med* 2:197–199, 1989.

128. Sydow M, Crozier TA, Zielmann S, et al: High-dose intravenous magnesium sulfate in the management of life-threatening status asthmaticus. *Intensive Care Med* 19:467–471, 1993.

129. Ciarallo L, Sauer AH, Shannon MW: Intravenous magnesium therapy for moderate to severe pediatric asthma: results from a randomized, placebo-controlled trial. *J Pediatr* 129:809–814, 1996.

130. Bloch H, Silverman R, Mancherje N, et al: Intravenous magnesium sulfate as an adjunct in the treatment of acute asthma. *Chest* 107:1576–1581, 1995.

131. Silverman R, Osborne H, Runge J, et al: Magnesium sulfate as an adjunct to standard therapy in acute severe asthma. *Acad Emerg Med* 3(5):467–468, 1996.

132. Nannini LJ, Hofer D: Effect of inhaled magnesium sulfate on sodium metabisulfite-induced bronchoconstriction in asthma. *Chest* 11:858–861, 1997.

133. Hill J, Britton J: Dose-response relationship and time-course of the effect of inhaled magnesium sulphate on airflow in normal and asthmatic subjects. *Br J Clin Pharmacol* 40:539–544, 1995.

134. Mangat HS, D'Souza GA, Jacob MS: Nebulized magnesium sulfate versus nebulized salbutamol in acute bronchial asthma: a clinical trial. *Eur Respir J* 12:341–344, 1998.

135. Haury VG. Blood serum magnesium in bronchial asthma and its treatment by the administration of magnesium sulfate. *J Lab Clin Med* 25:340–344, 1940.

136. Spivey WH, Skobeloff EM, Levin RM: Effect of magnesium chloride on rabbit bronchial smooth muscle. *Ann Emerg Med* 19:1107–1112, 1990.

137. Rolla G, Bucca C, Bugiani M, et al: Reduction of histamine-induced bronchoconstriction by magnesium in asthmatic subjects. *Allergy* 42:186–188, 1987.

138. Rolla G, Bucca C, Arossa W, Bugiani M: Magnesium attenuates methacholine-induced bronchoconstriction in asthmatics. *Magnesium* 6:201–204, 1987.

139. Molloy DW, Dhingra S, Solven F, et al: Hypomagnesemia and respiratory muscle power. *Am Rev Respir Dis* 129:497–498, 1984.

140. Green SM, Rothrock SG: Intravenous magnesium for acute asthma: failure to decrease emergency treatment duration or need for hospitalization. *Ann Emerg Med* 21:260–265, 1992.

141. Tiffany BR, Berk W, Todd IK, White S: Magnesium bolus or infusion fails to improve expiratory flow in acute asthma exacerbations. *Chest* 104:831–834, 1993.

142. Skobeloff EM, Spivey WH, McNamara RM: Estrogen alters the response of bronchial smooth muscle. *Ann Emerg Med* 21:647, 1992. Abstract.

143. Madison JM, Irwin RS: Heliox for asthma: A trial balloon. *Chest* 107:597–598, 1995.

144. Svartengren M, Anderson M, Philipson K, Camner P: Human lung deposition of particles suspended in air or in helium-oxygen mixture. *Exp Lung Res* 15:575–585, 1989.

145. Anderson M, Svartengren M, Bylin GB, et al: Deposition in asthmatics of particles inhaled in air or in helium-oxygen. *Am Rev Respir Dis* 147:524–528, 1993.

146. Melmed A, Hebb DB, Pohlman A, et al: The use of heliox as a vehicle for beta-agonist nebulization in patients with severe asthma. *Am J Respir Crit Care Med* 151:A269, 1995.

147. Henderson SO, Acharya P, Kilaghbian T, et al: Use of heliox-driven nebulizer therapy in the treatment of acute asthma. *Ann Emerg Med* 33:141, 1999. Abstract.

148. Manthous CA, Morgan S, Pohlman A, Hall JB: Heliox in the treatment of airflow obstruction: a critical review of the literature. *Respir Care* 42:1034–1042, 1997.

149. Curtis JL, Mahlmeister M, Fink JB, et al: Helium oxygen gas therapy: use and availability for the emergency treatment of inoperable airway obstruction. *Chest* 90:455, 1986.

150. Manthous CA, Hall JB, Melmed A, et al: The effect of heliox on pulsus paradoxus and peak flow in non-intubated patients with severe asthma. *Am J Respir Crit Care Med* 151:310–314, 1995.

150a. Kass JE, Terregino CA: The effect of heliox in acute severe asthma: a randomized controlled trial. *Chest* 116:296–300, 1999.

151. Verbeek PR, Chopra A: Heliox does not improve FEV1 in acute asthma patients. *J Emerg Med* 16:545, 1998.

151a. Rodrigo GJ, Rodrigo C, Pollack CV, Rowe BH: Heliox for nonintubated acute asthma patients. Cochrane review. In: *The Cochrane Library,* 2000 Oxford: Update Software.

152. Shiue ST, Gluck EH: The use of helium-oxygen mixtures in the support of patients with status asthmaticus and respiratory acidosis. *J Asthma* 26:177–180, 1989.

153. Kass JE, Castriotta RJ: Heliox therapy in acute severe asthma. *Chest* 107:757–760, 1995.

154. Kudukis TM, Manthous CA, Schmidt GA, et al: Inhaled helium-oxygen revisited: effect of inhaled helium-oxygen during the treatment of status asthmaticus in children. *J Pediatr* 130(2):217–224, 1997.

155. Gluck EH, Onorato DJ, Castriotta R: Helium-oxygen mixtures in intubated patients with status asthmaticus and respiratory acidosis. *Chest* 98:693–698, 1990.

155a. Schaeffer EM, Pohlman A, Morgans, Hall JB: Oxygenation in status asthmaticus improves during ventilation with helium-oxygen. *Crit Care Med* 27:2666–2670, 1999.

155b. Tassaux D, Jolliet P, Thouret JM, et al: Calibration of seven ICU ventilators for mechanical ventilation with helium-oxygen mixtures. *Am J Resp Crit Care Med* 160:22–32, 1999.

156. Teichtahl H, Buckmaster N, Pertnikovs E: The incidence of respiratory tract infection in adults requiring hospitalization for asthma. *Chest* 112:591–596, 1997.

157. Graham VAL, Knowles GK, Milton AF, Davies RJ: Routine antibiotics in hospital management of acute asthma. *Lancet* 1:418–420, 1982.

158. Berman SZ, Mathison DA, Stevenson DD, et al: Transtracheal aspiration studies in asthmatics in relapse with "infective" asthma and in subjects without respiratory disease. *J Allergy Clin Immunol* 56:206–214, 1975.

159. Saulnier FF, Durocher AV, Deturck RA, et al: Respiratory and hemodynamic effects of halothane in status asthmaticus. *Intensive Care Med* 16:104–107, 1990.

160. Echeverria M, Gelb AW, Wexler HR, et al: Enflurane and halothane in status asthmaticus. *Chest* 89:153–154, 1986.

161. Mori N, Nagata H, Ohta S, Suzuki M: Prolonged sevoflurane inhalation was not nephrotoxic in two

patients with refractory status asthmaticus. *Anesth Analg* 83:189–191, 1996.

162. O'Byrne PM, Israel E, Drazen JM: Antileukotrienes in the treatment of asthma. *Chest* 127:472–480, 1997.

163. Hogman M, Frostell CG, Hedenstrom H, Hedenstrierna G: Inhalation of nitric oxide modulates adult human bronchial tone. *Am Rev Respir Dis* 148:1474–1478, 1993.

164. Gaston B, Drazen JM, Loscalzo J, Stamler JS: The biology of nitrogen oxides in the airways. *Am J Respir Crit Care Med* 149:538–551, 1994.

165. Jatakon A, Lim S, Kharitonov SA, et al: Correlation between exhaled nitric oxide, sputum eosinophils, and methacholine responsiveness in patients with mild asthma. *Thorax* 53:91–95, 1998.

166. De Gouw HWFM, Hendriks J, Woltman AM, et al: Exhaled nitric oxide (NO) is reduced shortly after bronchoconstriction to direct and indirect stimuli in asthma. *Am J Respir Crit Care Med* 158:315–319, 1998.

167. Kanazawa H, Kawaguchi T, Shoji S, et al: Synergistic effect of nitric oxide and vasoactive intestinal peptide on bronchoprotection against histamine in anesthetized guinea pigs. *Am J Respir Crit Care Med* 155:747–750, 1997.

168. Takahashi Y, Kobayashi H, Tanaka N, Honda K, Kawakami T, Tomita T: Worsening of hypoxemia with nitric oxide inhalation during bronchospasm in humans. *Respir Physiol* 112:113–119, 1998.

169. Ricciardiolo FL, Geppetti P, Misretta A, et al: Randomized double-blind placebo-controlled study of the effect of inhibition of nitric oxide synthesis in bradykinin-induced asthma. *Lancet* 348:374–377, 1996.

170. Kaminsky DA, Janssen YMW: Evidence for peroxynitrite formation in severe human asthma. *Am J Respir Crit Care Med* 157:A876, 1998. Abstract.

171. Pendino JC, Nannini LJ, Chapman KR, et al: Effect of inhaled furosemide in acute asthma. *J Asthma* 35:89, 1998.

172. Karpel JP, Dworkin F, Hager D, et al: Inhaled furosemide is not effective in acute asthma. *Chest* 106:1396–1400, 1994.

173. Hunt LW, Swedlund HA, Gleich GJ: Effect of nebulized lidocaine on severe glucocorticoid-dependent asthma. *Mayo Clin Proc* 71:361–368, 1996.

174. Decco ML, Neeno TA, Hunt LW, et al: Nebulized lidocaine in the treatment of severe asthma in children: a pilot study. *Ann Allergy Asthma Immunol* 82:29–32, 1999.

175. Shono S, Higa K, Harasawa I, et al: Disappearance of wheezing during epidural lidocaine anesthesia in a patient with bronchial asthma. *Reg Anesth Pain Med* 24:463–466, 1999.

176. Kon H, Aokim, Yamamoto S, et al: A case of successfully managed acute asthma attack by cervical epidural block during mechanical ventilation. *Kokyu to Junkan* 38:1041–44, 1990.

177. Fish JE, Peterman VI: Effects of lidocaine on airway function in asthmatic subjects. *Respiration* 37:201–207, 1979.

178. Levtchenko E, Ramet J: Exogenous surfactant therapy for status asthmaticus. *Eur J Pediatr* 156:508, 1997.

179. Kurashima K, Ogawa H, Ohka T, et al: A pilot study of surfactant inhalation in the treatment of asthmatic attack. *Arerugi* 40:160–163, 1991.

Chapter 10

INHALED THERAPY IN NONINTUBATED PATIENTS

Carlos Rodrigo
Gustavo J. Rodrigo

INTRODUCTION

Inhalation allows drugs to be delivered directly to the large surface of the tracheobronchial tree and alveoli.[1] The value of this approach was recognized by ancient civilizations in India, China, and the Middle East, as well as by Hippocrates and Galen.[2] Since those times, aerosol delivery methods have been refined considerably and the advantages of this route for the delivery of specific drugs has become well recognized. In comparison to the systemic approach, inhalation is associated with a more rapid onset of action and fewer systemic side effects, due to the lower total dose required to reach a therapeutic drug concentration in the airway wall, and the fact that some inhaled bronchodilators are absorbed poorly into the circulation while maintaining a pharmacological effect in the airway.[3-5] For these reasons, inhaled pharmacological agents form the basis of therapy in obstructive airway disease. The purpose of this chapter is to analyze inhalation therapy in nonintubated acute severe asthma patients in the emergency department (ED) setting. Four areas will be emphasized: 1) factors that influence lower respiratory tract deposition of aerosol, 2) β-adrenergic agonists (dose, delivery methods, and drug toxicity), 3) anticholinergic drugs, and 4) inhaled corticosteroids.

FACTORS INFLUENCING LOWER RESPIRATORY TRACT DEPOSITION OF AEROSOL

Although a variety of medications have been delivered by aerosol, agents for treatment of airway obstruction constitute the greatest part of aerosol medicine. A variety of selective β agonists, anticholinergics, and corticosteroids are now available as aerosols and are frequently able to successfully treat acute asthma. These drugs have a higher therapeutic index (i.e., ratio of desired effects to side effects) when they are delivered as aerosols than when they are administered parenterally or enterally. Aerosol delivery methods have increased greatly in sophistication, but the mainstays of clinical aerosol generation in the ED setting are the *jet nebulizer* (NEB) and the *metered-dose inhaler* (MDI) with and without accessory or auxiliary devices (e.g., actuators, simple spacers, and holding chambers). Alternative propellants are being developed for MDIs, and other delivery techniques, such as dry powder formulations, have been investigated. For all these methods, several clinically important factors will determine the efficacy of aerosol delivery to the lower respiratory tract.[6]

1. Only the medication that is delivered to the lower respiratory tract is effective in the aero-

sol therapy of asthma.[7–9] This is a function of inertial impaction and sedimentation as a result of gravity and depends on the size of aerosol[10,11] and on the respiratory variables, namely, inspiratory flow rate, frequency, tidal volume, breath-holding time,[12,13] and airway caliber.[8] Aerosol generators used for therapeutic purposes are usually *heterodisperse,* that is, they generate particles of many different sizes (0.5 μm to 35 μm). Their behavior is probably best described by the mass median aerodynamic diameter (MMAD)[14–18]; 50% of the aerosol mass is contained in smaller particles and 50% is in larger particles than the MMAD. Only the particles with MMAD of 1 μm to 5 μm are efficiently deposited in the lower respiratory tract.[9] However, even under optimal inhalation conditions, only 10% to 15% of the output from an MDI, and 10% of that from most nebulizers, reach the lower respiratory tract.[19–22] Inhalation maneuvers that favor large inhaled volumes and prolong the contact time between aerosol and airway mucosa, have been shown to produce the greatest deposition.[22] Narrowed airways alter distribution and reduce the penetration of inhaled aerosols into the small airways because of enhanced aerosol deposition in the narrowed large airways. Not surprisingly, larger doses of aerosol must be administered during episodes of severe acute asthma to achieve the maximal effect, since high inspiratory flow rates, high frequencies, low tidal volumes, and pathologically narrowed airways all combine to reduce the effective dose of inhaled medication.

2.   A considerable number of patients have difficulty using MDIs effectively. The most important error is failure to coordinate firing the MDI with inhaling. This problem has been solved by the introduction of valved spacers and chambers that are interposed between the MDI and patient. Additionally, spacers reduce the size and velocity of aerosol particles leaving the MDI before aerosol inhalation. Hence, the improved patient-device interaction and the reduction in particle size and velocity optimize aerosol penetration into the lower airways and reduce aerosol deposition into upper airways.[6,23–25] This latter effect is particularly beneficial because drug absorption from the upper airway, although it contributes little to bronchodilation, can cause systemic side effects. The valved mouthpiece allows the patient to breathe aerosol from the spacer after the metered dose of aerosol has been discharged into it. On exhalation, the closed valve prevents breathing into the spacer as exhaled air enters the room.

3.   Dry powder inhalers (DPIs) are breath actuated, but usually they demand a higher inspiratory flow rate than is required for the MDI or NEB. Advantages include the ease of administration and the fact that they do not require chlorofluorocarbon propellants. When a DPI is used properly, deposition appears to be similar to that of a properly used MDI.[6] Disadvantages are 1) they usually are not particle-size selective, and thus, heavy oropharyngeal deposition may occur (similar to an MDI alone), 2) high humidity environments may cause clumping of the powder particles, and 3) DPIs cannot be used in ventilator circuits.

4.   *Helium-oxygen mixtures* (heliox), because of their low density with respect to air, have the potential for decreasing airway resistance and may benefit patients who suffer from acute severe asthma. Several studies have been published demonstrating benefit to heliox use in asthmatic patients.[26–30] Other studies have not demonstrated benefit.[31–33] Recently to determine the effect of the addition of heliox to standard medical care on the course of acute asthma, Rodrigo and colleagues performed a systematic review that included 4 randomized controlled trials with 288 acute asthma patients. The primary outcome variable was spirometry (FEV_1 or PEFR) in all trials. Pooling of the data demonstrated no significant benefit to heliox use.[34] Interestingly, several studies suggest that inhalation of drugs in heliox might be of therapeutic value when treating patients with severely obstructed airways.[35–37] The difference between inhalation with heliox and air was most prominent at high inhalation flow rates, and when airways were constricted. Deposition in mouth and throat was also significantly lower with heliox than with air. The differences in deposition between particles inhaled with heliox and air are probably

caused by differences in turbulent flow. Consequently, low-density gases such as heliox may reduce turbulent flow and could be employed to improve delivery of therapeutic aerosols.

β-ADRENERGIC AGONISTS

Specific short-acting β_2 agonists are the drugs of choice to treat acute severe asthma.[38–40] Human bronchial smooth muscle (mainly small airways) and submucosal glands contain β_2-adrenergic receptors,[41–42] and relaxation of bronchial smooth muscle depends on direct β_2-receptor stimulation.[43] In addition, stimulation of bronchial smooth muscle increases mucus secretion by submucosal glands, reduces microvascular hyperpermeability characteristic of tissue inflammation and inhibits the secretion of inflammatory mediators.

The α, β-adrenergic agonist, ephedrine, has been used in patients with airway problems for thousands of years. With the introduction of the β-adrenergic agonist isoproterenol in 1940, the clinical advantage of an agent with predominantly β-adrenergic action in patients with bronchoconstriction was quickly recognized.[44]

Three main groups of sympathomimetic bronchodilators have been described on the basis of their chemical structure.[45] The first group has mixed α and β effects. Epinephrine/adrenaline, isoproterenol, and isoetharine are members of this group. Their duration of action is short (30 to 90 minutes), because they are methylated rapidly by lung catechol-O-methyl-transferase. In addition to their short half-life, these agents lack β_2 specificity. The resorcinol group of sympathomimetic bronchodilators includes metaproterenol, orciprenaline, terbutaline, and fenoterol. These agents (except metaproterenol), are β_2-selective, and are not inactivated rapidly by methylatin, resulting in a duration of action from approximately 3 to 6 hours. Finally, the members of the salignin group are β_2-selective and have longer half-lives than isoproterenol (from 3 to 6 hours). This group includes salbutamol/albuterol, and pirbuterol. Bitolterol, an example of a pro-drug, is cleaved in

the lung by esterase to its active form, colterol. Isoproterenol, metaproterenol, isoetharine, and epinephrine are not recommended due to their potential for excessive extrapulmonary, unwanted effects, especially in high doses. Also, long-acting drugs, such as salmeterol, have a slow onset and cannot be recommended for emergency treatment.

Inhalation β-Agonist Dosing

The International Consensus on Clinical Aerosol Administration[6] emphasizes three principles pertaining to aerosol dosing, particularly with β agonists. First, rather than adhering to a standardized protocol, doses and dosing intervals should be individualized according to the severity of airway dysfunction, the response to the agent, and the delivery system used. Second, objective measurements of response (e.g., PEFR) to dosing strategy, particularly in patients with severe impairment, should be made. The response to initial treatment in the ED is a better predictor of the need for hospitalization than the severity of an exacerbation on presentation.[46,47] Third, in carrying out these guidelines, a substantial body of evidence supports *the use of considerably high, frequent, and cumulative doses.*[39]

The optimal doses of these agents in acute asthma have not been established.[48] The aim of the treatment is to induce maximal stimulation of β_2 receptors without causing significant side effects, and in many (but not all) patients there is a clear-cut dose response relationship.[5,49–55] Higher doses may be important because of the unpredictability of delivery systems, low tidal volumes, variable flow rates, increased frequency of breathing, peripheral dispersion of the inhaled medication and narrowed airways.[24] The cumulative technique produces greater bronchodilation than an equivalent single dose of aerosolized bronchodilator.[53] On the other hand, unwanted effects constitute the dose-limiting factor of β_2–adrenergic bronchodilators. These side effects generally are dose-dependent.[49–55]

There have been attempts to establish the optimal dose of β agonists in acute asthma. In one study, Rodrigo and Rodrigo analyzed 116 acute asthmatics treated with salbutamol/albuterol delivered by MDI with spacer at a dose of 400 μg (four puffs) every 10 minutes for 3 hours (Fig. 10-1).[56] Almost 81 of the 116 patients (70%) had a convincing response to increasing doses of salbutamol (67% obtained the discharge threshold after the administration of 2.4 mg of albuterol within 1 hour). At that time, they were asymptomatic, free of accessory muscle use, and they had a PEFR of 55% or more of the predicted value. In fact, 53% of responders met the discharge requirements after only 12 puffs (1.2 mg) (Fig. 10-2). In the remaining 35 patients in the study group (30%), treatment had little effect. Consequently, in this patient group, a 50% increase in dose to 600 μg every 10 minutes resulted in a slightly better therapeutic response, but with

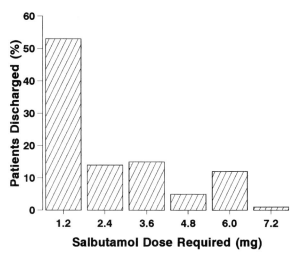

Figure 10-2
Dose of salbutamol required to attain discharge threshold. (From Rodrigo and Rodrigo[56])

Figure 10-1
Change in PEFR in response to cumulative doses of inhaled salbutamol in discharged and admitted patients. Values are shown as mean ± 1 SD (From Rodrigo and Rodrigo[56])

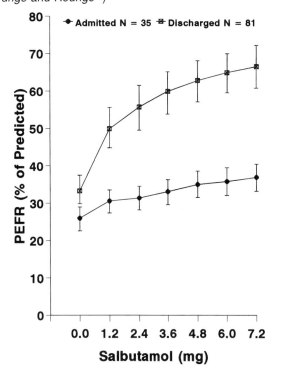

greater side effects related to higher serum albuterol levels.[55] Similarly, McFadden and colleagues found that 85% of patients who are discharged leave the ED with a PEFR greater than 60% of normal after receiving three aerosols of albuterol, 2.5 mg each, over 1 hour.[57] In another study, approximately 50% of patients reached maximal bronchodilation after a single dose of albuterol.[50] Finally, Strauss and colleagues found that 66% of acute asthma patients in their study responded to three doses of albuterol, 2.5 mg each, by nebulization every 20 minutes.[58] Of these 56% required 5 mg or less of drug to reach the discharge threshold.

These data demonstrate two different response patterns to inhaled high and cumulative doses of salbutamol. Approximately 66% of acute asthma patients respond to inhaled albuterol, and in this group, 2.4 mg to 3.6 mg delivered by MDI with spacer, or 5 mg to 7.5 mg delivered by NEB, represents optimal treatment. These findings support the recommendations found in the National Asthma Education and Prevention Program Expert Panel Report 2 (EPR-2), namely, salbutamol/albuterol 2.5 mg to 5 mg for three doses delivered by nebulization or 4 to 8 puffs (90 μg/puff to 100 μg/puff) every 20 minutes by MDI and spacer.[39]

In patients who do not respond to this treatment, salbutamol, even in high doses, has little effect. Accordingly, it is clear that there is little to be gained by prolonging treatment in ED. Immediate improvement following bronchodilator therapy appears to be due to resolution of smooth muscle contraction, and patients in whom this factor is the major contributor to disability do quite well following minimal treatment, even if the obstruction is severe.[59] Bronchodilator nonresponders probably have mucosal edema, airway wall inflammation, and intraluminal mucus, which portends a more protracted course.

The currently available β-adrenergic bronchodilators with relative β_2 selectivity (albuterol, terbutaline, pirbuterol, fenoterol, isoetharine) are all effective clinically, with similar pharmacologic features. Aerosolized isoetharine is as effective as fenoterol[60] and albuterol,[61–62] but has more possible side effects. In a similar way, fenoterol is as effective as albuterol, but with greater side effects.[46,63] However, when equimolar concentrations of both drugs are compared, there is μg equivalence with respect to bronchodilator effects and common side effects in the clinically relevant dose range. These effects are not age-dependent, as both old and young asthmatics respond similarly.[64]

Comparison Between MDI and NEB

Generally, hand-held NEBs are most commonly used in the ED setting, while MDIs are primarily used in the outpatient setting.[65] However, there is considerable evidence that MDI with spacer is as effective or better than NEB.[66–77] Radiolabeled studies have shown equivalent percentages of total lung deposition of salbutamol aerosolized by either an NEB or an MDI/holding chamber.[78] Furthermore, two systematic reviews concluded that MDI with holding chamber produced outcomes that were at least equivalent to NEB.[79–80] These studies did not allow for objective comparison of the aerosol delivery system independent of the doses of medication. Previous studies have reported equipotent dose ratios of β agonists delivered by MDI with spacer and by NEB, ranging

from 1:1 to 1:11. Blake and colleagues compared the effects of albuterol given by MDI or NEB on airway reactivity as assessed by histamine challenge, before and after albuterol administration.[81] This study design permitted evaluation of asthmatic patients with essentially normal baseline lung function and it also minimized the confounding influence of severity of airflow obstruction. Data from this study suggest that 10 puffs from the MDI, totaling 0.9 mg, would deliver approximately the same amount of albuterol to lung receptors as 2.5 mg of the nebulized solution. Similarly, two studies by Rodrigo and Rodrigo found that for every 1 mg of albuterol delivered by MDI with spacer, 2 mg to 2.5 mg are needed by nebulization to have an equal therapeutic response[76,82] (Fig. 10-3). Similar results are also seen when the mean MDI dose needed to reach a discharge threshold (2.4 mg albuterol)[56] is compared to the mean NEB dose required for discharge (1:2.1 dose ratio).[58] However, these therapeutically equivalent-dose ratios must be interpreted with caution because NEB output can be highly variable, both with respect to the rate of aerosol production and to the nature of the aerosol, specifically, the MMAD,[83–85] and

Figure 10-3
The relationship between FEV$_1$ (mean % of predicted) plotted against the cumulative dose of salbutamol. Bars represent mean ($\pm$ 1 SD). (From Rodrigo and Rodrigo[82])

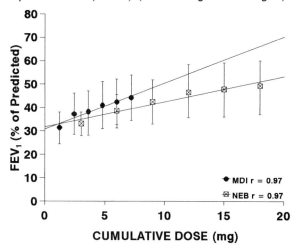

because of potential difference in patients among studies.

Continuous NEB is considered better than intermittent therapy in children,[86] but in adults the data are contradictory and do not allow for definite conclusions. Two studies do not show major differences among methods of administration.[87–88] Another recent study demonstrated that continuous delivery of albuterol at high (7.5 mg per hour) or standard (2.5 mg per hour) doses was superior to either dose given intermittently each hour for 2 hours.[89] There was no difference in improvement between the two groups treated with continuous NEB, but the standard-dose continuous treatment regimen had the fewest side effects.

Finally, with regard to the use of dry powder formulation for the treatment of acute severe asthma, little information is available. Tonnesen and colleagues have reported that terbutaline administered via the Turbuhaler caused a significantly better improvement in FEV_1, as compared to terbutaline administered via MDI attached to an aerosol holding chamber.[90] However, another prospective study of acute asthma patients showed a similar improvement in FEV_1 regardless of the three different delivery methods used (albuterol via NEB, MDI attached to a valved aerosol holding chamber and Rotahaler).[91] However, the major limitation of this study was that the authors did not demonstrate equivalence among the three therapeutic modalities. β agonist can be effectively delivered to patients with acute severe asthma by means of an MDI with spacer, or by NEB. The authors preferentially use MDI with spacer (Volumatic®), because it requires less time for drug administration and because cost and side effects are lower.[82] In addition, NEBs can be a source of pulmonary infections. Still, nebulizers may be used safely and effectively, and often with less patient supervision. The most important factor governing NEB performance is the flow of compressed air used to generate the aerosol. Aerosol size is inversely proportional to the compressed gas flow rate. For most jet NEBs a flow rate of ≥ 6 L per minute is necessary to insure that treatment times are acceptably short, and that the bulk of the aerosol mass is contained within particles of no more

than 5 μm aerodynamic diameter.[16] Also important is the fill volume. A combination of 4 ml volume fill and 6 L per minute gas flow rate is recommended to ensure a high aerosol output, small particle size, and short treatment time.

Drug Toxicity

Undesirable systemic side effects can occur during treatment with β agonists. These side effects are *dose-dependent* and can occur with all routes of drug administration, but for a given degree of bronchodilation, they are more pronounced with oral and intravenous administration.[92] For selective β_2-adrenergic agonists, the principal side effects are mediated via receptors on vascular smooth muscle (tachycardia and tachyarrhythmias[93,94]), skeletal muscle (tremor, hypokalemia due to potassium entry into muscle cells[95–99]), and cells involved in lipid and carbohydrate metabolism (increases in blood-free fatty acids, insulin, glucose, and pyruvate). Another unwanted effect is an increase in ventilation-perfusion mismatching, leading to an increased alveolar-arterial oxygen tension difference.[100–104] This has been attributed to differential regional vasodilator and bronchodilator effects. The resulting fall in arterial P_{O_2} is small, of short duration, and generally of negligible clinical significance. However, most of these studies have been conducted with healthy volunteers or in patients with stable asthma.

To study the feasibility of using high-dose continuously aerosolized albuterol in adults, Lin and colleagues treated seven acute asthma patients with a continuous nebulization of albuterol at a rate of 0.4 mg/kg per hour for 4 hours.[105] One patient withdrew at 3 hours after developing supraventricular tachycardia. Heart rate increases were observed in six of eight treatments, and serum albuterol levels at the end of treatment were greater than 25 ng/ml in all but one treatment (mean level, 37.7 ± 15.1 ng/ml). A mean increase in heart rate of 16.3% was observed for the entire group. Mean serum potassium was 4.07 ± 0.45 mg/dL at baseline and 3.3 ± 0.29 mg/dL after treatment. A significant improvement in FEV_1 was observed with a net increase of 37%. These data suggest that high-dose continuously aerosolized albuterol can result in markedly elevated serum albuterol levels and cardiac stimulation along with spirometric improvement.

In another study, Rodrigo and Rodrigo investigated the safety and efficacy of two cumulative doses of albuterol: 400 μg (37 μg/kg per hour) versus 600 μg (55 μg/kg per hour) at 10-minute intervals for 3 hours, delivered by MDI with spacer in the ED setting.[55] There were similar increases in FEV$_1$ in both groups, yet heart rate fell in the 400 μg group, and rose in the 600 μg group (Fig. 10-4). A moderate reduction in the serum potassium level was noted, with no significant difference between the groups. However, a reduction to less than 3.2 mg/dL, which may be considered a critical value, was seen once in the 400 μg group and four times in the 600 μg group. Additionally, there was

a significant increase in blood glucose in the 600 μg group, but not in the 400 μg group. Mean arterial oxygen saturation improved only in the 400 μg group. At the end of treatment, the albuterol plasma levels were 10.0 $\pm$ 1.67 ng/ml for the 400 μg group, and 14 $\pm$ 2.17 ng/ml for the 600 μg group.

These two studies suggest that there may be a dose or serum threshold level of albuterol that produces tachycardia. Initial tachycardia in acute asthma may be related to disease severity, which may be relieved with bronchodilator therapy.[106] However, albuterol treatment may increase or decrease heart rate, depending on the dose administered (particularly serum level obtained) and the therapeutic response. Schuh and colleagues demonstrated heart rate increases in asthmatic children with serum albuterol levels of 12.4 and 19.8 ng/ml.[107] In our study, heart rate decreased in improving patients with an albuterol level of approximately 10 ng/ml and increased in improving patients with an albuterol level of approximately 14 ng/ml. These data support the notion that the treatment of acute asthma patients in the ED with albuterol, 2.4 mg per hour (400 μg by MDI with spacer at 10-minute intervals), produces satisfactory bronchodilation, low serum albuterol levels, and minimal extrapulmonary effects. Additionally, no significant arrhythmias or other serious cardiovascular side effects were observed in these patients. On the other hand, high-dose continuous aerosolized albuterol may be associated with high serum albuterol levels and troublesome systemic effects.

Finally, interactions with other medications should be considered during β agonist administration. For instance, the addition of aminophylline plays no useful role in the ED treatment of acute asthma, because it provides no additional benefit to optimal inhaled β-agonist therapy and may increase adverse effects.[46,53,108–112]

In addition, combinations of high doses of β agonists and corticosteroids may cause significant hypokalemia. Taylor and colleagues demonstrated that the concomitant use of oral corticosteroids potentiates the hypokalemia of high-dose inhaled β agonist treatment.[113] In another trial, Lin and colleagues found that patients who reported corti-

Figure 10-4

Change in heart rate (HR) in response to cumulative doses of inhaled salbutamol. Values are shown as mean and SD. (From Rodrigo and Rodrigo[55])

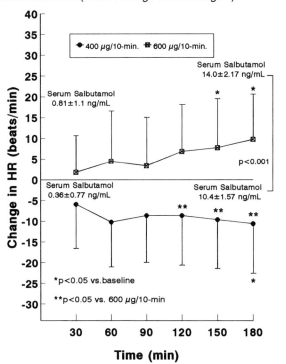

costeroid use before arrival to the ED had a higher heart rate during the second hour of β agonist treatment.[114] The significance of this finding is unclear.

ANTICHOLINERGIC DRUGS

The potential usefulness of anticholinergic drugs in the treatment of wheeze has long been recognized.[115] However, two developments in the past years have revived interest in anticholinergic bronchodilators. First, there has been an increasingly better understanding of the cholinergic mechanisms that control airway caliber in health and disease. Second was the development by pharmaceutical chemists of synthetic analogues of atropine that were not appreciably absorbed, but that still retained the anticholinergic properties of atropine. Currently, several anticolinergics are regularly prescribed by physicians worldwide, including atropine, ipratropium bromide, thiazinamium, oxitropium bromide, and glycopyrrolate. Of these, ipratropium bromide has been the most extensively studied.

Nonselective anticholinergic agents such as atropine, ipratropium bromide and oxitropium bromide block both prejunctional (M_2) and postjunctional (M_3) muscarinic receptors, producing smooth muscle relaxation in bronchial airways by competitively opposing the action of acetylcholine that is released at the effector surfaces of parasympathetic vagal nerve endings. Studies of the site of effect of anticholinergic agents suggest that bronchodilation occurs principally in the larger, central airways[116] in both normal controls,[117] and subjects with airway disease.[118] Atropine sulfate is not recommended in the treatment of acute asthma. However, despite having no FDA indication for this use, atropine sulfate has been used extensively as a nebulized solution by intensivists and ED specialists for years.[119] This drug is readily absorbed across the oral and respiratory mucosa and, when higher doses are used to maximize bronchodilation, the incidence of dry mouth, blurred vision, urinary retention, nausea, and tachycardia may limit atropine's usefulness. On the other hand,

when ipratropium bromide is inhaled, less than 1% of the administered dose is absorbed.[120] Additionally, in contrast to atropine, ipratropium bromide does not increase sputum viscosity or decrease mucociliary clearance, minimizing the concern that anticholinergic therapy will dry secretions in the critically ill patient.[121] Its half-life in the circulation is of the same order as atropine, approximately 3 hours. The onset of action is somewhat slower than that of a β-adrenergic agent, with peak bronchodilation typically occurring 30 to 90 minutes after administration. Another significant advantage to ipratropium bromide in the critically ill asthma patient is the lack of increase in heart rate, which does occur with β agonist use.[122]

The role of anticholinergic medications in the treatment of acute asthma is unclear. The use of ipratropium bromide as the initial bronchodilator has been consistently reported to be inferior to the use of a β-adrenergic agent in status asthmaticus.[123] However, the use of both classes of bronchodilators, either simultaneously or in sequence, has produced an almost equal number of positive[124–134] and negative trials.[135–142]

Recently, a series of systematic reviews were conducted to clarify this point. First, a review of 10 randomized controlled trials of children and adolescents[143] taking β_2 agonists for acute asthma with and without the addition of inhaled anticholinergics, showed significant group differences in lung function supporting combination treatment; additionally, multiple dose anticholinergic protocols, mainly in children and adolescents with severe exacerbations, reduced the risk of hospital admission by 30%. In a second meta-analysis (adult patients) of 10 randomized, double-blind, placebo-controlled trials[144] ipratropium was associated with a significant increase in pulmonary function (effect size = 0.38, 95% CI: 0.27 to 0.48) and a 27% reduction in hospital admissions. Finally, a third systematic review[145] that included 10 randomized, double-blind, controlled trials, with 1483 adults with acute asthma, showed a 10% increase in pulmonary function (the greatest improvement in patients with more severe obstruction) (Figure 10-5), and a 38% admission rate

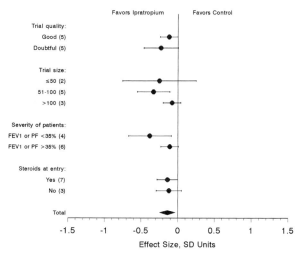

Figure 10-5
Sensitivity analysis comparing results of meta-analysis by quality of studies, severity of patients' asthma (mean pulmonary function), and use of corticosteroids. Effect size and 95% confidence intervals. Number in parenthesis = number of studies; FEV_1 = forced expiratory volume in 1 second; PF = peak expiratory flow. (From Rodrigo, Rodrigo, and Burschtin[145]).

reduction. Surprisingly, almost all these beneficial effects were obtained with the utilization of single dose protocols consisting in small doses of ipratropium bromide. However, only a few trials have administered high and cumulative doses of both β-adrenergics and anticholinergics. Rodrigo and Rodrigo[128] studied the effects of high and cumulative doses of salbutamol/albuterol and ipratropium bromide in the treatment of acute asthma. Subjects were entered in a double-blind, randomized manner into one of two treatment modalities. A regimen of albuterol alone was compared to albuterol combined with ipratropium. Albuterol and ipratropium were administered through MDI and spacer, 4 puffs each at 10-minute intervals over 3 hours. After 3 hours, the additional bronchodilation in the ipratropium group was 32.4% for PEFR and 41.2% for FEV_1. Finally, Rodrigo and Rodrigo conducted a larger, double-blind, randomized, prospective trial to test the hypothesis that acute asthma patients given combination high dose therapy with ipratropium bromide and

β_2 agonists will have greater improvement in pulmonary function and fewer hospital admissions than those given β_2 agonists alone.[146] One hundred eighty patients who consulted an ED for treatment of an exacerbation of asthma were assigned in a randomized, double-blind fashion to receive albuterol and placebo or albuterol and ipratropium. Both drugs were administered through a metered-dose inhaler and spacer at 10-min intervals for 3 hours (24 puffs each of albuterol and ipratropium each hour). Primary outcome measures were improvement in pulmonary function (FEV_1 or PEFR), and hospital admission rates. Both groups improved pulmonary function significantly over baseline values. Subjects who received ipratropium had an overall 20.5% (95% CI: 2.6 to 38.4%) (p = 0.02) greater improvement in PEFR and a 48.1% (95% CI: 19.8 to 76.4%) (p = 0.01) greater improvement in FEV_1 compared with controls. At the end of the protocol (3 hours), 39% of patients in the control group and 20% in the ipratropium group were admitted (p = 0.01). The use of high doses of ipratropium reduced the risk of hospital admission 49% (relative risk = 0.51, 95% CI: 0.31 to 0.83). Five (95% CI: 3 to 17) patients would need to be treated with high doses of ipratropium to prevent a single admission. A subgroup analysis showed that patients most likely to benefit from the addition of high doses of ipratropium were those with more severe obstruction (FEV_1 ≤30% of predicted) and long duration of symptoms before the ED presentation (≥24 hours).

Overall, these data suggest a significant advantage in the maximum bronchodilatation response when high doses of ipratropium bromide and albuterol administered by MDI and spacer are combined in the emergency treatment of acute severe asthma, specifically in patients with FEV_1 less than 30% and with long duration of symptoms before the ED presentation (≥24 h).

INHALED CORTICOSTEROIDS

Systemic glucocorticoids in the ED have been used for the treatment of asthma for more than 40 years. They have been recommended for patients who have moderate-to-severe exacerbations, and for patients who do not respond completely to initial β-agonist therapy.[39] The mechanisms of action of these drugs in asthma are unknown. They are not bronchodilators and their major utility appears to be related to reducing airway inflammation by influencing cell traffic and the metabolism of membrane-derived lipid mediators.[147–149] Several studies have suggested that glucocorticoids can acutely improve lung function during the course of several hours,[150,151] but these observations have not been confirmed.[152–159] Rather, the weight of evidence demonstrates that parenteral steroids in acute adult asthma require >6 to 24 hours to begin to achieve effect.[160] This time delay fits with the concept that beneficial effects require synthesis of new proteins through gene induction. While it appears quite likely that a minimum blood level is required before a therapeutic response will be seen, a threshold level has not been established.[161] Although it is commonly taught that high doses of glucocorticoids are more effective than small ones, a dose-response relationship does not clearly exist.[160]

Inhaled steroids are rarely mentioned[162] and generally considered ineffective in acute severe asthma.[163–166] Nevertheless, there is some evidence that suggests that inhaled corticosteroids offer an early therapeutic benefit. In a recent double-blind placebo-controlled trial, Scarfone and colleagues demonstrated that inhaled dexamethasone was as effective as oral prednisone in the ED treatment of children with acute asthma.[167] Indeed, inhaled drug was associated with a significantly greater proportion of discharges within 2 hours. Previous animal[168–169] and human research showed that inhaled topical corticosteroids have therapeutic effects as early as 2 hours. For example, Husby and colleagues observed a significant improvement 2 hours after administering 2 mg of nebulized budesonide to children hospitalized for croup.[170] Additionally, two recent studies concluded that 2 mg of nebulized budesonide resulted in prompt (within 2 hours) and important clinical improvement in children with mild-to-moderate croup in the ED.[171–172] Similarly, Gibson and colleagues demonstrated an acute effect on airway inflammatory

cells 6 hours after the administration of inhaled budesonide.[173] There are also data demonstrating suppression of exhaled nitric oxide 6 hours after a single dose of budesonide, suggesting an early effect of steroids on airway inflammation.[174]

Rodrigo and Rodrigo designed a randomized, double-blind controlled trial to determine the benefit of high and cumulative doses of flunisolide added to albuterol in patients with acute severe asthma.[175] Patients who presented to an ED for treatment of an acute exacerbation of asthma, were assigned to receive albuterol and placebo or albuterol combined with flunisolide. Both drugs were administered successively through MDI with spacer, at 10-minute intervals for 3 hours (400 μg of albuterol and 1 mg of flunisolide, every 10 minutes). Both groups improved FEV_1 and PEFR significantly over baseline values, but patients in the flunisolide group had significantly better airflow rates compared with placebo at 90, 120, 150, and 180 minutes. Data analyzed separately in accordance with the duration of the attack before ED presentation (<24 or $\geq$24 hours) showed that the placebo/$\geq$24 hours subgroup had a significantly lower FEV_1 at 120, 150, and 180 minutes, and a greater rate of admission than the remaining subgroups (Fig. 10-6).

Figure 10-6

FEV_1 (% of predicted) over time in 4 groups based on treatment and duration of attack before presentation ($P < .05$). (From Rodrigo and Rodrigo[175])

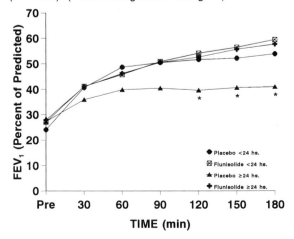

These findings support, for the first time, the notion that inhaled flunisolide administered in high dose offers a therapeutic benefit as early as 2 hours after ED presentation. This rapid response suggests a nonimmunologic topical anti-inflammatory effect,[176] or possibly inhibition of edema formation or constriction of the microcirculation.[177] In other investigations, cutaneous blanching has been used to measure corticosteroid activity of topical preparations,[178] an effect that can be seen within 2 hours. In conclusion, this study supports the assumption that high and cumulative doses of inhaled corticosteroids administered by MDI with spacer can be effective in patients with a prolonged duration of symptoms before ED presentation.

In contrast, in a recent randomized double-blind study by Afilalo and colleagues, 54 adults with mild to moderately severe asthma in the ED were assigned to two groups.[179] One group was administered 2.5 mg of nebulized salbutamol plus 1 mg (4 puffs) of beclomethasone dipropionate by MDI with spacer, and the other group was administered 2.5 mg of nebulized salbutamol by itself by MDI with spacer. The dose of corticosteroids was much lower than that used in the study by Rodrigo and Rodrigo. Treatments were given at baseline, 0.5, 1, 2, and 3 hours. Spirometry improved in both groups over the 6 hours of study, but there was no added benefit to the 5 mg of beclomethasone. However, there was a trend toward a difference in admission rates favoring the inhaled steroid group.

CONCLUSIONS

Compared to systemic administration, inhalation therapy offers more rapid onset of action with fewer systemic side effects, owing to the lower total dose required to reach a therapeutic drug concentration in the airway wall, and the fact that some inhaled bronchodilators are absorbed poorly into the circulation while maintaining a pharmacologic effect in the airway. For these reasons, inhaled pharmacologic agents form the basis of therapy in acute obstructive airway disease. A variety of selective β agonists, anticholinergic bronchodilators and corticosteroids are now available as aerosols and are frequently able (by themselves or in combination) to successfully treat acute severe asthma.

Specific short-acting β_2 agonists are the drugs of choice to treat acute severe asthma in nonintubated patients. The aim of treatment with these drugs is to induce maximal stimulation of β_2 receptors without causing significant side effects. A substantial body of evidence supports the use of considerably high, frequent, and cumulative doses. Available data also demonstrate two different response patterns to inhalation of high doses of albuterol. Approximately two-thirds of acute asthma patients respond to inhaled albuterol. In this group, treatment with 2.4 to 3.6 mg of albuterol delivered by MDI with spacer, or 5.0 to 7.5 mg delivered by NEB, delivered over the first hour, appears to be optimal. In the remainder of patients, albuterol, even in high doses, has little effect, and little is to be gained by prolonging treatment in the ED. β_2 agonists can be effectively delivered by means of an MDI with spacer, or by a nebulizer. However, there is considerable evidence that MDI with spacer is as effective (or better) than a nebulizer, allowing for quick, inexpensive, and simple therapy with minimal toxicity.

The role of anticholinergic medications is less well defined for patients with acute asthma. However, there are data that support a beneficial effect from the addition of ipratropium bromide to albuterol when both are administered in high doses, specifically in patients with more severe obstruction. Our approach is to administer ipratropium bromide combined with albuterol in high and cumulative doses by MDI with spacer until there is an acceptable clinical response or toxicity precludes further treatment.

Finally, there are data that suggest an early benefit to the use of high-dose inhaled corticosteroids. A therapeutic effect may occur as early as 2 hours after high-dose therapy is initiated, which indicates a nonimmunologic topical anti-inflammatory effect, inhibition of mucosal edema, or possible constriction of the microcirculation. Inhaled corticosteroids in high dose may prove to be particularly important in the management of patients who experience prolonged exacerbations before arriving at an ED.

REFERENCES

1. Newman SP, Clarke SW: Therapeutic aerosols 1- Physical and practical considerations. Editorial *Thorax* 38:881–886, 1983.
2. Ziment I: *Respiratory pharmacology and therapeutics.* Philadelphia, W B Saunders, 1–7, 1978.
3. Clark TJH: Factors influencing route of administration of airway therapy, in Sadoul P, Milic-Emili J: (eds): *Small airways in health and disease.* Amsterdam, Excerpta Medica, 1979, pp 170–178.
4. Toogood JH, Jennings B, Baskerville, Lefcoe NM: Personal observations on the use of inhaled corticosteroid drugs for chronic asthma. *Eur J Respir Dis* 65:321–328, 1984.
5. Rodrigo C, Rodrigo G: High-dose MDI salbutamol treatment of asthma in the ED. *Am J Emerg Med* 13:21–26, 1995.
6. American Respiratory Care Foundation and the American Association for Respiratory Care: Aerosol consensus statement. *Chest* 100:1106–1109, 1991.
7. Ruffin RE, Montgomery JM, Newhouse MT: Site of beta-adrenergic receptors in the respiratory tract: Use of fenoterol administered by two methods: *Chest* 74:256–260, 1978.
8. Santolicandro A, Giuntini C: Patterns of deposition of labeled monodispersed aerosols in obstructive lung disease. *J Nucl Med Allied Sci* 23:115–127, 1979.
9. Newman SP, Pavia D, Clarke SW: How should a pressurized β-adrenergic bronchodilator be inhaled? *Eur J Respir Dis* 62:3–21, 1981.
10. Morrow PE: Aerosol characterization and deposition. *Am Rev Respir Dis* 110:88–99, 1974.
11. Brain JD, Valberg PA: Deposition of aerosol in the respiratory tract. *Am Rev Respir Dis* 120:1325–1373, 1979.
12. Newhouse MT, Ruffin RE: Deposition and fate of aerosolized drugs. *Chest* 73:9365–942S, 1978.
13. Dolovich MB, Ruffin RE, Roberts R, Newhouse MT: Optimal delivery of aerosols from metered dose inhalers. *Chest* 80:911–915, 1981.
14. Morrow PE: An evaluation of the physical properties of monodisperse and heterodisperse aerosols

used in the assessment of bronchial function. *Chest* 80(suppl):809–813, 1981.
15. Clay MM, Pavia D, Newman SP, Clarke SW: Assessment of jet nebulizers for lung aerosol therapy. *Lancet* 2:592–594, 1983.
16. Clay MM, Pavia D, Newman SP, Clarke SW: Factors influencing the size distribution of aerosols from jet nebulizers. *Thorax* 38:755–759, 1983.
17. Clarke SW, Newman SP: Therapeutic aerosols: Two drugs available by the inhaled route. *Thorax* 39:1–7, 1984.
18. Kim CS, Eldridge MA, Sackner MA: Oropharyngeal deposition and delivery aspects of metered-dose inhaler aerosols. *Am Rev Respir Dis* 135:157–164, 1987.
19. Newman SP, Moren F, Pavia D, et al: Deposition of pressurized aerosols in the human respiratory tract. *Thorax* 36:52–55, 1981.
20. Newman SP, Pavia D, Garland N, Clarke SW: Effects of various inhalation modes on the deposition of radioactive pressurized aerosols. *Eur J Respir Dis* 119:57–65, 1982.
21. Newman SP: Aerosol deposition considerations in inhalation therapy. *Chest* 88:152S-160S, 1985.
22. Newhouse M, Dolovich M: Current concepts, control of asthma by aerosols. *N Engl J Med* 315:870–874, 1986.
23. Newman SP, Moren F, Pavia, D, et al: Deposition of pressurized suspension aerosols inhaled through extension devices. *Am Rev Respir Dis* 124:317–320, 1981.
24. Dolovich M, Eng P, Ruffin R, et al: Clinical evaluation of a simple demand inhalation MDI aerosol delivery device. *Chest* 84:36–41, 1983.
25. Newman SP, Millar AB, Lennard-Jones TR, et al: Improvement of pressurized aerosol deposition with nebuhaler spacer device. *Thorax* 39:935–941, 1984.
26. Manthous CA, Hall JB, Melmeda A, et al: Heliox improves pulsus paradoxus and peak expiratory flow in nonintubated patients with severe asthma. *Am J Respir Crit Care Med* 151:310–314, 1995.
27. Kass J, Terregino CA: The effect of heliox in acute severe asthma. A randomized controlled trial. *Chest* 116:296–300, 1999.
28. Gluck EH, Onorato DJ, Castriotta R: Helium-oxygen mixtures in intubated patients with status asthmaticus and respiratory acidosis. *Chest* 98:693–698, 1990.
29. Kudukis TM, Manthous CA, Schmidt GA, et al: Inhaled helium-oxygen revisited: Effect of helium-

oxygen during treatment of status asthmaticus in children. *J Pediatr* 130:217–224, 1997.

30. Kass JE, Castriotta RJ: Heliox therapy in acute severe asthma. *Chest* 107:757–760, 1995.

31. Carter ER, Webb CR, Moffit DR: Evaluation of heliox in children hospitalized with acute severe asthma. A randomized crossover trial. *Chest* 109:1256–1261, 1996.

32. Verbeek PR, Chopra A: Heliox does not improve FEV₁ in acute asthma patients. *J Emerg Med* 16:545, 1998.

33. Henderson SO, Acharya P, Kilaghbian T, et al: Use of heliox-driven nebulizer therapy in the treatment of acute asthma. *Ann Emerg Med* 33:141–146, 1999.

34. Rodrigo GJ, Rodrigo C, Pollack CV, Rowe BH: Heliox for nonintubated acute asthma patients. Cochrane review. In: *Cochrane Library,* 2000. Oxford: Update Software.

35. Anderson M, Svartengren M, Bylin O, et al: Deposition in asthetics of particles inhaled in air or in helium-oxygen. *Am Rev Respir Dis* 147:524–528, 1993.

36. Bateman JRM, Pavia D, Scheahan NF, et al: Impaired tracheobronchial clearance in patients with mild stable asthma. *Thorax* 38:463–467, 1983.

37. Pavia D, Bateman JRM, Scheahan NF, et al: Tracheobronchial mucociliary clearance in asthma: Impairment during remission. *Thorax* 40:171–175, 1985.

38. Rossing TH, Fanta CH, Goldstein DH, et al: Emergency therapy of asthma: Comparison of the acute effects of parenteral and inhaled sympathomimetics and infused aminophylline. *Am Rev Respir Dis* 122:365–371, 1980.

39. National Asthma Education and Prevention Program Expert Panel Report 2: *Guidelines For The Diagnosis And Management Of Asthma.* Bethesda, MD, NIH, Publication 55–4051, 1997.

40. British Asthma Guidelines Coordinating Committee: British Guidelines On Asthma Management, 1995 review and position statement. *Thorax* 52:S1–24, 1997.

41. Barnes PJ, Basbaum CB: Mapping of adrenergic receptors in mammalian trachea using an autoradiographic method. *Exp Lung Res* 5:183–192, 1983.

42. Barnes PJ, Basbaum CB, Nadel JA: Autoradiographic localization of autonomic receptors in airway smooth muscle: marked differences between large and small airways. *Am Rev Respir Dis* 127:758–762, 1983.

43. Zaagsma J, van der Heijden PJCM, van der Schaar MWG: Comparison of functional beta-adrenoreceptor heterogeneity in central and peripheral airway smooth muscle of guinea pig and man. *J Recept Res* 3:89–106, 1983.

44. Konzett H: Neue broncholytisch hochwirksame Korper der Adrenalin-reibe. *Arch Exp Pathol Pharmakol* 197:27–40, 1940.

45. Freedman BJ, Hill GB: Comparative study of duration of action and cardiovascular effects of bronchodilator aerosols. *Thorax* 26:46, 1971

46. Rodrigo G, Rodrigo C: Tratamiento de la crisis asmatica: comparación entre fenoterol y salbutamol en altas dosis administradas mediante inhalador de dosis medida con inhalocamara (Volumatic) y aminofilina intravenosa. *Pac Critico* 4:194–209, 1991.

47. Rodrigo G, Rodrigo C: Assessment of the patient with acute asthma in the emergency department: A factor analytic study. *Chest* 104:1325–1328, 1993.

48. Nowak RM: Inhaled beta-agonists and acute asthma. *Am J Emerg Med* 13:94–96, 1995.

49. Walters EH, Cockroft A, Griffiths T, et al: Optimal dose of salbutamol respiratory solution: Comparison of three doses with plasma levels. *Thorax* 36:625–628, 1981.

50. Lipworth BJ, Clark RA, Dhillon DP, et al: Beta-adrenoceptor responses to high doses of inhaled salbutamol in patients with bronchial asthma. *Br J Clin Pharmacol* 26:527–533, 1988.

51. Stanescu DC: High doses of sympathomimetics in severe bronchial asthma. *Eur Respir J* 2:597–598, 1989.

52. Colacone A, Afilalo M, Wolkove N, Kreisman H: A comparison of albuterol administered by metered dose inhaler (and holding chamber) or wet nebulizer in acute asthma. *Chest* 104:835–841, 1993.

53. Rodrigo C, Rodrigo G: Treatment of acute asthma: lack of therapeutic benefit and increase of the toxicity from aminophylline given in addition to high doses of salbutamol delivered by metered dose inhaler with a spacer. *Chest* 106:1071–1076, 1994.

54. Britton J, Tattersfield A: Comparison of cumulative and noncumulative techniques to measure dose-response curves for beta-agonists in patients with asthma. *Thorax* 39:597–599, 1984.

55. Rodrigo G, Rodrigo C: Metered dose inhaler salbutamol treatment of asthma in the ED: Comparison of two doses with plasma levels. *Am J Emerg Med* 14:144–150, 1996.

56. Rodrigo C, Rodrigo G: Therapeutic response patterns to high and cumulative doses of salbutamol in acute severe asthma. *Chest* 113:593–598, 1998.

57. McFadden Jr ER, Elsanadi N, Dixon L, et al: Protocol therapy for acute asthma: therapeutic benefits and cost savings. *Am J Med* 99:651–661, 1995.

58. Strauss L, Hejal R, Galan O, et al: Observations on the effects of aerosolized albuterol in acute asthma. *Am J Respir Crit Care Med* 155:545–458, 1997.

59. McFadden Jr ER, Kiser R, DeGroot WJ: Acute bronchial asthma: relations between clinical and physiologic manifestations. *N Eng J Med* 288:221–225, 1973.

60. Koning P, Hurst DJ: Nebulized isoetharine and fenoterol in acute attacks of asthma. *Arch Intern Med* 143:1361–1364, 1983.

61. Emerman CL, Cydulka RK, Efiron D, et al: A randomized, controlled comparison of isoetharine and albuterol in the treatment of acute asthma. *Ann Emerg Med* 20:1090–1093, 1991.

62. Shrestha M, Gourlay S, Robertson S, et al: Isoetharine versus albuterol for acute asthma: Greater immediate effect, but more side effects. *Am J Med* 100:323–327, 1996.

63. Newhouse MT, Chapman KR, McCallum AL, et al: Cardiovascular safety of high doses of inhaled fenoterol and albuterol in acute severe asthma. *Chest* 110:595–603, 1996.

64. Rodrigo G, Rodrigo C: Effect of age on bronchodilator response in acute severe asthma treatment. *Chest* 112:19–23, 1997.

65. Koning P: Spacer devices used with metered-dose inhalers: Breakthrough or gimmick? *Chest* 88:276–284, 1985.

66. Tarala RA, Madsen BJ, Paterson JW: Comparative efficacy of salbutamol by pressurized aerosol and wet nebulizer in acute asthma. *Br J Clin Pharmacol* 10:393–397, 1980.

67. Morgan MLD, Singh BV, Frame MH, Williams SJ: Terbutaline aerosol given through pear spacer in acute severe asthma. *Br Med J* 285:849–850, 1982.

68. Jasper AC, Mohsenifar Z, Kahan S, et al: Cost-benefit comparison of aerosol bronchodilator delivery methods in hospitalized patients. *Chest* 91:614–618, 1987.

69. Hodder RV, Calcutt LE, Leach JA: Metered dose inhaler with spacer is superior to wet nebulization for emergency room treatment of acute severe asthma. *Chest* 94:52S, 1988.

70. Morley TF, Marozsan E, Zappasodi SJ, et al: Comparison of beta-adrenergic agents delivered by nebulizer vs metered dose inhaler with inspirease in hospitalized asthma patients. *Chest* 94:1205–1210, 1988.

71. Turner JR, Corkery KJ, Eckman D, et al: Equivalence of continuous flow nebulizer and metered-dose inhaler with reservoir bag for treatment of acute airflow obstruction. *Chest* 93:476–481, 1988.

72. Salzman GA, Steele MT, Pribble W, et al: Aerosolized metaproterenol in the treatment of asthmatics with severe airflow obstruction: Comparison of two delivery methods. *Chest* 95:1017–1020, 1989.

73. Bowton DL, Goldsmith WM, Haponik EF: Substitution of metered-dose inhalers for hand-held nebulizers: Success and cost savings in a large, acute-care hospital. *Chest* 101:305–308, 1992.

74. Rodrigo G, Rodrigo C: Comparison of salbutamol delivered by nebulizer or metered-dose inhaler with a pear-shaped spacer in acute asthma. *Curr Ther Res* 54:797–808, 1993.

75. Idris AH, McDermott MF, Raucci JC, et al: Emergency department treatment of severe asthma: Metered-dose inhaler plus holding chamber is equivalent in effectiveness to nebulizer. *Chest* 103:665–672, 1993.

76. Gambriolo E, Levitt MA, Fink J: A comparative trial of continuous nebulization versus metered dose inhaler in acute bronchospasm. *Acad Emerg Med* 1:A38, 1994.

77. Mandelberg A, Chen E, Noviski N, Priel IE: Nebulized wet aerosol treatment in emergency department—is it essential? *Chest* 112:1501–1505, 1997.

78. Wildhaber JH, Dore ND, Wilson JM, et al.: Inhalation therapy in asthma: nebulizer or pressurized metered-dose inhaler with holding chamber? In vivo comparison of lung deposition in children. *J Pediatr* 136:28–33, 1999.

79. Turner MO, Patel A, Ginsburg S, FitzGerald JM: Bronchodilator delivery in acute airflow obstruction. A meta-analysis. *Arch Int Med* 157:1736–1744, 1997.

80. Cates CJ: Holding chambers versus nebulizers for beta-agonist treatment of acute asthma (Cochrane Review). In: *The Cochrane Library,* Issue 2, 1999. Oxford: Update Software.

81. Blake KV, Hoppe M, Harman E, Hendeles L: Relative amount of albuterol delivered to lung receptors from a metered-dose inhaler and nebulizer solution: Bioassay by histamine bronchoprovocation. *Chest* 101:309–315, 1992.

82. Rodrigo C, Rodrigo G: Salbutamol treatment of acute severe asthma in the ED: a comparison of metered-dose inhaler and spacer versus hand-held nebulizer with plasma levels. *Am J Emerg Med,* 16:637–642, 1998.

83. Alvine GF, Rodgers P, Fitzsimmons M, Ahrens RC: Disposable jet nebulizers: How reliable are they? *Chest* 101:316–319, 1992.

84. Todd Loffert D, Ikle D, Nelson HS: A comparison of commercial jet nebulizers. *Chest* 106:1788–1793, 1994.

85. Coates AL, MacNeish CF, Meisner D, et al: The choice of jet nebulizer, nebulizing flow, and addition of albuterol affects the output of tobramycin aerosols. *Chest* 111:1206–1212, 1997.

86. Papo MC, Frank J, Thompson, AE: A prospective, randomized study of continuous versus intermittent nebulized albuterol for severe status asthmaticus in children. *Crit Care Med* 21:479–486, 1993.

87. Colacone A, Wolkove N, Stern E, et al: Continuous nebulization of albuterol (salbutamol) in acute severe asthma. *Chest* 97:693–697, 1990.

88. Lin RY, Sauter D, Newman T, et al: Continuous versus intermittent albuterol nebulization in the treatment of acute asthma. *Ann Emerg Med* 22:71–77, 1993.

89. Shrestha M, Bidadi K, Gourlay S, Hayes J: Continuous vs intermittent albuterol, at high and low doses, in the treatment of severe acute asthma in adults. *Chest* 110:42–47, 1996.

90. Tonnesen F, Laursen LC, Evald T, et al: Bronchodilating effect of terbutaline powder in acute severe bronchial obstruction. *Chest* 105:697–700, 1994.

91. Raimondi AC, Schottlender J, Lombardi D, Molfino NA: Treatment of acute severe asthma with inhaled albuterol delivered via jet nebulizer, metered dose inhaler with spacer, and dry powder. *Chest* 112:24–28, 1997.

92. Larsson S, Svedmyr N: Bronchodilating effect and side effects of beta-adrenoreceptor stimulants by different modes of administration (tablets, metered aerosol, and combination thereof). *Am Rev Respir Dis* 116:861–869, 1977.

93. Kung M, Croley SW, Phillips BA: Systemic cardiovascular and metabolic effects associated with the inhalation of an increased dose of albuterol: Influence of mouth rinsing and gargling. *Chest* 91:382–387, 1987.

94. Jerrard DA, Olshaker J, Welebob E, et al: Efficacy and safety of a rapid-sequence metaproterenol

protocol in the treatment of acute adult asthma. *Am J Emerg Med* 13:392–395, 1995.

95. Clausen T, Flatman JA: Beta₂-adrenoreceptors mediate the stimulating effect of adrenaline on active electrogenic Na-K transport in rat soleus muscle. *Br J Pharmacol* 68:749–755, 1980.

96. Brown MI, Brown DC, Murphy MB: Hypokalemia from beta₂-receptor stimulation by circulating epinephrine. *N Engl J Med* 309:1414–1419, 1983.

97. Scheinin M, Koulu M, Larikainene E, Mlonene H: Hypokalemia and other nonbronchial effects on inhaled fenoterol and salbutamol: A placebo controlled dose-response study in healthy volunteers. *Br J Clin Pharmacol* 24:645–653, 1987.

98. Burgess CD, Flatt A, Seibers R, et al: A comparison of the extent and duration of hypokalemia following nebulized beta 2-adrenoceptor agonists. *Eur J Clin Pharmacol* 36:415–417, 1989.

99. Crane J, Burguess C, Beasley R: Cardiovascular and hypokalaemic effects of inhaled salbutamol, fenoterol, and isoprenaline. *Thorax* 44:136–140, 1989.

100. Tal A, Pasterkamp H, Leahy F: Arterial oxygen desaturation following salbutamol inhalation in acute asthma. *Chest* 86:868–869, 1984.

101. Roca J, Ramis LI, Rodriguez-Roisin R, et al: Serial relationships between ventilation-perfusion inequality and spirometry in acute severe asthma requiring hospitalization. *Am Rev Respir Dis* 137:1055–1061, 1988.

102. Ballester E, Reyes A, Roca J, et al: Ventilation-perfusion mismatching in acute severe asthma: effects of salbutamol and 100% oxygen. *Thorax* 44:258–267, 1989.

103. Rodriguez-Roisin R, Ballester E, Torres A, et al: Mechanisms of abnormal gas exchange in patients with status asthmaticus needing mechanical ventilation. *Am Rev Respir Dis* 139:732–739, 1989.

104. Rodriguez-Roisin R: Acute severe asthma: pathophysiology and pathobiology of gas exchange abnormalities. *Eur Respir J* 10:1359–1371, 1997.

105. Lin RY, Smith AJ, Hergenroeder P: High serum albuterol levels and tachycardia in adult asthmatics treated with high-dose continuously aerosolized albuterol. *Chest* 103:221–225, 1993.

106. McFadden Jr ER: Clinical physiological correlates in asthma. *J Allergy Clin Immunol* 77:1–5, 1986.

107. Schuh S, Parkin P, Rajan A, et al: High versus low-dose, frequently administered nebulized albuterol in children with severe, acute asthma. *Pediatrics* 83:513–518, 1989.

108. Rossing TH, Fanta CH, Goldstein DH, et al: Emergency therapy of asthma: Comparison of the acute effects of parenteral and inhaled sympathomimetics and infused aminophylline. *Am Rev Respir Dis* 122:365–371, 1980.

109. Fanta CH, Rossing TH, McFadden Jr ER: Treatment of acute asthma: Is combination therapy with sympathomimetics and methyxanthines indicated? *Am J Med* 80 5–10, 1986.

110. Siegel D, Sheppard D, Gelb A, Weinberg PF: Aminophylline increases the toxicity but not the efficacy of an inhaled beta-adrenergic agonist in the treatment of acute exacerbations of asthma. *Am Rev Respir Dis* 132:283–286, 1985.

111. Murphy DO, McDermott MF, Rydman RI, et al: Aminophylline in the treatment of acute asthma when beta$_2$-adrenergic and steroids are provided. *Arch Intern Med* 153:1784–1788, 1993.

112. Coleridge J, Cameron P, Epstein J, Teichtahl H: Intravenous aminophylline confers no benefit in acute asthma treated with intravenous steroids and inhaled bronchodilators. *Aust N Z J Med* 23:348–354, 1993.

113. Taylor DR, Wilkins OT, Herbison OP, Flannery EM: Interaction between corticosteroid and β-agonist drugs: Biochemical and cardiovascular effects in normal subjects. *Chest* 102:519–524, 1992.

114. Lin RY, Newman TO, Sauter D, et al: Association between reported use of inhaled triamcinolone and differential short-term responses to aerosolized albuterol in asthmatics in an emergency department setting. *Chest* 106:452–457, 1994.

115. Gross NJ, Skorodin MS: Anticholinergic, antimuscarinic bronchodilators. *Am Rev Respir Dis* 129:856–870, 1986.

116. Barnes PJ, Basbaum CB, Nael JA: Autoradiographic localization of autonomic receptors in airway smooth muscle: Marked differences between large and small airways. *Am Rev Respir Dis* 127:758–762, 1983.

117. Ingram RH, Wellman JJ, McFadden Jr ER, Mead J: Relative contributions of large and small airways to flow limitation in normal subjects before and after atropine and isoproterenol. *J Clin Invest* 59:696–703, 1977.

118. Ashutosh K, Mead O, Dickey Jr DC, et al: Density dependence of expiratory flow and bronchodilator response in asthma. *Chest* 77:68–75, 1980.

119. Siefkin AD: Optimal phamacologic treatment of the critically ill patients with obstructive airways disease. *Am J Med* 100(suppl):545–615, 1996.

120. Deckers W: The chemistry of new derivates of tropane alkaloids and the pharmacokinetics of a new quaternary compound. *Postgrad Med J* 51(Suppl 7):76–81, 1975.

121. Ghafouri MA, Patil KD, Kass I: Sputum changes associated with the use of ipratropium bromide. *Chest* 86:387–393, 1984.

122. Chapman KR, Smith DL, Rebuck AS, Leenen FHH: Hemodynamic effects of inhaled ipratropium bromide alone and combined with an inhaled beta-agonist. *Am Rev Respir Dis* 132:845–847, 1985.

123. Leahy BC, Gomm SA, Allen SC: Comparison of nebulized salbutamol with nebulized ipratropium bromide in acute asthma. *Br J Dis Chest* 77:159–163, 1983.

124. Bryant DH: Nebulized ipratropium bromide in the treatment of acute asthma. *Chest* 88:24–29, 1985.

125. Rebuck AS, Chapman KR, Abboud R, et al: Nebulized anticholinergic and sympathomimetic treatment of asthma and chronic obstructive airway disease in the emergency room. *Am J Med* 82:59–64, 1987.

126. Higgins RM, Stradling JR, Lane DJ: Should ipratropium bromide be added to beta-agonist in treatment of acute severe asthma? *Chest* 94:718–722, 1988.

127. ODriscoll BR, Taylor RJ, Horsley MG, Chambers DK: Nebulized salbutamol with and without ipratropium bromide in acute airflow obstruction. *Lancet* i:1418–1420, 1989.

128. Rodrigo C, Rodrigo G: Treatment of acute asthma: administration of high dose of salbutamol and ipratropium bromide delivered by metered dose inhaler with spacer. *Am J Respir Crit Care Med* 153:A60, 1996. Abstract.

129. FitzGerald JM, Orunfeld A, Pare PD, Levy RD, et al: The clinical efficacy of combination nebulized anticholinergic and adrenergic bronchodilators vs nebulized adrenergic bronchodilator alone in acute asthma. *Chest* 111:311–315, 1997.

130. Kamei T, Nakamura H, Kishimoto T, et al: Comparison between fenoterol inhalation and fenoterol plus oxitropium bromide inhalation to relief acute asthma attack. *Am J Respir Crit Care Med* 155:A530, 1997. Abstract.

131. Lanes SF, Garret JE, Wentworth CE, FitzGerald JM, Karpel JP: The effect of adding ipratropium bromide to albuterol in the treatment of acute asthma. A pooled analysis of three trials. *Chest* 114:365–372, 1998.

132. Garret JE, Town GI, Rodwell P, Kelly AM: Nebulized salbutamol with and without ipratropium bromide in the treatment of acute asthma. *J Allergy Clin Immunol* 100:165–170, 1997.

133. Lin RY, Pesola OR, Bakalchuk L, et al: Superiority of ipratropium plus albuterol over albuterol alone in the emergency department management of adult asthma: A randomized clinical trial. *Ann Emerg Med* 31:208–213, 1998.

134. Weber EJ, Levitt M, Covington JK, Gambrioli E: Effect of continuously nebulized ipratropium bromide plus albuterol on emergency department length of stay and hospital admission rates in patients with acute bronchospasm. A randomized, controlled trial. *Chest* 115:937–944, 1999.

135. Ward MI, Fentem PH, Roderick WH, Davies D: Ipratropium bromide in acute asthma. *Br Med J* 282:598–600, 1981.

136. Summers QA, Tarala RA: Nebulized ipratropium in the treatment of acute asthma. *Chest* 97:425–429, 1990.

137. Owens M, George RB: Nebulized atropine sulfate in the treatment of acute asthma. *Chest* 99:1084–1087, 1991.

138. Whyte KF, Gould GA, Jeffrey AA, et al: Dose of nebulized ipratropium bromide in acute severe asthma. *Respir Med* 85:517–520, 1991.

139. Karpel JP, Schacter EN, Fanta C, et al: A comparison of ipratropium and albuterol vs albuterol alone for the treatment of acute asthma. *Chest* 110:611–616, 1996.

140. Agoro A, Smith PR, Nampoothiri M, et al: Nebulized albuterol plus ipratropium bromide vs alone in the treatment of acute asthma. *Am J Respir Crit Care Med* 155:A530, 1997.

141. Diaz JE, Dubin R, Gaeta TJ, et al: Efficacy of atropine sulfate in combination with albuterol in the treatment for acute asthma. *Acad Emerg Med* 4:107–113, 1997.

142. McFadden Jr ER, ElSanadi N, Strauss L, et al: The influence of parasympatholytics on the resolution of acute attacks of asthma. *Am J Med* 102:7–13, 1997.

143. Plotnick LH, Ducharme FM: Should inhaled anticholinergics be added to β_2 agonists for treating acute childhood and adolescent asthma? A systematic review. *BMJ* 317:971–977, 1998.

144. Stoodley RG, Aaron SD, Dales RE: The role of ipratropium bromide in the emergency management of acute asthma exacerbations: a metaanalysis of randomized clinical trials. *Ann Emerg Med* 34:8–18, 1999.

145. Rodrigo GJ, Rodrigo C, Burschtin O: Ipratropium bromide in acute adult severe asthma: a meta-analysis of randomized controlled trials. *Am J Med* 107:363–370, 1999.

146. Rodrigo GJ, Rodrigo C: First-line therapy for adult acute asthma patients with a multiple dose protocol of ipratropium bromide plus albuterol on the emergency department. *Am J Respir Crit Care Med,* in press, 2000.

147. Munk A, Mendel DB, Smith LI, Orti E: Glucocorticoid receptors and actions. *Am Rev Respir Dis* 141:52-S10, 1990.

148. Barnes NC: Effects of corticosteroids in acute severe asthma. *Thorax* 47:582–583, 1992.

149. McFadden Jr ER: Dosages of corticosteroids in asthma. *Am Rev Respir Dis* 147:1306–1310, 1993.

150. Ellul-Micallef R, Borthwick RC, McHardy GJR: The time-course of response to prednisolone in chronic bronchial asthma. *Clin Sci Molec Med* 47:105–117, 1974.

151. Klaustermeyer WB, Hale FC: The physiologic effect of an intravenous glucocorticoid in bronchial asthma. *Ann Allergy* 37:80–86, 1976.

152. Collins W, Clark TJH, Brown D, Townsend J: The use of corticosteroids in the treatment of acute asthma. *Quart J Med* 174:259–273, 1975.

153. Britton MG, Collins JV, Brown D, et al: High-dose corticosteroids in severe acute asthma. *BR Med J* 2:73–74, 1976.

154. McFadden Jr ER, Kiser R, deGroot WJ, et al: A controlled study of the effects of single doses of hydrocortisone on the resolution of acute attacks of asthma. *Am J Med* 60:52–59, 1976.

155. Fanta CH, Rossing TH, McFadden Jr ER: Glucocorticoids in acute asthma critical controlled trial. *Am J Med* 74:845–851, 1983.

156. Haskell RI, Wong BM, Hansen JE: A double-blind, randomized clinical trial of methylprednisolone in status asthmaticus. *Arch Intern Med* 143:1324–1327, 1983.

157. Sue MA, Know FK, Klaustermeyer WB: A comparison of intravenous hydrocortisone, methylprednisolone and dexamethasone in acute bronchial asthma. *Ann Allergy* 56:406–409, 1986.

158. Stein LM, Cole RP: Early administration of corticosteroids in emergency room treatment of acute asthma. *Ann Intern Med* 112:822–827, 1990.

159. Rodrigo C, Rodrigo G: Early administration of hydrocortisone in the emergency room treatment

of acute asthma: A controlled trial. *Respir Med* 88:755–761, 1994.

160. Rodrigo G, Rodrigo C: Corticosteroids in the emergency department therapy of acute adult asthma. An evidence-based evaluation. *Chest* 116:285–295, 1999.

161. Britton MG, Collins JV, Brown D, et al: High dose corticosteroids in severe acute asthma. *BMJ* 2:73–74, 1976.

162. Leatherman J: Life-threatening asthma. *Clin Chest Med* 15:453–479, 1994.

163. Barnes PJ: A new approach to the treatment of asthma. *N Engl J Med* 321:1517–1527, 1989.

164. Reed CE: Aerosol glucocorticoid treatment of asthma. *Am Rev Respir Dis* 141:S82–588, 1990.

165. Hall JB, Wood LDH: Management of the critically ill asthmatic patient. *Med Clin North Am* 74:779–96, 1990.

166. Guttman A, Afilalo M, Colacone A et al: The effects of combined intravenous and inhaled steroids (beclomethasone dipropionate) for the emergency treatment of acute asthma. *Acad Emerg Med* 4:100–106, 1997.

167. Scarfone RI, Loiselle JM, Wiley JF, et al: Nebulized dexamethasone versus oral prednisone in the emergency treatment of asthmatic children. *Ann Emerg Med* 26:480–486, 1995.

168. Erlansson M, Svensjo E, Bergqvist D: Leukotriene B-4 induced permeability increase in postcapillary venules and its inhibition by three different antunflammatory drugs. *Inflammation* 13:693–705, 1989.

169. Miller-Larsson A, Brattsand R: Topical anti-inflammatory activity of the glucocorticoid budesonide on airway mucosa: evidence for a "hit and run" type of activity. *Agents Actions* 29:127–129, 1990.

170. Husby S, Agertoft L, Mortesen S, Pedersen S:

Treatment of croup with nebulized steroid (budesonide): A double blind, placebo controlled study. *Arch Dis Child* 68:352–355, 1993.

171. Klassen TP, Feldman ME, Watters LK, et al: Nebulized budesonide for children with mild-to-moderate croup. *N Engl J Med* 331:285–289, 1994.

172. Klassen TP, Watters LK, Feldman ME, et al: Efficacy of nebulized budesonide in dexamethasone-treated outpatients with croup. *Pediatrics* 97:463–466, 1996.

173. Gibson PG, Saltos N, Carty K, et al: Acute effect of budesonide on airway eosinophils and airway responsiveness in asthma. *Am J Respir Crit Care Med* 155:A289, 1997.

174. Kharitonov SA, Barnes PJ, O'Connor BJ: Reduction in exhaled nitric oxide after a single dose of nebulized budesonide in patients with asthma. *Am J Respir Crit Care Med* 153:A799, 1996.

175. Rodrigo G, Rodrigo C: Inhaled flunisolide for acute severe asthma. *Am J Respir Crit Care Med* 157:698–703, 1998.

176. McFadden ER: Inhaled glucocorticoids and acute asthma: therapeutic breakthrough or nonspecific effect? *Am J Respir Crit Care Med* 157:677–678, 1998. Editorial.

177. Phillips OH: Structure-activity relationship of topically active steroids: the selection of fluticasone propionate. *Respir Med* 84:19–23, 1990.

178. Brown PH, Teelucksingh S, Matusiewicz SP, et al: Cutaneous vasoconstrictor response to glucocorticoids in asthma. *Lancet* 337:576–580, 1991.

179. Afilalo M, Guttman A, Colacone A, et al: Efficacy of inhaled steroids (beclomethasone dipropionate) for treatment of mild to moderately severe asthma in the emergency department: A randomized clinical trial. *Ann Emerg Med* 33:304–309, 1999.

Chapter 11

THERAPEUTIC AEROSOLS IN MECHANICALLY VENTILATED PATIENTS

Constantine A. Manthous
Jesse B. Hall

INTRODUCTION

Aerosolized bronchodilators are primary therapy for the management of acute exacerbations of asthma. The endotracheal tube and ventilator circuitry provide potential impediments to the delivery of aerosolized particles in mechanically ventilated patients and thus may limit the effectiveness of this important treatment modality. This chapter briefly reviews clinically relevant concepts of aerosol science and emphasizes clinical studies that illuminate methods of using aerosolized bronchodilators to effectively treat bronchospasm.

BASIC PRINCIPLES OF AEROSOL SCIENCE

An abundance of clinical data demonstrate that aerosol effectiveness depends on getting the bronchodilator to the airways which is, in turn, dependent upon utilizing appropriate techniques of aerosol generation and administration. Clinicians can increase the likelihood of successful treatment by understanding and applying principles of aerosol science. Administration of therapeutic aerosols can be separated into two steps: production and delivery of the formed droplets or particles to the airways.

Aerosol Production

Aerosols are solid particles suspended in a gaseous medium and are produced for clinical application by several devices.

1. *Nebulizers* (NEB) pass a stream of gas over, or ultrasonic waves through, a reservoir of dissolved medication, forming small droplets that are entrained by a breath to the airways of the patient (Fig. 11-1). In mechanically ventilated patients, NEBs are most often driven by oxygen from a wall source.

2. *Metered dose inhalers* (MDI) are chlorofluorocarbon-pressurized cannisters of suspended micronized crystals of medication. When the cannister is actuated, a cloud of aerosolized medication is produced which is then entrained by a breath. Each actuation produces a predetermined amount of medication.

3. *Dry powder inhalers* (DPI) are tablets that are emulsified and the dust inhaled.

The size of the particles or droplets is termed the mean mass aerodynamic diameter (MMAD) and varies from 0.1 to >10 μm depending on the method of aerosol production. Particles of larger MMAD (>10 μm) are more likely to deposit on the nebulizer side-wall[1] and ventilator/endotracheal tubing[1,3–8] never reaching the airways of the patient. Particles delivered to the end of the endotracheal tube are deposited in the airways or alveoli, based upon size (see below). Particle size during nebulization varies significantly (0.1 to 10 μm) among specific nebulizers, while MDIs generate particles between 1 and 7 μm.[1,2] Nebulizers and MDIs have been studied in mechanically ventilated patients, while DPIs have thus far only been utilized in ambulatory patients.

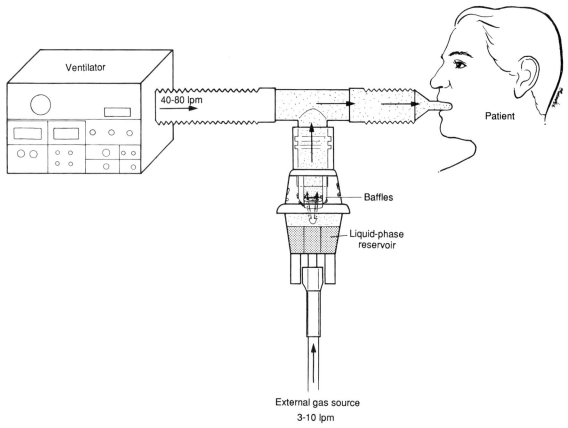

Figure 11-1
A common jet nebulizer system. Extrinsic gas flow, either from a compressed air source or from the ventilator. The gas flow passes through a Venturi and is accelerated, which leads to a pressure gradient that causes diluent/solubilized drug in the reservoir to be aerosolized and then entrained in another stream of gas (tidal volume) that goes to the patient. (With permission, from Manthous CA, Hall JB: Administration of therapeutic aerosols to mechanically ventilated patients. Chest 106:560–571, 1994.)

Aerosol Delivery

General Considerations   The delivery of aerosol to the airways is dependent upon the physical characteristics of the aerosol and the gaseous vehicle/flow regimes used to entrain them. The efficiency of aerosol delivery can be defined as: (amount of drug deposited on the airways)/(amount of drug administered).

1. *Aerosol physical properties.* The most important physical characteristic determining the site of aerosol deposition is droplet size. Droplets less than 0.5 μm are inhaled and exhaled and those 0.5 to 2 μm penetrate and deposit in alveoli; droplets in the range of 2 to 10 μm are deposited on the upper airways, including trachea, bronchi and bronchioles.[1] In mechanically ventilated patients, droplets larger than 10 μm are most likely to deposit on ventilator/endotracheal tubing. Other physical factors including electrical properties are not believed to dramatically alter clinical efficacy.[1,2]

2. *Carrier gas properties.* When inhaled gas traverses narrow orifices, turbulent flow regimes

result and increase the likelihood that aerosolized particles suspended in the gaseous phase will deposit on airways.[1] Deposition of aerosols can be affected by both the velocity of flow of a breath (↑ flow→ ↑ turbulence) and the density of the inspired gas (↑ density→ ↑ turbulence). In mechanically ventilated patients, high (frequently >1 L/s) inspired flow rates tend to increase aerosol deposition in ventilator circuit tubing and upper airways. This is particularly true in asthma patients for whom higher inspiratory flow rates are chosen in order to reduce inspiratory time, thus effecting a reduction in dynamic hyperinflation.

Intubated, Ventilated Patients   The ventilator circuit and endotracheal tube can be thought of as potential barriers to airway aerosol delivery (Table 11-1) Variables affecting delivery and efficacy include:

1.   The device used to create the aerosol (nebulizer versus MDI)

2.   The size and shape of aerosol spacers (when they are used with MDI)

3.   The position of the device in the ventilator circuit

4.   Parameters of mechanical ventilation, including inspiratory flow rate, tidal volume, respiratory rate, humidification of the inspired gases, and timing of aerosol production (inspiratory/expiratory)

Table 11-1
Potential determinants of aerosol delivery in intubated, mechanically ventilated patients

Ventilator/circuit-related factors	Patient-determined factors

Ventilator settings
  1. Inspiratory flow rate
  2. Respiratory rate
  3. Tidal volume
  4. Flow waveform
  5. Ventilator cycling—volume vs pressure
  6. Delivery by manual bag inflations
Circuit determinants
  1. Characteristics of the delivery device
      NEB
        Volume of fill
        Frequency selection for ultrasonic devices
        Specifications of the NEB device used including MMAD
        Flow rates for jet nebulization
      MDI
        Timing of the actuation
        Spacer device
        Actuator
        Intraendotracheal tube catheters
  2. Amount of drug administered
  3. Humidification of inspired gases
  4. Where in circuit MDI/NEB is administered
  5. Length and diameter of ventilator tubing
  6. Diameter and length of the endotracheal tube
  7. Use of low-density gas (heliox)
	Airway determinants
	  1. Bronchoconstriction
	  2. Secretions
	  3. Mucosal function
	
	Patient's effects on gas flow
	  1. Spontaneous respiratory pattern
	  2. Generation of intrinsic PEEP

SOURCE: With permission, from Brain and Valberg.[1]

5.   The characteristics of the endotracheal tube.

STUDIES ASSESSING AEROSOL DELIVERY

Quantitative and physiologic response studies have been performed to assess the adequacy of aerosol delivery in in vivo and in vitro models.

Quantification Studies

Numerous studies have examined the quantity of aerosol delivered to lung models[5,6,9–15] and patients.[4,7,8,16] Many of these studies have demonstrated reduced aerosol delivery/deposition to lung (or models) when compared to deposition studies in spontaneously breathing non-intubated patients. Nebulizers deliver between 1% and 37% of the administered dose with *significant variability* among devices.[6,8] Delivery is enhanced by increasing the volume of fill (amount of diluent)[5] and by manipulating ventilator parameters[5,6] (see below). MDI without spacer delivers between 5% and 7%[7,12]; addition of a spacer increases delivery up to 35%[12]; actuation into an intraendotracheal tube catheter (ETTC) delivers between 20% and 90%[13–15] of the administered dose. Delivery is enhanced by low inspiratory flow rates[5,6] and increased ventilator duty cycle.[5,6,17] It is reduced by humidification of inspired gases.[6,17]

A more recent study has illuminated where in the patient-ventilator circuit aerosolized particles are trapped.[18] Fink and colleagues noted that in vitro measurements regularly demonstrated that 5–7% more particles reach lung models than reach human lungs in vivo. Seeking to reconcile the in vitro and in vivo data, these investigators also examined the effects of various techniques and ventilator parameters on delivered doses of MDI-spacer albuterol. In 10 mechanically ventilated patients, 4.8% of the administered dose was *exhaled*. When 4.8% (exhaled in vivo) is subtracted from 16.2% noted in their bench model, the value of 11.4% deposited in patients' airways is similar to that reported in previous

in vivo studies.[16] This study also demonstrated that:

1.   Humidification of the circuit reduced (roughly by half) the efficiency of delivery

2.   Hydrofluoroalkane-propelled MDI was (24%) less efficient than MDI driven by chlorofluorocarbons

3.   15 seconds in between MDI actuations was as effective as 60 seconds

4.   Lower inspiratory flows (40 L/min vs. 80 L/min) and longer duty cycles (0.50 vs. 0.25) yielded better aerosol delivery to the airways.

Quantification studies can be distilled to the following conclusions: 1) both NEB and MDI *can* deliver aerosolized particles to the lungs, 2) delivery varies significantly among devices, 3) some systems such as MDI with spacer or MDI with ETTC are more efficient than others, 4) inefficient delivery can be clinically effective if more medication is administered, and 5) ventilator circuit characteristics and settings significantly impact the efficiency of delivery. Since the precise methodologies (particular devices and ventilator circuit/lung model) vary considerably among studies, clinicians should remain cautious when extrapolating these in vitro data to bedside use. Delivery and deposition of radiolabeled particles to a lung model (or even human lungs) *do not* necessarily prove that the method is effective in vivo. Quantification studies have aided in the identification of potentially useful techniques and devices that can be tested for clinical physiologic effect.

Physiologic Studies

In past 3 to 4 years, investigations were initiated to examine the physiologic effects of various aerosol delivery methods in intubated patients[19–31] (Table 11-2). These studies were performed in a heterogenous group of critically ill patients, very few of whom had severe status asthmaticus. The end points that have been studied include respiratory system resistance, respiratory system compliance (both dynamic and static), intrinsic positive end-expiratory pressure, and toxicities (tachycardia

Table 11-2

Studies examining the physiologic effects of nebulized and MDI-delivered bronchodilators to intubated mechanically ventilated patients ([a] signifies that the report is in abstract form).

Reference	n	Patient population	Intervention	Endpoints	Conclusions
MDI efficacy					
Gold[19]	12	Heterogenous anesthetized	250 μg isoproterenol MDI by manual bag inflation	Peak airway pressure	Peak pressure decreased in all 12 patients
Sprague[20]	16	Bronchospastic anesthetized	680 μg isoetharine/140 μg phenylephrine MDI by Y-piece adapter, with inspir pause	Peak airway pressure	Peak pressure decreased in all 16 patients
Fernandez[28]	20	COPD	.2 mg salbutamol vs .04 mg MDI ipratropium by slow manual inflation and 10% insp pause	Peak, static airway pressures, resistance	Both MDI drugs decreased airway resistance and pressure
Manthous[29]	10	Heterogenous	5, 15, 35 cumulative puffs of MDI/spacer albuterol	Peak, static pressures	5 and 15 puffs reduced resistive pressure, no further reduction beyond 15 puffs
Dhand[30]	7	COPD	10 puffs of MDI/spacer albuterol	Inspiratory resistance, I-PEEP	Both resistance and I-PEEP decreased
Moulondi[33]	9	COPD	6 puffs of MDI/spacer salbutamol	Peak, static pressures, inspiratory resistance, compliance, I-PEEP	Airway pressures, resistance and I-PEEP decreased.
Dhand[30]	12	COPD	4, 12, 28 cumulative puffs of MDI/spacer albuterol	Airway resistance	Resistance decreased maximally by 4 puffs
NEB efficacy					
MacIntyre[4]	7	Heterogenous	NEB metaproterenol	Peak, static airway pressure, heart rate	No changes after NEB metaproterenol
MDI v NEB					
Fuller[7]	21	"Airflow limitation"	MDI with spacer vs NEB fenoterol	Peak airway pressure	Neither MDI nor NEB decreased peak airway pressure
Gay[21]	18	"Suspected airflow obstruction"	3 puffs MDI by slow manual inflation vs 2.5 mg of NEB albuterol	Airway resistance by occlusion technique	Both NEB and MDI albuterol decreased airway resistance
[a]Farhangfar[22]	12	COPD	2 puffs of MDI (no spacer) vs 2.5 mg of NEB albuterol	Peak, static airway pressures	Both MDI and NEB improved resistive airway pressures
[a]Gutierrez[23]	20	COPD	2 puffs of MDI (with spacer) vs 2.5 mg NEB metaproterenol	Peak, static, resistive pressures	Both MDI and NEB improved airway resistance
[a]Hess[24]	16	Heterogenous	360 μg MDI (into ETT with insp pause) vs 2.5 mg albuterol	Expiratory resistive pressure	Both MDI and NEB improved expiratory resistive pressure
Bakow[25]	30	Heterogenous	MDI vs NEB both in proximal and distal positions in the inspir limb (few specifics)	Peak and plateau airway pressures, R_{aw}	Equal improvement in both groups
Manthous[26]	10	Heterogenous	100 puffs of MDI via adapter vs 2.5, 7.5, 15.0 mg NEB albuterol	Peak-static airway pressure (resistive pressure)	MDI had no effect; NEB reduced airway pressure at 2.5 and 7.5 mg with limited toxicity
[a]Fort[27]	9	Heterogenous	NEB albuterol via ETTC	Peak, static pressures, expiratory resistance	NEB with ETTC reduced resistance and increased compliance more than MDI

[a] NOTE: These reports are in abstract form with permission from *J Crit Illness*.

and hypotension). Most newer ventilators possess software and hardware to analyze respiratory mechanics. In the absence of these capabilities, respiratory system resistance can be measured during volume ventilation with a square inspiratory flow pattern as: (peak airway pressure-plateau pressure)/inspiratory flow rate, when patients are ventilated passively (Fig. 11-2). When there is a constant inspiratory flow of 60 L/m, respiratory system resistance (in units of cm H_2O/L per second) is simply the difference between peak and plateau pressure. The ventilator and endotracheal tubing contribute 5 to 20 cm H_2O/L per second depending upon size of the endotracheal tube and the duration of intubation. Values greater than

15 cm H_2O/L per second are considered elevated; with values as high as 60 to 80 cm H_2O/L per second in severe status asthmaticus. Total respiratory system static compliance (Δvolume/Δpressure) can be easily measured as: tidal volume/(plateau pressure–total positive end-expiratory pressure), where total positive end-expiratory pressure (PEEP) is defined as machine-set PEEP plus auto-PEEP. Dynamic compliance (Crs,dyn) is calculated similarly, except that pressure is computed as peak airway pressure-total PEEP. Respiratory system compliance decreases with dynamic hyperinflation and is another parameter that can be used to gauge successful bronchodilation. Intrinsic PEEP is not readily detected by examining

Figure 11-2

Superimposed pressure and volume curves during mechanical ventilation. The addition of an end-inspiratory pause (shown in breaths 3–5) causes airway pressure to plateau at a level representing the pressure required to expand the lung and chest wall at the given tidal volume (static airway pressure). The difference between peak (dynamic) and static airway pressures is related to flow and airway resistance. In intubated patients, resistive pressure includes contributions from the ventilator circuit, the endotracheal tube, and the airways of the patient. The 5th breath (dotted lines) demonstrates the effects of increased airway resistance on mechanics: peak airway pressure increases while static pressure remains unchanged. In situations of inadequate expiratory time, trapped gas at end-expiration may lead to intrinsic positive end-expiratory pressure which increases peak pressure through increases in static pressure. (Courtesy of Richard Samsel, MD, who used the Critical Concepts Inc.® Human Physiology Simulator™) (With permission, from Manthous CA, Hall JB: Administration of therapeutic aerosols to mechanically ventilated patients. Chest 106:560–71, 1994.)

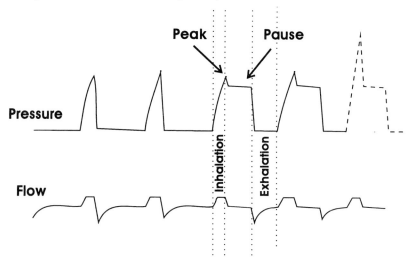

the inspiratory airway pressures and must be sought by special maneuvers. When patients are being passively ventilated, a brief end-expiratory pause allows equilibration of distal airway pressures with the ventilator-pressure monitors, thus revealing "intrinsic PEEP" or "auto-PEEP" (Fig. 11-3).

Assessment of Nebulizer Efficacy Nebulizers have been used extensively to deliver aerosolized medications to mechanically ventilated patients. Gay and colleagues demonstrated that 2.5 mg of nebulized albuterol reduced airway resistance.[21] Data from several studies published in abstract form also suggest that nebulized bronchodilators reduce airway resistance in mechanically ventilated patients.[22–25] Manthous and colleagues demonstrated that cumulative doses of 2.5 and 7.5 mg of jet NEB albuterol delivered by conventional ventilator parameters reduced airways resistance.[26] Fort and colleagues demonstrated improved lung compliance and reduced resistance

when 2.5 mg of albuterol was nebulized through an ETTC.[27] Thus, when proven devices and administration techniques are utilized, nebulized bronchodilators *can be* effective in treating bronchospasm in mechanically ventilated patients. The administered dose-response curves vary significantly among patients; some patients experience clinically significant improvement in physiologic parameters after 2.5 mg of albuterol whereas others experience no improvement after 7.5 mg.[26]

MDI Efficacy Gay and colleagues demonstrated that 3 puffs of MDI albuterol actuated into a bag and delivered by slow manual inflations significantly reduced airway resistance and was equivalent to nebulization of 2.5 mg of albuterol.[21] Fernandez demonstrated that salbutamol was equivalent to ipratropium (both delivered by MDI) in reducing airway resistance.[28] Manthous and colleagues showed that 100 puffs of albuterol delivered by MDI without spacer was ineffective[26] and later demonstrated that cumulative doses of

Figure 11-3
Determination of intrinsic PEEP. At end-expiration, the alveolar pressure is normally atmospheric. In the presence of significant airflow obstruction, however, exhalation is incomplete and the alveolar pressure may still be positive. Since the expiratory limb of the ventilator is open to atmosphere (or the PEEP valve) during expiration, the airway pressure gauge shows only atmospheric pressure (or the set PEEP), not the abnormally elevated alveolar pressure. By closing the expiratory limb of the ventilator at end-expiration, the alveolar pressure can be measured.

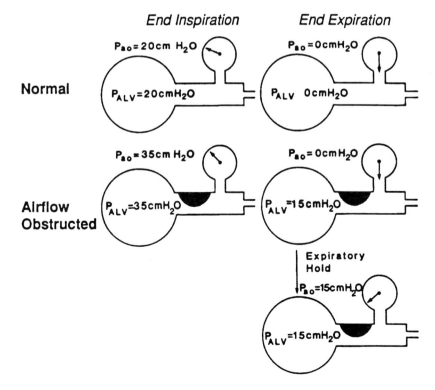

5 and 15 puffs of albuterol delivered by MDI with spacer significantly reduced airway resistance.[29] Dhand and colleagues demonstrated that 10 puffs of albuterol delivered by MDI with an in-line spacer significantly reduced airway resistance.[30] A subsequent study found that maximal response was reached after 4 puffs of albuterol delivered by MDI with spacer; no additional improvement was noted at cumulative doses of 12 and 28 puffs.[31] These investigators used nearly optimal aerosol techniques. MDI were actuated into a spacer just before inspiration at 20 to 30 second intervals and patients were sedated to achieve ventilator synchrony with increase of the respiratory rate "until all spontaneous breathing efforts were suppressed" and "negative deflections of airway pressures (were ablated) and uniformity of the pressure contour and breath cycle duration had been achieved." Toxicity, as manifested by a statistically significant increase in heart rate (from 81 to 89/min with no patient >110/min), occurred after 28 cumulative puffs of albuterol. These investigators also demonstrated that serum levels of albuterol increased similarly after administration in 9 ventilated patients compared to 10 non-intubated controls.[32] A recent study also demonstrated reduced airway pressures and resistance following administration of MDI salbutamol via an in-line spacer. This study also examined the effects of two tidal volumes used to deliver the salbutamol; V_T of 8 mL/kg yielded similar results to delivery with 12 mL/kg.[33] These studies decisively prove that MDI bronchodilators administered through an in-line spacer can be physiologically effective in this setting.

CLINICAL RECOMMENDATIONS

The following conclusions and suggestions can be reached from the available data:

1. *Nebulized bronchodilators are effective and higher than conventional doses can be administered safely to achieve maximal bronchodilation.* Nebulization devices clearly differ with regard to their efficiencies.[6] Placement of a device close to the ventilator manifold and use of larger than normal (>3 mL) amounts of diluent improve the efficiency of delivery.[5,6]

2. *MDIs are effective when administered into a spacing device.*[28,29,31] Some concern has been raised that MDI medications may cause tracheal cytotoxic effects when administered by ETTC. Thus, the use of intraendotracheal tube catheters to enhance delivery remains experimental.

3. *Although no studies have examined clinical end points, the available in vitro data suggest that certain ventilator techniques enhance delivery.* More aerosol particles are delivered when humidification systems are turned off during treatments,[6,17,18] ventilation occurs with low inspiratory flow (40 lpm), and duty cycle is increased.[5,6,17,18] These approaches should be considered in mechanically ventilated patients with bronchospasm, using physiologic end points to assess efficacy. Great care must be exercised if inspiratory flow rates are reduced during ventilation of patients with severe asthma. Since low inspiratory flow rate contributes to dynamic hyperinflation, intrinsic PEEP can rise to dangerous levels. Inspiratory flow rates should only be reduced transiently during treatments and with experienced personnel at the bedside to monitor for increasing intrinsic PEEP.

4. *The only data regarding the efficacy of atropine derivatives in mechanically ventilated patients with COPD demonstrated benefit,*[28] although there are no data to support any benefit when *added* to β-agonist therapies in ventilated asthma patients. However, atropine derivatives should be superior to β agonists in the treatment of ventilated patients with COPD.[34,35]

5. *No studies have assessed the use of alternative carrier gases for aerosol delivery in mechanically ventilated patients.* One study examining radio-label deposition in asthma patients,[36] and a preliminary report examining physiologic end points suggested that heliox may improve aerosol delivery in non-intubated patients.[37] Since heliox therapy adds to the cost of treatment, and aerosols can be delivered to the airways without it, heliox is unlikely to become a routine vehicle for aerosol

delivery in intubated patients. However, it is possible that heliox will be useful in maximizing aerosol delivery to intubated patients with very severe exacerbations of asthma.

Summary

Both jet nebulization and MDI with spacer can be effective delivery devices. No device should be used without quantification data and preferably, physiologic data, to assure that aerosol *can be* delivered to airways. Since the optimal delivery and deposition of therapeutic aerosolized medications is affected by numerous variables, one formula is unlikely to maximize therapy for all patients. Accordingly, *aerosolized therapies should be titrated to physiologic effect.* It is reasonable to begin therapy with conventional doses of nebulized medications, for instance, 2.5 mg of albuterol *or* 5 puffs of MDI delivered with an in-line spacer placed 10 cm from the wye on the inspiratory limb. Airway resistance and/or intrinsic PEEP should be measured immediately before and 15 minutes after treatment. If resistance remains greater than 25 cm H_2O/L per second or intrinsic PEEP remains greater than 10 cm H_2O, a second dose should be administered and parameters should be remeasured 15 minutes later. If resistance still remains greater than 25 cm H_2O/L per second, initiation of continuously nebulized bronchodilator until airway resistance falls below 25 cm H_2O/L per second, should be considered.[38] This value (i.e., 25 cm H_2O/L per second) is arbitrary (clinicians might disagree with this threshold by ± 10 cm H_2O), but once it is reached, the frequency of aerosolized treatments can be reduced to every 2 hours and as resistance continues to fall, it can be reduced to every 4 to 6 hours. It is important to note that some asthma patients will manifest β-agonist toxicity while airway pressures remain dangerously high (i.e., refractory bronchospasm/airway inflammation). In these situations, it is difficult to decipher whether the tachycardia and hypotension are related to severe asthma or to medications. If β-agonist serum assays[32] were to become more widely available, they could be employed to differentiate refractory asthma patients with β-agonist toxicity (those with high serum concentrations of β agonist and persistently elevated airway pressures) from patients in whom the administered dose is not delivered efficiently to the airways (those with low serum concentrations).

In patients with asthma who do not improve on continuously nebulized agonist, an inhaled atropine derivative (e.g., ipratropium bromide) can be considered, although few data demonstrate additive effect in mechanically ventilated patients.

Ventilator parameters can be changed during treatments, in all intubated patients with asthma as a matter of ICU policy, or they can be reserved for patients who are not responding to aerosols with standard ventilation. In non-responding patients, in-line humidifiers should be temporarily stopped during aerosol treatments. However, reducing the humidity of inspired gases may contribute to dessication of secretions, which may be a problem in some asthma patients. Thus, the humidifier should only be turned off for brief intervals (<20 to 30 minutes at a time) during aerosol administration. When nebulizers are used, the available data support their installation near the ventilator manifold. Flows and inspiratory rates should be reduced, when possible, to maximize delivery. Note, however, that patients with asthma who are on mechanical ventilators are particularly susceptible to dynamic hyperinflation when the duty cycle is increased; whenever flow rates are reduced, great care should be taken to watch for the development of dangerous levels of lung hyperinflation with possible hemodynamic compromise. Accordingly, ventilator changes initiated to improve aerosol deposition should be of brief duration, and a skilled technician or physician should be present. Intrinsic PEEP (or plateau airway pressure) should be monitored during these treatments to avoid excessive hyperinflation. Increments in plateau airway pressure 5 cm H_2O or decrements of systolic blood pressure 10 mm Hg should prompt discontinuation of the treatment, return to previous ventilatory parameters and reassessment to assure return of airway and/or arterial pressures to pretreatment values.

COSTS

Insofar as the literature suggests that both NEB and MDI β agonist can be equally effective in mechanically ventilated patients, the choice of treatment modality frequently is dictated by cost considerations. Patients with status asthmaticus require frequent or continuous aerosol treatments until airway pressures decrease to safer levels. In the experience of the authors, nebulized treatments are the most cost-effective means of providing treatment at the beginning of hospitalization, when very frequent or continuous therapy is used, when compared to the high cost and impractibility of stationing a respiratory therapist at the bedside to continually actuate the MDI. However, once therapies are reduced to every 3 to 4 hours, the most cost-effective route is largely determined by which method takes less time to administer, since labor comprises the majority of the overall cost of aerosol therapies. Table 11-3 delineates representative costs assuming that the time involved is 1 minute to prepare for MDI administration, 1 puff is actuated every 15 seconds,[30] followed by 2 minutes for documentation. For nebulization, we assumed 3 minutes of preparation time for initiation of a dose and an extra minute when an additional single volume dose is added to the nebulizer. These values likely vary considerably among practitioners and can depend upon the specific devices used. However, assuming equal effectiveness of 2.5 mg and five puffs of albuterol, nebulizers are less expensive in our hospital (labor costs are roughly equal but the cost of the spacer makes MDI slightly more expensive). However, differences in cost depend upon assumptions regarding labor time and, regardless, are very small. However, if respiratory therapists do not use effective techniques (and demonstrate that they have obtained the intended physiologic effects) significant resources can be wasted (i.e., aerosol treatments ineffectively administered impose cost with no benefit).

CONCLUSIONS

Aerosolized bronchodilators and intravenous corticosteroids are the mainstays of therapy for pa-

Table 11-3

Cost estimates for initial equipment and each treatment of albuterol MDI delivered by a commercially available spacer versus small volume nebulizer

	MDI	Nebulizer
Equipment	$3.95/chamber	$0.69/nebulizer
Medication	0.01 × 5 puffs = $0.05/5 puffs 0.01 × 10 puffs = $0.10/10 puffs	$0.22/2.5 mg $0.44/5.0 mg
Labor	4.25 minutes × $22.0/hour = $1.56/5 puffs 5.5 minutes × $22.0/hour = $2.02/10 puffs	5 minutes × $22.0/hour = $1.83/one 2.5 mg treatment 5 minutes × $22.0/hour = $1.83/one 5.0 mg treatment
Totals	$3.95 start-up plus: $1.61/5 puffs $2.12/10 puffs	$0.69 start-up plus: $2.05/1 treatment of 2.5 mg $2.27/1 treatment of 5.0 mg

These are estimated costs (in U.S. $) of treatments at Bridgeport, Hospital (Bridgeport Connecticut), February 2000 using the following assumptions: Labor times for MDI are 1 minute for initial set-up, then 15 seconds for each puff (see reference 33) followed by 2 minutes of documentation time. Labor times for nebulizer are 3 minutes for set-up and administration of the first dose of small volume nebulizer followed by 2 minutes for documentation. We assumed roughly 1 minute of set-up time for subsequent nebulizer treatments and no time for set-up of subsequent MDIs. Note that nebulizers are slightly less expensive for up to 36 treatments in our hospital because labor costs are similar for the two methods of administration, the cost of NEB solution is slightly higher/treatment ($0.22 vs. 0.05) and the cost of the MDI spacer is greater than the small volume nebulizer. This analysis will vary depending upon local prices and assumptions about labor time, but the difference in cost is relatively trivial.

tients with status asthmaticus. Recent investigations have elucidated effective methods of delivering aerosol therapies to intubated patients. It has been common practice to administer therapeutic aerosols without measuring physiologic end points. In all patients, but particularly patients with severe asthma, bronchodilators should be titrated to either reduced airway pressures or to toxicity. Hospital protocols should be scrutinized and, when necessary, redesigned to achieve optimal efficacy of these therapies. Finally, a thorough understanding of the pathophysiology of asthma and the principles of aerosol science allows the clinician to customize delivery approaches and troubleshoot problems that may arise in the treatment of the patient with severe asthma and respiratory failure.

REFERENCES

1. Brain JD, Valberg PA: Deposition of aerosol in the respiratory tract. *Am Rev Respir Dis* 120(6):1325–1373, 1979.
2. Newman SP: Aerosol generators and delivery systems. *Respir Care* 36(9):939–951, 1991.
3. Heyder J: Mechanisms of aerosol particle deposition. *Chest* 80:820–823, 1981.
4. MacIntyre NR, Silver RM, Miller CW, et al: Aerosol delivery in intubated, mechanically ventilated patients. *Crit Care Med* 13(2):81–84, 1985.
5. O'Doherty MJ, Thomas SHL, Page CG, et al: Delivery of a nebulized aerosol to a lung model during mechanical ventilation. *Am Rev Respir Dis* 146(2):383–388, 1992.
6. O'Riordan TG, Greco MJ, Perry RJ, Smaldone GC: Nebulizer function during mechanical ventilation. *Am Rev Respir Dis* 145:1117–1122, 1992.
7. Fuller HD, Dolovich MB, Posmituck G, et al: Pressurized aerosol versus jet aerosol delivery to mechanically ventilated patients. *Am Rev Respir Dis* 141(2):440–444, 1990.
8. O'Riordan TG, Palmer LB, Smaldone GC: Aerosol deposition in mechanically ventilated patients. Optimizing nebulizer delivery. *Am J Respir Crit Care Med* 149:214–219, 1994.
9. Crogan SJ, Bishop MJ: Delivery efficiency of metered dose aerosols given via endotracheal tubes. *Anesthesiology* 70(6):1008–1010, 1989.
10. Bishop MJ, Larson RP, Buschman DL: Metered dose inhaler aerosol characteristics are affected by the endotracheal tube actuator/adapter used. *Anesthesiology* 73(6):1263–1265, 1990.
11. Hodder RV, Calcutt LE, Leech JA, et al: Metered dose inhaler with spacer is superior to wet nebulization during mechanical ventilation. *Crit Care Med* 17(4):S153, 1989.
12. Rau JL, Harwood RJ, Groff JL: Evaluation of a reservoir device for metered-dose bronchodilator delivery to intubated adults. *Chest* 102(3):924–930, 1992.
13. Taylor RH, Lerman J: High-efficiency delivery of salbutamol with a metered dose inhaler in narrow tracheal tubes and catheters. *Anesthesiology* 74(2):360–363, 1991.
14. Taylor RH, Lerman J, Chambers C, Dolovich M: Dosing efficiency and particle size characteristics of pressurized metered-dose inhaler aerosols in narrow catheters. *Chest* 103:920–924, 1993.
15. Niven RW, Kacmarek RM, Brain JD, Peterfreund RA: Small bore nozzle extensions to improve the delivery efficiency of drugs from metered dose inhalers: Laboratory evaluation. *Am Rev Respir Dis* 147(6):1590–1594, 1993.
16. Fuller HD, Dolovich MB, Turpie FH, Newhouse MT: Efficiency of bronchodilator aerosol delivery to the lungs from the metered dose inhaler in mechanically ventilated patients. A study comparing four different actuator devices. *Chest* 105:214–218, 1994.
17. Fink JB, Dhand R, Duarte AG, et al: Aerosol delivery from a metered-dose inhaler during mechanical ventilation: An in vitro model. *Am J Respir Crit Care Med* 154:382–387, 1996.
18. Fink JB, Dhand R, Grychowski J, et al: Reconciling in vitro and in vivo measurements of aerosol delivery from a metered-dose inhaler during mechanical ventilation and defining efficiency-enhancing factors. *Am J Respir Crit Care Med* 159:63–68, 1999.
19. Gold MI: Treatment of bronchospasm during anesthesia. *Anesth Analg* 54(6):783–786, 1975.
20. Sprague DH: Treatment of intraoperative bronchospasm with nebulized isoetharine. *Anesthesiology* 46(3):222–224, 1977.
21. Gay PC, Patel HG, Nelson SB, et al: Metered dose inhalers for bronchodilator delivery in intubated, mechanically ventilated patients. *Chest* 99(1):66–71, 1991.
22. Farhangfar R, Safirstein B, Khan MA: Comparison of the efficacy of albuterol delivered as metered-dose inhaler (MDI) with that of a nebulizer in me-

chanically ventilated patients with chronic obstructive pulmonary disease (COPD). *Am Rev Respir Dis* 145(4):A60, 1992. Abstract.

23. Gutierrez CJ, Nelson R: Short-term bronchodilation in mechanically ventilated patietns receiving metaproterenol via small volume nebulizer (SVN) or metered-dose inhaler (MDI). *Respir Care* 33(10):910, 1988.

24. Hess D, Fillman D, Daugherty A, et al: Use of metered dose inhalers in intubated patients. *Respir Care* 34(11):1027, 1989.

25. Bakow ED, Galgon P, Bachman V, Lucke J: Beta-agonist delivery in-line with a ventilator circuit by either metered dose inhaler or updraft nebulizer in a distal or proximal position. *Respir Care* 34(11):1027–1029, 1989.

26. Manthous CA, Hall JB, Schmidt G, Wood LDH: Metered-dose inhaler versus nebulized albuterol for treatment of bronchospasm in intubated patients. *Am Rev Respir Dis* 148:1567–1570, 1993.

27. Fort P, Dolan S, Morales C, Derdak S: Delivery of nebulized albuterol through intratracheal catheters in mechanically ventilated patients. *Am J Respir Crit Care Med* 149:A1037, 1995. Abstract.

28. Fernandez A, Lazaro A, Garcia A, et al: Bronchodilators in patients with chronic obstructive pulmonary disease on mechanical ventilation. Utilization of metered-dose inhalers. *Am Rev Respir Dis* 141(1):164–168, 1990.

29. Manthous CA, Chatila W, Schmidt GA, Hall JB: Treatment of bronchospasm by metered-dose inhaler albuterol in mechanically ventilated patients. *Chest* 107:210–213, 1995.

30. Dhand R, Jubran A, Tobin MJ: Bronchodilator delivery by metered-dose inhaler in ventilator-supported patients. *Am J Respir Crit Care Med* 151:1827–1833, 1995.

31. Dhand R, Duarte A, Jubran A, et al: Dose-response to bronchodilator delivered by metered-dose inhaler in ventilator-supported patients. *Am J Respir Crit Care Med* 154:388–393, 1996.

32. Duarte AG, Dhand R, Reid R, et al: Serum albuterol levels in mechanically ventilated patients and healthy subjects after metered dose inhaler administration. *Am J Respir Crit Care Med* 154:1658–1663, 1996.

33. Mouloudi E, Katsanoulas K, Anastasaki M, et al: Bronchodilator delivery by metered-dose inhaler in mechanically ventilated COPD patients: Influence of tidal volume. *Intensive Care Med* 25:1215–1221, 1999.

34. Nisar M, Earis JE, Pearson MG, Calverley PM: Acute bronchodilator trials in chronic obstructive pulmonary disease. *Am Rev Respir Dis* 146(3):555–559, 1992.

35. Karpel JP, Pesin J, Greenberg D, Gentry E: A comparison of the effects of ipratropium bromide and metaproterenol sulfate in acute exacerbations of COPD. *Chest* 98(4):835–839, 1990.

36. Anderson M, Svartengren M, Bylin G, et al: Deposition in asthmatics of particles inhaled in air or in helium-oxygen. *Am Rev Respir Dis* 147(3):524–528, 1993.

37. Melmed A, Hebb DB, Pohlman A, et al: The use of heliox as vehicle for β-agonist nebulization in patients with severe asthma. *Am J Respir Crit Care Med* 151:A269, 1995. Abstract.

38. Shrestha M, Khalil B, Gourlay S, Hayes J: Continuous vs intermittent albuterol, at high and low doses, in the treatment of severe acute asthma in adults. *Chest* 110:42–47, 1996.

Chapter 12

NONINVASIVE POSITIVE PRESSURE VENTILATION IN PATIENTS WITH ASTHMA

G. Umberto Meduri

INTRODUCTION

The incidence and severity of asthma have increased in recent years, and the number of asthma patients who developed acute respiratory failure (ARF) and were admitted to the intensive care unit (ICU) has also increased. ARF in asthma is called *status asthmaticus* (SA)[1] and refers to a severe deterioration in gas exchange that may require mechanical ventilation (MV) for life support. If conservative treatment fails, MV is instituted to correct the pathophysiology of ARF, reduce the work of breathing, and ameliorate dyspnea while concomitant pharmacologic intervention is directed at correcting the condition that resulted in ARF.

The purpose of this chapter is to provide a review of data dealing with the application of noninvasive ventilation (NIV) in patients with obstructive airway disease (OAD) and hypercapnic ARF. A description of the pathophysiology of status asthmaticus is followed by a review of physiological data explaining the mechanisms of action of NIV in asthma and chronic obstructive pulmonary disease (COPD). Correct application and monitoring of NIV in patients with ARF is critical to its success, and methodology is covered at length at the end of the chapter.

PATHOPHYSIOLOGY OF STATUS ASTHMATICUS AND NEED FOR MECHANICAL VENTILATION

The pathophysiology of SA includes airflow obstruction of both large and small airways, inhomo-geneous lung inflation, considerable dynamic hyperinflation (PEEPi, 9 to 19 cm H_2O), ventilation/perfusion mismatch, and respiratory muscle fatigue.[2–4]

The pathogenesis of airflow obstruction involves airway wall inflammation, smooth muscle-mediated bronchoconstriction, and intraluminal mucus.[1] Mucous plugs, consisting of mucus, fibrin, desquamated epithelium, and inflammatory cells may lead to occlusion of peripheral airways and may be difficult to remove. However, the alveolar units distal to these obstructed airways may be slightly ventilated through collateral pathways from relatively less affected neighboring lung units.[3]

In spontaneously breathing asthma patients, progressive reductions in FEV_1 are associated with proportional increments in the inspiratory work of breathing (WOBi).[2] A fall in FEV_1 to 50% of baseline is associated with a 10.7-fold increase in the inspiratory muscle work.[2] At any level of bronchoconstriction, increased inspiratory muscle work is largely the result of hyperinflation and, to a lesser extent, increased airway resistance.[2] Dynamic hyperinflation causes substantial shortening of the diaphragm and the inspiratory intercostal and accessory muscles, thereby reducing their mechanical efficiency and endurance.[2] In addition, the presence of intrinsic positive end-expiratory pressure (PEEPi) results in an inspiratory threshold load.[5]

With the progression of asthma, mean pleural pressure becomes more negative as patients breath against increased airway resistance and increased intrathoracic pressure from air trapping. When pleural pressures drop to oppose airway closure, interstitial pressures are also lowered, but vascular pressure is maintained, promoting pulmonary interstitial edema and peribronchial cuffing which may further increase airway resistance.[6] In severe asthma, large negative swings in intrapleural pressure can significantly impair right ventricular function.[7]

As airway obstruction becomes more severe (FEV_1 <25% of predicted), the load on the respiratory muscle pump becomes excessive and muscle fatigue can develop. Respiratory muscle fatigue is defined as a condition in which the respiratory muscle fibers that are repeatedly contracting under load cannot generate enough force and velocity; the condition is reversible by rest.[8,9] Patients with exacerbation of OAD (COPD and asthma) present with dyspnea and a high respiratory frequency. However, most of the breaths are shallow and much of the tidal volume is wasted as dead space ventilation, resulting in retention of carbon dioxide and respiratory acidosis.[10] Acute respiratory acidosis itself impairs the contractility of the diaphragm in humans.[11] Hypercapnia correlates with hyperinflation,[12] and usually does not occur unless the FEV_1 is <25% of predicted.[13]

Asthma patients with hypercapnia, in comparison to patients without CO_2 retention, are more dyspneic and tachypneic, have a larger pulsus paradoxus, and a significantly higher incidence of quiet chest on auscultation.[14] During medical therapy, the timing of correction of hypercarbia is variable, and is affected by premorbid hypercapnic drive and duration of exacerbation.[14] Mountain and Sahn reported a mean time to normalization of Pa_{CO_2} of 5.9 hours, ranging from 30 minutes to 16 hours.[14] During β-adrenergic agonist aerosol treatment, respiratory rate, heart rate, and blood pressure do not improve as rapidly as peak expiratory flow rate (PEFR).[15] Failure to improve Pa_{CO_2} may require institution of mechanical ventilation (MV).[16]

Endotracheal intubation (ETI) and MV are required for a minority of patients with asthma and hypercapnia, but rarely for patients without hypercapnia.[14] In assessing the need for MV,

Table 12-1
Advantages of Noninvasive Ventilation

1. Noninvasiveness
   Application[a]
     Is easy to implement
     Is easy to remove
     Allows intermittent application
     Improves patient comfort
     Reduces need for sedation
   Oral patency
     Preserves speech and swallowing
     Reduces the need for nasoenteric tubes

2. Avoids the resistive work imposed by the endotracheal tube

3. Avoids the complications of endotracheal intubation
   Early
     Local trauma
     Aspiration
   Late
     Injury to the hypopharynx, larynx, and trachea
     Nosocomial infections

[a]NOTE: In comparison to endotracheal intubation.
SOURCE: Modification from Meduri.[15]

changes in response to therapy appear to be as important as absolute values.[16] Mountain and Sahn found that among 61 patients with SA presenting with hypercarbia (46% with pH < 7.30), only 5 (8%) required MV.[14] Because intubation is an invasive procedure resulting in increased airflow resistance[17,18] and a high rate of complications,[19] it is used only as a last resort in SA when patients develop exhaustion of the ventilatory muscles or life-threatening complications (hypotension, arrhythmias, decreased level of consciousness, etc.).[16]

The potential advantages of MV in patients with SA, however, cannot be denied or postponed if MV can be delivered effectively and safely without requiring ETI. The advantage of noninvasive positive pressure ventilation (NPPV) is that it avoids the complications of invasive procedures such as endotracheal intubation and other related instrumentation (Table 12-1). The disadvantages of NPPV include the system, the mask, and the lack of airway access (Table 12-2). Noninvasive ventilation (NIV) includes various techniques of

Table 12-2
Disadvantages of Noninvasive Ventilation

System	Comments
Slower correction of gas exchange abnormalities	Dependent on type of mask and mode
Increased initial time commitment by staff	Time involvement similar to ETI/MV
Gastric distention	Incidence 2%[a]
Mask	
Facial skin necrosis	Incidence 9%[a]
Eye irritation	Incidence 2%[a]
Air leakage	
Transient hypoxemia from accidental removal	Rare occurrence
Lack of airway access and protection	
Suctioning of secretions	NPPV is highly effective in patients
Aspiration pneumonia	Incidence 1%[a]

[a]NOTE: Data obtained from 15 studies involving 541 patients treated with NPPV and reporting on complications.

ABBREVIATION: ETI/MV, mechanical ventilation via endotracheal tube.

SOURCE: Modified from Meduri.[15]

augmenting alveolar ventilation without an endotracheal airway, and has been extensively investigated in regard to various forms of hypercapnic ARF.[15] Clinical application of NIV using continuous positive airway pressure (CPAP) alone is referred to as *mask CPAP*. NIV using intermittent positive pressure ventilation (IPPV) with or without CPAP is referred to as *noninvasive (intermittent) positive pressure ventilation* (NPPV).

NONINVASIVE POSITIVE PRESSURE VENTILATION IN ASTHMA

In patients with OAD and acute exacerbation, the inspiratory effort is divided into two components: an isometric contraction of the inspiratory muscles to counterbalance PEEPi (inspiratory threshold load) followed by an isotonic contraction to generate inspiratory flow and tidal volume.[20] Studies evaluating the effects of mechanical ventilation delivered by mask on the work of breathing and gas exchange in patients with OAD (COPD and asthma) indicate that low-level CPAP (5 cm H_2O) can offset one of the detrimental effects of PEEPi. CPAP can reduce the magnitude of the inspiratory effort to resume spontaneous breathing (alveolar pressure needs to be lowered to the CPAP pressure rather than to ambient pressure to begin inspiration),[20–22] while IPPV improves tidal volume, gas exchange, respiratory rate, and diaphragmatic activity in proportion to the amount of pressure applied.[20,23–26]

Physiologic Response to Mask Ventilation

Continuous Positive Airway Pressure   The pathophysiology of SA can be improved by application of mask CPAP, which causes bronchodilation, decreasing airway resistance. It also reexpands atelectasis and promotes removal of secretions, rests the inspiratory muscles and offsets PEEPi, and decreases the adverse hemodynamic effects of large negative peak and mean inspiratory pleural pressures.

In 1939, bronchography demonstrated bronchial dilation during CPAP.[27] In seven asthma patients, CPAP (7 cm H_2O) increased the diameter of smaller bronchi by 1 mm and moderate-sized bronchi by 2 mm (Fig. 12-1). Three recent studies have shown that the use of mask CPAP (8 to 12 cm H_2O) in exercise-, histamine-, or methacholine-induced asthma significantly decreased airflow obstruction (FEV_1, PEFR, and pulmonary resistance).[28–30]

As mentioned above, mask CPAP is also useful to reexpand atelectasis and to promote removal of secretions by increasing collateral flow (through collateral channels) to obstructed lung regions.[31] In excised human lungs, experimentally collapsed lung regions can be recruited by CPAP through collateral channels with pressures less than or equal to those needed for reinflation through the ordinary bronchial route.[31] Collateral reinflation also has a potential secretion clearing effect; the pressure behind the obstruction rises,

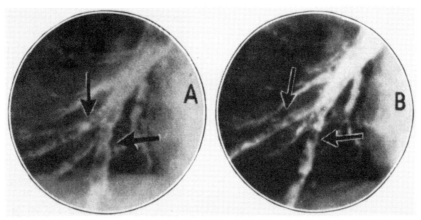

Figure 12-1
A branch of the bronchial tree after injection of iodized poppyseed oil at the end of expiration. **A.** *Patient breathing air without pressure.* **B.** *Patient breathing under positive pressure. (With permission, from Barach and Swenson[27])*

forcing secretions centrally to larger bronchi where they are more easily removed.[31]

Similar to COPD patients,[20] several case reports have suggested that in intubated asthma patients, externally applied positive end-expiratory pressure (PEEP) may offset PEEPi,[32–35] although one study of four asthma patients [using a tidal volume (V_T) of 15 ± 3 mL/kg] did not confirm this finding.[36] In COPD patients, applying mask CPAP at a level slightly lower (80 to 90%) than PEEPi significantly reduces inspiratory workload (by offsetting PEEPi) without worsening pulmonary hyperinflation.[20] Application of CPAP (15 cm H_2O),[37] and the combination of CPAP (5 cm H_2O) with an inspiratory pressure of 10 cm H_2O[20] generated a similar reduction (from 20 to 11 cm H_2O) in the tidal excursion of the Pdi (Δ Pdi). In acute asthma, mask CPAP reduced transdiaphragmatic pressure (Pdi), pressure-time product for the inspiratory muscles and diaphragm, and fractional inspiratory time (T_I/T_{TOT}).[22,29] When increasing levels of CPAP (0, 5, 7.5, 10, and 12 cm H_2O) were applied by face mask in severe acute asthma (peak flow <200 L/min), patients were most comfortable at a CPAP level of 5.3 ± 2.8 cm H_2O, which corresponded to a significant reduction (by 8.65%, $P < 0.1$) in T_I/T_{TOT} (Fig. 12-2).[22]

In asthma, CPAP also decreases the adverse hemodynamic effects of large negative swings in mean inspiratory pleural pressures that compromise right and left ventricular ejection.[6,7,33]

Intermittent Positive Pressure Ventilation
Although there is a lack of physiological studies evaluating IPPV in asthma, there are data avail-

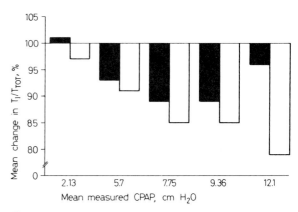

Figure 12-2
Changes in T_I/T_{TOT} with increasing levels of CPAP in 21 patients with acute asthmatic exacerbation **(black bar)** *and 19 controls* **(white bar)**. *The reduction was statistically significant ($P < 0.01$) in both groups compared to values at zero CPAP. (With permission, from Shivaram et al[22])*

able for patients with COPD. Applying mask IPPV (without CPAP) in acute exacerbations of COPD has been associated with reduced diaphragmatic activity, increased V_T, decreased respiratory rate, and improved gas exchange.[20,23,24] Of clinical importance, similar to intubated patients,[38] short-term (15 to 20 min) application of mask IPPV alone (without CPAP) did not offset PEEPi.[20,24] Increments in applied inspiratory pressure led to a progressive reduction in diaphragmatic electromyographic (EMG) activity.[23,24] A significant change has been observed when inspiratory pressure was increased from 12 cm H_2O to either 15 cm H_2O[23] or 20 cm H_2O.[24] NPPV suppressed the activity of the inspiratory muscles uniformly, rather than simply altering the pattern of recruitment among different inspiratory muscle groups.[23] The response to IPPV was rapid; suppressed phasic EMG activity occurred within six delivered breaths.[23] EMG changes were more significant in patients with lower FEV_1 (<0.55 L).[39] It should be noted that mouth opening during nasal ventilation results in air leakage and decreased effectiveness. In one study, diaphragmatic activity increased from 15% (mouth closed) to 98% (mouth open) of values recorded during spontaneous breathing.

When adequate pressure is applied, improvements in gas exchange are rapid and proportional to the increments in respiratory minute volume (V_E). As the level of inspiratory pressure is increased, V_E increases through an increase in tidal volume (V_T) and a reduction in respiratory rate.[20,24,25] In one study, increased applied inspiratory pressure from 12 cm H_2O to 20 cm H_2O resulted in significant additional reduction of the respiratory rate (16 $\pm$ 9 vs 3 $\pm$ 2 breaths per minute, $P < .05$) and Pa_{CO_2} (a decrease of 21 $\pm$ 10 vs 4 $\pm$ 3 mm Hg, $P < .05$).[24] Table 12-3 shows the effects of CPAP and IPPV delivered by mask, alone or in combination, in patients with obstructive and restrictive lung disease.

Clinical Application of Mask Ventilation

Mask CPAP   The use of positive pressure as an aid to breathing in the treatment of severe asthma was first reported by Oertel in 1878.[40] In 1936, the clinical efficacy of mask CPAP for acute asthmatic exacerbation was reported by two groups.[41,42] In 1981, the work of Wilson and colleagues in patients with exercise-induced asthma[28] stimulated a reappraisal of mask CPAP in acute asthma. Recently, Shivaram and colleagues studied nasal mask CPAP in 27 asthma patients presenting to the emergency department (ED) with severe (peak flow <150 L/min) exacerbation, comparing them to six control patients.[43] CPAP was applied for 30-minute intervals at the levels (5 and 7.5 cm H_2O) previously found to produce maximal improvement in dyspnea.[22] CPAP resulted in a significant reduction in dyspnea and respiratory rate, without changes in Pa_{O_2}, Pa_{CO_2}, or PET_{CO_2}. The magnitude of improvement was proportional to the degree of initial abnormality. CPAP eliminated cough. Two patients left the study because their dyspnea increased with CPAP. Seventeen (81%) patients slept while on CPAP therapy but awoke when CPAP was removed. None of the six control patients had improved dyspnea, respiratory rate, or sleep pattern. Similarly, Mansel and colleagues reported a patient with acute severe asthma and metabolic acidosis who was able to forgo intubation by use of face mask CPAP (5 cm H_2O) and continuous sodium bicarbonate infusion.[44] Nocturnal nasal CPAP may benefit asthma patients with coexisting sleep apnea;[45,46] however, it is associated with disrupted sleep architecture in nonapneic asthmatics.[47]

Noninvasive Positive Pressure Ventilation   In 1935, Barach first described a method to increase pressure during inspiration with a motor blower in synchrony with respiration in asthma patients receiving a helium-oxygen mixture.[48] Relief was experienced after six to ten breaths, and use of the accessory muscles diminished. In three patients who were refractory to adrenalin and were unconscious, treatment for 1 to 2 hours was followed by resolution of asthma and return of consciousness.

Six randomized studies have confirmed the benefits of NPPV in patients with acute exacerbation of COPD.[49] Overall NPPV was associated with decreased mortality (odds ratio = 0.29; 95%

Table 12-3

Effects of CPAP and PSV Delivered by a Mask, Alone and in Combination, on Gas Exchange and Transdiaphragmatic Pressure[a]

	Obstructive		Restrictive	
	Gas exchange	Transdiaphragmatic pressure	Gas exchange	Transdiaphragmatic pressure
CPAP	↑	↓	↑	↓
PSV	↑	↓	↑	↓
CPAP + PSV	↑	↓ ↓	↑ ↑	↓ ↓

[a]NOTE: In patients with obstructive and restrictive lung disease. Data obtained from references 20, 21, 23–26.

ABBREVIATIONS: CPAP, continuous positive airway pressure; PSV, pressure support ventilation; ↑ improved, ↓ decreased.

SOURCE: Modified from Meduri.[15]

CI, 0.15 to 0.59) and decreased need for endotracheal intubation (odds ratio, 0.20; 95% CI, 0.11 to 0.36).[49] The recent experience with NPPV (CPAP+IPPV) in SA is limited but encouraging.[50–53] One study recently reported on 17 patients with SA (pH 7.25 ± 0.01, Pa_{CO_2} 65 ± 2).[52] NPPV with CPAP (4 ± 2 cm H_2O) and pressure support ventilation (14 ± 5 cm H_2O) achieved rapid correction of gas exchange abnormalities (Fig. 12-3). The mean (± 1 SD) peak inspiratory pressure to ventilate the NPPV-treated patients was 18 ± 5 cm H_2O and was always <25 cm H_2O. Oral patency for intake (liquid diet) or expectoration was preserved. There was no problem with secretion re-

tention. The effects of positive pressure[31] (previously described) in nonsedated patients with patent upper airways and intact cough reflex may have facilitated removal of secretions. Only one patient required some sedation during NPPV. Two patients required intubation (35 minutes and 89 hours after initiation of NPPV, respectively) for worsening Pa_{CO_2}. Duration of NPPV was 16 ± 21 hours. All patients survived and were discharged from the hospital between 1 and 5 days.

NPPV was also evaluated as a modality to deliver aerosolized β_2 agonist in the ED.[54] Patients with mild-to-moderate asthma exacerbation were randomized to receive two doses of aerosolized

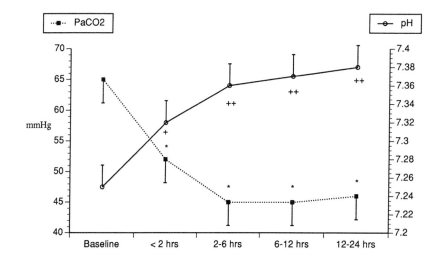

Figure 12-3

*Pa_{CO_2} and pH response during noninvasive positive pressure ventilation in seventeen patients with status asthmaticus. +, P = .0012; ++, P < .001; *, P = .002 (With permission, from Meduri et al[52])*

Table 12-4
Criteria for Selecting Patients for NPPV

- Alert and cooperative patient[a]
- Hemodynamic stability
- No need for endotracheal intubation to protect the airways[b] or remove excessive secretions
- No acute facial trauma
- Properly fitted mask

[a]NOTE: Patients with COPD and CO_2 narcosis are an exception (see text).
[b]NOTE: Mental obtundation, impaired swallowing, or active upper gastrintestinal bleeding.
SOURCE: Modified from Meduri.[15]

albuterol delivered via small-volume nebulizer (40 patients) or nasal BiPAP® set at IPAP 10 cm H_2O and EPAP 5 cm H_2O (60 patients). Treatment with BiPAP was associated with greater increase in percent of peak expiratory flow rate ($57 \pm 21\%$ vs $69 \pm 19\%$; $P = 0.002$).[54]

In conclusion, physiological studies indicate a positive effect for mask CPAP at low pressure levels in acute asthma. Similar to patients with COPD and ARF, short-term application of mask CPAP does not improve gas exchange. However, when IPPV is added to mask CPAP, gas exchange rapidly improves. In a recent consensus conference on NPPV, it was concluded that level III studies (nonrandomized with concurrent cohort comparison) provide supportive evidence indicating that NPPV may avert endotracheal intubation in SA.[55]

METHODOLOGY

Patient Selection

It is essential that the patient is alert and cooperative for initiating NPPV or mask CPAP (Table 12-4). For NPPV, patients must be able to voluntarily synchronize respiratory efforts with the ventilator, allow fully controlled ventilation in the intermittent mechanical ventilation (IMV), or assist control ventilation (ACV) mode. Patients with COPD and CO_2 narcosis, however, are an excep-

tion. In our and others'[56] experience, most of these patients exhibited improved mentation within 15 to 30 minutes of effective NPPV, and only a minority required intubation. Although extremely anxious patients may be better served by sedation and endotracheal intubation, moderate degrees of anxiety were frequently overcome once ventilatory needs were met. During NPPV, patients achieved a level of control and independence that differed totally from intubation, and sedation was infrequently required. When necessary, we have found intravenous administration of a small dose (2 mg) of morphine sulphate to be very effective.

NPPV should be avoided in patients with cardiovascular instability (hypotension or life-threatening arrhythmia), in those who require an endotracheal tube to protect the airways (coma, acute abdominal processes, impaired swallowing), or have life-threatening refractory hypoxemia (Pa_{O_2}, <60 mm Hg on 1.0 $F_{I_{O_2}}$). Patients with morbid obesity ($>200\%$ of ideal body weight) or with unstable angina or acute myocardial infarction should be closely managed by experienced personnel only.

Interface

Mask CPAP studies have almost exclusively used a facial mask, while a nasal mask was used more often in NPPV studies. Nasal masks add less dead space, cause less claustrophobia (a rare occurrence), minimize potential complications if vomiting occurs (a rare occurrence), and allow for both expectoration and oral intake without removing the mask. With a nasal mask, patients can vocalize more clearly and voluntarily discontinue ventilation by opening the mouth. On the other hand, a facial mask is preferable in severe respiratory failure because dyspneic patients are mouth-breathers, mouth breathing bypasses resistances of the nasal passages, and mouth opening during nasal mask ventilation results in air leakage and decreased effectiveness.[23,57,58] With nasal masks, an elastic chin strap is often sufficient to control mask leaks, although this is rarely successful in edentulous patients. Preliminary studies in normal adults suggest that nasal ventilation is of limited effectiveness when nasal resistance exceeds 5 cm H_2O/ L per second.[59]

Although no study has directly compared their efficacy, one group has reported a higher success rate with face mask NPPV versus their institutional historical control with NPPV nasal mask.[60] Improvement in arterial blood gas (ABG) appears to be slower in some of the studies using a nasal mask[23,51,61-63] in comparison to those using a face mask.[24,64-67] In one study, CPAP via face mask was superior to CPAP via endotracheal tube in improving oxygen saturation.[68] This author believes that a face mask is best suited for patients with severe ARF and dyspnea. The dead space volumes of a facial and a nasal mask are 250 ml and 105 ml, respectively.[69] Dead space volume from the mask and the oropharynx does not appear to affect the effectiveness of ventilation. In mild forms of ARF, a nasal mask could be tried first, switching to a facial mask if necessary. Recently, a new full-face mask prototype (TFM, Respironics Inc., Monroeville, PA) for NPPV was described; it has fewer leaks ($P < 0.003$) and improved comfort ($P < .02$) when compared to a nasal or regular face mask.[69] Among 12 patients (11 with COPD, one with pneumonia) with ARF who failed NPPV with a conventional facial or nasal mask (due to leaks or discomfort), the use of the new full-face mask improved gas exchange and avoided ETI in 10 (84%) patients.[70]

A mask with a transparent dome is preferred because it allows visual monitoring of the oral airway for presence of secretions. The mask should be lightweight to aid in its application and have a soft, pliable, adjustable seal to reduce trauma and leakage.[71] Types of available seals include contoured cushion, air bladder cushion, foam cushion, and double spring.[15] The mask is secured with head straps and has four prongs for attaching these straps. Masks with prongs positioned peripherally allow for a more uniform distribution of pressure on the facial surface (Benefit™, Puritan-Bennett Co., Lenexa, KS). The nasal masks by Respironics have a spacer to fill the space between the forehead and the mask to reduce pressure on the nasal bridge.

Aerophagia during NPPV is unusual when

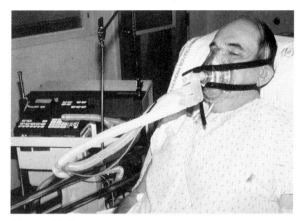

Figure 12-4
Patient with face mask connected to a mechanical ventilator.

the applied pressure is <25 cm H_2O (see below for details);[72,73] thus, routine placement of a nasogastric tube is not required. The mask is connected to the ventilator (Fig. 12-4), similar to an endotracheal tube. To prevent drying of the nasal passages and oropharynx, a humidifier should be connected with the heater turned off because the upper airways, which naturally warm inspired gas, are not bypassed with noninvasive ventilation.

Comfort

Because patient tolerance is essential to the success of NPPV, a tight, uncomfortable fit should be avoided when possible.[74,75] Even in patients with hypoxemic respiratory failure who receive mask CPAP alone, a small leak will not cause airway pressure to drop.[71,75,76] When securing the mask, enough space should be allowed to pass two fingers beneath the head straps. Masks with an air cushion fit most facial contours and do not require tight strapping. Small degrees of air leakage are well tolerated if the returned tidal volume is adequate ($\geq$7 mL/kg). When necessary, a skin patch (Restore®, Hollister, Libertyville, IL or Duoderm®, Bristol-Myers Squibb, Princeton, NJ) can be used to plug air leaks. It has often been found that proper fitting of the mask is difficult in edentulous patients and in those with a beard (in the latter, a nasal mask may be more effective).[77] In one report, edentulous patients on NPPV by nasal mask had persistent leaks despite using a chin strap.[58] Placing a nasogastric tube is indicated only for patients developing gastric distention (see below) or to provide access for enteral feeding. In the experience of the author, patients in the ICU can be best fed by mouth with a liquid diet, while other investigators allow patients on nasal pressure ventilation to eat small meals.[62] Enteral feeding by tube can be provided during the night for patients who do not achieve required caloric intake during the daytime.

Mode Of Ventilation

Most NPPV studies have used pressure-limited ventilation delivered by a broad range of ventilators. Pressure-limited ventilation improves the efficacy of spontaneous breathing by allowing an optimal synchrony between patient effort and delivered assistance. Inspiration is initiated when the inspiratory muscles and the inspiratory glottic abductors (with consequent glottis widening) are activated by the patient. During pressure support ventilation, the volume and duration of inspiration is determined by the effort of the patient. Gas flow begins after the inspiratory effort reduces pressure in the inspiratory circuit of the ventilator by a predetermined value, usually 1 to 2 cm H_2O. Pressure control ventilation has a preset inspiratory time and respiratory rate and may more effectively ventilate patients with low ventilatory drive. In comparison to volume-cycled ventilation, pressure-limited ventilation minimizes peak inspiratory mask pressure and air leakage. Although tidal volume may vary as a function of change in airway resistance and compliance, extreme variation has been rare, in our experience. In three comparison studies in patients with hypercapnic ARF pressure support ventilation in comparison to assist control ventilation was equally effective in reducing work of breathing[78] and improving gas exchange,[60,78] but was better tolerated[60,78,79] and associated with fewer complications.[60] During NPPV of stable COPD patients, flow triggering reduces the respiratory effort and PEEPi during both pressure support and assist control ventilation when compared to pressure triggering.[80] No differences were found between 1 and 5 L/min flow triggers.[80] Two reports found nasal ventilation with assist control ventilation to be ineffective and time consuming in end-stage obstructive lung disease.[81,82] Patients may inform the physician as to which mode of ventilation is most effective in ameliorating dyspnea.[56] Portable units have frequently been used in patients with less severe forms of ARF. Recent reviews of the characteristics of pressure-targeted ventilators used for NPPV can be found in references 15 and 83.

Glottic aperture is influenced by vocal cord angle and is the main factor regulating effective ventilation in healthy subjects subjected to NPPV. A positive correlation ($r = 0.945$; $P < .0001$) exists between vocal cord angle and effective V_T reaching the lung.[84] In healthy volunteers, mechanical factors (pressure and flow) influenced glottic behavior during passive (control mode) NPPV. With volumetric respirators, increments in effective ventilation were achieved by increasing flow up to 0.9 L/sec and respiratory rate up to 20 breaths per min. Further increases in flow and respiratory rate, or increases in delivered V_T above 10 to 15 ml/kg resulted in no change or a reduction in effective ventilation.[85] With passive two-level positive pressure ventilation, effective ventilation was found to be less predictable, especially when IPAP was kept below 15 cm H_2O.[84] Two-level positive pressure ventilation in spontaneous mode may obviate this problem.[84]

Mechanical Ventilation

The physiologic effects of NPPV with PSV were previously described. With NPPV, V_T, gas exchange, respiratory rate, and diaphragmatic activity are improved in proportion to the amount of pressure applied.[20,23,24] The methodology for NPPV at the University of Tennessee is shown in Table 12-5. The initial ventilator settings are CPAP, 0 cm H_2O and pressure support ventilation, 10 cm H_2O; the mask is gently held on the patient's face until the patient is comfortable and in synchrony with the ventilator. F_{IO_2} is titrated to

Table 12-5
Methodology for Noninvasive Positive Pressure Ventilation in Patients with Acute Respiratory Failure[a]

- Position the head of the bed at a 45° angle.
- Choose the correct size mask and connect the mask to the ventilator.
- Turn the ventilator on and silence the alarms. The initial ventilatory settings are CPAP, 0 cm H_2O, with pressure support 10 cm H_2O. $F_{I_{O_2}}$ is titrated to achieve an oxygen saturation over 90%.
- Explain the modality to the patient and provide reassurance.
- Hold the mask gently on the patient's face until the patient is comfortable and in full synchrony with the ventilator.
- If necessary, apply wound care dressing on the nasal bridge and other pressure points.
- Secure the mask with the headgear, avoiding a tight fit. Allow enough space to pass two fingers beneath the head straps.
- Slowly increase CPAP to ≥5 cm H_2O.
- Increase pressure support to obtain an exhaled tidal volume ≥7 mL/kg, a respiratory rate ≤25 breaths/min, and patient comfort.
- In hypoxic patients, increase CPAP in increments of 2 to 3 cm H_2O until $F_{I_{O_2}} \le 0.6$.
- Avoid peak mask pressure above 30 cm H_2O. Allow minimal air leaks if exhaled tidal volume is adequate.
- Set the ventilator alarms and apnea backup parameters.
- Ask the patient to call for needs (repositioning of the mask, pain or discomfort, expectoration), or if complications occur (respiratory difficulties, abdominal distention, nausea, vomiting).
- Monitor with oximetry and adjust ventilator settings following arterial blood gas results.

[a]NOTE: At the University of Tennessee, Memphis.
SOURCE: Modified from Meduri.[15]

achieve an oxygen saturation over 90%. After the mask is secured, CPAP is slowly increased to 3 to 5 cm H_2O, and pressure support ventilation is increased to obtain the largest (>7 mL/kg) exhaled V_T, a respiratory rate <25 breaths/min, and patient comfort. These objectives may not be achieved in patients with severe lung disease or with a leaky interface. In intubated patients with OAD criteria of optimal pressure support ventilation level has varied.[38] It is important to recognize that excessive pressure support ventilation levels can cause excessive inflation with consequent patient-ventilator dysynchrony and activation of expiratory muscles during inspiration.[38] To avoid gastric distention, peak mask pressure should be kept ≤30 cm H_2O. In one study, patients noticed the best sensation of comfort at a mask CPAP level of 5.3 ± 2.8 cm H_2O.[22] When intubated patients on mechanical ventilation were given the option of choosing their V_T without mechanical constraints, they frequently chose a lower V_T (7.1 mL/kg, range 3.0 to 10.4 mL/kg) than conventionally targeted (10 to 12 mL/kg).[86] In patients with hypoxemia, CPAP is increased in increments of 2 to 3 cm H_2O until a preselected end point is achieved ($F_{I_{O_2}} \le 0.6$ or $Pa_{O_2}/F_{I_{O_2}} \ge 300$.[56] CO_2 rebreathing can occur during BiPAP ventilatory assistance using the standard exhalation device (Whisper-Swivel) and can be eliminated with a new plateau exhalation device or a non-rebreather valve.[87] Application of EPAP (≥4 cm H_2O) decreases inhaled CO_2 which is eliminated at a level of 8 cm H_2O.[87]

Few studies have remarked on patient positioning during NPPV.[64,65] The author suggests that the head of the bed should be elevated at ≥45° angle at all times during NPPV (see Fig. 12-4). Although the original purpose of this elevation was to facilitate manipulation of the mask and to minimize the risk of aspiration in patients without airway protection, it has been demonstrated that in some patients, NPPV may be more effective (larger delivered V_T) in the upright position, in which there is increased deployment of inspiratory muscles acting directly on the rib cage and decreased abdominal compliance (gravitationally induced), increasing rib cage expansion.[88]

Portable units, such as the Respironics' BiPAP, the Puritan-Bennett's PB-335®, and the Healthdyne's Quantum™ PSV automatically compensate for mask leaks and mouth opening. A pressure and flow sensor in the ventilator monitors system pressure and total system flow. As the system flow fluctuates, the control valve changes position to release either more or less flow. This will compensate for changes in flow and the system pressure to maintain the set pressure despite leaks. With conventional critical care ventilators, leaks large enough to compromise achievement of set pressure support ventilation may cause an inspiratory plateau. During this plateau, increased patient efforts are not recognized by the ventilator and the work of exhalation is increased. Delivered respiratory rate slows and minute ventilation may be reduced substantially. Modifications in ventilator settings that improve responsiveness to all simulated patient efforts as well as preserved V_T delivery are possible. These strategies were compiled into a leak algorithm that was evaluated with a leak model (Fig. 12-5).[89] If air leakage is not improved, despite manipulations of the mask and application of a skin patch, first CPAP and then applied pressure (or V_T) are decreased to reduce peak mask pressure.

In most studies, mechanical ventilation was delivered continuously until ARF resolved. Intermittent 5- to 15-minute periods without NPPV were provided for oral intake or expectoration. Some clinicians, treating less severe forms of respiratory failure, have delivered NPPV for a few hours per day over extended periods of time.[90,91] After the initial stabilization period on NPPV (4 to 6 hours), patients with hypercapnic respiratory failure or with hypoxemia on low level CPAP (≤ 5 cm H_2O) can safely remove the mask for 5 to 15 minutes, during which time they can talk, drink small amounts of liquid, expectorate, or receive nebulized bronchodilator therapy. Because mask ventilation provides a great degree of flexibility, it can be adjusted to meet individual patient needs. In some patients with COPD and mild forms of respiratory acidosis, nocturnal ventilation is continued for a few days following resolution of respiratory failure.

Monitoring

Continuous oximetry with alarm should be provided. In patients with severe hypercapnia, it is advisable to have an arterial line in place. Ventila-

tor settings should be adjusted based on results of arterial blood gases obtained within 1 hour and, as necessary, at 2- to 6-hour intervals. Patients with status asthmaticus ventilated via an endotracheal tube are routinely heavily sedated. Patients receiving NPPV or mask CPAP need not be heavily sedated; relief of dyspnea and resolution of signs of respiratory distress are usually achieved soon after adequate positive pressure is provided. Correction of acidosis may be slow with NPPV depending on the mode of ventilation, amount of applied pressure, and severity of underlying disease. Patients showing improved gas exchange in the first hour of NPPV are more likely to avoid intubation (see below). In the authors' experience, the first 30 to 60 minutes of NPPV is labor intensive. The bedside presence of a respiratory therapist or nurse who is familiar with this mode of ventilation is essential for adjusting the mask and the settings.

In addition to gas exchange response of the patient, the following clinical parameters should be monitored: subjective response (dyspnea, comfort, and mental status), objective response (respiratory rate, heart rate, and use of accessory muscle of respiration), and possible complications (abdominal distention, facial pressure necrosis, retention of secretions). Use of the accessory muscles of respiration (respiratory load)[67] and contraction of the transversus abdominis muscle (activated with excessive inflation)[92] can be monitored by visual inspection or palpation. Providing reassurance and adequate explanation to the patient about what to expect is of the utmost importance. Patients are instructed to call the nurse if they have needs or develop complications. Needs include repositioning the mask for comfort or leaks or removal of the mask for oral intake or expectoration. Complications include respiratory difficulties, development of abdominal distention, or nausea/vomiting.

It has been found that, after the first hour of uncomplicated NPPV, most patients do not require continuous bedside observation; ventilator and oximetry alarms provide warnings for early intervention, if necessary. Time involvement with NPPV is proportional to the level of experience,

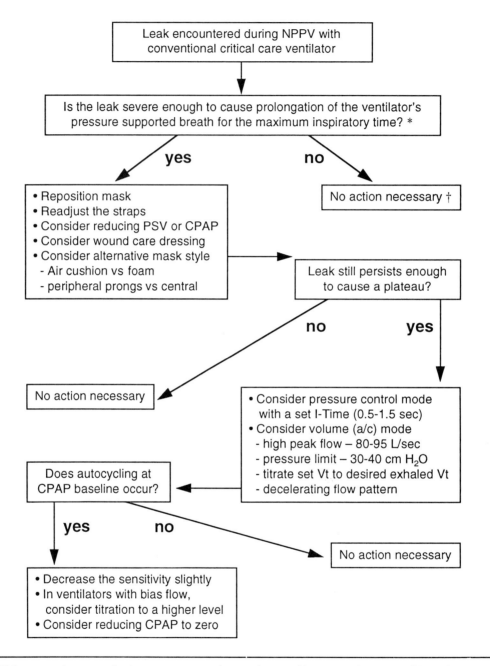

* This can reduce respiration rate, cause air trapping, and increase the work of breathing.
† Tidal volume remains constant as long as the leak does not cause plateauing of inspiration.

Figure 12-5
Sequential approach to the patient with mask leak. (From Foust et al[89])

Table 12-6
Criteria to Discontinue NPPV

- Inability to tolerate the mask due to discomfort or pain
- Inability to improve gas exchange or dyspnea
- Need for endotracheal intubation to manage secretions or protect the airways
- Hemodynamic instability
- Electrocardiographic instability with evidence of ischemia or significant ventricular arrhythmias
- Failure to improve mental status, within 30 min of initiating noninvasive ventilation, of patients who are lethargic from CO_2 retention or agitated from hypoxemia

SOURCE: Modified from Meduri.[15]

which may explain the findings described by one group.[81] In two randomized studies and one prospective control trial, bedside time commitment by nurses and therapists was similar for patients receiving NPPV or conventional treatment.[63,93,94] Criteria to abandon NPPV are shown in Table 12-6. When patients have to be transitioned from NPPV to endotracheal intubation, they must be considered as very unstable, with airway control and initial stabilization on the ventilator achieved by senior, experienced clinicians.

Education and Implementation

Understanding this method of mechanical ventilation by the respiratory therapy team is an extremely important adjunct to ensuring the safety of this technique and its proper use on patients with acute respiratory failure. A dedicated team (therapist and intensivist) should provide inservice training to respiratory therapists, critical care nurses, and house staff prior to implementing this method of ventilation. Continuous supervision is required until providers are fully comfortable in all aspects of noninvasive ventilation. Two studies have shown that with proper training, NPPV can be transferred to clinical practice with results similar to those of small studies conducted by researchers.[74,95]

CONCLUSION

Noninvasive ventilation with either mask CPAP or NPPV can be a safe and effective means of recruiting alveoli and augmenting ventilation in patients with status asthmaticus if physicians and hospital respiratory technicians acquire expertise with this method. Patient selection is essential to avoid complications. Although most patients improve with noninvasive ventilation, the response to treatment and the duration of mechanical ventilation cannot be clearly predicted by the severity of the underlying lung disease or by the arterial blood gas values obtained before initiating mechanical ventilation. Noninvasive ventilation is well tolerated, principally because it allows the patient to be in control and to continue verbal communication. NIV, however, is not uniformly successful. Patients with ARF placed on NIV should be closely monitored to avoid dangerous delays if intubation becomes necessary. When NIV is effective, the duration of mechanical ventilation and its associated complications are decreased. For these reasons, pulmonologists should become familiar with this modality and consider implementation for eligible patients. Future randomized studies should clarify whether NPPV is better than conventional ventilation in patients with acute asthma, as it has already been demonstrated to be for patients with acute exacerbation of COPD.[49]

ACKNOWLEDGMENT

The author wishes to thank Greg Foust, RRT, for his assistance in the preparation of the section on leak compensation and Figure 12-5, and Lee A. Thompson for editorial revision.

REFERENCES

1. Corbridge TC, Hall JB: The assessment and management of adults with status asthmaticus. *Am J Respir Crit Care Med* 151:1296–1316, 1995.
2. Martin JG, Shore SA, Engel LA: Mechanical load

and inspiratory muscle action during induced asthma. *Am Rev Respir Dis* 128:455–460, 1983.

3. Rodriguez-Roisin R, Ballester E, Roca J, et al: Mechanisms of hypoxemia in patients with status asthmaticus requiring mechanical ventilation. *Am Rev Respir Dis* 139:732–739, 1989.

4. Roca J, Ramis L, Rodriguez-Roisin R, et al: Serial relationships between ventilation perfusion inequality and spirometry in acute severe asthma requiring hospitalization. *Am Rev Respir Dis* 137:1055–1061, 1988.

5. Smith T, Marini J: Impact of PEEP on lung mechanics and work of breathing in severe airflow obstruction. *J Appl Physiol* 65:1488–1499, 1988.

6. Stalcup S, Mellins RB: Mechanical forces producing pulmonary edema in acute asthma. *N Engl J Med* 297:592–596, 1977.

7. Jardin F, Dubourg O, Margairaz A, et al: Inspiratory impairment in right ventricular performance during acute asthma. *Chest* 92:789–795, 1987.

8. Roussos C, Macklem PT: The respiratory muscles. *N Engl J Med* 307:786–797, 1982.

9. National Heart, Lungs, and Blood Institute: Workshop Summary: Respiratory muscle fatigue. Report of the Respiratory Muscle Fatigue Workshop Group. *Am Rev Respir Dis* 142:474–480, 1990.

10. Derenne JP, Fleury B, Pariente R: Acute respiratory failure of chronic obstructive pulmonary disease. *Am Rev Respir Dis* 138:1006–1033, 1988.

11. Juan G, Calverey P, Talamo C, et al: Effect of carbon dioxide on diaphragmatic function in human beings. *N Engl J Med* 310:874–879, 1985.

12. Pitcher WD, Cunningham HS: Oxygen cost of increasing tidal volume and diaphragmatic flattening in obstructive pulmonary disease. *J Appl Physiol* 74:2750–2756, 1993.

13. Nowak RM, Tomlanovich MC, Sarker DD, et al: Arterial blood gases an pulmonary function testing in acute bronchial asthma: predicting patient outcomes. *JAMA* 249:2043–2046, 1983.

14. Mountain RD, Sahn SA: Clinical features and outcome in patients with acute asthma presenting with hypercapnia. *Am Rev Respir Dis* 138:535–539, 1988.

15. Meduri GU: Noninvasive positive-pressure ventilation in patients with acute respiratory failure. *Clin Chest Med* 17(3):513–553, 1996.

16. Finfer SR, Garrard CS: Ventilatory support in asthma. *Brit J Hosp Med* 49:357–360, 1993.

17. Shnider SM, Papper EM: Anesthesia for the asthmatic patient. *Anesthesiology* 22:886–889, 1961.

18. Tuxen DV, Trevor JW, Scheinkestel CD, et al: Use of a measurement of pulmonary hyperinflation to control the level of mechanical ventilation in patients with acute severe asthma. *Am Rev Respir Dis* 146:1136–1142, 1992.

19. Zimmerman JL, Dellinger RP, Shah AN, Taylor RW: Endotracheal intubation and mechanical ventilation in severe asthma. *Crit Care Med* 21:1727–1730, 1993.

20. Appendini L, Patessio A, Zanaboni S, et al: Physiologic effects of positive end-expiratory pressure and mask pressure support during exacerbations of chronic obstructive pulmonary disease. *Am J Respir Crit Care Med* 149:1069–1076, 1994.

21. de Lucas P, Taranco'n C, Puente L, et al: Nasal continuous positive airway pressure in patients with COPD in acute respiratory failure. *Chest* 104:1694–1697, 1993.

22. Shivaram U, Donath J, Khan FA, Juliano J: Effects of continuous positive airway pressure in acute asthma. *Respiration* 52:157–162, 1987.

23. Carrey Z, Gottfried SB, Levy RD: Ventilatory muscle support in respiratory failure with nasal positive pressure ventilation. *Chest* 97:150–158, 1990.

24. Brochard L, Isabey D, Piquet J, et al: Reversal of acute exacerbations of chronic obstructive lung disease by inspiratory assistance with a face mask. *N Engl J Med* 323:1523–1530, 1990.

25. Ambrosino N, Nava S, Bertone P, et al: Physiologic evaluation of pressure support ventilation by nasal mask in patients with stable COPD. *Chest* 101:385–391, 1992.

26. Elliott MW, Aquilina R, Green M, et al: A comparison of different modes of noninvasive ventilatory support: effects on ventilation and inspiratory muscle effort. *Anaesthesia* 49:279–283, 1994.

27. Barach AL, Swenson P: Effect of breathing gases under positive pressure on lumens of small and medium sized bronchi. *Arch Intern Med* 63:946–948, 1939.

28. Wilson BA, Jackson PJ, Evans J: Effects of positive end-expiratory breathing on exercise-induced asthma. *Int J Sports Med* 2:27–30, 1981.

29. Martin JG, Shore S, Engel LA: Effect of continuous positive airway pressure on respiratory mechanics and pattern of breathing in induced asthma. *Am Rev Respir Dis* 126:812–817, 1982.

30. Horng-Chyuan L, Chun-Hua W, Cheng-Ta Y, et al: Effect of nasal continuous positive airway pressure on methacholine-induced bronchoconstriction. *Am J Respir Crit Care Med* 151:A398, 1995. Abstract.

31. Andersen JB, Qvist J, Kann T: Recruiting collapsed

lung through collateral channels with positive end expiratory pressure. *Scand J Respir Dis* 60:260–266, 1979.

32. Qvist J, Anderson JB, Pemberton M, Bennike KA: High-level PEEP in severe asthma. *N Engl J Med* 307:1347–1348, 1982.

33. Tenaillon A, Salmona JP, Burdin M: Continuous positive airway pressure in asthma. *Am Rev Respir Dis* 127:658, 1983.

34. Mathieu M, Tonneau MC, Zarka D, Sartene R: Effect of positive end-expiratory pressure in severe acute asthma. *Crit Care Med* 15:1164, 1987.

35. Maltais F, Sovilj M, Goldberg P, Gottfried SB: Respiratory mechanics in status asthmaticus. *Chest* 106:1401–1406, 1994.

36. Tuxen DV: Detrimental effects of positive end-expiratory pressure during controlled mechanical ventilation of patients with severe airflow obstruction. *Am Rev Respir Dis* 40:5–9, 1989.

37. Gottfried S, Simkovits P, Skaburskis M: Effect of constant positive airway pressure (CPAP) on breathing pattern and respiratory muscle function in chronic obstructive pulmonary disease (COPD). *Chest* 92:127S, 1987.

38. Jubran A, Van De Graaff WB, Tobin MJ: Variability of patient-ventilator interaction with pressure support ventilation in patients with chronic obstructive pulmonary disease. *Am J Respir Crit Care Med* 152:129–136, 1995.

39. Lien T, Wang J, Chang M, Kuo D: Comparison of BiPAP nasal ventilation and ventilation via iron lung in severe stable COPD. *Chest* 104:460–466, 1993.

40. Oertel MJ: Von Ziemssen's Handbook of Therapeutics, Translated from the German by J. B. Yeo. Wm. Wood & Co, 1885:iii, p 547.

41. Barach AL: The therapeutic use of helium. *JAMA* 107:1273, 1936.

42. Poulton EP, Oxon DM: Left-sided heart failure with pulmonary edema—its treatment with the "pulmonary plus pressure machine." *Lancet* 231:981–983, 1936.

43. Shivaram U, Cash ME, Beal A: Nasal continuous positive airway pressure in decompensated hypercapnic respiratory failure as a complication of sleep apnea. *Chest* 104:770–774, 1993.

44. Mansel JK, Stogner SW, Norman JR: Face-mask CPAP and sodium bicarbonate infusion in acute, severe asthma and metabolic acidosis. *Chest* 96:943–944, 1989.

45. Chan CS, Woolcock AJ, Sullivan CE: Nocturnal asthma: Role of snoring and obstructive sleep apnea. *Am Rev Respir Dis* 137:1502–1504, 1988.

46. Guilleminault C, Quera-Salva MA, Powell N, et al: Nocturnal asthma: snoring, small pharynx and nasal CPAP. *Eur Respir J* 1:1902–1907, 1988.

47. Martin RJ, Pak J: Nasal CPAP in nonapneic nocturnal asthma. *Chest* 100:1024–1027, 1991.

48. Barach AL: The use of helium in the treatment of asthma and obstructive lesions in the larynx and trachea. *Ann Intern Med* 9:739–765, 1935.

49. Keenan SP, Kernerman PD, Cook DJ, et al: The effect of noninvasive positive pressure ventilation on mortality in patients admitted with acute respiratory failure: A meta-analysis. *Crit Care Med* 25(10):1685–1692, 1997.

50. Pontopiddan H, Geffin B, Lowenstein E: *Acute Respiratory Failure in the Adult*, part III. Boston, Little Brown, 1973, p 801.

51. Benhamou D, Girault C, Faure C, Portier F, Muir JF: Nasal mask ventilation in acute respiratory failure. Experience in elderly patients. *Chest* 102:912–917, 1992.

52. Meduri GU, Cook TR, Turner RE, et al: Noninvasive positive pressure ventilation in status asthmaticus. *Chest* 110:767–774, 1996.

53. Pollack CV, Jr., Torres MT, Alexander L: Feasibility study of the use of bilevel positive airway pressure for respiratory support in the emergency department. *Ann Emerg Med* 27:189–192, 1996.

54. Pollack CV, Fleisch KB, Dowsey K: Treatment of acute bronchospasm with Beta-adrenergic agonist aerosols delivered by a nasal bilevel positive airway pressure circuit. *Ann Emerg Med* 26:552–557, 1995.

55. American Respiratory Care Foundation: Consensus conference: noninvasive positive pressure ventilation. *Respir Care* 42(4):364–369, 1997.

56. Fernandez R, Blanch LI, Valles J, et al: Pressure support ventilation via face mask in acute respiratory failure in hypercapnic COPD patients. *Intensive Care Med* 19:456–461, 1993.

57. Soo Hoo GW, Santiago S, Williams AJ: Nasal mechanical ventilation for hypercapnic respiratory failure in chronic obstructive pulmonary disease: determinants of success and failure. *Crit Care Med* 22:1253–1261, 1994.

58. Chiang AA, Lee KC: Use of nasal mask BiPAP in patients with respiratory distress after extubation. *Chest* 104(2):135S, 1993.

59. Ohi M, Chin K, Tsuboi T, et al: Effect of nasal resistance on the increase in ventilation during non-

invasive ventilation. *Am J Respir Crit Care Med* 149:A643, 1994.

60. Vitacca M, Rubini F, Foglio K, et al:. Non-invasive modalities of positive pressure ventilation improve the outcome of acute exacerbations in COLD patients. *Intensive Care Med* 19:450–455, 1993.

61. Elliott MW, Steven MH, Phillips GD, Branthwaite MA: Non-invasive mechanical ventilation for acute respiratory failure. *Br Med J* 300:358–360, 1990.

62. Pennock BE, Kaplan PD, Carlin BW, et al: Pressure support ventilation with a simplified ventilatory support system administered with a nasal mask in patients with respiratory failure. *Chest* 100:1371–1376, 1991.

63. Bott J, Carroll MP, Conway JH, et al: Randomized controlled trial of nasal ventilation in acute ventilatory failure due to chronic obstructive airways disease. *Lancet* 341:1555–1558, 1993.

64. Meduri GU, Conoscenti CC, Menashe P, Nair S: Noninvasive face mask ventilation in patients with acute respiratory failure. *Chest* 95:865–870, 1989.

65. Meduri GU, Abou-Shala N, Fox RC, et al: Noninvasive face mask mechanical ventilation in patients with acute hypercapnic respiratory failure. *Chest* 100:445–454, 1991.

66. Meduri GU, Mauldin GL, Wunderink RG, et al: Causes of fever and pulmonary densities in patients with clinical manifestations of ventilator-associated pneumonia. *Chest* 106:221–235, 1994.

67. Wysocki M, Tric L, Wolff MA, et al: Noninvasive pressure support ventilation in patients with acute respiratory failure. *Chest* 103:907–913, 1993.

68. Jousela I: Endotracheal tube versus face mask with and without continuous positive airway pressure (CPAP). *Anaesthesiol Scand* 37:381–385, 1993.

69. Criner GJ, Travaline JM, Brennan KJ, Kreimer DT: Efficacy of a new full face mask for noninvasive positive pressure ventilation. *Chest* 106:1109–1115, 1994.

70. Roy B, Kreimer DT, Mullarkey J, et al: Noninvasive positive pressure ventilation with a total face mask for acute respiratory failure. *Am J Respir Crit Care Med* 153(4):A608, 1996.

71. Branson RD, Hurst JM, DeHaven CB: Mask CPAP: State of the art. *Respir Care* 30:846–857, 1985.

72. Linton DM, Potgieter PD: Conservative management of blunt chest trauma. *S Afr Med J* 61:917–919, 1982.

73. Dodds WJ, Hogan WJ, Lyden SB, et al: Quantitation of pharyngeal motor function in normal human subjects. *J Appl Physiol* 39:692–696, 1975.

74. Pennock BE, Crawshaw L, Kaplan PD: Noninvasive nasal mask ventilation for acute respiratory failure. *Chest* 105:441–444, 1994.

75. Covelli HD, Weled BJ, Beekman JF: Efficacy of continuous positive airway pressure administered by face mask. *Chest* 81:147–150, 1982.

76. DeVita MA, Friedman V, Petrella V: Mask continuous positive airway pressure in AIDS. *Crit Care Clin* 9:137–151, 1993.

77. Gregg RW, Friedman BC, Williams JF, et al: positive airway pressure by face mask in *Pneumocystis carinii* pneumonia. *Crit Care Med* 18:21–24, 1990.

78. Girault C, Bonmarchand G, Richard JC, et al: Physiologic assessment of ventilatory mode during non invasive ventilation in acute hypercapnic respiratory failure (AHRF): assist-control (ACV). *Am J Respir Crit Care Med* 151:A426, 1995. Abstract.

79. Richard JC, Molano C, Tengang B, et al: Nasal intermittent positive pressure ventilation vs bilevel pressure ventilation during acute respiratory failure in patients with COPD. *Am J Respir Crit Care Med* 153(4):A609, 1996.

80. Nava S, Bruschi C, Ambrosino N, Paturno V, Confalonieri M: Inspiratory effort during non-invasive mechanical ventilation with flow and pressure triggers in COPD patients. *Intensive Care Med* 21:S120, 1995.

81. Chevrolet JC, Jolliet P, Abajo B, et al: Nasal positive pressure ventilation in patients with acute respiratory failure. Difficult and time-consuming procedure for nurses. *Chest* 100:775–782, 1991.

82. Soo Hoo GW, Williams AJ: Noninvasive face-mask mechanical ventilation in patients with acute hypercapnic respiratory failure. *Chest* 103:1304, 1993.

83. Kacmarek RM: Characteristics of pressure-targeted ventilators used for noninvasive positive pressure ventilation. *Respir Care* 42(2):380–388, 1997.

84. Parreira VF, Jounieaux V, Aubert G, et al: Nasal two-level positive-pressure ventilation in normal subjects. Effects on the glottis and ventilation. *Am J Respir Crit Care Med* 153:1616–1623, 1996.

85. Parreira V, Jounieaux V, Delguste P, et al: Effects of systematic changes in delivered tidal volume, inspiratory flow and respirator frequency on effective ventilation (VI) during intermittent positive pressure ventilation applied through a nasal mask (NIPPV), in healthy subjects awake and asleep. *Am J Respir Crit Care Med* 153(4):A762, 1996.

86. Marantz S, Webster K, Patrick W, et al: Respiratory responses to different levels of proportional assist

ventilation (PAV) in ventilator dependent patients. *Am Rev Respir Dis* 145:A525, 1992.

87. Ferguson GT, Gilmartin M: CO_2 rebreathing during BiPAP ventilatory assistance. *Am J Respir Crit Care Med* 151:1126–1135, 1995.

88. Druz WS, Sharp JT: Activity of respiratory muscles in upright and recumbent humans. *J Appl Physiol: Respirar Environ Exercise Physiol* 51(6):1552–1561, 1981.

89. Foust G, Reader C, Potter W, Meduri GU: Leak compensation during NPPV. *Am J Respir Crit Care Med* 155(4):A408, 1997. Abstract.

90. Leger P, Jennequin J, Gaussorgues P, Robert D: Acute respiratory failure in COPD patient treated with noninvasive intermittent mechanical ventilation (control mode) with nasal mask. *Am Rev Respir Dis* 137:A63, 1988.

91. Marino W: Intermittent volume cycled mechanical ventilation via nasal mask in patients with respiratory failure due to COPD. *Chest* 99:681–684, 1991.

92. Ninane V, Yernault JC, DeTroyer A: Abdominal muscles, active expiration and intrinsic PEEP ($PEEP_1$) in stable patients wtih chronic airflow limitation (CAO). *Eur Respir J* 5:421s, 1992.

93. Kramer N, Meyer TJ, Meharg J, et al: Randomized, prospective trial of noninvasive positive pressure ventilation in acute respiratory failure. *Am J Respir Crit Care Med* 151:1799–1806, 1995.

94. Nava S, Bruni M, Evangelisti I, et al: Is non-invasive mechanical ventilation (NIMV) really time-consuming procedure compared to invasive mechanical ventilation (IMV)? *Am J Respir Crit Care Med* 153(4):A607, 1996. Abstract.

95. Meduri GU, Turner RE, Abou-Shala N, et al: Noninvasive positive pressure ventilation via face mask: first-line intervention in patients with acute hypercapnic and hypoxemic respiratory failure. *Chest* 109:179–193, 1996.

Chapter 13

MECHANICAL VENTILATION FOR SEVERE ASTHMA

David V. Tuxen
Michael B. Anderson
Carlos D. Scheinkestel

INTRODUCTION

Asthma is a common condition that is increasing in frequency in the community.[1–7] In the majority of patients, asthma can be easily controlled by appropriate therapy; however, if it is poorly controlled or if an unusual allergen exposure occurs, it can lead to a serious or even life-threatening episode. The frequency of life-threatening events depends on their definition, but has been estimated to affect 5 per 1000 patients with asthma per year.[8] The definition of a life-threatening event varies from an unscheduled asthma presentation to the occurrence of hypercapnic respiratory failure. The latter group has a high risk of respiratory decompensation and requires aggressive treatment with observation in a facility capable of providing ventilatory assistance should this be required.

The frequency of reported asthma deaths varies between communities[9,10] and had been increasing[11] until the last decade when improved asthma treatment may have reversed the trend in some communities.[12–15] The majority of asthma deaths occur in the community prior to hospitalization; however, some asthma deaths occur despite the instigation of mechanical ventilatory assistance that was intended to be life saving. In several studies, 18 to 40% of reported deaths occurred after medical treatment, usually including positive pressure ventilation, had been initiated.[10,16]

The overall mortality from 1261 episodes of mechanical ventilation for asthma reported in 37 papers published over four decades was 12.4%.[17] Although the reported mortality has significantly decreased, from 16% in these first two decades (1960 to 1979) to 11% in the last two decades (1980 to 1997, $P < .05$), the reported mortality in different series in the 1990s still ranged from 0% to as high as 38%. The most frequently reported cause of death was cerebral hypoxia, most commonly as a result of cardiorespiratory arrest before initiation of ventilation.[17] Other important causes of mortality were hypotension or circulatory failure, pneumonia, and septicemia. Studies utilizing hypoventilation strategies to minimize dynamic hyperinflation[18–21] reported no or low mortality (0 to 8%) that was usually due to preexisting cerebral ischemic injury. Studies not specifying a hypoventilation strategy have reported higher mortality rates. The latter were rarely attributed to complications of mechanical ventilation; many of the causes of death were not reported in series using hypoventilation. It must be suspected that complications of mechanical ventilation have been significant contributors to mortality (apart from cerebral ischemic injury) especially where the cause of death involved or could have involved circulatory failure or barotrauma.

Severe asthma is a condition that challenges the clinician because of the potential for rapid deterioration in patient status and the necessity for aggressive early treatment. Adequate initial and ongoing clinical assessment is critical to identifying and appropriately managing patients with potentially more fulminating episodes.

Despite early aggressive treatment, some patients either fail to respond, continue to deteriorate, or present with an attack that is immediately life-threatening. In these situations, ventilatory support may be required. It can be difficult to predict which patients will reach this point.

Mechanical ventilation can be life-saving for patients with severe asthma. It can also contribute to morbidity and mortality both by the complications of excessive dynamic hyperinflation (pulmonary barotrauma, circulatory failure or cardiac tamponade),[17,22–27] and myopathy.[28] Similarly, delayed instigation of mechanical ventilation, allowing risk of respiratory arrest and cerebral ischemic injury, is also undesirable. Thus, every attempt should be made to avoid mechanical ventilation, but it should be instigated when avoidance is unsafe.

The aim of mechanical ventilation is to maintain adequate oxygenation and prevent respiratory arrest without circulatory compromise or lung injury until response to bronchodilators enables ventilatory assistance to be withdrawn.

The findings of a number of studies[18–22] now suggest that a strategy of mechanical ventilation that aims to reduce dynamic hyperinflation will result in the best outcomes. This involves the use of low minute volumes, short inspiratory times, and long expiratory time, with the consequence of permissive hypercapnia. This is intended to provide the most efficacious balance between supporting the patient and maintaining oxygenation while diminishing dynamic hyperinflation and the potential for ventilator-associated morbidity and mortality.

CLINICAL BACKGROUND

Although the severity and characteristics of an asthma attack vary considerably among individual patients, two clinical patterns of life-threatening asthma have been recognized[1,29–35] identifiable primarily by the rate of deterioration in clinical status and responsiveness to bronchodilator therapy.

Acute severe asthma is more common, occurring in approximately 70% of patients, more often female,[30] and requires mechanical ventilation. It is characterized by a gradual, progressive onset over several days prior to hospital presentation. It is associated with a high level of chronic bronchial inflammation, persisting moderate airflow obstruction and, as a result, often has a slow response to therapy. Hypercapnia is a late feature. Arterial CO_2 tension may be low, normal, or only mildly elevated[36] on presentation. Although a corresponding degree of dynamic hyperinflation must be present, ventilation is probably occurring below total lung capacity (TLC). An increasing Pa_{CO_2}, despite full aggressive treatment, usually represents fatigue with the capacity to transiently increase minute ventilation but not to sustain that increase.

The development of moderate hypercapnia despite full treatment is an important clinical indicator of deterioration in this group. Under these circumstances, ventilatory assistance may be required.

Sudden asphyxic asthma,[30] also known as hyperacute asthma,[37] is characterized by a rapidly progressive course associated with a high level of bronchial hyperreactivity[30,34,38] and often profound hypercapnia. Patients can develop severe life-threatening respiratory insufficiency within several hours and, uncommonly, within minutes[35] of symptom onset. It tends to occur in younger male patients and is more likely to result in respiratory arrest prior to, or shortly after, hospital admission.[23,32] This group of patients tends to have less chronic airflow changes, a high level of bronchial reactivity,[34] and airflow obstruction with a large component of bronchospasm. As a result, this group may respond rapidly to therapy. Prompt aggressive treatment may avoid mechanical ventilation despite the presence of much higher levels of hypercapnia on presentation.

This patient group may develop respiratory arrest before or shortly after arrival at the hospital[23,39] or present significant with respiratory distress and a markedly elevated Pa_{CO_2} (60 to 110 mm Hg). Severe dynamic hyperinflation will be present, with ventilation occurring at, or marginally above, total lung capacity (TLC). At this lung volume, inspiration is limited by the inability to inspire further and expiration is limited by severe airflow obstruction. The ventilatory capacity is low (i.e., 6 to 10 L per minute) whereas the ventilatory requirement for normocapnia in severe asthma may be quite high (i.e., 15 to 20 L per minute) because of increased dead space and increased CO_2 production.[39] CO_2 production is increased due to increased work of breathing and increased skeletal muscle activity associated with anxiety and distress. Thus, a high Pa_{CO_2}, usually before full aggressive treatment, represents a physical limitation of ventilation without fatigue necessarily being present. Since this patient group may also have a rapid response to treatment, intubation may not be immediately required.

The different mechanisms leading to hypercapnia, together with the different airway pathologies and different responses to treatment, make it inappropriate to establish criteria for intubation and ventilation based on specific numeric values of Pa_{CO_2}, pH, respiratory rate, peak expiratory flow (PEF), pulsus paradoxus, or other indicators of severity.

Although not all patients fall neatly into these two categories, the background pattern of asthma is an important consideration when assessing the need for ventilatory support and an important determinant of the likely duration of mechanical ventilation, should it be required.

PREVENTION OF MECHANICAL VENTILATION

Preventable morbidity and mortality may also result from failure to recognize and adequately manage a deterioration in patient status,[32,40,41] primarily due to inadequate observation and assessment.[42] For these reasons, patients with severe asthma need to remain in an environment with an appropriate level of skilled and organized staff. Regular assessments of asthma severity in such patients should include patient appearance, respiratory rate, PEF if appropriate,[43] pulse oximetry, blood gases, and assessment of any treatment side effects.

All attempts should be made to avoid mechanical ventilation. Full aggressive drug therapy should include continuous or nebulized salbutamol or an equivalent inhaler every 1 to 2 hours,[44] ipratropium bromide nebulized four times per hour,[45,46] early commencement of intravenous steroids, and possibly nebulized budesonide.[47] The use of intravenous salbutamol and aminophylline in refractory patients should also be considered (see Chapter 9).

If a patient with severe asthma is not responding appropriately or is deteriorating despite the above treatment, then other promising but unproven therapies should be considered. Epinephrine has the theoretical benefit of mucosal shrinkage, in addition to its bronchodilator properties, and there have been anecdotal reports suggesting its superiority to β agonists.[48] Systematic studies comparing the two agents have failed to demonstrate this advantage,[49-51] but there have been no randomized studies (to our knowledge) to assess whether epinephrine provides additional benefit in the presence of full β agonist therapy. Although additional benefit from epinephrine has not been established, it has been increasingly used and recommended[43,52] for patients who do not respond to standard bronchodilator therapy. A combination of helium and oxygen (heliox) has no bronchodilator properties but may improve airflow, gas exchange, and inhaled bronchodilator delivery in patients with severe asthma[53,54] because its low density and high viscosity reduces turbulent gas flow and gas flow resistance. This may avert the need for mechanical ventilation by allowing more time for bronchodilators to work before fatigue occurs.

Noninvasive positive pressure ventilation (NPPV) is a more recent modality that offers limited mechanical support to ventilation without endotracheal intubation and with the potential for fewer side effects. It warrants detailed consideration (see Chapter 12).

INDICATIONS FOR NONINVASIVE POSITIVE PRESSURE VENTILATION AND INTUBATION WITH VENTILATION

Severe asthma is a medical emergency with the potential for respiratory arrest and death. Patients with acute severe asthma may not need ventilatory assistance, may benefit from NPPV, or may require intubation and mechanical ventilation. Patients who have undergone respiratory arrest, who are obtunded or comatose, or who have rapidly deteriorating respiratory function despite medical treatment should be intubated and ventilated as a matter of urgency.

It is important to remember that cerebral hypoxia as a result of a prior cardiorespiratory arrest is the leading cause of mortality in patients who require mechanical ventilation.[17] The decision to intubate requires careful consideration of potential reversible disease in patients with severe asthma and significant impairment of respiratory function, but who are not ''in extremis'' (as above).

Intubation and ventilation of the patient with severe asthma has the potential for significant morbidity[23,28] and mortality.[17] Although much of this can be minimized, it is more desirable to avoid mechanical ventilation whenever possible. This desire must be balanced against allowing patients to deteriorate to a point where intubation becomes urgent or a respiratory arrest occurs.

The most important single guide to patient status that determines the need for intubation is the assessment of clinical appearance by an experienced clinician. The patient with the clinical appearance of exhaustion, severe respiratory distress and clinically tiring with a decline in respiratory rate, respiratory effort, level of awareness and ability to cooperate, requires intubation and ventilation. A patient's own assessment of their level of fatigue is a useful adjunct to guide the decision to undertake ventilation. Although patients may underestimate their asthma severity, they will seldom overestimate the degree of respiratory difficulty. Thus self-assessment of near exhaustion or collapse by a patient should be taken seriously.

An important adjunct to this assessment is a deterioration in measured values such as PEF (or FEV_1), respiratory rate, or Pa_{CO_2}[55] despite maximal treatment. Deterioration is a more serious clinical sign than any absolute numeric value as a guide to the necessity for intervention with mechanical ventilation.

Patients with labored breathing but who are

cooperative and state that they are coping and not yet exhausted need very close observation and aggressive treatment (including NPPV), but not immediate intubation. Recently presented patients who are tachypneic and have the appearance of a high respiratory workload but who are not severely distressed may continue to be closely monitored despite marked hypercapnia (i.e., $Pa_{CO_2} > 80$ mm Hg). Such patients may respond to aggressive therapy sufficiently rapidly to avoid the need for intubation and mechanical ventilation. Increasing hypercapnia and deteriorating clinical status despite full aggressive medical therapy is a reasonable indicator for instituting ventilatory assistance. Reassurance is vital during this period to ensure that the patient is aware that sufficient expertise is readily available to provide ventilatory assistance should the patient tire, but that ventilation will not be undertaken without an adequate indication; this is often more acceptable to the patient.

There is now limited but increasing evidence that NPPV may assist patients with acute severe asthma and possibly reduce the requirement for intubation.[56] NPPV appears to be well tolerated and without serious side effects. Although it appears desirable to avoid mechanical ventilation wherever possible, NPPV may be used more readily. It may be appropriate to administer NPPV to all patients who are acutely hypercapnic, have the clinical appearance of a high respiratory workload, or who are moderately distressed. Patients who are severely distressed, obtunded, or who have a rapidly deteriorating respiratory status despite NPPV should proceed to endotracheal intubation and ventilation.

NONINVASIVE POSITIVE PRESSURE VENTILATION

Following limited success with continuous positive airway pressure (CPAP) as a noninvasive respiratory support modality, NPPV, delivered via nasal or full-face mask, has developed in recent years as a more advanced, more successful support modality. NPPV refers to the application of positive pressure ventilation to a patient without the mandatory requirement of establishing an invasive artificial airway (usually an endotracheal tube). NPPV requires the use of a mechanical device that provides, in addition to CPAP, either pressure- or volume-cycled inspiratory assistance via a nasal or face mask, using a relatively simple purpose-built device or a full adult ventilator. An appropriate level of CPAP reduces the negative intrathoracic pressure required to initiate inspiration and thereby reduces the work of breathing.[57–59] Volume or pressure support during the inspiratory phase appears to further assist inspiration by enhancing tidal volume (V_T) and thereby further reducing work of breathing.[60,61]

A major goal of NPPV is to avoid the necessity for intubation and mechanical ventilation, with its inherent associated risks. These include the respiratory and cardiovascular risks of establishment of an artificial airway in an acutely ill patient, the necessity for sedation, and subsequent loss of protective airway reflexes. In patients with severe asthma, these risks also include the complications of dynamic hyperinflation[17,22,23] and neuromuscular blockade[28,62,63] (see Chapters 5 and 14).

NPPV has been shown to reduce the requirement for intubation, improve oxygenation, decrease dyspnea, and respiratory rate in patients with acute exacerbations of chronic obstructive pulmonary disease (COPD),[61,64–67] and is probably superior to CPAP alone in the treatment of other causes of respiratory failure.[68,69] At present there have been no published randomized controlled clinical trials demonstrating the efficacy of the use of NPPV in acute asthma. Studies have demonstrated that the use of low to medium levels of CPAP in acute asthma reduces respiratory rates, inspiratory work and subjective sensations of dyspnea.[58,59,70–72] A case series describing the use of NPPV via face mask in asthma patients[56] demonstrated improved gas exchange and speculated that the need for mechanical ventilation was reduced. In this series, NPPV appeared to be safe and well tolerated. Complications normally attributed to dynamic hyperinflation (hypotension and barotrauma) have not been reported during NPPV.[56,61,64]

NPPV also has advantages of lower cost and greater convenience compared with invasive mechanical ventilation. An uncontrolled study suggesting that NPPV was associated with a significantly increased workload in terms of nursing hours[73] has not been supported by subsequent studies,[64,65] particularly once the patient has been settled and stabilized on NPPV.[64]

NPPV by face mask may be initiated in patients with severe asthma who are at risk of intubation and who are not responding adequately to bronchodilator therapy. A key factor for successful application of NPPV in this group is to identify appropriate patients early and commence NPPV before deterioration to a point where NPPV will be less well tolerated and hence less effective. NPPV is usually initiated with an expiratory positive airway pressure (EPAP) setting of 5 to 7 cm H_2O and an inspiratory positive airway pressure (IPAP) setting of 10 to 20 cm H_2O. These pressure settings are then adjusted according to patient tolerance, the sensation of dyspnea, and the observed clinical response. Patient tolerance and acceptability of NPPV may be improved by cycling periods of NPPV with periods of oxygen therapy by conventional face mask.

Nebulized bronchodilator therapy should continue at the required frequency while asthma patients are treated with NPPV. The delivery of nebulized bronchodilators to the airways was shown to be reduced during CPAP therapy compared with conventional oxygen masks, but there was no difference in the clinical response to nebulized bronchodilators.[74]

Patients whose acute asthma is sufficiently severe to warrant a trial of support with NPPV should be managed in a high-dependency or intensive care setting so that they may be carefully monitored and readily intubated if needed.

NPPV should be continued until there is clear clinical improvement that is sustained after removal of NPPV.

While NPPV has the potential to be a highly effective respiratory support and to avert the need for mechanical ventilation in some patients with acute severe asthma, it is not suitable for use in all patients. The success of NPPV depends upon both the selection of patients with an appropriate level of asthma severity and upon patient tolerance of the technique.

NPPV is not safe in patients who lack airway protection, especially if NPPV also causes gastric distention, increasing the risk of aspiration. Patients who are obtunded, apneic, profoundly exhausted, uncooperative, have excessive secretions, are hypotensive, or have manifestations of shock should be intubated and mechanically ventilated.

Poor patient tolerance, usually as a result of mask discomfort, patient anxiety, claustrophobia, or failure to relieve dyspnea, can cause failure of NPPV as a ventilatory support mode. Inappropriate levels of CPAP or inspiratory assistance, inadequate flow responses in the ventilator circuit, or staff inexperience with the use of NPPV will adversely affect the ability of a patient with respiratory failure to tolerate NPPV.

INTUBATION

Whenever possible, intubation should be performed by a clinician experienced in airway procedures and ventilation. Unskilled airway manipulation in asthma patients may produce laryngospasm and an exacerbation of bronchospasm, whereas an experienced airway proceduralist may minimize these phenomena. Also, these patients often have little physiological reserve by the time ventilatory support is required. Consequently, it is important that intubation be performed as smoothly and expeditiously as possible.

The approach to intubation should follow standard and well-accepted clinical guidelines for the intubation of any seriously ill patient. Initial preparation is vital and includes ensuring that appropriate intubation equipment, a selection of endotracheal tubes, suction, and a minimum of one experienced assistant are available prior to undertaking the procedure. A pre-intubation inspection of the patient for potential difficulties with airway visualization and intubation is vital to avoid the catastrophic situation of a failed or unnecessarily prolonged intubation in patients who may have minimal physiological reserve. A rapid sequence induction using an intravenous sedative/anesthetic agent in combination with succinylcholine is the preferred choice to secure the airway while protecting against potential aspiration of gastric contents.

Unless technical difficulties prevail, patients should be intubated via the oral route using an appropriately sized endotracheal tube (i.e., 8 mm ID for adult females, 8 to 9 mm ID for adult males). Such large endotracheal tubes minimize resistance to airflow, particularly when high inspiratory flow rates are used, and facilitate the suction of tracheal secretions. These considerations are particularly important in the patient with asthma since the tube will be placed in series with obstructed airways and during the recovery phase of acute asthma. Mobilization of large tenacious mucous plugs is common, causing a risk of acute occlusion of the endotracheal tube.

Although nasal intubation is better tolerated than oral intubation, there are potential disadvantages in the asthma patient including: 1) the need to insert an endotracheal tube smaller in diameter with an inherently greater airflow resistance; 2) the increased risk of a slightly more complex and time consuming procedure in a hypercapnic and hypoxic patient; 3) the increased risk of nasal bleeding due to the higher incidence of mucosal edema and nasal polyps in the atopic asthmatic population; and 4) the increased risk of sinusitis.

Sedation is an important adjunct to mechanical ventilation in severe asthma since it provides patient comfort, allows tolerance of controlled hypoventilation, minimizes the potentially asynchronous respiratory efforts of the patient, reduces CO_2 production and O_2 consumption, and facilitates procedures. Sedation preferably is administered by intravenous infusion titrated to individual requirements. Sedatives used most commonly include benzodiazepines (midazolam, lorazepam), narcotics (morphine), propofol, and ketamine. As a significant number of ventilated asthma patients improve to a safe weaning point relatively quickly, (within 18 to 30 hours),[39] shorter-acting agents, such as midazolam and propofol allow more rapid awakening and facilitate weaning.

Ketamine, an intravenous anesthetic and analgesic agent, has been shown to have bronchodilator properties[75–78] through an unknown mechanism of action. It has been described in isolated cases as alleviating intractable bronchospasm in mechanically ventilated asthmatics with severe bronchospasm refractory to conventional bronchodilator therapy.[79,80] However, a randomized control trial of low-dose ketamine in the treatment of asthma in an emergency department failed to demonstrate any benefit compared with conventional bronchodilator therapy.[81] Although the efficacy of ketamine remains to be clearly demonstrated in severe asthma, it may have a useful adjunctive role as a sedative agent in the ventilated asthma patient who remains refractory to maximal conventional bronchodilator therapy.

Similarly, volatile anesthetic agents (halothane, enflurane, and isofluorane) have been reported to successfully treat patients with severe refractory asthma,[82,83] probably acting as direct relaxants of bronchial smooth muscle. Administration of halothane to a group of 12 mechanically ventilated asthma patients produced an improvement in gas exchange and a reduction in peak airway pressures without untoward cardiovascular effects.[84] Enflurane and isoflurane have also been shown to be efficacious in similar patients.[85,86] Despite these encouraging reports, these drugs are not widely used; and the role of the volatile anesthetic agents in the management of the mechanically ventilated patient with asthma is unclear. Technical difficulties with administration of these agents in the intensive care setting and the potential for untoward cardiovascular complications, particularly hypotension and arrhythmias, suggest that their role may best be reserved for last-resort therapy of refractory life-threatening asthma.

FACTORS INFLUENCING VENTILATOR MANAGEMENT

The primary role of mechanical ventilation in acute severe asthma is to maintain oxygenation and ventilation and prevent respiratory arrest. It is essential that ventilator management is conducted with the aim of minimizing both immediate and delayed morbidity and mortality. Mechanical ventilation provides no inherent therapeutic benefit to airflow obstruction in asthma. Thus, the mechanical ventilator must safely support the patient until bronchodilator therapy improves airflow obstruction sufficiently for independent ventilation to occur. A clear understanding of the immediate and delayed risks is required to balance their impact on the mechanical ventilation strategy.

Immediate and short-term risks of mechanical ventilation are primarily hypotension, pulmonary barotrauma, and occasionally, severe circulatory compromise with risk of death.[24,25,31] The time immediately following intubation, when mechanical ventilation is first applied, can be crucial for the patient with severe bronchospasm. Considerable care is required to manage this phase safely, including judicious use of sedation, neuromuscular blockade, fluid loading, bronchodilators, mechanical ventilation assessments, and management strategies. Furthermore, airflow obstruction may continue to deteriorate during the first 24 hours of mechanical ventilation,[19,23] possibly due to the irritating effects of lower airway instrumentation. This, or injudicious ventilator adjustments, can lead to pneumothoraces or further circulatory impairment.

These immediate and short-term risks of mechanical ventilation primarily relate to the complications of dynamic hyperinflation. Dynamic hyperinflation is a direct consequence of airflow obstruction and results in tidal ventilation occurring well above the normal functional residual capacity (FRC). FRC is the passive relaxation volume that is reached following an expiratory time long enough to allow all expiratory airflow to cease. In severe asthma, FRC is considerably elevated above normal due to airway closure during expiration as lung volume decreases.[39] Dynamic hyperinflation is superimposed on this elevated baseline. Expiratory times that are long enough for all expiratory airflow to cease are commonly 40 to 90 seconds in severe asthma.[22,39] During either spontaneous or mechanical ventilation, expiratory times are always considerably shorter than this and, thus, dynamic hyperinflation must occur owing to incomplete exhalation of the previous breath. Since this dynamic gas trapping occurs with every breath, it is cumulative, but fortunately self-limiting. It is self-limiting because as lung volume increases, so too does lung elastic recoil pressure and small airway caliber. Both of these factors improve expiratory airflow, and the lungs inflate to a lung volume in which exhalation of the inspired tidal volume (V_T) can be completed (Fig. 13-1).

During spontaneous ventilation with mild airflow obstruction, this process is adaptive as it allows the desired minute ventilation to be achieved, albeit at a higher lung volume, without serious compromise of inspiratory muscle capacity.

During spontaneous ventilation with severe asthma, dynamic hyperinflation is limited by inability of the patient to inspire much beyond TLC; tidal ventilation occurs immediately below this lung volume (Fig. 13-1). The physical limit to minute ventilation at this lung volume results in hypercapnia, even in the absence of fatigue. Although inspiratory muscles are acting at a severe mechanical disadvantage and ventilation at this lung volume can only be sustained for a short time before fatigue ensues, this prevents the more serious problems of lung volumes increasing beyond this safe limit.

Figure 13-1

Comparison of the effects of maximum spontaneous ventilation and excessive mechanical ventilation on dynamic hyperinflation and lung volumes in a patient with severe asthma. The functional residual capacity (FRC) reached following a period of apnea is shown relative to predicted normal FRC and total lung capacity (TLC) levels. V_T, tidal volume; Vtr, volume of gas trapped by dynamic hyperinflation. (Adapted from Tuxen et al[39])

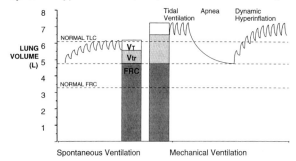

During mechanical ventilation of patients with severe airflow obstruction, the limitation of lung inflation to TLC does not apply as it does during spontaneous ventilation (Fig. 13-1). Mechanical ventilation can easily continue inspiration beyond TLC. The lung volumes required to achieve the equilibrium point, where expired and inspired V_T equalize, can be considerably above TLC.[22,39] Although a new equilibrium with less hypercapnia can be established at lung volumes above TLC, doing so risks cardiac tamponade and pneumothorax[19,23] and probably contributes to mechanical ventilation morbidity and mortality.[17] TLC has been shown[19,23] to be the safety limit at which these complications are prevented.

The level of dynamic hyperinflation is primarily determined by three factors: 1) the inspired tidal volume, 2) the expiratory time, and 3) the severity of airflow obstruction.[22] If bronchodilator therapy has been maximized, it is likely that airflow obstruction is not immediately alterable during initial mechanical ventilation and thus, the regulation of dynamic hyperinflation will depend primarily on the use of small tidal volumes and long expiratory times. The latter is achieved by the use of low respiratory rates and high inspiratory flow rates. High inspiratory flow rates shorten inspiratory time and thereby increase expiratory time at any given ventilator rate.

High inspiratory flow rates have been recommended by some researchers.[39,87–92] However, this remains controversial[18,20,93–95] because of theoretical concerns that high inspiratory flow rate and high airway pressure may redistribute excessive ventilation to low-resistance lung units, risking barotrauma. These concerns are based on early mechanical and mathematical lung models,[96,97] but have no supporting clinical data. The only clinical data comparing different flow rates suggest that less dynamic hyperinflation[22] (Fig. 13-2) and improved gas exchange[89] result from high inspiratory flow rates.

The use of low tidal volumes and low ventilator rates necessarily results in a low minute ventilation and significant hypercapnic acidosis. To enable patients to tolerate this during mechanical

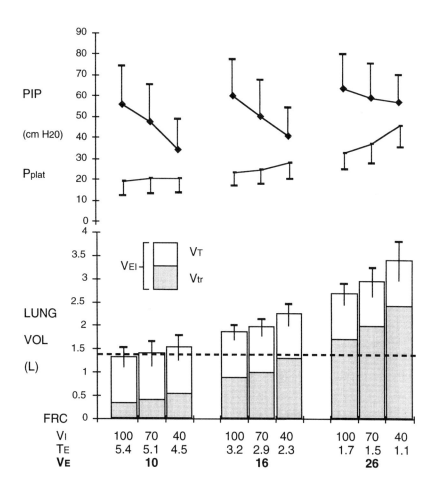

Figure 13-2
The effect of V_E and V_I (and expiratory time, T_E) on V_{EI}, V_{tr}, P_{plat}, and PIP (mean ± SD) at a constant V_T. in patients receiving mechanical ventilation for severe asthma. A reference line for the safe level of V_{EI} (1.4 L, 20 ml/kg) is shown. Only the lowest V_E and the highest V_I achieved a mean V_{EI} below the safe limit (a V_E of 8 L/min and a lower V_T would have achieved all patients in this study below the safe V_{EI}). Notice also that every mean PIP below 50 cm H_2O was associated with an unsafe level of DHI, whereas the only V_{EI} below the safe limit (with V_I 100 L/min) was associated with a mean PIP of 55 cm H_2O and a range >70 cm H_2O. PIP, peak inspiratory pressure; P_{plat}, plateau airway pressure; V_T, tidal volume (L); V_{tr}, trapped volume above FRC due to dynamic hyperinflation; V_I, inspiratory flow rate (L/min); T_E, expiratory time (sec); V_E, minute ventication (L/min). (Adapted from Tuxen et al[22])

ventilation, heavy sedation and initial neuromuscular blockade are often required.

Because the severity of airflow obstruction may vary considerably among patients with severe asthma, a fixed ventilatory pattern results in a range of dynamic hyperinflation, that may or may not be safe (below TLC). Thus, although a ventilatory pattern that suits the majority of patients with severe asthma may be chosen, it is essential that the level of dynamic hyperinflation be assessed so that the level of minute ventilation can be adjusted to suit the severity of airflow obstruction. Numerous methods have been proposed. Keeping peak inspiratory pressure (PIP) below an arbitrary limit

(usually 50 to 60 cm H_2O) has been suggested. This has been shown by Tuxen[22] to be illogical and potentially dangerous because of the paradoxical effects of inspiratory flow on PIP and dynamic hyperinflation. Decreasing inspiratory flow decreases PIP (potentially to within a "safe" limit) but concurrently increases dynamic hyperinflation (to potentially beyond a safe limit) by decreasing expiratory time. Williams and colleagues have demonstrated that the volume of gas released during a period of prolonged apnea is the best discriminator for the occurrence of dynamic hyperinflation complications (hypotension and pneumothorax).[23] This gas volume has been termed the lung volume at end-inspiration above FRC (V_{EI}). Although this has been shown[39] to be a useful and safe tool to regulate the level of mechanical ventilation, it is technically complex since it requires volumetric bellows for its measurement and it also requires the patient to be paralyzed to accept a period of apnea. For these reasons it is not widely used.

Measurement of auto-PEEP has been widely advocated to detect the presence of dynamic hyperinflation. Auto-PEEP is reliable for this purpose and a high level of auto-PEEP does indicate a danger. However, the auto-PEEP maneuver only assesses those lung units remaining in communication at the end of expiration and not those that have undergone airway closure at higher alveolar pressures. This has been shown to underestimate total auto-PEEP and to be insensitive to changes in airflow obstruction.[98] For these reasons, auto-PEEP cannot be recommended as a reliable sole guide to assess dynamic hyperinflation.

A simpler, easier alternative may be P_{plat}. Although this has not been shown to be as good a discriminator as V_{EI} for the occurrence of complications,[23] it has the advantage of simplicity and ready availability. A P_{plat} measurement of <25 cm H_2O may be a better discriminator of a safe level of ventilation.[23] It is important to remember that P_{plat} should be measured following a single breath only. An end-inspiratory pause left in place for a series of breaths will shorten expiratory time and increase the severity of dynamic hyperinflation during that period which is not safe and will falsely elevate the value of P_{plat}. Williams and colleagues[23] have speculated that the reduced predictive value of P_{plat} for complications when compared with V_{EI} is due to the variation in chest-wall compliance among patients with asthma. This is not surprising when mechanical ventilation is occurring with lung volumes close to TLC, at which point chest wall compliance may decrease dramatically. Thus, it is possible that transpulmonary pressure, enabled by the measurement of esophageal pressure, would be a better indicator of the safe level of dynamic hyperinflation; however this remains purely speculative.

Thus, ventilator strategies aimed at, or permitting, aggressive normalization of Pa_{CO_2} should

not be initiated until airflow obstruction improves, and P_{plat} decreases sufficiently for them to be safe.

The most important delayed risk of mechanical ventilation is the occurrence of acute necrotizing myopathy.[28,62] It is, as reported by many investigators, most directly associated with the combination of steroids and neuromuscular blocking agents (NMBAs).[63] It ranges in severity from mild weakness to functional quadraparesis[63,99] and can delay weaning from mechanical ventilation, prolong intensive care and hospital stay, require rehabilitation and, in a small number of patients, result in permanent disability. Acute necrotizing myopathy is currently the major complication threatening a patient who requires mechanical ventilation for severe asthma. It is characterized by non-uniform, non-inflammatory myonecrosis which may be extensive. This is almost always accompanied by an increase in creatine kinase, which may be large (>5000 IU/L) or small (<800 IU/L) and prolonged.[100] Patients with a small creatine kinase increase may have substantial weakness because small patches of necrosis adjacent to neuromuscular junctions may functionally denervate a larger amount on non-necrotic muscle.

In one study, creatine kinase increases were found in 75% and weakness in 35% of patients who routinely received parenteral steroids and NMBAs during mechanical ventilation for asthma.[28] All patients received a similar dose of steroids and the extent of creatine kinase increase and the incidence and severity of myopathy was proportional to the dose of NMBA. The etiology of this condition is uncertain. Dubois has demonstrated increased expression of glucocorticoid receptors on skeletal muscle following denervation and has speculated that this may play a role in muscle injury from steroids in the presence of neuromuscular blockade.[101]

Measures to detect and minimize the occurrence of myopathy include:

- Daily measurement of creatine kinase levels.

- Minimization of systemic steroid dose by institution of relatively low initial parenteral steroid dose (e.g., 60 mg methylprednisolone IV, 6 hourly),[102] commencement of steroid dose reduction after 24 hours, provided there has been some improvement in airflow obstruction, and early use of nebulized steroids[47] to facilitate reduction in parenteral steroids.

- NMBA minimization, including avoiding any use of NMBAs in patients whose asthma is rapidly recovering and use of one or two initial bolus doses of NMBA instead of infusions. Where infusions are necessary, use of regular nerve stimulation assessment to minimize the infusion level, and cessation of infusions every 24 hrs to reassess need are advisable. Minimization of NMBAs can necessitate high levels of sedation to facilitate hypoventilation. Sedation used to the point of profound immobility may also contribute to myopathy.

- The need to minimize NMBAs and to avoid profound inactivity has had a significant impact both on the assessment of dynamic hyperinflation and on the ventilatory strategy used to reduce it. Initially, profound empirical hypoventilation was proposed.[18] This ensured minimal risk from dynamic hyperinflation, but produced the highest risk of myopathy. Prolonged neuromuscular blockade to ensure careful measurement and regulation of dynamic hyperinflation[39] also carried significant risk of myopathy.[28] Alternatively, series that did not specifically regulate dynamic hyperinflation had a high mortality.[55,103–105] Ventilatory strategies that maintain the safety of hypoventilation in combination with minimal NMBA and modest sedative use are probably the best compromise.[21] In these strategies, it is important to carefully assess dynamic hyperinflation so that minute ventilation can be regulated to provide the best compromise between the risks of excessive or inadequate hypoventilation. Such strategies can indirectly contribute to myopathy depending on the amount of NMBA employed.

MECHANICAL VENTILATION STRATEGY

Initial Mechanical Ventilation

The most established mode for mechanical ventilation is volume cycle. Mechanical ventilation should be commenced in synchronized intermittent mechanical ventilation (SIMV) mode using a V_T of 8 mL/kg and a respiratory rate of 10 to 12 breaths per minute, resulting in a minute ventilation <115 mL/kg/min.[23] Tuxen has recommended that the V_T be delivered at a high inspiratory flow rate (80 to 100 L per minute) to ensure a short inpiratory time (<0.5 sec) and a long expiratory time ($\geq$4 seconds)[22,39] (Fig. 13-2). This level of minute ventilation has been shown by Williams and colleagues to be appropriate for 80% of patients who required mechanical ventilation for severe asthma and resulted in only mildly excessive dynamic hyperinflation in the remaining 20%.[23] Rarely, patients with exceptionally severe airflow obstruction may develop a dangerous level of dynamic hyperinflation, despite this low initial minute ventilation.[24–27,106,107] However, this is usually recognized immediately by the occurrence of severe hypotension and should be diagnosed with an apnea test (see below) and treated with a low V_T and a lower respiratory rate (4 to 6 breaths per minute).[24]

Initial mechanical ventilation should not be accompanied by any significant pressure support as this may enable a patient to elevate his minute ventilation beyond a safe limit, and it usually needs to be accompanied by heavy sedation to assist tolerance of hypoventilation. Infusions of midazolam or propofol are suitable and may cause less hypotension than bolus doses. Concurrent infusion of morphine is commonly used to assist suppression of spontaneous ventilation. Despite the use of heavy sedation, adequate suppression of spontaneous ventilation is often incomplete, resulting in inadequate hypoventilation and risk of barotrauma and hypotension. An initial one or two bolus doses of an NMBA (e.g., cis-atracurium) allows stabilization of ventilation without the use of excessive sedation which could result in significant hypotension.[23] Initial neuromuscular blockade is commonly required and should be used in the majority of patients who require mechanical ventilation except those whose asthma is rapidly recovering.

The vasodilatory effects of sedation and hypercapnia, when combined with positive pressure ventilation, may lead to mild hypotension and require a positive fluid balance of 1 to 2 L during the first 24 hours of mechanical ventilation. Occasionally, patients will have much larger fluid requirements.[23] If pulse pressure (the difference between systolic and diastolic blood pressures) rises with brief cessation (~60 sec) of mechanical ventilation, it is likely further fluid resuscitation is required (see below).

Assessment of Dynamic Hyperinflation

P_{plat} and auto-PEEP should be measured as soon as mechanical ventilation has been stabilized, during initial paralysis. P_{plat} should be measured during a 0.5 second end-inspiratory pause[22,23] applied following a single breath only. If possible, V_{EI} should be measured using a volumetric measuring device during 60 seconds of apnea. Even in the absence of a volumetric measuring device, it is worthwhile to apply a period of apnea in order to observe the circulatory response. Any significant increase in blood pressure, accompanied by a decrease in central venous pressure, suggests significant dynamic hyperinflation affecting the circulation.

Initial Ventilator Adjustments

If P_{plat} exceeds 25 cm H_2O, auto-PEEP exceeds 10 cm H_2O, or if there is a significant improvement in the circulation during a period of apnea, then the ventilator rate should be reduced by 2 to 4 breaths per minute, depending on the magnitude of the change required. Sedation and paralysis should be continued and reassessment undertaken. If P_{plat} is <20 cm H_2O, auto-PEEP is <5 to 7 cm H_2O, and there is no significant hemodynamic improvement during a period of apnea, then the ventilator rate can be increased by 2 breaths per minute and reassessment undertaken. Paralysis should not be continued and sedation may be decreased, depending on the degree of hypercapnia present.

Asthma Time Course

The majority of patients with severe asthma have a large chronic component that can take several days to improve sufficiently to allow weaning. These patients may have slow improvement in air-

flow obstruction despite aggressive therapy. Under these circumstances, a high level of sedation may need to be continued, but paralysis should cease after 1 or 2 bolus doses unless mechanical ventilation without paralysis is a significant problem. Whether asthma improvement is rapid or slow, it can be recognized by a reduction in P_{plat} and auto-PEEP in addition to a reduction in wheeze and increased expectoration of secretions.[39] When liberalizing ventilation in response to these improvements results in a minimal degree of hypercapnic acidosis, then sedation should be reduced or discontinued and a small amount of pressure support introduced.

Pressure Control Ventilation

The use of pressure support or pressure control ventilation as a primary support mode in asthma is less well established. Successful use of pressure support ventilation has been reported[108–110] without apparent side effects, despite the use of high levels of initial minute ventilation (13 L per minute), tidal volumes (10 mL/kg) and ventilation rates (21 breaths per minute). All of these settings exceeded commonly recommended limits.[18,23,39,52,90–92] Pressure control ventilation has the theoretical advantages of maintaining dynamic hyperinflation within a safe limit (e.g., 25 cm H_2O) when airflow obstruction is severe and of automatically increasing minute ventilation as airflow obstruction improves. However, pressure control ventilation also has a theoretical disadvantage. Because severe airflow obstruction is present, alveolar pressure is slow to rise and will not equilibrate with the extrinsic control pressure during the short inspiratory time that should be in use. Thus, if pressure control is set to a safe limit (e.g., 25 cm H_2O), this will result in a lower V_T and more hypoventilation than would occur with an equivalent volume control mode. This can increase the need for sedation and paralysis and increase the risk of myopathy. Attempts to overcome this problem by increasing inspiratory time either reduce expiratory time and increase dynamic hyperinflation or mandate a rate reduction to maintain expiratory time, which will still result in increased hypercapnia. If the pressure control level is set above the safe limit to offset the reduced V_T, then lung overinflation may occur when airflow obstruction improves and inspiratory airway resistance decreases. At present, there is little data to support the use of pressure control ventilation and there are some theoretical concerns regarding its use. Careful assessment of this mode of ventilation must be made before its use is recommended.

MANAGEMENT OF HYPOTENSION

Mild hypotension may result from vasodilation due to hypercapnia and sedation, in combination with positive pressure ventilation. Severe hypotension is almost always due either to excessive dynamic hyperinflation or a tension pneumothorax (usually due to excessive dynamic hyperinflation). When hypotension occurs during mechanical ventilation of a patient with severe airflow obstruction, dynamic hyperinflation should be assessed, fluid loading undertaken, and a chest radiograph obtained. Dynamic hyperinflation should be assessed by measuring P_{plat} (and if possible, auto-PEEP and V_{EI}) and by conducting an apnea test.[24]

An apnea test consists of disconnecting the patient from the ventilator for a minimum of 60 to 90 seconds and observing the effects on blood pressure, heart rate, and central venous pressure over 3 to 4 minutes, both during apnea and following resumption of mechanical ventilation.[24] Prior to undertaking this test, 100% O_2 should be in place. A positive test (suggesting excessive dynamic hyperinflation was present) will show a significant increase in blood pressure with concurrent reductions in heart rate and central venous pressure at the end of the period of apnea, and the reverse 1 to 2 minutes after mechanical ventilation has been resumed. An alternative to the apnea test is a profound hypoventilation test[92] which consists of 2 to 3 breaths per minute with a longer period of observation. Another more cautious assessment method is a rate reduction test, which may both diagnose and resolve mild hypotension but requires a longer period of more careful observation, and the results are not always as clear.

If P_{plat} is excessive or if hypotension resolves during apnea or rate reduction, then it is strongly suggestive that excessive dynamic hyperinflation is present and the respiratory rate should be reduced. Fluid loading should be undertaken to overcome any component of relative hypovolemia resulting from vasodilation. A chest radiograph should be taken to ensure no pneumothoraces are present.

Rare patients with exceptionally severe airflow obstruction may develop profound hypotension to the point of circulatory collapse,[24–27,106,107] apparent electromechanical dissociation and the need for external cardiac massage. It has been reported that delayed recognition of excessive dynamic hyperinflation in a number of patients has lead to severe circulatory compromise, ineffective resuscitation, and cerebral injury,[24,25] all of which could have been averted if dynamic hyperinflation had been promptly diagnosed and relieved. When profound hypotension or circulatory collapse occurs during the mechanical ventilation of a patient with severe asthma, an immediate apnea test (as above) or profound hypoventilation test[92] should be undertaken. Such maneuvers are both diagnostic and therapeutic if dynamic hyperinflation is the cause of hypotension. When conducting an apnea test, it is important that at least 1 minute of apnea is given. This is the time it takes for lung deflation to occur and for subsequently improved venous return to result in an improvement in both left ventricular output and blood pressure. Although 1 to 1.5 minutes of apnea may be hard to administer to a patient in extremis, Pa_{CO_2} will not rise by more than 5 to 6 mm Hg during this time period and mild or moderate arterial desaturation, if it occurs, is preferable to severe hypotension. Patients whose asthma is sufficiently severe to cause profound hypotension despite initial hypoventilation (V_E <115 mL/kg/min, with 10 to 12 breaths per minute) will frequently require a marked reduction in respiratory rate to 4 to 6 breaths per minute for circulatory stability.[24] This may result in marked hypercapnia (i.e., Pa_{CO_2} >100 mm Hg) and marked acidemia (i.e., pH <7.05). The use of slow intravenous bicarbonate[111] has not been shown to be of benefit in patients with moderate hypercapnic acidosis, but may increase patient tolerance of hypercapnia by reducing acidemic drive to ventilation, and may be warranted in patients with more severe acidemia.

Very rarely, patients with exceptionally severe airflow obstruction may have persisting hypotension despite profound hypoventilation (as above), fluid loading, and the use of inotropes. Under these circumstances, extracorporeal membrane oxygenation may be used;[26,27,106,107] however, heliox may be a preferable alternative since it has been used successfully under similar circumstances (unpublished communication). The highest helium content compatible with adequate oxygenation should be used. Heliox containing 60% helium and 40% oxygen is a suitable first choice.[54] Concentrations of helium below 60% are unlikely to be of any benefit; and if oxygenation permits, helium concentration should be increased to 80%. Mechanical ventilators must be adapted for the oxygen inlet to receive gas from a nonstandard cylinder, must be bench-tested to ensure they function with heliox, and must be calibrated with a volumetric measuring device to compensate for the altered volume delivery that occurs with heliox.[107a] Such patients with extreme hypercapnia and acidemia may also benefit from measures to reduce CO_2 production, such as cooling and low-carbohydrate feeding.

MANAGEMENT OF PNEUMOTHORACES

Although pneumothoraces may occur in patients with asthma, they rarely occur spontaneously during an acute exacerbation. In one series of patients admitted to the intensive care unit (ICU) for severe asthma, pneumothoraces occurred exclusively in those patients who required mechanical ventilation.[23] During the mechanical ventilation of a patient with severe asthma, pneumothoraces result from either a complication of central venous catheter placement or from excessive dynamic hyperinflation. Central venous catheters are useful in both the assessment and management of patients with severe asthma. To reduce the risk of pneumothorax, the internal jugular approach should be used.

The presence of airflow obstruction results in a high probability of a pneumothorax being under tension and an increased risk that bilateral pneumothoraces will occur. The risk of tension is increased because dynamically hyperinflated lungs rarely collapse when a pneumothorax occurs. The airflow obstruction acts as a one-way valve that continues to admit air to the ruptured alveolus during inspiration but provides very slow exhalation of gas, which can occur far more rapidly through the rupture. The net effect of this is often the development of considerable tension in a pneumothorax with a lung that is only moderately collapsed. When a tension pneumothorax occurs, the minute ventilation to this lung must be substantially reduced. During volume cycle ventilation, this must result in an increased level of ventilation to the contralateral lung, with a consequent increase in its dynamic hyperinflation. Since the cause of the initial pneumothorax may have been excessive dynamic hyperinflation, a further increase in dynamic hyperinflation to the second lung greatly increases its risk of developing a second tension pneumothorax.

Pneumothoraces are commonly reported during the mechanical ventilation of patients with severe asthma[17,23] when mechanical ventilation is not being carefully controlled. Tension pneumothoraces may have been responsible for >6% of deaths of patients who required mechanical ventilation for severe asthma.[17]

Tension pneumothoraces may be recognized by a sudden or unexplained increase in airway pressures, a hemodynamic deterioration (increased heart rate and central venous pressure, and decreased blood pressure), a deterioration in gas exchange, or increasing patient restlessness or distress. Clinical signs of pneumothorax are not always clear. Hyperinflation, soft breath sounds, and increased percussion resonance are commonly already present in severe asthma and further exaggeration of these signs due to a pneumothorax can be hard to detect. Despite considerable tension, only moderate lung collapse may occur and, during mechanical ventilation, breath sounds may be maintained. Tracheal shift may not be clearly apparent. Thus, a confident clinical diagnosis is not always easy. Furthermore, the use of blind intercostal catheters in the absence of a pneumothorax risks lung injury, which may cause the problem that it was intended to treat.

Thus, as soon as pneumothorax is suspected, the ventilator rate should be immediately decreased by 2 to 4 breaths, to reduce the risk of excessive hyperinflation to the contralateral lung. This may require an increase in sedation and possibly, the use of paralysis. To minimize the risk of catheter-induced lung injury, it is preferable that an urgent chest radiograph be obtained prior to undertaking intercostal catheter placement. If hypotension is mild (systolic blood pressure >80 mm Hg) then an urgent chest radiograph with preparation for an intercostal catheter is preferable to blind intercostal catheter insertion. If hypotension is severe (systolic blood pressure <70 mm Hg) *and dynamic hyperinflation is not apparent by APNEA test,* then careful blind intercostal catheter insertion should be undertaken immediately on the suspected side of the pneumothorax. If an intercostal catheter is necessary, it is essential that catheter insertion be undertaken using blunt dissection without the use of a stilette to minimize the risk of lung injury.

MECHANICAL VENTILATION DURING CEREBRAL ISCHEMIC INJURY

Mechanical ventilation follows cardiorespiratory collapse in approximately 20% of episodes.[19,23] In patients in whom cardiorespiratory collapse has occurred outside a hospital, significant delays in resuscitation are common. In other instances, prolonged resuscitation following instigation of mechanical ventilation has been required.[24,25,112] Under either circumstance, significant cerebral ischemic injury may be present and the brain is at risk of cerebral edema and further injury from hypotension. Approximately 40% of deaths in patients who have received mechanical ventilation for severe asthma are due to cerebral hypoxic injuries sustained as a result of cardiorespiratory arrest prior to mechanical ventilation.[17] This creates a dilemma during mechanical ventilation of such patients.

Use of hypoventilation is important to limit

dynamic hyperventilation and thereby maintain cerebral perfusion pressure[113,114] by reducing the risk of hypotension. However, hypoventilation frequently results in hypercapnic acidosis, which can increase the severity of cerebral edema. If cerebral injury is severe, increasing cerebral edema can cause the brain injury to become worse and, in some instances, can lead to death due to coning. As heavy sedation and sometimes paralysis can be in place, deterioration in conscious state may be hard to detect.

If a patient has had a prolonged cardiorespiratory arrest and has a poor conscious state prior to sedation, then the risk of significant cerebral injury is present. Under these circumstances, intracranial pressure monitoring should be undertaken so that the effects of hypercapnic acidosis on intracranial pressure during the first 48 to 72 hours can be judged. If significant intracranial hypertension is present, then active measures to combat cerebral edema should be undertaken. The extent of hypercapnic acidosis should be minimized by administering small increases in minute ventilation. Small excesses in dynamic hyperinflation can be tolerated under these circumstances provided they do not cause hypotension, impede cerebral venous drainage, or increase the intracranial pressure.

TIME COURSE FOR ASTHMA RECOVERY

In patients requiring mechanical ventilation for asthma, 16 to 20% have rapid improvement in the airflow obstruction, which allows the withdrawal of sedation, weaning, and extubation within 24 hours.[19,23] Such patients are predominately those with hyperacute asthma[30] whose pathology is dominated by bronchospasm. Those patients who do not have rapid improvement may require prolonged mechanical ventilation (2 to 7 days) as a result of slow resolution of severe airflow obstruction, presumably dominated by acute or chronic airway inflammation. We have studied the time course for asthma recovery in the slower recovery group in detail,[19] and it was found that resolution of asthma was signaled by both a reduction in the minute ventilation required for normocapnia and an improvement in airflow obstruction enabling a high minute ventilation to be safely undertaken. The reduction in minute ventilation required for normocapnia was presumably due to both a reduction in CO_2 production and to a reduction in dead space as airflow obstruction improved.[19] Initial resolution of airflow obstruction was slow, but then entered an accelerated phase prior to weaning that was accompanied by increased secretions from the lungs.

LONG-TERM OUTCOME

Most, if not all, episodes of mechanical ventilation for asthma have been judged as preventable had there been the opportunity for prior appropriate therapy.[115] Following a life-threatening event that resulted in mechanical ventilation, it would be expected that patients would receive full asthma treatment and the risk of recurrence would be minimal. In contrast to this assumption, 9% of episodes of mechanical ventilation for asthma are recurrent episodes in the same patient.[17] Long-term follow-up studies in the patients who have been mechanically ventilated for asthma showed surprisingly high mortality rates,[40,104,116–118] ranging between 7 and 25% depending on age and duration of follow-up. Factors identified as contributing to these poor outcomes included poor compliance with treatment, denial, low socioeconomic status, under-estimation of asthma severity by both patients and clinicians, and inadequate follow-up and treatment.

These findings highlight the need for aggressive patient management following an episode of mechanical ventilation (see Chapter 18). Patients need to be educated regarding their asthma severity, their risk of recurrent events, their need for regular assessment, their measurement of airflow obstruction, and their need to respond to minor deterioration. These patients should have regular follow-up, regular assessment of lung function, and aggressive bronchodilator therapy, which almost invariably includes long-term adequate doses of inhaled corticosteroids. Patients also need to have management plans that include possible deteriora-

tion that may range from mild to severe. These plans may include increases in inhaler or nebulized bronchodilators, inhaled corticosteroids, commencement of oral corticosteroids, and early medical attendance.[119] In case of severe deterioration, they should have rapid access to a doctor and/or hospital planned. Patients with very brittle asthma may need additional instructions regarding administration of subcutaneous epinephrine, commencement of immediate high-dose oral steroids, and their capacity to alert an emergency ambulance.

CONCLUSION

Despite increasing community prevalence, reports of significant improvements in asthma mortality during the last decade are now emerging[12–15] accompanied by decreasing numbers of patients requiring mechanical ventilation for severe asthma. These improvements have been attributed to a number of factors, including the more widespread use of inhaled corticosteroids.[12,15] However, some series have reported increasing hospital presentations for asthma patients,[6,7] which may reflect increasing recognition and therapy.[12]

While the overall number of patients that require mechanical ventilation for asthma may be decreasing, patients who continue to require mechanical ventilation appear to be those with more severe refractory asthma; they also present the greatest management problems. Thus, fewer patients with asthma are mechanically ventilated, but those that are require an increased level of vigilance.

REFERENCES

1. Pingleton S: Asthma mortality has increased not only in the United States but also across the world. *JAMA* 273(21):1717–1718, 1997.
2. National Heart, Lung, and Blood Institute: Data Fact Sheet: Asthma Statistics. Bethesda, U.S. Dept of Health and Human Services, Public Health Service, National Institute of Health, 1989.
3. Bauman A, Young L, Peat J, et al: Asthma underrecognition and undertreatment in an Australian community. *Aust NZ Med J* 22:36–40, 1992.

4. Musk A, Ryan G, Perera D, et al: Mortality from asthma in Western Australia. *Med J Aust* 147:423–427, 1987.

5. Fleming D and Crombie D: Prevalence of asthma and hay fever in England and Wales. *Br Med J* 294:279–283, 1987.

6. Anderson H, Butland B, Strachan D: Trends in prevalence and severity of childhood asthma. *Br Med J* 308:1600–1604, 1994.

7. Peat J, Van der Berg R, Green W, et al: Changing prevalence of asthma in Australian children. *Br Med J* 308:1591–1596, 1994.

8. Seale J: Asthma deaths: where are we now? *Aust NZJ Med* 21:678–679, 1991.

9. O'Donnell T: Asthma—Australia and New Zealand. *Aust N Z J Med* 18:303–310, 1988.

10. Sears M, Rea H, Beaglehole R, et al: Asthma mortality in New Zealand: a two-year national study. *NZ Med J* 98:271–275, 1985.

11. Sly M: Changing asthma mortality. *Ann Allergy* 73:259–268, 1994.

12. Wilson J, Jenkins C: Asthma mortality: where is it going? *Med J Aust* 164:391–392, 1996.

13. Kemp T, Pearce N: The decline in asthma hospitalizations in persons aged 30–40 years in New Zealand. *Aust N Z J Med* 27:578–581, 1997.

14. Causes of death. Australia, 1989–94. *Australian Bureau of Statistics*, Catalogue No 3303.0.

15. Comino E, Bauman A: Trends in asthma-mortality in Australia. 1960–1996. *Med J Aust* 168:525–527, 1998.

16. Sutherland D, Beaglehole R, Fenwick J, et al: Deaths from asthma in Auckland: Circumstances and validation of causes. *N Z Med J* 97:845–8, 1984.

17. Tuxen D: Mechanical ventilation in asthma, in T. Evans, Hinds C, (eds): *Recent Advances in Critical Care Medicine* 4th ed. London, Churchill Livingstone, 1996, pp 165–189.

18. Darioli R, Perret C: Mechanical controlled hypoventilation in status asthmaticus. *Am Rev Respir Dis* 129:385–387, 1984.

19. Tuxen D, Williams T, Scheinkestel C, et al: Limiting dynamic hyperinflation in mechanically ventilated patients with severe asthma reduces complications. *Anaesth Intensive Care* 21(5):718, 1993 Abstract.

20. Limthongkul S, Udompanich V, Wongthim S, et al: Status asthmaticus: an analysis of 560 episodes and comparison between mechanical and non-mechanical ventilation groups. *J Med Assoc Thai* 73:321–327, 1990.

21. Bellomo R, McLaughlan P, Tai E, Parkin G: Asthma requiring mechanical ventilation. A low morbidity approach. *Chest* 105:891–896, 1994.

22. Tuxen D, Lane S: The effects of ventilatory pattern on hyperinflation, airway pressures, and circulation in mechanical ventilation of patients with severe airflow obstruction. *Am Rev Respir Dis* 136:872–879, 1987.

23. Williams T, Tuxen D, Scheinkestel C, et al: Risk factors for morbidity in mechanically ventilated patients with acute severe asthma. *Am Rev Respir Dis* 146(3):607–615, 1992.

24. Rosengarten P, Tuxen D, Dziukas L, et al: Circulatory arrest induced by intermittent positive pressure ventilation in a patient with severe asthma. *Anaesth Intensive Care* 19:118–121, 1990.

25. Kollef M: Lung hyperinflation caused by inappropriate ventilation resulting in electromechanical dissociation: a case report. *Heart Lung* 21:74–77, 1992.

26. Shapiro M, Kleaveland A, Bartlett R: Extracorporeal life support for status asthmaticus. *Chest* 103:1651–1654, 1993.

27. King D, Smales C, Arnold A, Jones O: Extracorporeal membrane oxygenation as emergency treatment for life threatening acute severe asthma. *Postgrad Med J* 62:555–557, 1986.

28. Douglass J, Tuxen D, Horne M, et al: Myopathy in severe asthma. *Am Rev Respir Dis* 146(2):517–519, 1992.

29. Johnson A, Nunn A, Somner A, et al: Circumstances of death from asthma. *Br Med J* 288:1870–1872, 1984.

30. Wasserfallen J, Schaller M, Feihl F, Perret C: Sudden asphyxic asthma: a distinct entity? *Am Rev Respir Dis* 142:108–111, 1990.

31. Kallenbach J, Frankel A, Lapinski S, et al: Determinants of near fatality in acute severe asthma. *Am J Med* 95:265–272. 1993.

32. Molfino N, Nannini L, Martelli A, Slutsky A: Respiratory arrest in near-fatal asthma. *N Engl J Med* 324(5):285–288, 1991.

33. Sur S, Crotty T, Kephart G: Sudden-onset fatal asthma: a distinct entity with few eosinophils and relatively more neutrophils in the airway submucosa. *Am Rev Respir Dis* 148:713–719, 1993.

34. Hetzel M, Clark T, Branthwaite M: Asthma: analysis of sudden deaths and ventilatory arrests in hospital. *Br Med J* 1:808–811, 1977.

35. Robin E, Lewiston N: Unexpected, unexplained

sudden death in young asthmatic subjects. *Chest* 96:790–793, 1989.

36. Rees H, Millar J, Donald J: A study of the clinical course and arterial blood gas tensions of patients in status asthmaticus. *Quart J Med* 37:234–243, 1968.

37. Tuxen D, Oh T: Acute severe asthma, in Oh T (ed): *Intensive Care Manual.* Sydney, Butterworths, 1990, pp 192–199.

38. Strunk R: Death due to asthma: new insights into sudden unexpected deaths but the focus remains on prevention. *Am Rev of Respir Dis* 148:550–552, 1993.

39. Tuxen D, Williams T, Scheinkestel C, et al: Use of a measurement of pulmonary hyperinflation to control the level of mechanical ventilation in patients with severe asthma. *Am Rev Respir Dis* 146(5):1136–1142, 1992.

40. Westerman D, Benatar S, Potgieter P, Ferguson A: Identification of the high-risk asthmatic patient. Experience with 39 patients undergoing ventilation for status asthmaticus. *Am J Med* 66:565–572, 1979.

41. Karetzky M: Asthma mortality associated with pneumothorax and intermittent positive pressure breathing. *Lancet* 1:828–829, 1975.

42. Williams MJ: Life-threatening asthma. *Arch Intern Med* 140:1604, 1980.

43. Beveridge R, Grunfeld A, Hodder R, Verbeek P: Guidelines for the emergency management of asthma in adults. *Can Med Assoc* 155(1):25–37, 1996.

44. Mandelberg A, Chen E, Noviski N, Priel I: Nebulized wet aerosol treatment in emergency department—is it essential? *Chest* 112(6):1501–1505, 1997.

45. Schuh S, Johnson D, Callahan S, et al: Efficacy of frequent nebulized ipratropium bromide added to frequent high-dose albuterol therapy in severe childhood asthma. *J Pediatr* 126(4):639–645, 1995.

46. Karpel J, Schacter E, Fanta C, et al: A comparison of ipratropium and albuterol versus albuterol alone for the treatment of acute asthma. *Chest* 110:611–6, 1996.

47. Rodrigo G, Rodrigo C: Inhaled flunisolide for acute severe asthma. *Am J Respir Crit Care Med* 157:698–703, 1998.

48. Appel D, Karpel J, Sherman M: Epinephrine improves expiratory flow rates in patients with asthma who do not respond to inhaled metaproterenol sulfate. *J Allergy Clin Immunol* 84:90–98, 1989.

49. Baughman R, Ploysongsang Y, James W: A comparative study of aerosolized terbutaline and subcutaneously administered epinephrine in the treatment of acute bronchial asthma. *Ann Allergy* 53:131–134, 1984.

50. Tinkelman D, Webb C, Vanderpool G, et al: The use of ketotifen in the prophylaxis of seasonal allergic asthma. *Ann Allergy* 56:213–217, 1986.

51. Spiteri M, Millar A, Pavia D, Clarke S: Subcutaneous adrenaline vs terbutaline in the treatment of acute severe asthma. *Thorax* 43:19–23, 1988.

52. Levy B, Kitch B, Fanta C: Medical and ventilatory management of status asthmaticus. *Intensive Care Med* 24(2):105–117, 1998.

53. Manthous C, Hall J, Caputo M, et al: The effect of heliox on pulsus paradoxus and peak flow in non-intubated patients with severe asthma. *Chest* 104:29S, 1992.

54. Gluck E, Onorato D, Castriotta R: Helium-oxygen mixtures in intubated patients with status asthmaticus and respiratory acidosis. *Chest* 98:693–698, 1990.

55. Ferrer A, Torres A, Roca J, et al: Characteristics of patients with soybean dust-induced acute severe asthma requiring mechanical ventilation. *Eur Respir J* 3:429–433, 1990.

56. Meduri G, Cook T, Turner R, et al: Noninvasive positive pressure ventilation in status asthma. *Chest* 110(3):767–774, 1996.

57. Martin J, Shore S, Engel L: Effect of continuous positive airway pressure on respiratory mechanics and pattern of breathing in induced asthma. *Am Rev Respir Dis* 126:812–817, 1982.

58. Tenaillon A, Salmona J, Burdin M: Continuous positive airway pressure in asthma. *Am Rev Respir Dis* 127:658, 1983.

59. Shivaram U, Donath J, Khan F, Juliano J: Effects of continuous positive airway pressure in acute asthma. *Respiration* 52(3):157–162, 1987.

60. Renston J, DiMarco A, Supinski S: Respiratory muscle rest using nasal BiPaP Ventilation in patients with stable severe COPD. *Chest* 105:1053–1060, 1990.

61. Brochard L, Mancebo J, Wysocki M, et al: Noninvasive ventilation for acute exacerbations of chronic obstructive pulmonary disease. *N Engl J Med* 333(13):817–22, 1995.

62. Hansen-Flaschen J, Cowen J, Raps E: Neuromuscular blockade in the Intensive Care Unit. More than we bargained for. *Am Rev Respir Dis* 147:234–236, 1993.

63. Nates J, Cooper D, Tuxen D: Acute weakness syn-

dromes in critically ill patients—a reappraisal. *Anaesth Intensive Care* 25(5):502–513, 1997.

64. Kramer N, Meyer T, Meharg J, Cece R, Hill N: Randomized prospective trial of noninvasive positive pressure ventilation in acute respiratory failure. *Am J Respir Crit Care Med* 151:1799–806, 1995.

65. Bott J, MP C, Conway J, Keilty S, Ward E: Randomized controlled trial of nasal ventilation in acute ventilatory failure due to chronic obstructive airways disease. *Lancet* 341:1555–1557, 1993.

66. Vitacca M, Rubini F, Foglio K, et al: Noninvasive modalities of positive pressure ventilation improve the outcome of acute exacerbations in COLD patients. *Intensive Care Med* 19:450–455, 1993.

67. Fernandez M, Blanch L, Valles J, et al: Pressure support ventilation via face mask in acute respiratory failure in hypercapnic COPD patients. *Intensive Care Med* 19:456–461, 1993.

68. Meduri G, Abou-Shala N, Fox R: Noninvasive face mask mechanical ventilation in patients with acute hypercapnic respiratory failure. *Chest* 100:445–454, 1991.

69. Mehta S, Gregory D, Woolard R, et al: Randomized prospective trial of bilevel versus continuous positive airway pressure in acute pulmonary edema. *Crit Care Med* 25(4):620–628, 1997.

70. Weng J, Smith D, Graybar G, Kirby R: Hypotension secondary to air trapping treated with expiratory flow retard. *Anesthesiology* 60:350–353, 1984.

71. Mathieu M, Tonneau M, Zarka D, Sartene R: Effects of positive end-expiratory pressure in severe acute asthma. *Crit Care Med* 15:1164, 1987.

72. Shivaram U, Miro A, Cast M, et al: Cardiopulmonary responses to continuous positive airway pressure in acute asthma. *J Crit Care* 8(2):87–92, 1993.

73. Chevrolet J, Jolliet P, Abajo B, et al: Nasal positive pressure ventilation in patients with acute respiratory failure. *Chest* 100:775–782, 1991.

74. Parkes S, Bersten A: Aerosol kinetics and bronchodilator efficacy during continuous positive airway pressure delivered by mask. *Thorax* 52(2):171–175, 1997.

75. Sato N, Matsuki A, Zsigmond E, Rabito S: Ketamine relaxes and airway smooth muscle contracted by endothelium. *Anesth Analg* 84(4):900–906, 1997.

76. Hirota N, Hashimoto Y, Sakai T, et al: In vivo spasmolytic effect of ketamine and adrenaline on histamine-induced airway constriction. Direct visualization method with a superfine fiber optic bronchoscope. *Acta Anaesthesiol Scand.* 42(2):184–188, 1998.

77. Betts E, Parkin C: Use of ketamine in an asthmatic child. *Anesth Analgesia. Curr Res* 50(3):420–421, 1971.

78. Fisher M: Ketamine hydrochloride in severe bronchospasm. *Anaesthesia* 32:771–772, 1977.

79. Hemming A, MacKenzie I, Finfer S: Response to ketamine in status asthamaticus resistant to maximal medical treatment. *Thorax* 49(1):90–91, 1994.

80. Sarma V: Use of ketamine in acute severe asthma. *Acta Anaesthesiol Scand* 36:106–107, 1992.

81. Houton J, Rose J, Daffy S, et al: Randomized double-blind placebo-control trial of intravenous ketamine in acute asthma. *Am Emerg Med* 27(2):170–175, 1996.

82. Rosseel P, Lauwers L, Bawte L: Halothane treatment in life threatening asthma. *Intensive Care Med* 11(5):241–246, 1985.

83. Bayliff C, Koch J, Fadier S: The use of halothane in the treatment of status asthmatics. *Drug Intell Clin Pharm* 19(4):307–309, 1985.

84. Saulnier F, Durocher A, Deturck R, et al: Respiratory and hemodynamic effects of halothane in status asthmaticus. *Intensive Care Med* 16:104–107, 1990.

85. Escheverria M, Gelb A, Wexler H, et al: Enflurane and halothane in status asthmaticus. *Chest* 89:152–154, 1986.

86. Johnston R, Nosworthy T, Frieser F, et al: Isoflurorane therapy for status asthmaticus in children and adults. *Chest* 97:698–701, 1990.

87. Tuxen D: Detrimental effects of positive end-expiratory pressure during controlled mechanical ventilation of patients with severe airflow obstruction. *Am Rev Respir Dis* 140:5–9, 1989.

88. Petty T: Oxygen and mechanical ventilation in status asthmaticus, in Eb W (ed): *Status Asthmaticus.* Baltimore, University Park Press, 1978, pp 285–292.

89. Connors A, McCaffree D, Gray B: Effect of inspiratory flow rate on gas exchange during mechanical ventilation. *Am Rev Respir Dis* 124:537–543, 1981.

90. Bone R, Burch S: Management of status asthmaticus. *Ann Allergy* 67:461–469, 1991.

91. Hall J, Wood L: Management of the critically ill asthmatic patient. *Med Clin N Am* 74(3):779–96, 1990.

92. Corbridge T, Hall J: The assessment and management of adults with status asthmaticus. *Respir Crit Care Med* 151(2):1296–1316, 1995.

93. Williams N, Crook J: The practical management of severe status asthmaticus. *Lancet* 108:1081–1083, 1968.

94. Lissac J, Labrousse J, Tenaillon A, et al: Traitment des asthmes aigus graves de l'adulte. *Ann Med Interne* 137(1):34–37, 1986.

95. Lukska A, Smith P, Coakley J, et al: Acute severe asthma treated by mechanical ventilation: 10 years' experience from a district general hospital. *Thorax* 41:459–463, 1986.

96. Otis A, McKerrow C, Bartlett R, et al: Mechanical factors in distribution of pulmonary ventilation. *J Appl Physiol* 8:427–443, 1956.

97. Bates J, Rossi A, Milic-Emili J: Analysis of the behavior of the respiratory system with constant inspiratory flow. *J Appl Physiol* 58(6):1840–1848, 1985.

98. Leatherman J, Ravenscraft S, Iber C, Davies S: Does measured auto-PEEP accurately reflect the degree of dynamic hyperinflation during mechanical ventilation of status asthma? *Am Rev Respir Dis* 147:877A, 1993.

99. Williams T, O'Hehir R, Czarny D, et al: Acute myopathy in severe asthma treated with intravenously administered corticosteroids. *Am Rev Respir Dis* 137:460–463, 1988.

100. Douglass J, Tuxen D, Horne M, et al: Acute myopathy following treatment of severe life threatening asthma (SLTA). *Am Rev Respir Dis* 141:A397, 1990.

101. DuBois D, Almon R: A possible role for glucocorticoids in denervation atrophy. *Muscle Nerve* 4:370–373, 1981.

102. McFadden E: Dosages of corticosteroids in asthma. *Am Rev Respir Dis* 147:1306–1310, 1993.

103. Lam K, Mow B, Chew L: The profile of ICU admissions for acute severe asthma in a general hospital. *Singapore Med J* 33(5):460–462, 1992.

104. Marquette C, Saulnier F, Leroy O, et al: Long-term prognosis of near-fatal asthma. *Am Rev Respir Dis* 146:76–81, 1992.

105. Mansel J, Stogner S, Petrini M, Norman J: Mechanical ventilation in patients with acute severe asthma. *Am J Med* 89:42–48, 1990.

106. Mabuchi N, Takasu H, Ito S, et al: Successful extracorporeal lung assist (ECLA) for a patient with severe asthma and cardiac arrest. *Clin Intensive Med* 2:292–294, 1991.

107. Tajimi K, Kasai T, Nakatani T, Kobayashi K: Extracorporeal lung assist (ECLA) for a patient with hypercapnia due to status asthmaticus. *Intensive Care Med* 14:588–589, 1988.

107a. Tassaux D, Jolliet P, Thouret JM, et al: Calibration of seven ICV ventilators for mechanical ventilation with helium-oxygen mixtures. *Am J Respir Crit Care Med* 160:22–32, 1999.

108. Luger T, Putensen C, Baum M, et al: Weaning an asthmatic with biphasic positive airway pressure together with continuous sufentanil administration. *Anaesthetist* 39:557–560, 1990.

109. Tokioka S, Saito S, Takahashi T, et al: Effectiveness of pressure support ventilation for mechanical ventilatory support in patients with status asthmaticus. *Acta Anaesthesiol Scand* 36:5–9, 1992.

110. Tokioka S, Saito S, Saeki S, et al: The effect of pressure support ventilation on auto-PEEP in a patient with status asthmaticus. *Chest* 101:285–286, 1992.

111. Cooper D, Cailes J, Scheinkestel C, Tuxen D: Acute severe asthma and acidosis—effect of bicarbonate on cardiac and respiratory function. *Anaesth Intensive Care* 22(2):212–213, 1993.

112. Rogers P, Schlichtig R, Miro A, Pinsky M: Auto-PEEP during CPR. An "occult cause of electromechanical dissociation. *Chest* 99:492–493, 1991.

113. Lange E, Chesnut R: Intracranial pressure and cerebral perfusion pressure in severe head injury. *New Horizons* 3:400–409, 1995.

114. Rosner M, Rosner S, Johnson A: Cerebral Perfusion Pressure; Management protocol and clinical results. *J Neurosurg* 83:948–962, 1995.

115. Petty T: Treat status asthmaticus three days before it occurs. *J Intensive Care Med* 4:135–136, 1989.

116. Maynard R, Hillman K: Intensive care admission as a predictor of asthma mortality. *Anaesth Intensive Care* 21(5):712, 1993.

117. Richards G, Kolbe J, Fenwick J, Rea H: Demographic characteristics of patients with severe life threatening asthma: comparison with asthma deaths. *Thorax* 48:1105–1109, 1993.

118. Seddon P, Heaf D: Long term outcome of ventilated asthmatics. *Arch Dis Childhood* 65:1324–1328, 1990.

119. *Asthma Management Handbook 1998.* Melbourne: National Asthma Campaign Ltd, 1998.

Chapter 14

SEDATION, PARALYSIS, AND ACUTE MYOPATHY

William A. Marinelli
James W. Leatherman

INTRODUCTION

Acute respiratory failure in status asthmaticus is associated with increased physiologic dead space due to alveolar overdistention. As a consequence of the large amount of wasted ventilation, most patients with asthma who require mechanical ventilation have significant acute respiratory acidosis at conventional levels of minute ventilation.[1] Efforts to correct hypercapnia by increasing minute ventilation expose the patient to greater risk of barotrauma and hypotension.[2] An alternative approach, termed *controlled hypoventilation*, seeks to minimize dynamic hyperinflation and allows Pa_{CO_2} to remain elevated.[3] This strategy is associated with very low mortality and a low incidence of ventilator-related complications; it is currently recommended by many experts.[4–6] Because acidemia markedly increases the drive to breathe, pharmacologic suppression of minute ventilation, either by use of intensive sedation by itself or by sedation and neuromuscular paralysis, assumes a crucial role during controlled hypoventilation. Serious complications may arise during mechanical ventilation of the severely ill asthma patient from either inadequate sedation or side effects of the drugs used to achieve muscle relaxation.[7–10] Achieving a degree of muscle relaxation that is both safe and effective may prove challenging.

In this chapter, we first review the principal drugs used for sedation, analgesia, and neuromuscular paralysis during mechanical ventilation. Second, the use of these agents in the context of mechanical ventilatory support of patients with status asthmaticus is addressed. Finally, the problem of diffuse muscle weakness due to acute myopathy is discussed, since diffuse muscle weakness is a common cause of morbidity affecting asthma patients who undergo mechanical ventilation and it is believed to be caused, in large part, by the agents used to achieve muscle relaxation.

SEDATION AND ANALGESIA

Various sedative and analgesic agents have been used to facilitate mechanical ventilation for patients with status asthmaticus. The most commonly used drugs are the benzodiazepines, propofol, and narcotics. Other agents, including barbiturates, ketamine, and general anesthetics have also been used but have little role in managing the critically ill patient with asthma.

Benzodiazepines

The benzodiazepines are the sedatives most often used in the ICU. The three benzodiazepines available as intravenous preparations suitable for use in the ICU are midazolam, lorazepam, and diazepam.

General Properties   The pharmacologic effects of benzodiazepines result from binding to a specific high-affinity "supramolecular receptor complex" located in the neuronal membrane. This complex also binds the inhibitory neurotransmitter gamma-aminobutyric acid (GABA) that results in the opening of chloride channels and hyperpolarization of the neuronal membrane.[11–14] Benzodiazepines act by potentiating the inhibitory influence of GABA; however, they do not affect its maximal achievable inhibitory effects[14,15] (Fig. 14-1). A number of other agents, including ethanol, barbiturates, propofol, and etomidate also act through this supramolecular receptor complex, thereby allowing synergistic effects when used with benzodiazepines. These agents can act independently of GABA to directly open chloride channels and may therefore lead to greater maximal neuronal inhibition than occurs with benzodiazepines.

All benzodiazepines have some degree of anxiolytic, sedative-hypnotic, anticonvulsant, and muscle relaxant properties. Of considerable relevance to the management of the mechanically ventilated patient, benzodiazepines also produce anterograde amnesia. However, they have no intrinsic analgesic properties. Two important physiologic effects of benzodiazepines that have particular relevance to the mechanically ventilated asthma patient are a reduction in respiratory drive and a decrease in blood pressure, which is mediated through a direct relaxant effect on vascular smooth muscle and by a reduction in sympathetic activity (see below).[11,16,17]

The concentration of any drug at its target tissue is determined by the factors that govern its absorption, distribution, and elimination. In the ICU, sedative agents are almost always given by intravenous injection, thereby insuring complete absorption. After intravenous injection of a benzodiazepine, initially there is a substantial decline from peak plasma levels due to redistribution from the central to the peripheral compartment; in time, there is a more gradual decline due to metabolic elimination.[12] When analyzing the overall decline in the plasma concentration of a drug, the α half-life refers to the rate of decline due to redistribution, and the β half-life to the rate of decline due to metabolism to inactive conjugated forms, and urinary excretion. Hepatic biotransformation via hepatic oxidation and glucuronide conjugation accounts for essentially all of the benzodiazepine clearance in humans; factors such as old age or liver disease have a much greater effect on oxidation than conjugation.[18–20]

One of the most important aspects of benzodiazepine pharmacokinetics is their lipid solubility. Although all of the benzodiazepines are lipophilic, there are clear differences between the various agents (Table 14-1).[12] High lipid solubility results in rapid entry of drug into the brain, resulting in a short onset of action after intravenous injection. In addition, the more lipophilic the drug, the greater the distribution into peripheral tissues and the shorter the duration of action after a bolus injection. Furthermore, with repeated doses or use of continuous infusions, accumulation of lipophilic drugs in peripheral tissues may result in a prolonged duration of action after sedation is discontinued, especially in obese patients.[12,18,20] Indeed, the duration of effect of a drug may depend more on its lipid solubility than on its metabolism. As such, classification of benzodiazepines as short-, intermediate-, or long-acting, based solely on metabolism and terminal β half-life of an individual drug may be misleading. Another pharmacologic property of benzodiazepines is their significant protein binding, accounting for the fact that patients with hypoalbuminemia or malnutrition may demonstrate an increased drug effect.[11,21]

Tolerance and dependence can occur with prolonged use of benzodiazepines. Tolerance is evidenced by a progressive increase in the dose

Figure 14-1
The effect of benzodiazepine on GABA-induced neuronal inhibition. (With permission, from Teboul and Chouinard[14])

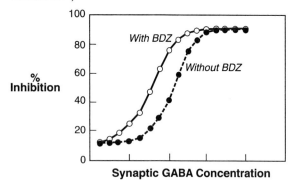

Table 14-1
Properties of Benzodiazepines

	Lipid solubility index (vs Diazepam)	Distribution, $t_{\frac{1}{2}} \alpha,^a$ min	Elimination, $t_{\frac{1}{2}} \beta,^a$ h	Equipotent dose	Active metabolites
Midazolam	1.54	1–2	1–4	2.5	Yes–limited
Lorazepam	0.48	3	10–15	1	No
Diazepam	1.00	1–2	20–80	5	Yes

^{a}NOTE: $t_{\frac{1}{2}} \alpha$ and β values reflect a single intravenous administration.
SOURCE: Adapted from Murray, et al[11]; Greenblatt[12]; Levine[15]; Pohlman.[29]

of drug required to produce the desired effect. Tolerance is less of a problem in status asthmaticus than in many other causes of respiratory failure, because most asthma patients can be extubated within a few days. However, patients who have more refractory airflow obstruction may develop a degree of tolerance to the sedative effects of benzodiazepines. The mechanisms of tolerance are not well understood, but may involve changes at the GABA-benzodiazepine receptor complex. In addition, patients who require prolonged sedation may occasionally develop clinically significant withdrawal reactions after abrupt discontinuation of benzodiazepines.[22,23]

Specific Benzodiazepines   *Midazolam* is a potent and rapid-acting benzodiazepine whose duration of action after a single dose is relatively short (usually less than 2 hours).[18] Its rapid onset of action and relatively short elimination half-life after bolus administration make it an attractive agent for short-term sedation[24] (Table 14-1). As packaged, the drug is water soluble in a buffered acidic medium (pH 3.5), but undergoes a transformation to a highly lipid soluble form at a pH above 4. Since midazolam does not require a preservative such as ethylene glycol, there is no phlebitis during intravenous administration.[12] Midazolam is highly lipophilic, accounting for its rapid onset and short duration of action after bolus injection (Table 14-1), and its peak effects are typically observed within 2 to 5 minutes of bolus administration. From a practical point of view, this means that boluses may be repeated every few minutes until

the desired effect is achieved, allowing rapid titration to the appropriate level of sedation. The major risk of repeated boluses of midazolam in the nonintubated patient is respiratory depression, however, respiratory depression is a desired effect in the mechanically ventilated asthma patient. Overly rapid and excessive dosing of midazolam may contibute to hypotension. As with other drugs used for sedation and analgesia in the ICU, hypotension is more likely in patients who are hypovolemic or elderly, and most often occurs at the time of intiation of mechanical ventilation (see below).[23,25]

The metabolism of midazolam occurs almost completely by hepatic biotransformation, including hydroxylation by hepatic microsomal enzymes and conjugation with glucuronic acid. Thus, the clearance of midazolam depends on hepatic perfusion and microsomal enzyme activity. After conjugation with glucuronic acid, its metabolites are excreted in the urine. Midazolam metabolites have significantly less affinity for receptor binding and central nervous system (CNS) uptake than does the parent compound.[12,26,27] Even in the absence of hepatic dysfunction or advanced age, prolonged recovery rates may be seen after midazolam infusions, presumably due to its high lipid solubility, which encourages accumulation in peripheral tissues.[23,28]

Lorazepam is a benzodiazepine whose pharmacokinetic properties differ in a number of important ways from those of midazolam. The onset of sedation after a single dose of intravenous lorazepam is somewhat slower than that of midazolam, most likely because lorazepam is less lipophilic and therefore enters the brain less readily[12,18] (see Table 14-1). Its lower lipid solubility also results in less redistribution into peripheral tissues, and the duration of action after a single dose is typically longer than with midazolam. Lorazepam is eliminated principally by glucuronide conjugation, and its elimination should therefore be less influenced by advanced age and liver disease than would the clearance of midazolam, but there are no clinical data to support this supposition. The major lorazepam metabolite does not appear to have pharmacologic activity.[12,18]

Due to its slower onset of action and longer elimination half-life, lorazepam may be less desirable than midazolam when short-term sedation and amnesia are desired, as with various ICU procedures. However, lorazepam is much less expensive than midazolam and is therefore a more attractive agent for long-term use in the ICU (Table 14-2). Long-term sedation with lorazepam may be achieved by the intravenous route through use of

intermittent boluses or a continuous infusion, or by the less expensive enteral route. During the initial period of management, it is much easier to titrate the dose of lorazepam using the intravenous route. However, once a stable dose of lorazepam has been reached, conversion to the same rate of drug administration given enterally is reasonable and represents an effective and inexpensive option for long-term sedation of the mechanically ventilated patient. Since most patients with status asthmaticus do not require prolonged mechanical ventilation, enteral lorazepam does not play a major role in this setting.

Diazepam was the first benzodiazepine used in the ICU when it became available for clinical use in 1961. Diazepam is not water-soluble and must be dissolved in an ethylene glycol preservative, which accounts for the thrombophlebitis that may occur with peripheral vein injection.[12] Continuous infusion of diazepam is impractical, because of the large volumes of fluid required for dilution.[24] Diazepam is an inexpensive agent with high lipid

Table 14-2

Comparison of Sedative and Narcotic Costs

	Dosage, mg/h	Avg. wholesale price pharmacy cost per day,[a] $	HCMC cost,[a] $
Midazolam	5	216	162
	10	432	322
	20	864	644
Lorazepam	2	132	21
	4	263	42
	8	526	85
Propofol	100 ($\sim$1.4 mg/kg/h)[b]	225	164
	200 ($\sim$2.9 mg/kg/h)	375	273
	400 ($\sim$5.7 mg/kg/h)	750	545
Fentanyl	0.05 mg	14	2
	0.10 mg	21	4
	0.20 mg	39	8
Morphine	5	5	3
	10	10	5
	20	20	9

[a]NOTE: Approximate costs as of 1/99.

[b]NOTE: For 70 kg individual.

ABBREVIATION: HCMC, Hennepin County Medical Center.

solubility, a large volume of distribution, and slow hepatic metabolism. It is similar to midazolam in that its high lipid solubility permits rapid transfer across the blood-brain barrier and its onset of action is seen at the end of an infusion[12,20] (see Table 14-1). This rapid onset of action allows for an almost immediate dose-response titration. When given as a single bolus, diazepam has a shorter duration of action than lorazepam, because of a greater degree of redistribution into peripheral tissues. However, diazepam has an active metabolite (N-desmethyldiazepam) that has a greater affinity for receptor binding than the parent compound, and both the parent compound and the active metabolite have a relatively long elimination half-life. Their rate of elimination may become especially prolonged in the elderly or in patients with hepatic dysfunction.[11] When large doses are given over time, the combination of accumulation in peripheral tissues and the relatively slow hepatic clearance may sometimes result in very long recovery times.

Several studies have compared the different benzodiazepines for sedation of the mechanically ventilated patient. These studies have shown that clinically relevant outcomes may not be reliably predicted with the above-mentioned differences in the pharmacologic properties of the various benzodiazepines. For example, Pohlman and colleagues examined continuous infusions of lorazepam and midazolam in a prospective randomized study of 20 medical ICU patients who received mechanical ventilatory support.[29] The infusion rate was adjusted to achieve and maintain a Ramsay sedation level of 2 to 3. One might predict that onset of sedation would be faster with midazolam and time to recovery would be longer with lorazepam. However, the time to achieve adequate sedation was not statistically different between the lorazepam and midazolam groups. Furthermore, the time to recovery was similar after discontinuation of the two agents, with enormous variability among patients (Fig. 14-2). Of interest, three of the six midazolam-treated patients who ultimately returned to baseline mental status required more than 24 hours for recovery after discontinuation of midazolam. In contrast, all seven patients in

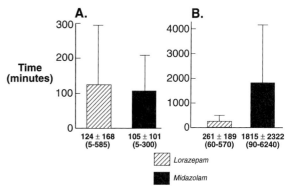

FIGURE 14-2
A. *Time to achieve sedation.* **B.** *Time to return to baseline mental status (mean ± 1 SD). Numbers in parentheses represent the range of values. No significant difference between lorazepam and midazolam with regard to time to achieve sedation and time to return to baseline mental status. (With permission, from Pohlman, et al[29])*

the lorazepam-treated group who regained their baseline mental status recovered in less than 12 hours. The mean initial sedative infusion rate was 0.06 mg/kg per hour for lorazepam and 0.15 mg/kg per hour for midazolam.[29] These doses were higher than what had often been recommended in earlier literature. Because the infusion rates required were often high, the volume of fluid needed to deliver benzodiazepines by continuous infusion was often large (up to 3.6 L per day for midazolam and 2.4 L per day for lorazepam). No adverse outcomes, including hemodynamic impairment, were identified in these study patients. The results of this study suggest that midazolam has no clinical advantage over lorazepam for continuous sedation during mechanical ventilation. Lorazepam achieves the same level of sedation as midazolam at much less cost. Therefore, lorazepam is preferable to midazolam for continuous intravenous sedation of the mechanically ventilated patient.

A second study compared the use of lorazepam and midazolam over 8 hours in 95 mechanically ventilated patients with right heart catheters.[30] Lorazepam was given by intermittent intravenous injection and midazolam by continuous infusion. Both drug regimens were well tolerated and achieved effective sedation. Furthermore, hemodynamic and oxygen delivery parameters were similarly affected by both treatment regimens, and limited changes were demonstrated in the hemodynamic and oxygen delivery parameters measured. Similar to the findings of Pohlman and colleagues,[29] the dose required to achieve adequate sedation was significantly greater for midazolam than for lorazepam.

A number of different studies have compared midazolam and diazepam as sedative agents. In a recent review, Ariano and colleagues analyzed eight trials that reported data on rate of recovery from short-term sedation.[31] Of interest, most of these studies found no significant differences in the sedative recovery rate and when a difference was found, it often favored diazepam. Thus, as was suggested by the above-cited study,[29] the sedative recovery rates of benzodiazepines may not parallel their elimination half-lives. Half-life data are readily available, but unfortunately do not give a complete picture of the pharmacodynamic actions of benzodiazepines. As mentioned earlier, lipophilicity is a crucial factor in time to recovery, but recovery is also influenced by the size of the dose, blood versus central nervous system concentration, and receptor site tolerance or adaptation.

Propofol

Propofol, an ultrashort-acting alkylphenol, is a potent and rapidly acting intravenous sedative with a short duration of effect after discontinuation. It has been available for use in the United States since 1993.[32] Despite its high cost, propofol has become a very popular agent for short-term sedation of the intubated patient (Table 14-2). In addition to its sedative effects, propofol has significant hypnotic, anxiolytic, and amnestic effects when administered in subanesthetic doses. At higher doses, propofol is an effective anesthetic and is commonly used in the operating room. Of possible relevance to the management of patients with airflow obstruction, propofol has been shown to have bronchodilator properties in intubated patients with COPD.[33]

Although the mechanism of propofol action has not been fully defined, it appears to potentiate GABA-mediated inhibitory effects.[34,35] Propofol has been shown to be highly protein bound and its marked lipophilicity results in a large volume of distribution.[32] In one study, propofol was rapidly cleared, and serum levels declined by approximately 50% only 10 minutes after discontinuation of infusion.[22,36] This markedly high clearance rate appeared to exceed hepatic blood flow, suggesting extrahepatic mechanisms.[32,37] The clearance of propofol was not significantly changed in patients with advanced renal or hepatic disease. However, clearance may be reduced in elderly patients.[32]

Serious adverse effects of propofol infusions are relatively uncommon. However, transient hypotension has been reported in up to 20% to 30% of ICU patients who receive it.[32] Hypotension appears to be significantly more common after a large bolus injection of propofol, especially in patients who have underlying hypovolemia, vasodilation, or significant myocardial dysfunction. Propofol may result in bradycardia.[32,38] A reduction or discontinuation of the propofol infusion usually results in a rapid return of the heart rate to baseline.

The lipid emulsion commercially used to deliver propofol has been associated with several potential complications. Hypertriglyceridemia may be seen, particularly in patients prediposed to hypertriglyceridemia, including diabetics.[32,39] When high doses are used, problems associated with overfeeding may occur; the lipid-related calories provided by propofol infusions should be considered when prescribing nutritional support. Lastly, the lipid emulsion supports rapid microbial growth at room temperature and has been associated with bacteremia, dictating the need for strict aseptic technique.[40]

Of greatest concern, propofol has been associated with lethal complications in pediatric patients. Fatal cases of propofol toxicity have been associated with unexplained severe lactic acidosis, rhabdomyolysis, and multisystem organ failure.[41-45] Uniformly, affected children had received prolonged infusions of propofol at very high doses. Although large doses of propofol are used to safely provide anesthesia for brief periods, each of the patients who died as a result of propofol had received high-dose infusion for at least 30 hours.[41–45] At this time, it is not clear whether these fatalities were related to a greater inherent susceptibility of children to the toxic effects of propofol, or to the use of much higher doses (on a per-kg basis) in children than in adults. Some of the fatalities were adolescents who may have been physiologically similar to adults. Lethal toxicity from propofol could be a consequence of prolonged infusion at high doses rather than a special sensitivity in children. Based on the above concerns, we currently limit the infusion rate of propofol to 80 μg/kg per minute (approximately 5 mg/kg per hour) when it is used for more than a few hours.

Several investigators have compared propofol and midazolam as sedative agents during mechanical ventilation.[46–50] In general, these studies demonstrated that both drugs produced reliable sedation with few adverse effects, including a low incidence of hypotension that was similar for both agents. One important difference found between propofol and midazolam was that sedation with propofol was associated with a much more rapid wake-up time and a significantly shorter time to extubation.[46–48] Recovery from propofol was always rapid; failure to awaken after 2 hours of discontinuation suggests an alternative reason for reduced level of consciousness.[47] In contrast, the time to awaken from midazolam was often quite prolonged, depending in part on duration of sedation. For example, in one study, the average time to extubation after cessation of a midazolam infusion was 14 hours when sedation had been maintained for 1 to 7 days, and 37 hours when patients had been sedated for more than 1 week.[48]

Both propofol and midazolam are costly, but at equally effective doses propofol is somewhat more expensive. However, when the cost of delayed extubation was considered, economic analysis in some studies favored propofol.[46,48] There have been no similar studies comparing propofol and lorazepam. Lorazepam may also be associated with prolonged recovery times,[29] but it is much less expensive than either midazolam or propofol (see Table 14-2). Lorazepam may enjoy a cost

advantage over propofol, even when the cost of delayed extubation is considered.

Recently, the combination of propofol and midazolam has been compared with the use of either agent alone.[51] This prospective randomized study of patients who had undergone coronary bypass grafting found that use of the combined regimen permitted a significant reduction in the maintenance dose of both agents, yielding a cost savings of 28% for midazolam and 68% for propofol. The patients who received synergistic sedation also had greater hemodynamic stability (Fig. 14-3). The effectiveness of sedation was similar in all three groups studied, but the propofol and combination groups demonstrated more rapid awakening and earlier extubation than did patients who received midazolam by itself.[51]

Narcotics

Narcotics are the most effective analgesic agents available for use in the ICU. A number of different narcotics are manufactured for intravenous use, including both pure agonists and agonist-antagonists. The two narcotic agents most often used in the ICU are morphine and fentanyl.

General Properties   In addition to their potent analgesic properties, narcotics also have sedative effects. However, their limited amnestic effects may be associated with frequent recall when these agents are used alone.[20,52,53] As a rule, when narcotics are given to critically ill patients undergoing mechanical ventilation, they should be used in combination with drugs that have potent sedative-hypnotic and amnestic properties, such as benzodiazepines or propofol.

Narcotics exert their pharmacologic effects by binding to at least three classes of receptors that are located in both the CNS and peripheral tissue.[11] Pure agonists act primarily at the mu (μ) receptor, which is primarily responsible for pain relief and respiratory depression. Depression of respiratory drive, including significant blunting of hypercapnic and hypoxic response curves, is a notable property of all narcotic agents.[54,55] The effect on respiration by narcotics is potentiated by use of

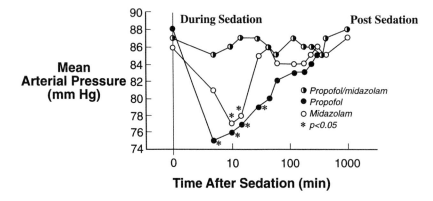

FIGURE 14-3
Effect of different sedative regimens on blood pressure of patients who had undergone coronary artery bypass surgery. Through combined use of lower doses of midazolam and propofol, acceptable sedation was achieved with less effect upon hemodynamics. (With permission, from Carrasco et al[51])

benzodiazepines or propofol. Through their ability to reduce respiratory drive, narcotics may be particulary helpful when controlled hypoventilation with permissive hypercapnia is used in patients with severe asthma receiving mechanical ventilation. Combining the analgesic and respiratory depressant effects of narcotics with the sedative-hypnotic, amnestic, and respiratory depressant properties of either a benzodiazepine or propofol offers obvious benefits.

The principal adverse effects of narcotic agents in the intubated asthma patient include hypotension, depression of gastrointestinal motility, and prolonged sedative and respiratory depressant effects.[11,20,54] The mechanism of narcotic-related hypotension is related to both a direct vasodilatory effect on arterial and venous smooth muscle, and an indirect reduction in sympathetic output (see below).[20,56] Morphine and meperidine administration may also result in histamine release, another potential cause of hypotension.[11,57] Fentanyl has less direct cardiovascular effects than morphine, but may nonetheless produce hypotension through indirect mechanisms. As is the case with benzodiazepines and propofol, the hemodynamic effect of narcotics is accentuated in patients who are hypovolemic or elderly. Furthermore, the hypotensive effects of narcotics are synergistic with those of benzodiazepines and propofol, increasing the risk of hypotension with co-administration.[18] Depression of gastrointestinal motility due to narcotics may interfere with successful enteral feeding. Lack of adequate nutrition is likely not of

great importance in patients who can be extubated within a few days, but may become an important issue when more prolonged ventilatory support is required. Lastly, an unusual syndrome of reduced chest wall compliance has been reported after administration of high doses of intravenous fentanyl in elderly patients.[20]

As with the benzodiazepines, tolerance to the effects of narcotics and the appearence of withdrawal symptoms after their discontinuation are problems that must be addressed when prolonged use is required.[18,22] Tolerance generally can be overcome by increasing the dose of narcotic. Since the narcotics most often used in the ICU are very inexpensive, the economic impact of tolerance is minimal (Table 14-2).

A number of different factors besides tolerance can influence the degree or duration of opioid effect, including age, protein binding, obesity, and hepatic and renal function. The important caveat from a clinical standpoint is that many different factors may act to increase or decrease the intensity and duration of opioid effect. As with other drugs used to facilitate mechanical ventilation, dosing should be targeted to the desired clinical response rather than to a predetermined infusion rate. Even when a desired dose is achieved, the latter must be re-evaluated and adjusted accordingly as the clinical course evolves.

Specific Narcotics *Morphine* and *fentanyl* are the narcotic agents most widely used in the ICU.[24] These two agents have many similar pharmaco-

Table 14-3
Properties of Narcotics

	Lipid solubility	Distribution, $t_{\frac{1}{2}} \alpha,^a$ min	Elimination, $t_{\frac{1}{2}} \beta,^a$ h	Equipotent dose	Active metabolites
Morphine	Low	4–11	2–5	10	Yes
Fentanyl	High	10	2–4	0.05–0.1	No

^{a}NOTE: $t_{\frac{1}{2}} \alpha$ and β values reflect a single intravenous administration.
SOURCE: Adapted from Murray, et al[11]; Levine[15]; Mirski.[34]

logic effects, but differ greatly with regard to their lipid solubility. Morphine is distributed rapidly after intravenous injection, but is much less lipid soluble than fentanyl; therefore it crosses the blood-brain barrier less readily and its onset of action is slower than that of fentanyl (Table 14-3). Because of its lower lipid solubility, the duration of effect appears to be determined more by the rate of hepatic metabolism than by distribution into peripheral tissues. However, hepatic metabolism of morphine through glucuronic acid conjugation ultimately generates a metabolite that is significantly more potent than the parent compound, morphine-6-glucuronide. This active metabolite is renally excreted and has a markedly prolonged elimination half-life in patients with abnormal renal function.[58] Thus, the use of morphine should be avoided in patients with compromised renal function. Lastly, the ability of morphine to increase the severity of bronchospasm via histamine release offers a theoretical argument against its use in the critically ill asthma patient; however, the clinical significance of this observation has not been clarified.

Fentanyl is a highly potent narcotic, with approximately 100 times the potency of morphine[54] (Table 14-3). Fentanyl is 7000 times as lipophilic as morphine, allowing rapid CNS penetration and onset of action within minutes. Rapid redistribution into the peripheral tissues results in a short duration of action. As with other highly lipid-soluble drugs (e.g., midazolam), prolonged infusions may be associated with significant tissue accumulations and extended clinical effects, especially in obese individuals.[11] The pharmacologic

properties of fentanyl and its cardiovascular tolerance profile make this agent useful for short-term use in the ICU for percutaneous or endoscopic procedures. Fentanyl is also given as a continuous infusion to patients who require prolonged mechanical ventilation, usually in combination with a benzodiazepine or propofol. Like morphine, fentanyl is quite inexpensive, and the economic impact of long-term use of this agent is minimal (see Table 14-2). It should be noted that tissue accumulation can occur, which leads to unwanted prolongation of intubation due to persistent sedation after the drug is discontinued; however, this may be partly offset by the development of tolerance and may be dealt with, in part, by appropriate dose reduction during prolonged infusions. Therefore, fentanyl appears to be a reasonable choice for longer-term sedation and analgesia.

Alfentanil and *sufentanil* are derivatives of fentanyl that are used primarily in the operating-room setting, and are rarely used in the ICU.[54] Alfentanil is less potent than fentanyl, but has a more rapid onset and a shorter duration of action. Sufentanil also has a rapid onset of action and is significantly more potent than fentanyl, requiring careful dose determination and clinical assessment. Both of these derivatives are significantly more expensive than fentanyl and appear to offer few advantages compared to fentanyl for use in the ICU.

Meperidine is an effective narcotic for intermittent use. However, hepatic metabolism generates normeperidine, a metabolite with potent CNS stimulatory effects. Prolonged use of meperidine, or use in patients with renal failure, may result in toxicity and may induce seizures.[54,59] In addition, meperidine also has vagolytic and histamine-releasing properties that may cause tachycardia and hypotension.[20] Thus, meperidine would not be an ideal agent to use in the management of the patient with severe asthma.

Miscellaneous Agents

Ketamine is a dissociative anesthetic with unique properties.[60] After administration of ketamine, patients appear to be in a cataleptic state with their eyes open, but will not have recall of events that occur during anesthesia. Ketamine crosses the blood-brain barrier rapidly and reaches a peak effect within 1 minute. It does not have significant effects on respiratory drive and has bronchodilator properties, owing largely to catecholamine release. This release results in an increase in blood pressure, heart rate, and cardiac output. Ketamine has been used in the treatment of refractory status asthmaticus, but it is not clear that patients who are receiving maximal inhaled bronchodilator therapy would derive additional benefit from ketamine.[61] Side effects include hallucination and delirium, although the incidence of the latter may be mitigated by concomitant use of benzodiazepines. Other potential side effects include an increase in salivation and airway secretions and an increase in cerebral blood flow, cerebral metabolism, and intracranial pressure. It is contraindicated in patients with psychiatric disorders, ischemic heart disease, or intracranial pathology that may increase in severity owing to an increase in intracranial pressure. Ketamine would seem to have a minimal role in the overall treatment of life-threatening asthma, and is not a good choice for continuous sedation of the mechanically ventilated asthma patient.

Barbiturates have CNS effects that progress from sedation to hypnosis to anesthesia. They are effective at suppressing seizure foci and reducing intracranial pressure, issues that are rarely of concern in the mechanically ventilated asthma patient. Barbiturates have profound effects on both respiration and cardiovascular function. They cause central respiratory depression, which is a potentially desirable effect when controlled hypoventilation is used. However, they also have marked effects on blood pressure, especially when cardiac function or fluid status is marginal. Because they are highly lipophilic, they may accumulate in tissues, resulting in marked prolongation in half-life. Although barbiturates have been used in the management of patients with severe asthma, they offer no advantage over the use of benzodiazepines, narcotics, or propofol for sedation during mechanical ventilation and are not recommended.

Numerous anecdotal reports have described a benefit from the use of inhalational anesthetics in severe refractory asthma.[62–66] The purpose of using these anesthetics was not sedation, but rather to achieve additional bronchodilation. Many of the inhalational anesthetics have bronchodilator properties; *halothane* and *isoflurane* are the agents used most often in severe asthma. The bronchodilator effects of isoflurane are similar to those of halothane, but it is less arrhythmogenic in the setting of respiratory acidosis, which is typical of severe asthma, and thus is a better choice. However, isoflurane may cause hypotension due to arterial and venous dilation, but this effect can usually be counteracted by increased fluid administration. When used by experienced personnel, isoflurane is reasonably safe and can be administered in the ICU setting, most conveniently through ventilators that permit direct attachment of a vaporizer.[65] An important question is whether such an approach is necessary. Although the actual benefit derived from use of general anesthetics is difficult to determine from data in many published reports, at least one small study showed a convincing reduction in airway resistance and degree of dynamic hyperinflation when isoflurane was administered to asthma patients who were already receiving high doses of inhaled β_2 agonists.[66] Nonetheless, while general anesthetics may acutely lower airway pressures and improve arterial blood gases, they have no effect on the ultimate resolution of status asthmaticus. Given the generally good patient tolerance of hypercapnia, and the excellent outcomes associated with the use of a strategy of controlled hypoventilation, inhalational anesthetics would seem to have a minimal role in the management of the intubated asthma patient. Low-dose isoflurane has also been used for the purpose of achieving long-term sedation in the ICU,[67] but does not appear to offer any advantages when compared to more conventional approaches.

NEUROMUSCULAR PARALYSIS

Neuromuscular paralysis is sometimes useful in managing the critically ill patient with asthma. When administered by individuals who are highly skilled in airway management, the use of a short-acting neuromuscular blocking agent (NMBA) may help facilitate endotracheal intubation using a rapid-sequence approach. Furthermore, the addition of an NMBA may be necessary for mechanically ventilated asthma patients in whom adequate muscle relaxation is not achieved with a sedative-narcotic regimen. Because NMBAs lack any sedative or analgesic properties, they must only be used with the co-administration of a sufficient dose of an amnestic sedative-hypnotic agent to prevent awareness. Despite some benefits of neuromuscular paralysis in the management of the critically ill asthma patient, the potential role for NMBAs in the development of neuromuscular weakness syndromes has tempered enthusiasm for their routine use.[68–71]

Transmission at the neuromuscular junction (NMJ) involves binding of the acetylcholine released from the presynaptic terminal to a postsynaptic nicotinic receptor, a complex composed of five subunits.[69,71,72] The binding of acetylcholine to its receptor alters the permeability of the postsynaptic striated muscle membrane, leading to depolarization. After its binding to the receptor, acetylcholine is rapidly degraded by acetylcholinesterase, an enzyme present within the junctional space. On the basis of their action at the NMJ, NMBAs are divided into two groups, depolarizing and nondepolarizing drugs. Depolarizing drugs directly bind to the NMJ, resulting in sustained depolarization and neuromuscular blockade. In contrast, nondepolarizing agents compete with acetylcholine for binding to the receptor.

Acetylcholine receptors are normally concentrated at the NMJ. However, disease states characterized by impaired muscle fiber innervation exhibit the presence of multiple fetal-subtype receptors diffusely distributed across the striated muscular surface.[69,73] These include cerebral vascular accidents, spinal cord trauma, poliomyelitis, severe burns, extensive muscle trauma, crush injuries, and prolonged immobilization. Fetal-subtype receptors appear to be more sensitive to depolarizing agents, as evidenced by reports of life-threatening hyperkalemia after succinylcholine administration in some patients with the above-mentioned disease states. In addition, the fetal-variant receptors exhibit a greater resistance to the competitive effects of nondepolarizing agents. Furthermore, the prolonged use of NMBAs appears to result in denervation-like changes with up-regulation in the number of acetylcholine receptors. Dodson and colleagues examined autopsy specimens of the rectus abdominis muscle in patients who received NMBAs prior to death and found a correlation between the density of nicotinic cholinergic receptors and the average daily vecuronium dose.[74] This observation offers a potential mechanism for the progressive increase in NMBA dose requirements seen in some patients receiving long-term neuromuscular blockade. Of practical importance, succinylcholine should not be used in patients who have recently received long-term therapy with a nondepolarizing agent because of the potential for life-threatening hyperkalemia secondary to an acquired denervation-like syndrome.[75]

Depolarizing Agents

Succinylcholine, composed of two acetylcholine molecules, is the only depolarizing agent available for clinical use[69,71,72] (Table 14-4). After an intravenous dose of 1.0 to1.5 mg/kg, succinylcholine results in rapid (30 to 90 second) paralysis preceded by muscle fasciculations from the initial depolarization of the NMJ (Table 14-4). Paralysis occurs after the prolonged depolarization and neuromuscular

Table 14-4

Neuromuscular Blocking Agents

	Loading dose, mg/kg	Onset, min	Duration, min	Infusion, μg/kg/min
Succinylcholine	1–1.5	≤1.5	4–10	not used
Vecuronium	0.08–0.1	2–3	20–45	0.8–1.2
Atracurium	0.4–0.6	2–3	20–40	4–12
Pancuronium	0.06–0.1	2–3	45–100[a]	0.3–0.5

[a]NOTE: Variable dependent on renal funciton.

SOURCE: Adapted from Coursin and Prielipp[69]; Isenstein[70]; Shapiro[75]; Aguilera.[91]

blockade, leaving the receptor refractory and un-excitable. Rapid redistribution and metabolism by pseudocholinesterase results in a short duration of action (4 to 10 minutes). These characteristics have made succinylcholine a commonly used agent for rapid-sequence intubation.

The duration of neuromuscular blockade by succinylcholine may be prolonged in patients with reduced levels of plasma pseudocholinesterase, which is an enzyme synthesized by the liver. Reduction in pseudocholinesterase levels may be found in patients with malnutrition, advanced liver disease, myxedema, chronic renal failure, a rare homozygous recessive trait for pseudocholinesterase synthesis, and during pregnancy.[69,71,72] Furthermore, several drugs may inhibit pseudocholinesterases, including anticholinesterases, cytotoxic drugs, and monoamine oxidase inhibitors. Succinylcholine has been associated with other potentially serious complications. As described above, one of the most notable of these complications is the possibility of life-threatening hyperkalemia in patients with denervation syndromes secondary to an exaggerated release of intracellular potassium.[69,70,72] In contrast, the serum potassium concentration increases by no more than 0.5 to1.0 mEq/L in patients without a pre-existing denervation syndrome. After muscarinic receptor binding, succinylcholine may result in either tachycardia or bradycardia, suggesting the use of an alternative agent in patients with cardiac dysrrhythmias. Succinylcholine has also been associated with elevation in intraocular, intragastric, and intracranial

pressures, and is not recommended in clinical situations where this would likely be important. Lastly, succinylcholine has been associated rarely with the development of malignant hyperthermia.[69,70]

Nondepolarizing Agents

Nondepolarizing agents bring about neuromuscular blockade by competively blocking the NMJ.[69] Because of this mechanism of action, they may be reversed with the use of acetylcholinesterase inhibitors, including neostigmine, physostigmine, and edrophonium.[70,76] Nondepolarizing agents are derived from either aminosteroid or benzylisoquinoline compounds, and their duration of neuromuscular blockade may be classified as short-, intermediate-, or long-acting.[69,71,72] Typically, short-acting agents are used for brief procedures or interventions, while intermediate- and long-acting agents are reserved for intermittent or continuous dosing in the ICU. The recommended dosages, onset, and duration of action of the nondepolarizing agents most commonly used in the ICU are included in Table 14-4.

Short-acting nondepolarizing agents available for use in the mechanically ventilated asthmatic include rocuronium and mivacurium.[70,71] *Rocuronium* is a recently approved aminosteroid-derived NMBA with a rapid onset and short duration of action when administered in low doses, and has an intermediate-acting profile when administered in higher doses. *Mivacurium* is a costly short-acting agent whose expense likely precludes it from long-term use in the ICU.

Intermediate-acting nondepolarizing agents include vecuronium, atracurium, and cisatracurium.[69,71,72] *Vecuronium* is an aminosteroid-derived agent that is structurally related to pancuronium. However, vecuronium lacks the vagolytic effects commonly seen with pancuronium and does not result in either tachycardia or hemodynamic instability. Less than 50% of vecuronium undergoes hepatic metabolism, thus generating three active metabolites that are excreted in the urine.[77] The remaining vecuronium is eliminated in the bile and urine without metabolic change. Due to the accumulation of active metabolites, the use of vecuronium in patients with renal failure may result in prolonged paralysis after the drug is discontinued.[78] Some studies also suggest a prolongation of paralysis in the setting of hepatic disease. Recently published task-force recommendations on neuromuscular blockade advocated use of vecuronium for patients with either cardiac disease or hemodynamic instability.[75]

Atracurium is an intermediate-acting benzyl-isoqiunolinium-derived agent that undergoes a nonenzymatic breakdown by Hoffman elimination into nonactive metabolites.[69,71,72] Its duration of effect is unaffected by either liver or kidney failure and it may be particularly well suited for patients who have either hepatic or renal disease. One of the metabolites of atracurium, laudanosine, is a CNS stimulant that is excreted in the urine and has been associated with seizures in animal models. However, there have been no well-documented cases of laudanosine toxicity in humans, and it appears unlikely that toxic concentrations of laudanosine are achieved during clinical use of atracurium.[69,71,79] Similar to vecuronium, atracurium has minimal direct hemodynamic effect. Rapid bolus injection of atracurium has been associated with histamine release, but this may be avoided by slow administration.[69,80] *Cisatracurium* is a derivative of atracurium with very similar properties. The principal theoretical benefits of cisatracurium compared with atracurium are that it results in lower levels of laudanosine[81] and less histamine release.

Long-acting NMBAs include d-tubocurarine, pancuronium, doxacurium, metocurine, and pipecuronium.[69,71] Although *d-tubocurarine* has the longest history of use, having been discovered in poisoned arrow tips used by native Indian tribes of South America in the sixteenth century, this benzylisoquinolinium-derived long-acting NMBA is no longer used clinically because newer agents have better safety profiles.

Pancuronium is a long-acting aminosteroid agent and is the least expensive NMBA available for use in the ICU. Pancuronium has vagolytic effects and may also block the reuptake of norepinepherine by adrenergic nerves, resulting in tachycardia and hypertension. Hemodynamic effects of pancuronium can be mitigated by slow injection and are not usually a concern when the drug is given by continuous infusion. It may also result in histamine release from mast cell degranulation. The histamine-releasing properties of pancuronium could potentially increase airway constriction, but the clinical relevance of this theoretical disadvantage is not clear. Like all aminosteroid agents, pancuronium is metabolized in the liver, resulting in the potential for prolonged effect in patients with liver disease. The active metabolites of pancuronium are excreted in the urine, prolonging the effect in patients with renal insufficiency.[69,71,72] Despite these concerns, pancuronium is the least expensive of the NMBAs that are commonly used in the ICU and it has been recommended as the preferred agent for most critically ill patients.[75]

Doxacurium is a long-acting NMBA derived from benzylisoquinolinium and has no adverse cardiovascular effects.[82] It is excreted renally after limited metabolism. Prolongation of its effect has been reported in patients with significant hepatic or renal impairment. *Metocurine* is a long-acting derivative of tubocurarine with significantly less histamine release and ganglionic blockade than tubocurarine, which is renally excreted in an active form. Although this agent has been available for years, it is rarely used in the ICU. *Pipecuronium* is a long-acting NMBA without adverse cardiovascular or histamine-releasing effects. Experience with pipecuronium in the ICU is limited.

Monitoring Neuromuscular Blockade

The goal of neuromuscular paralysis should be defined for each patient, since a complete blockade is usually not required. In the mechanically ventilated asthma patient, the principal goals of paralysis are to 1) limit the degree of hyperinflation by controlling the respiratory rate and 2) eliminate vigorous respiratory efforts or patient-ventilator asynchrony despite sedation and analgesia. Monitoring the degree of neuromuscular blockade involves assessing both clinical status and the response of the patient to electrical stimulation.[83,84]

The degree of paralysis should be clinically monitored by noting the presence of active respiratory efforts and whether the patient responds to physical stimuli such as repositioning and oropharyngeal or endotracheal suctioning. The response to electrical stimulation may be an important component in monitoring the degree of blockade.[70,75,83] In part because of its accessibility during surgery, the visible twitch of the adductor pollicus muscle of the thumb is the most common site for monitoring the response to electrical stimulation.

The most frequently used technique of electrical stimulation is a series of four electrical stimuli at 0.5-second intervals, termed a *train-of-four*.[70,83] One recommended protocol is to administer an intermediate- or long-acting NMBA with intermittent boluses while following the response to electrical stimulation at frequent intervals.[83] Initially, the train-of-four response is monitored every 20 to 30 minutes and then reduced to every 8 to 12 hours after a steady-state condition has been achieved. With this approach, subsequent boluses of NMBAs should not be administered unless at least one muscle twitch appears. When an NMBA is given by continuous infusion, the infusion is titrated to the appearance of at least 1 to 2 twitches. Importantly, experience with NMBAs has shown that the degree of neuromuscular blockade varies significantly among different muscle groups. For example, the diaphragm and laryngeal muscles appear more resistant to neuromuscular blockade than the adductor pollicis muscle.[85,86] Small muscle groups (e.g., hand and extraocular muscles) recover neuromuscular function earlier than respiratory muscles.[72] Thus, a comprehensive assessment of clinical parameters is necessary, especially when extubation is considered.

The routine use of train-of-four monitoring during the administration of NMBAs has been recommended by a recent critical-care task force.[75] However, surveys of the prevalence of train-of-four monitoring reveal a pattern of infrequent use, with only 4% of ICUs in the in the United States. and 8% of ICUs in the United Kingdom regularly using this assessment.[87,88] Recently, two prospective studies examined whether the use of train-of-four monitoring offered a benefit compared with standard clinical assessment during the use of NMBAs. In a prospective randomized study, the regular use of train-of-four monitoring was associated with a significant reduction in the total cumulative dose of vecuronium and a more rapid recovery of neuromuscular function, as compared with clinical assessment only.[77] In this study, the clinical assessment group was determined to have an adequate dose of vecuronium when the patient was observed to be "no longer moving or breathing spontaneously." In contrast, another prospective nonrandomized study compared regular train-of-four monitoring with clinical assessment in patients receiving atracurium.[89] This study did not demonstrate a significant difference in the dose of atracurium delivered or the neuromuscular recovery time between the two groups of patients. However, patients in the clinical assessment group were evaluated at least every 12 hours when reducing the dose of atracurium until patient movement was identified, after which the dose was increased until the patient was "slightly more paralyzed."[89] Although these studies had different designs, both their results suggested a benefit was derived from the regular use of either a train-of-four assessment or reduction of the dose of NMBA until a return in neuromuscular function was identified. Thus, assessment after a reduction or removal of neuromuscular blockade, termed a *drug holiday*, is recommended to allow neurologic examination and assessment of the adequacy of concomitant sedation and analgesia.[75]

Unfortunately, there are a number of complications associated with neuromuscular paralysis.[73] Obviously, the paralyzed patient is at grave risk should accidental extubation or ventilator disconnection/malfunction occur and continuous observation is required to avoid these possible accidents. Although less common during the usual short-term use of NMBAs, mechanically ventilated asthma patients are also at greater risk for skin breakdown and pressure sores, corneal ulceration, nerve compression syndromes, thromboembolic disease, and nosocomial pneumonia. Potential adverse cardiovascular effects are most common with pancuronium and are less common with vecuronium or atracurium. The relationship of neuromuscular paralysis to the development of neuromuscular weakness syndromes is reviewed below. As mentioned previously, inadequate sedation during neuromuscular blockade may result in an extremely frightening experience for the patient and must be prevented.

Numerous drugs may potentiate the effects of NMBAs, including halogenated anesthetics, lidocaine, aminoglycosides, clindamycin, vancomycin, procainamide, bretylium, calcium-channel blockers, β blockers, dantrolene, diuetics, lithium, and cyclosporine.[72,73,75] Electrolyte disorders may also potentiate the effect of NMBAs, particularly in the presence of hypermagnesemia, hypokalemia, hypocalcemia, and hyponatremia.[72,90] Finally, acidosis may enhance the effects of NMBAs.[91] Thus, a lower dose of NMBA may be required in the mechanically ventilated asthma patient with severe respiratory acidosis.

SEDATION AND PARALYSIS IN STATUS ASTHMATICUS

Mechanical ventilation of the patient with severe asthma presents some special issues that must be taken into account when devising a strategy for sedation and paralysis. To minimize serious adverse effects of extreme pulmonary hyperinflation, it is usually necessary to limit minute ventilation and to accept the presence of hypercapnia.[2-6] The often profound acute respiratory acidosis of severe asthma serves as a potent stimulus for respiration, and large doses of sedatives may be required to

keep the patient sufficiently relaxed and minute ventilation at a safe level. Unfortunately, when large doses of benzodiazepines, narcotics, or propofol are used, there is the potential for hemodynamic instability because of direct effects on vascular smooth muscle and indirect effects from a reduction in sympathetic activation. Of particular importance is the effect on venous capacitance vessels that leads to a reduction in the stressed vascular volume and a consequent decrease in the mean systemic pressure that drives venous return.[56,92,93] When there is marked increase in intrathoracic pressure (seen with positive pressure ventilation of patients with severe airflow obstruction) along with a mean systemic pressure decrease, there is the potential for large reductions in cardiac output and life-threatening hypotension.

Hypotension that follows administration of sedatives to a patient with severe airflow obstruction most often occurs at the time of intubation, when the sedative agents are typically given as a rapid bolus, there is a marked increase in mean intrathoracic pressure, lung volume may increase significantly, and sympathetic activity may acutely decrease as a result of sedation, reduced work of breathing, and a fall in Pa_{CO_2}.[94] While the peri-intubation period is a high-risk time with regard to cardiovascular instability, as long as the above physiologic effects are appreciated and appropriate measures taken to anticipate and minimize the hemodynamic consequences of intubation, hypotension should be able to be managed without much difficulty. The most important measures to ensure peri-intubation hemodynamic stability are to 1) limit the dose of sedative to that required to provide adequate intubating conditions, 2) use a low frequency of manual ventilation with an Ambu bag after intubation, and 3) rapidly administer intravenous saline if there is any evidence of hemodynamic instability. Even though hypotension is related primarily to the direct and indirect vascular effects of sedatives on vascular compliance and dynamic hyperinflation rather than hypovolemia per se, rapid infusion of saline will increase the stressed vascular volume and thereby increase the driving pressure for venous return.[92,93] Occasionally, short-term administration of dopamine or another vasoactive agent is required to achieve hemodynamic stability. Hypotension can also occur as a consequence of maintenance infusion of sedative agents, but is much less common.

The most important adverse effects of continuous administration of sedatives in status asthmaticus are persistent sedation after drug discontinuation and prolonged muscle inactivity that may increase the risk of acute myopathy (see below). With the exception of propofol, the agents used for continuous sedation of the mechanically ventilated asthma patient may result in prolonged sedation after they are discontinued.[25,29,48] The large drug doses often required to achieve adequate sedation and suppression of respiratory drive in the critically ill asthma patient may increase the potential for prolonged recovery time. For certain types of respiratory failure (e.g., adult respiratory distress syndrome), resolution is very gradual and prolonged recovery from sedation does not often delay extubation. In contrast, patients with status asthmaticus may undergo a transition from life-threatening alterations in respiratory mechanics to near-normal lung function over a relatively short period of time. Sometimes the patient who requires a very deep level of sedation for initially extreme airflow obstruction can be extubated the following day, provided he or she is awake and cooperative. Therefore, delayed extubation due to prolonged sedative recovery time may be particularly problematic in patients with status asthmaticus.

An attractive feature of propofol is that it permits rapid titration to a deep level of sedation, with a guarantee of recovery within 1 to 2 hours after its discontinuation.[47] Therefore, despite its relatively high cost, propofol would be a reasonable choice for initial sedation of the intubated asthma patient. As discussed previously, we believe that the maximal dose of propofol should be limited to 80 μg/kg per minute (approximately 5 mg/kg per hour) when administered for more than a few hours. Even though there is a greater chance of prolonged sedation, a benzodiazepine would be a reasonable alternative to propofol for initial sedation. Midazolam offers no advantage over lorazepam with regard to rate of recovery from seda-

tion[29] and is much more expensive. Diazepam is less expensive, but may sometimes be associated with very prolonged recovery times, due to a high lipid solubility that may lead to tissue accumulation and to the long terminal half-life of both the parent drug and active metabolite. Also, constant infusion of diazepam is impractical. Lorazepam would seem to be the preferred benzodiazepine for sedation of the mechanically ventilated asthma patient, considering the cost, ease of administration via constant infusion, and sedative recovery time.

The duration of intubation in severe asthma may be predicted in part by the speed of onset of exacerbation.[95] Those individuals who have a very rapid and explosive onset usually have relatively pure bronchospasm and are likely to improve very quickly, making propofol an excellent choice for sedation in such cases. However, when the asthma exacerbation has been in progress for several days, the likelihood of significant airway edema and mucous plugging is high and resolution is often slow. In this case, sedation with lorazepam as opposed to propofol may be a more rational and cost-effective approach. However, precise details regarding the mode of onset are not always available and, even if they are, the mode of onset does not invariably predict the rate of resolution. Therefore, the authors generally prefer to use propofol initially and to observe the patient's course during the first 24 hours. Many patients with status asthmaticus can be extubated within one or two days. If airflow obstruction appears to be more refractory to therapy, then patients initially managed with propofol during the initial 24 to 48 hours may be converted to lorazepam, a more cost-effective means of providing ongoing sedation.

Propofol and benzodiazepines may not provide sufficient suppression of ventilatory drive in the acidemic patient with status asthmaticus in whom controlled hypoventilation is being used. When suppression of respiratory drive is a major goal, the addition of fentanyl (or morphine) to either propofol or a benzodiazepine may provide better control over minute ventilation than a narcotic-free regimen would. Indeed, a propofol-narcotic or benzodiazepine-narcotic combination may offer the greatest likelihood of meeting the goals of providing adequate amnesia, hypnosis, analgesia, and respiratory depression. As mentioned previously, recent data also suggest a possible benefit of synergistic sedation with a propofol-benzodiazepine combination.[51]

Short-term paralysis may be a useful adjunct in managing patients with very severe airflow obstruction in whom it is difficult to quickly achieve adequate muscle relaxation with sedation by itself, or in whom escalation of sedation leads to hemodynamic compromise. Of course, whenever an NMBA is given, the patient must receive sufficient doses of a benzodiazepine or propofol to ensure amnesia. Intermittent bolus of an NMBA is preferable to a continuous infusion. Intermittent boluses of a paralytic agent reduce the likelihood of unnecessarily prolonged paralysis and force the clinician to repetitively re-evaluate the adequacy of sedation. Between boluses of the NMBA, the dose of sedatives should be increased, to try to avoid the need for subsequent paralysis. Although short-term paralysis may be useful in the early management of the critically ill asthma patient, few patients need prolonged paralysis, which may be associated with increased risk of acute myopathy.

ACUTE MYOPATHY IN SEVERE ASTHMA

One of the more common complications of mechanical ventilation for severe asthma is the development of profound muscle weakness as the result of acute myopathy. First described more than twenty years ago,[96] acute myopathy, in the setting of status asthmaticus, has been the focus of numerous case reports, a number of clinical studies[8,9,97,97a] and several literature reviews.[7,10,98] Although important risk factors for its development have been identified, the pathogenesis of this syndrome is not well understood, in part because of the lack of adequate experimental models that would allow manipulation of the various factors that may be relevant to acute muscle injury. As such, the available literature is largely descriptive, accounting for the variety of names used to describe this clinical syndrome. The following terms have all been used in reference to the syndrome of diffuse muscle weakness associated with mechnical ventilation for acute asthma: *acute corticosteroid (or hydrocortisone) myopathy*,[97,99–103] *acute quadriplegic myopathy*,[10,104,105] *acute myopathy with myosin deficiency*,[106–108] *acute necrotizing myopathy*,[109–110] *disuse atrophy related to neuromuscular blockade*,[111] and the *floppy-person syndrome*.[112] Although the following discussion focuses on acute myopathic weakness seen in status asthmaticus, it is important to realize that an identical myopathy may be seen in other critical care settings.[113–115]

Clinical Features

Acute myopathy complicating status asthmaticus is almost invariably associated with the use of mechanical ventilation for at least 4 to 5 days, and usually for more than 1 week.[7] Therefore, patients with severe asthma are at very low risk for acute myopathy if they do not require intubation, or if they can be extubated within a few days. Often, the presence of muscle weakness is first appreciated after withdrawal of sedation, generally at the time the patient is being assessed for possible extubation. Weakness is usually diffuse and is often quite profound, and the ability of patients to perform activities of daily living is usually profoundly impaired.[9] Deep tendon reflexes may be absent if weakness is severe, but sensory deficits are not seen. Many affected individuals are unable to walk unassisted, and a significant minority are unable to lift their limbs against gravity or to turn in bed. Although upper-extremity weakness may prevent self-feeding, bulbar function is not impaired and swallowing is typically unaffected. The patient often needs help with bathing, dressing, grooming, and other aspects of personal hygiene.

Although the literature emphasizes the more severe near-quadriplegic presentations of acute myopathy, less severe and more regional weakness may be seen, and it is likely that patients with milder weakness have been reported less often. Interestingly, acute myopathy differs from many chronic myopathies, including chronic steroid myopathy, in that distal muscles are commonly involved as much as (or more than) proximal muscles. In some cases, wrist drop or foot drop may be a dominant clinical feature. Although weakness of the limb muscles is often the most striking clinical feature of acute myopathy, involvement of other skeletal muscles may give rise to a variety of clinical syndromes. For example, facial weakness has been reported, as has complete external ophthalmoplegia.[116] Eyelid muscles may also be affected. When weakness is profound and the patient is unable to open his or her eyes, it may appear that the patient is comatose because of lack of response to verbal stimulation.

One of the more interesting aspects of the acute myopathy of severe asthma is that clinically severe involvement of the respiratory muscles is unusual. In one study, the average maximal inspiratory pressure was -35 cm H_2O and in only 1 of 20 cases did respiratory muscle weakness contribute to prolonged ventilatory assistance.[9] Even in cases in which there was profound involvement of nearly all skeletal muscles, the patient usually was able to breathe comfortably without ventilatory assistance, provided that the underlying asthma was resolved.

Weakness due to acute myopathy resolves completely, but the time to recovery may be quite variable. Often, recovery occurs over a period of a few weeks. In a minority of cases, it may take several months for an individual to regain normal muscle strength. At the other extreme, disabling weakness sometimes resolves quite rapidly, progressing from profound quadriparesis to near-normal function in 7 to 10 days.[117] The occasionally rapid recovery from very profound weakness may offer some insights into the pathogenesis of this disorder (see below).

Diagnostic Studies

A diagnosis of acute myopathy is very likely when diffuse muscle weakness occurs during the course of mechanical ventilation for severe asthma. Measuring serum CK level, obtaining an electromyogram (EMG), and performing a biopsy of involved muscle have been used to help confirm a myopathic etiology of muscle weakness. Most patients

have an elevation in serum CK, but some do not,[105] and even when CK is increased, the degree of abnormality is often relatively modest. In two series, the average peak CK elevation was 1,575 and 1,168 IU/L, respectively.[8,9] Furthermore, the degree of CK elevation correlates poorly with the severity of muscle weakness, and patients with profound weakness may have CK levels that are minimally elevated, or even normal.[105]

There are limited data on the pathologic features of the actue myopathy observed in mechanically ventilated asthma patients. In some cases, focal myonecrosis has been described.[9,101,110] However, massive muscle necrosis is probably not typical, since extreme elevations of serum CK are seldom observed. Indeed, pathologic findings are sometimes surprisingly minimal.[105] One consistent pathologic feature has been the absence of inflammatory infiltrate, which suggests that immune or infectious processes are not involved.

The EMG is perhaps the most useful diagnostic tool for differentiating the various causes of weakness in the ICU. In acute myopathy, there is a rather consistent myopathic pattern without evidence for either significant neuropathy or NMJ block. A cardinal finding in myogenic weakness was early recruitment of short-duration, low-amplitude polyphasic motor units during voluntary muscle contraction.[9] In addition, some patients show abnormal spontaneous activity, including fibrillation potentials, positive sharp waves, and complex repetitive discharges. Nerve conduction studies revealed a marked reduction in the compound muscle action potential (CMAP) amplitude with normal sensory nerve conduction.[9,113,117] Recently, direct muscle stimulation has been used to test muscle excitability and findings suggested that the cause of the reduced CMAP amplitude may be inexcitibilty of muscle.[104,105]

Pathogenesis

The pathogenesis of the acute myopathy seen during status asthmaticus is not completely understood. This is due in part to a paucity of prospective clinical studies and, more importantly, to a lack of available animal models; thus, there has been minimal investigation into the various factors that may contribute to skeletal muscle injury during status asthmaticus. Despite this lack of unequivocal data, clinical studies of patients with status asthmaticus have identified certain factors that appear to increase risk for acute myopathy.[8,9] In addition, animal studies that have examined the synergistic effect of corticosteroids and denervation in causing acute muscle injury may have relevance to the clinical setting of severe asthma.[118–121]

Clinical Studies: Risk Factors Acute myopathy in status asthmaticus has been addressed retrospectively[9,97a] and by several reviews of the literature.[7,10,98] Only one prospective study has attempted to define risk factors for clinical myopathy.[8] To date, no randomized clinical trials have manipulated the putative risk factors to ascertain their effect on the incidence of myopathy. As a result, the available clinical data prevent firm conclusions regarding the importance of the various factors responsible for muscle injury. Nonetheless, there is a consistency in the findings reported in most of the retrospective reviews and in the lone prospective study that, coupled with the results of the experimental studies, permits some tentative conclusions and a reasonable hypothesis regarding the factors that are most likely responsible for muscle injury.

Corticosteroids Corticosteroids are perhaps the most strongly implicated etiologic factor in the acute myopathy associated with status asthmaticus. Indeed, in the original report that described this complication, the researchers felt that use of high doses of intravenous corticosteroids was probably responsible.[96] A strong emphasis on the putative myotoxic effects of corticosteroids has been evident in most subsequent reports.[7,100,101] It is somewhat difficult to ascertain with certainty that corticosteroids are a primary etiologic factor for acute myopathy in status asthmaticus because essentially all patients with acute severe asthma receive systemic corticosteroids. Nonetheless, due to the known toxic effects of corticosteroids on muscle, together with corroborative data from animal studies,[118–121] it seems highly likely that corti-

costeroids are a crucial factor in the acute myopathy seen with status asthmaticus.

Whether the dose of cortisteroids is important is not clear. This question was examined in several small studies. One study found that although the daily dose did not seem to be a factor, the total overall dose given during the entire ICU stay may have been since the overall dose was greater in those patients who developed muscle weakness than in those who did not.[97] However, this observation may simply serve to point out the risk associated with prolonged mechanical ventilation (see below). Two subsequent studies concluded that there did not appear to be any clear relationship to corticosteroid dose and clinically evident myopathy,[8,9] but this issue remains unresolved because of lack of controlled data.

Neuromuscular Paralysis Even if corticosteroids are a key factor in the pathogenesis of acute myopathy in status asthmaticus, there must clearly be additional processes involved, since corticosteroids are universally given to patients with acute asthma but acute myopathy occurs in only a small fraction of patients. One of the most strongly implicated cofactors for acute myopathy in status asthmaticus is the prolonged use of neuromuscular blocking agents. In a review of the literature published in 1993, 33 of 35 (94%) asthma patients with acute myopathy received a nondepolarizing NMBA.[7] The duration of paralysis was reported in most cases and was almost always 3 or more days.[7] In the only prospective evaluation of acute myopathy associated with mechanical ventilation for status asthmaticus, duration of paralysis was found to be the most important risk factor; the duration of paralysis in patients with clinically evident myopathy was 5.4 ± 2.0 days.[8] In a subsequent retrospective analysis of more than 100 mechanically ventilated patients with asthma, those who developed myopathy had uniformly been paralyzed.[9] Furthermore, of the patients who had been managed with an NMBA, the duration of paralysis was significantly longer in those who developed myopathy than in those who were not clinically weak (Fig. 14-4).[9] Recent retrospective data similarly demonstrate that the duration of

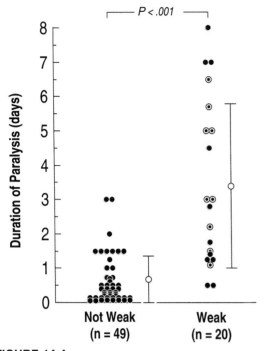

FIGURE 14-4
Duration of paralysis in patients with and without weakness. (With permission, from Leatherman, et al[9])

paralysis is a predictor for the development of myopathy.[97a]

The relative risk of myopathy with different NMBAs has been debated. Initially, it was thought that steroidal agents (e.g., vecuronium and pancuronium) carried greater risk than nonsteroidal agents (e.g., atracurium, cisatracurium). However, there have been reports of acute myopathy with nonsteroidal agents,[122] and one study found no difference in the incidence of myopathy with atracurium and vecuronium.[9] Although this issue has not been settled conclusively, current evidence suggests that the chemical structure of the NMBA is of little importance in determining the risk of myopathy.

If prolonged neuromuscular paralysis does indeed substantially enhance the myotoxic effects of cortisteroids, what is the mechanism of this effect? Simply put, is the potentiation of myotoxicity directly related to loss of muscle innervation per se or to the resulting inactivity of muscle? Animal models using surgical denervation cannot answer this question, and the only study that used pinning of the hindlimb in preference to denervation evaluated only the effect on corticosteroid receptors,[117] and did not examine other aspects of muscle physiology, biochemistry, or ultrastructure. At present, there are limited human data to help distinguish the effects of denervation per se and prolonged muscle inactivity. However, the data that do exist suggest that prolonged inactivity may be the most critical factor. For example, in several of the earlier anecdotal reports of severe acute myopathy, the affected patient received either no NMBA or was paralyzed only briefly.[99,100] More recently, a report described four patients who developed acute myopathy after treatment with corticosteroids and deep sedation with propofol.[103] A recent unpublished experience of the authors has also shown that asthma patients who required prolonged deep sedation were at risk for myopathy, even when the use of NMBAs was minimized or avoided altogether. Therefore, while the evidence regarding mechanism of action is not yet conclusive, the authors believe that neuromuscular paralysis increases acute corticosteroid myotoxicity by rendering muscle completely inactive. When administration of large doses of sedative agents results in prolonged and near-complete muscle inactivity, the patient is probably at risk for acute corticosteroid-related myopathy, even when paralysis has been avoided.

Prolonged Intubation One of the most consistent findings in reported cases of acute myopathy after mechanical ventilation for severe asthma is a prolonged duration of intubation. In one review of the literature, the duration of intubation was found to be 14 ± 11 days.[7] In the prospective study by Douglass and colleagues, patients with acute myopathy underwent 12.6 ± 6.6 days of mechanical ventilation, as compared to only 3.1 ± 3.1 days of intubation when myopathy did not develop.[8] In our experience, asthma patients who developed severe myopathy have universally been intubated for more than 5 days and, in the great majority of cases, the duration of intubation was greater than one week.

The strong association between prolonged intubation and myopathy is not explained by difficulty in weaning owing to involvement of respiratory muscles. While this issue has not been clearly addressed in most reports, our experience has been that respiratory muscle weakness is rarely a reason for prolonged intubation; patients typically have acceptable measurements of negative inspiratory force even when nonrespiratory musculature is profoundly weak.[9] Rather, the prolonged duration of intubation is nearly always due to refractory asthma with very slow resolution of airways obstruction. The slow course of resolution is most consistent with airways obstruction due primarily to airway edema and mucous plugging rather than bronchospasm per se. In those instances of status asthmaticus in which airflow obstruction results from relatively pure bronchospasm, as is often the case in patients who present with so-called sudden asphyxic asthma, the duration of intubation is much shorter. When rapid reversal of bronchospasm permits extubation within a few days, the risk of myopathy appears to be extremely low, even if the patient was initially treated with high doses of corticosteroids and NMBAs.

There is no plausible reason why intubation in and of itself should predispose to myopathy. It is likely that a long duration of intubation is a marker for prolonged muscle inactivity, thus predisposing the patients to corticosteroid-induced muscle injury. Patients with asthma do not need to be gradually "weaned" from the ventilator. Once airflow obstruction has improved sufficiently so that the load on unsupported breathing is not excessive, the patient can be safely extubated. However, while severe airflow obstruction persists, the patient is often kept heavily sedated, reducing the opportunity for active contraction of the skeletal musculature. This practice, which is done to prevent patient restlessness and agitation and to avoid potentially dangerous levels of dynamic hyperinflation, may predispose the patient to developing residual muscle weakness. In other words, the risk of myopathy may, to a considerable extent, be dictated by the severity and refractoriness of the status asthmaticus episode.

Although prolonged muscle inactivity may be important in the pathogenesis of the acute myopathy, acute myopathy is not simply disuse atrophy. With disuse atrophy, patients do not develop the profound degree of muscle weakness often seen with acute myopathy. Furthermore, the EMG findings in disuse atrophy and acute myopathy are different.[123] Lastly, the sometimes rapid recovery of muscle strength and normal muscle size seen in acute myopathy would not be consistent with near-quadriplegic weakness caused by muscle atrophy.

It is not known whether regular passive range-of-motion exercises would reduce the risk of myopathy in corticosteroid-treated patients who are paralyzed or deeply sedated for many days, but anecdotal experience indicates that this does not prevent myopathy. Preservation of active muscle contraction seems to have a greater likelihood of preventing myopathy, but given the risks inherent in using only light sedation in managing the mechanically ventilated patient with life-threatening airflow obstruction, this goal may be hard to achieve. Nonetheless, a temporary reduction in the level of sedation to a point where some muscle activity can be encouraged, without exposing the patient to undue risks of extreme restlessness or excessive minute ventilation, could be beneficial.

Experimental Studies A number of experimental studies have examined the short-term effects of corticosteroids on skeletal muscle, and several have specifically examined the interaction of corticosteroid administration and denervation.[120,121] Even though these investigations have been designed primarily to explore the process of corticosteroid-induced muscle atrophy, a problem primarily associated with long-term corticosteroid administration, they may well have relevance to the development of acute myopathy seen in the mechanically ventilated asthma patient.

As noted earlier, it is believed that the systemic corticosteroids universally used to treat patients with acute asthma are a major factor in the development of acute myopathy and clinical muscle weakness. However, while virtually all patients with acute asthma receive corticosteroids, only those who require mechanical ventilation appear to be at risk for acute myopathy, and in the great majority of cases, myopathy has followed the administration of high doses of corticosteroids to a patient who has undergone neuromuscular paralysis for several days.[7-9] No published animal studies have explored the synergistic effects of corticosteroids and paralysis on skeletal muscle. However, several experiments have addressed various effects of surgical denervation (or immobilization) and its relationship to corticosteroid myotoxicity.

Almost 20 years ago it was observed that immobilized muscles of rats showed a marked increase in the number of cytosolic glucocorticoid receptors.[118] Similar findings were noted when the affected muscle was surgically denervated.[119] In the latter model, there was a progressive increase in the number of glucocorticoid receptors as a function of time after denervation; the ratio of receptors in denervation:control limbs increased to 1.5:1 by day 5 and more than 2:1 by day 15.[119] The marked increase in the number of corticosteroid receptors in denervated or immobilized skeletal muscle could be a major reason for the previously noted observation that the catabolic effects of corticosteroids on skeletal muscle was much more pronounced when muscles were less active.[124]

Subsequent experiments have further examined the interaction of denervation and corticosteroids on biochemical, physiologic, and ultrastructural changes in skeletal muscle. In one elegant study, the isolated effects of corticosteroids and denervation were compared with the effects of both denervation and corticosteroid administration.[120] The results clearly showed a dramatic synergistic effect of denervation and corticosteroids. Physiologic assessment revealed that absolute twitch amplitude was not significantly affected by isolated treatment with steroids or denervation, but was markedly diminished when the two interventions were combined.[120] Ultrastructurally, there were signficant changes in the combined corticosteroid-denervation group, including considerable loss of thick filaments (myosin) in most fibers. In contrast, electron microscopy revealed no abnormalities in animals treated with steroids alone

and minimal changes with denervation.[120] Biochemical evaluation also demonstrated a striking effect on myosin content resulting from combined treatment with steroids and denervation. Whereas neither actin (light chain) nor myosin (heavy chain) content was greatly reduced when rats were treated with either steroids or denervation, combining the two interventions led to a dramatic loss of myosin and a much lesser reduction in actin.[120] As such, the myosin:actin ratio was markedly decreased by combined steroids and denervation. The preferential loss of myosin is highly unusual in myopathology, since it is seen in very few disorders.[107] Of interest, selective myosin depletion has been described in asthma patients treated with high doses of corticosteroids while undergoing neuromuscular paralysis.[106-109] Myosin depletion may be the result of both increased catabolism of muscle protein and decreased skeletal muscle myosin heavy-chain synthesis. Infusion of glutamine, an essential amino acid that plays a pivotal role in the metabolic activity of muscle, has been shown to help prevent the corticosteroid-induced downregulation of myosin heavy-chain synthesis and mitigate the degree of steroid-induced muscle atrophy.[125] It is unknown whether glutamine might have benefit to patients at risk for acute myopathy.

Mechanism of Muscle Weakness

One might assume that the profound muscle weakness seen in typical cases of acute corticosteroid myopathy might simply be explained by extensive damage to the contractile apparatus within muscle fibers. However, this explanation may not be sufficient to account for some of the findings often seen in this syndrome. For example, while some patients may have evidence of widespread myonecrosis, others show relatively minor changes in muscle architecture and have normal or minimally elevated serum CK levels, despite profound clinical weakness. Perhaps an even more striking observation is that some profoundly weak patients may undergo extraordinarily rapid recovery and have near- normal muscle strength within 1 to 2 weeks. Clearly, near-quadriplegic weakness due to severe atrophy or massive necrosis of muscle fibers would not be expected to resolve so quickly.

Recently, electrophysiologic findings have provided an alternative explanation for profound muscle weakness: inexcitable muscle.[104,105] In their initial report, Rich and colleagues described three patients who had no response to direct muscle stimulation after receiving high doses of corticosteroids combined with prolonged paralysis or deep sedation.[104] Restoration of normal excitability paralleled clinical recovery. In a subsequent study, 11 of 14 patients with acute myopathy were found to have muscle inexcitibility.[105] The authors concluded that while loss of contractile proteins (especially myosin) may contribute to muscle weakness, this would not lead to the typically profound decrease in the CMAP with direct muscle stimulation. While the mechanisms of muscle weakness in acute myopathy are not fully understood, temporary muscle inexcitibility would seem to be a more cogent explanation than loss of contractile proteins. Of interest, in the latter studies demonstrating muscle inexcitibility, a number of affected patients developed acute myopathy in the setting of severe sepsis without having received either corticosteroids or NMBAs.[105] Therefore, a clinically and electrophysiologically similar pattern may be seen in patients with sepsis and those with asthma who receive corticosteroids and undergo prolonged mechanical ventialtion while paralyzed or deeply sedated. This raises the question of whether certain patients with sepsis and multiorgan system failure in whom weakness is attributed to critical illness polyneuropathy may in fact have acute myopathy.

REFERENCES

1. Tuxen DV, Williams TJ, Scheinkestel CD: Use of a measurement of pulmonary hyperinflation to control the level of mechanical ventilation in patients with acute severe asthma. *Am Rev Respir Dis* 146:1136–1142, 1992.
2. Williams TJ, Tuxen DV, Scheinkestel CD: Risk factors for morbidity in mechanically ventilated patients with acute severe asthma. *Am Rev Respir Dis* 146:607–615, 1992.
3. Darioli R, Perret C: Mechanical controlled hypoventilation in status asthmaticus. *Am Rev Respir Dis* 129:385–387, 1984.
4. Corbridge TC, Hall JB: The assessment and management of adults with status asthmaticus. *Am J Respir Crit Care Med* 15:296–1316, 1995.
5. Feihl F, Perret C: Permissive hypercapnia. How permissive should we be? *Am J Respir Crit Care Med* 150:1722–1737, 1994.
6. Tuxen DV: Permissive hypercapnic ventilation. *Am J Respir Crit Care Med* 150:870–875, 1994.
7. Shapiro JM, Condos R, Cole RP: Myopathy in status asthmaticus: Relation to neuromuscular blockade and corticosteroid administration. *J Intensive Care Med* 8:144–152, 1993.
8. Douglass J, Tuxen D, Horne, M, et al: Myopathy in severe asthma. *Am Rev Respir Dis* 146:517–519, 1992.
9. Leatherman J, Fluegel W, David W, et al: Muscle weakness in mechanically ventilated patients with severe asthma. *Am J Resp Crit Care Med* 153:1686–1690, 1996.
10. Hirando M, Ott B, Raps F., et al: Acute quadriplegic myopathy. *Neurology* 42:2082- 2087, 1992.
11. Murray MJ, DeRuyter ML, Harrison BA: Opioids and benzodiazepines. *Critical Care Clinics* 11:849–873, 1995.
12. Greenblatt DJ: Sedation: Intravenous benzodiazepines in critical care medicine, in Chernow B (ed): *The Pharmacologic Approach to the Critically Ill Patient.* Baltimore, Williams & Wilkins, 1994, pp 321–326.
13. Zorumski CF, Isenberg KE: Insights into the structure and function of GABA-benzodiazepine receptors: Ion channels and psychiatry. *Am J Psychiatry* 143:162–173, 1991.
14. Teboul E, Chouinard G: Current perspectives. A guide to benzodiazepine selection. Part 1: Pharmacological aspects. *Can J Psychiatry* 35:700–710, 1990.
15. Levine RL: Pharmacology of intravenous sedatives and opioids in critically ill patients. *Critical Care Clinics* 10:709–731, 1994.
16. Alexander CM, Gross JB: Sedative doses of midazolam depress hypoxic ventilatory responses in humans. *Anesth Analg* 67:377–382, 1988.
17. Forster A, Gardaz JP, Suter PM, et al: Respiratory depression by midazolam and diazepam. *Anesthesiology* 53:494–497, 1980.
18. Barr J, Donner A: Optimal intravenous dosing

strategies for sedatives and analgesics in the intensive care unit. *Crit Care Clin* 11:827–847, 1995.

19. MacGilchrist AJ, Birnie GG, Cook A, et al: Pharmacokinetics and pharmacodynamics of intravenous midazolam in patients with severe alcoholic cirrhosis. *Gut* 27:190–195,1986.

20. Wheeler AP: Sedation, analgesia, and paralysis in the intensive care unit. *Chest* 104:566–577, 1993.

21. Vinik HR, Reves JG, Greenblatt DJ, et al: Pharmacokinetics of midazolam in chronic renal failure patients. *Anesthesiology* 59:390–394, 1983.

22. Cammarano WB, Pittet JF, Weitz S, et al: Acute withdrawal syndrome related to the administration of analgesic and sedative medications in adult intensive care unit patients. *Crit Care Med* 26:676–684, 1998.

23. Shafer A: Complications of sedation with midazolam in the intensive care unit and a comparison with other sedative regimens. *Crit Care Med* 26:947–956, 1998.

24. Shapiro BA, Warren J, Egol AB, et al: Practice parameters for intravenous analgesia and sedation for adult patients in the intensive care unit: An executive summary. *Crit Care Med* 23:1596–1600, 1995.

25. Chamorro C, de Latorre FJ, Montero A, et al:, Comparative study of propofol versus midazolam in the sedation of critically ill patients: Results of a prospective, randomized, multicenter trial. *Crit Care Med* 24:932–938, 1996.

26. Reves JG, Fragen RJ, Vinik HR, et al: Midazolam: Pharmacology and uses. *Anesthesiology* 62:310–324, 1985.

27. Arendt RM, Greenblatt DJ, Liebiseh DC, et al: Determinants of benzodiazepine brain uptake: Lipohilicity versus binding affinity. *Psychopharmacology* 93:72–76, 1987.

28. Malacrida R, Fritz ME, Suter PM, et al: Pharmacokinetics of midazolam administered by continuous intravenous infusion to intensive care patients. *Crit Care Med* 20:1123–1126, 1991.

29. Pohlman AS, Simpson KP, Hall JB: Continuous intravenous infusions of lorazepam versus midazolam for sedation during mechanical ventilatory support: A prospective, randomized study. *Crit Care Med* 22:1241–1247, 1994.

30. Cernaianu AC, DelRossi AJ, Flum DR, et al: Lorazepam and midazolam in the intensive care unit: A randomized, prospective, multicenter study of hemodynamics, oxygen transport, efficacy, and cost. *Crit Care Med* 24:222–228, 1996.

31. Ariano RE, Kassum DA, Aronson, KJ: Comparison of sedative recovery time after midazolam versus diazepam administration. *Crit Care Med* 22:1492–1496, 1994.

32. Mirenda J, Broyles G: Propofol as used for sedation in the ICU. *Chest* 108:539–548, 1995.

33. Conti G, Dell'Utri D, Vilardi V, et al: Propofol induces bronchodilation in mechanically ventilated chronic obstructive pulmonary disease (COPD) patients. *Acta Anaesth Scand* 37:105–109, 1993.

34. Mirski MA, Muffelman B, Ulatowski JA, et al: Sedation for the critically ill neurologic patient. *Crit Care Med* 23:2038–2053, 1995.

35. Hara M, Yoshihisa K, Ikemoto Y: Propofol activates GABAA receptor-chloride ionophore complex in dissociated hippocampal pyramidal neurons of the rat. *Anesthesiology* 79:781–788, 1993.

36. Bailie G, Cockshott I, Douglass E, et al: Pharmacokinetics of propofol during and after long-term continuous infusion for maintenance of sedation in ICU patients. *Br J Anaesth* 68:486–491, 1992.

37. White PF: Propofol: Pharmacokinetics and pharmacodynamics. *Semin Anesth* 7(Suppl):4–20, 1988.

38. Baraka A: Severe bradycardia following propofol-suxamethonium sequence. *Br J Anaesth* 61:482–483, 1988.

39. Eddleston JM, Shelly MP: The effect on serum lipid concentrations of a prolonged infusion of propofol: Hypertriglyceridemia associated with propofol administration. *Intensive Care Med* 17:424–426, 1991.

40. Bennett SN, McNeil MM, Bland LA, et al: Postoperative infections traced to contamination of an intravenous anesthetic, propofol. *N Engl J Med* 333:147–154, 1995.

41. Trotter C, Serpell MG: Neurological sequelae in children after prolonged propofol infusion. *Anaesthesia* 47:340–342, 1992.

42. Parke TJ, Stevens JE, Rice ASC, et al: Metabolic acidosis and fatal myocardial failure after propofol infusion in children: Five case reports. *Br Med J* 305:613–616, 1992.

43. Strickland RA, Murray MJ: Fatal metabolic acidosis in a pediatric patient receiving an infusion of propofol in the intensive care unit: Is there a relationship? *Crit Care Med* 23:405–410, 1995.

44. van Straaten EA, Hendriks JJE, Ramsey G, et al: Rhabdomyolysis and pulmonary hypertension in a child, possibly due to long-term high-dose propofol infusion. *Intensive Care Med* 22:997–1001, 1996.

45. Hanna JP, Ramundo ML: Rhabdomyolysis and

hypoxia associated with prolonged propofol infusion in children. *Am Acad Neurol* 50:301–303, 1998.

46. Barrientos-Vega R, Sanchez-Soria MM, Morales-Garcia C, et al: Prolonged sedation of critically ill patients with midazolam or propofol: Impact on weaning and costs. *Crit Care Med* 25:33–40, 1997.

47. Kress JP, O'Connor MF, Pohlman AS, et al: Sedation of critically ill patients during mechanical ventilation. *Am J Respir Crit Care Med* 153:1012–1018, 1996.

48. Carrasco G, Molina R, Costa J, et al: Propofol vs. midazolam in short-, medium-, and long-term sedation of critically ill patients. A cost-benefit analysis. *Chest* 103:557–564, 1993.

49. Chamorro C, de Latorre FJ, Montero A, et al: Clinical investigations. Comparative study of propofol versus midazolam in the sedation of critically ill patients: Results of a prospective, randomized, multicenter trial. *Crit Care Med* 24:932–938, 1996.

50. Ronan KP, Gallagher TJ, George B, et al: Comparison of propofol and midazolam for sedation in intensive care unit patients. *Crit Care Med* 23:286–292, 1995.

51. Carrasco G, Cabre L, Sobrepere, et al: Clinical investigations. Synergistic sedation with propofol and midazolam in intensive care patients after coronary artery bypass grafting. *Crit Care Med* 26:844–851, 1998.

52. Wong KC: Narcotics are not expected to produce unconsciousness and amnesia. *Anesth Analg* 62:625–626, 1983.

53. Stanford TJ, Smith NT, Dec-Silver H, et al: A comparison of morphine, fentanyl and sufentanil anesthesia for cardiac surgery: Induction, emergence and extubation. *Anesth Analg* 65:259–266, 1986.

54. Balestrieri FJ, Fisher S: Analgesics, in Chernow B (ed): *The Pharmacologic Approach to the Critically Ill Patients.* Baltimore, Williams & Wilkins, 1994, pp 640–650.

55. Weil J, McCullough R, Kline J, et al: Diminished ventilatory response to hypoxia and hypercapnia after morphine in normal man. *N Engl J Med* 295:1103–1106, 1975.

56. Green JF, Jackman AP, and Parsons G: The effects of morphine on the mechanical properties of systemic circulation in the dog. *Circ Res* 42:474–478, 1978.

57. Roscow CE, Moss J, Philbin DM, et al: Histamine release during morphine and fentanyl anesthesia. *Anaesthesiology* 56:83–97, 1982.

58. Osborne RJ, Joel SP, Slevin ML: Morphine intoxication in renal failure: The role of morphine-6-glucuronide. *Br Med J* 292:1548–1549, 1986.

59. Szeto HH, Inturrisi CE, Houde R, et al: Accumulation of normeperidine, an active metabolite of meperidine, in patients with renal failure or cancer. *Ann Intern Med* 86:738–741, 1977.

60. White PF, Way WL, Trevor AJ: Ketamine: Its pharmacology and therapeutic uses. *Anaesthesiology* 56:119–136, 1982.

61. Rock MJ, DeLaRocha SR, L'Hommedieu CS, Truemper E: Use of ketamine in asthmatic children to treat respiratory failure refractory to conventional therapy. *Crit Care Med* 14:514–516, 1986.

62. Schwartz SH: Treatment of status asthmaticus with halothane. *JAMA* 251:2688–2689, 1984.

63. Parnass SM, Feld JM, Chamberlin WH, Segil LJ: Status asthmaticus treated with isoflurane and enflurane. *Anesth Analg* 66:1193–1195, 1987.

64. Saulnier FF, Durocher AV, Deturck RA, et al: Respiratory and hemodynamic effects of halothane in status asthmaticus. *Intensive Care Med* 16:104–107, 1990.

65. McIndoe AK, Stewart P, Wilson IH: Drawover vaporizers for sedation in intensive care. *Intensive Care Med* 23:704–707, 1997.

66. Maltais F, Sovilj M, Goldberg P, et al: Respiratory mechanics in status asthmaticus: Effects of inhalational anesthesia. *Chest* 105:1401–1406, 1994.

67. Spencer EM and Willatts SM: Isoflurane for prolonged sedation in the intensive care unit, efficacy and safety. *Intensive Care Med* 18:415–421, 1992.

68. Nates JL, Cooper DJ, Day B, Tuxen DV: Acute weakness syndromes in critically Ill patients—A reappraisal. *Anesth Intensive Care* 25:502–513, 1997.

69. Coursin DB, Prielipp RC: Use of neuromuscular blocking drugs in the critically ill patient. *Crit Care Clin* 11:957–981, 1995.

70. Isenstein DA, Venner DS, Duggan J: Neuromuscular blockade in the intensive care unit. *Chest* 102:1258–1266, 1992.

71. Hunter JM: New neuromuscular blocking drugs. *Drug Therapy* 332:1691–1698, 1995.

72. Hanson CW: Pharmacology of neuromuscular blocking agents in the intensive care unit. *Crit Care Clin* 10:779–797, 1994.

73. Prielipp RC, Coursin DB, Wood KE, et al: Complications associated with sedative and neuromuscu-

lar blocking drugs in critically ill patients. *Crit Care Clin* 11:983–1003, 1995.

74. Dodson BA, Kelly BJ, Braswell LM, et al: Changes in acetylcholine receptor number in muscle from critically ill patients receiving muscle relaxants: An investigation of the molecular mechanism of prolonged paralysis. *Crit Care Med* 23:815–820, 1995.

75. Shapiro BA, Warren J, Egol AB, et al: Practice parameters for sustained neuromuscular blockade in the adult critically ill patient: An executive summary. *Crit Care Med* 23:1601–1605, 1995.

76. Rupp SM, McChristian JW, Miller RD, et al: Neostigmine and edrophonium antagonism of varying intensity neuromuscular blockade induced by atracurium, pancuronium or vecuronium. *Anaesthesiology* 64:711–717, 1986.

77. Rudis MI, Sikora CA, Angus E, et al: A prospective, randomized, controlled evaluation of peripheral nerve stimulation versus standard clinical dosing of neuromuscular blocking agents in critically ill patients. *Crit Care Med* 25:575–582, 1997.

78. Segredo V, Caldwell J, Matthay M, et al: Persistent paralysis in critically ill patients after long-term administration of vecuonium. *N Engl J Med* 327:524–528, 1992.

79. Grigore AM, Brusco L, Jr, Kuroda M, et al: Laudanosine and atracurium concentrations in a patient receiving long-term atracurium infusion. *Crit Care Med* 26:180–183, 1998.

80. Basta SJ: Modulation of histamine release by neuromuscular blocking drugs. *Curr Opin Anaesth* 5:572–576, 1992.

81. Newman PJ, Quinn AC, Grounds RM, et al: A comparison of cisatracurium (51W89) and atracurium by infusion in critically ill patients. *Crit Care Med* 25:1139–1142, 1997.

82. Basta SJ, Savarest JJ, Ali HH, et al: Clinical pharmacology of doxacurium chloride: A new long acting non-depolarizing muscle relaxant. *Anaesthesiology* 69:478–486, 1988.

83. Strange C: Peripheral neuromuscular function, in Tobin MJ (ed): *Principles and Practice of Intensive Care Monitoring.* New York, McGraw-Hill, 1998, pp 1047–1055.

84. Dulin PG, Williams CJ: Monitoring and preventive care of the paralyzed patient in respiratory failure. *Crit Care Clin* 10:815–826, 1994.

85. Helbo-Hansen H, Nielsen HK, Skovgaard LT: The accuracy of train-of-four monitoring at varying stimulating currents. *Anaesthesiology* 76:199–203, 1992.

86. Tschida SJ, Loey LL, Bryan KV: Inconsistency with train-of-four monitoring in a critically ill paralyzed patient. *Pharmacotherapy* 15:540–545, 1995.

87. Hansen-Flaschen JH, Brazinsky S, Basile C, et al: Use of sedating drugs and neuromuscular blocking agents in patients requiring mechanical ventilation for respiratory failure: A national survey. *JAMA* 266:2870–2875, 1991.

88. Appadu BL, Greiff JM, Thompson JP: Postal survey on the long-term use of neuromuscular block in the intensive care. *Intensive Care Med* 22:862–866, 1996.

89. Strange C, Vaughan L, Franklin C, et al: Comparison of train-of-four and best clinical assessment during continuous paralysis. *Am J Respir Crit Care Med* 156:1556–1561, 1997.

90. Stannard CF, Jones JG: Neuromuscular blockade, sedation, and pain control, in Tobin MT (ed): *Principles and Practice of Mechanical Ventilation.* New York, McGraw-Hill, 1994, pp 1125–1147.

91. Aguilera L, Alonso J, Arizaga A, et al: Sedation and paralysis during mechanical ventilation, in Marini JJ, Slutsky AS (eds): *Physiological Basis of Ventilatory Support.* New York, Marcel Dekker, 1998, pp 601–621.

92. Magder S: Shock Physiology, in Pinsky MR, Dhainaut JF (eds): *Physiological Foundations of Critical Care Medicine.* Baltimore, Williams & Wilkins, 1992, pp 140–160.

93. Magder S, De Varennes, B: Clinical death and measurement of stressed vascular volume. *Crit Care Med* 26:1061–1064, 1998.

94. Franklin C, Samuel J, and Hu T: Life-threatening hypotension associated with emergency intubation and the initiation of mechanical ventilation. *Am J Emerg Med* 12:425–428, 1994.

95. Wasserfallen JB, Schaller MD, Feihl F, Perre CH: Sudden asphyxic asthma: A distinct entity? *Am Rev Respir Dis* 142:108–111, 1990.

96. MacFarlane I, Rosenthal F: Severe myopathy after status asthmaticus. *Lancet* 2:615, 1977.

97. Shee CD: Risk factors for hydrocortisone myopathy in acute severe asthma. *Respir Med* 84:229–233, 1990.

97a. Behbehani NA, Al-Mane F, D'yachkova Y, et al: Myopathy following mechanical ventilation for acute severe asthma: the role of muscle relaxants and corticosteroids. *Chest* 115:1627–1631, 1999.

98. Lacomis D, Smith T, Chad D: Acute myopathy and neuropathy in status asthmaticus: Case report and literature. *Muscle Nerve* 16:84–90, 1993.

99. Van Marle W, Woods K: Acute hydrocortisone myopathy. *Br Med J* 281:271–272, 1980.

100. Knox A, Mascie-Taylor B, Muers M: Acute hydrocortisone myopathy in acute severe asthma. *Thorax* 41:411–412, 1986.

101. Williams T, O'Hehir R, Czarny D, et al: Acute myopathy in severe acute asthma treated with intravenously administered corticosteroids. *Am J Rev Respir Dis* 137:460–463, 1988.

102. Kaplan PW, Rocha W, Sanders DB, et al: Acute steroid-induced tetraplegia following status asthmaticus. *Pediatrics* 78:121–123, 1986.

103. Hanson P, Dive A, Brucher J-M, et al: Acute cortisteroid myopathy in intensive care patients. *Muscle Nerve* 20:1371–1380, 1997.

104. Rich M, Teener J, Raps E, et al: Muscle is electrically inexcitable in acute quadriplegic myopathy. Neurology 46:731–736, 1996.

105. Rich MM, Bird S, Raps, et al: Direct muscle stimulation in acute quadriplegic myopathy. Neurology 20:665–673, 1997.

106. Sher JH, Shafiq SA, Schutta HS: Acute myopathy with selective lysis of myosin filaments. *Neurology* 29:100–106, 1979.

107. Danon MJ and Carpenter S: Myopathy with thick filament (myosin) loss following prolonged paralysis with vecuronium during steroid treatment. *Muslce Nerve* 14:1131–1139, 1991.

108. Waclazwik AJ, Sufit RL, Beinlich BR, Schutta HS: Acute myopathy with selective degeneration of myosin filaments following status asthmaticus treated with methylprednisolone and vecuronium. *Neuromusc Disord* 2:19–26, 1992.

109. Al-lozi MT, Pestronk A, Yee WC, et al: Rapidly evolving myopathy with myosin-deficient muscle fibers. *Ann Neurol* 35:275–279, 1994.

110. O'Leary MJ, Honavar M, Coakley JH: Acute necrotizing myopathy and acute renal failure in association with acute severe asthma. *Anaesth Intensive Care* 22:729–732, 1994.

111. Kupfer Y, Okrent DG, Twersky RA, Tessler S: Disuse atrophy in a ventilated patient with status asthmaticus receiving neuromuscular blockade. *Crit Care Med* 19:1125–1131, 1991.

112. Knox S, Sheridan P, Venna N: The floppy person syndrome with prolonged Norcuron infusion. *Neurology* 40:119, 1990.

113. Lacomis M, Guiliani M, Van-Cott A, Kramer D: Acute myopathy of intensive care: Clinical electromyographic, and pathological aspects. *Ann Neurol* 40:645–654, 1996.

114. Zochodne D, Ramsey D, Saly V, et al: Acute necrotizing myopathy of intensive care: Electrophysiological studies. *Muscle Nerve* 17:285–292, 1994.

115. Showalter CJ, Engel AG: Acute quadriplegic myopathy: Analysis of myosin isoforms and evidence for calpain-mediated proteolysis. *Muscle Nerve* 20:316–322, 1997.

116. Sitwell LD, Weinshenker BG, Monpetit V, Reid D: Complete opthmalmoplegia as a complication of acute cortisteroid-and pancuronium-associated myopathy. *Neurology* 41:921–922, 1991.

117. David WS, Roehr CL, Leatherman JW: EMG findings in acute myopathy with status asthmaticus, steroids, and paralytics. Clinical and electrophysiologic correlation. *Electromyogr Clin Neurophysiol* 38:371–376, 1988.

118. Dubois DC, Almon RR: Disuse atrophy of skeletal muscle is associated with an increase in number of glucocorticoid receptors. *Endocrinology* 107:1649–1651, 1980.

119. Dubois DC, Almon RR: A possible role for glucocorticoids in denervation atrophy. *Muscle Nerve* 4:370–373, 1981.

120. Rouleau G, Karpati G, Carpenter S, et al: Glucocorticoid excess induces preferential depletion of myosin in denervated skeletal muscle fibres. *Muscle Nerve* 10:428–438, 1987.

121. Massa R, Carpenter S, Holand P, Karpel G: Loss and renewal of thick myofilaments in glucocorticoid-treated rat soleus after denervation and reinnervation. *Muscle Nerve* 15:1290–1298, 1992.

122. Manthous CA, Chatila W: Prolonged weakness after the withdrawal of atracurium. *Am J Resp Crit Care Med* 150:1441–1443, 1994.

123. Booth FW: Effect of limb immobilization on skeletal muscle. *J Appl Physiol* 52:1113–1118, 1982.

124. Goldberg AL, Goodman HM: Relationship between cortisone and muscle work in determining muscle size. *J Physiol* 200:667–675, 1969.

125. Hickson RC, Czerwinski SM, Wegrzyn LE: Glutamine prevents downregulation of myosin heavy chain synthesis and muscle atrophy from glucocorticoids. *Am J Physiol* 268 (*Endocrinol Metab* 31): E730–E734, 1995.

CHAPTER 15

ACUTE ASTHMA IN CHILDREN

Okan Elidemir
Giuseppe N. Colasurdo
Leland L. Fan

INTRODUCTION

Asthma is the most common chronic pediatric disease and affects an estimated 4.5 million children in the United States.[1] Recent increases in both pediatric hospitalizations and deaths from asthma[2-7] have led to global initiatives that provide comprehensive guidelines to diagnose and manage asthma in an attempt to reverse these trends.[8-11] Despite appropriate emphasis on asthma prevention and control, exacerbations of asthma remain common and rescue therapy is often needed.

Acute severe asthma (ASA) develops from bronchoconstriction and airway inflammation, and the inflammation causes airway wall edema and luminal mucus plugging. The resulting airway obstruction leads to increased work of breathing and hypoxemia from ventilation-perfusion mismatch. With increasing airway obstruction, intrapulmonary shunting may develop through regions of the lung that are atelectatic, worsening hypoxemia. Interestingly, early studies in which arterial blood gases were measured demonstrated that hypoxemia was present in virtually all children with ASA.[12-14] Severe hypoxemia may lead to metabolic acidosis, myocardial depression, cardiac arrhythmias, mental status changes, and seizures.[15-17] When airway obstruction becomes more severe, hypoventilation with hypercapnia ensues as a result of respiratory muscle fatigue. Children, particularly infants, are vulnerable to these changes because of several anatomic and functional characteristics including lower cross-sectional area of the small airways, more compliant airway walls, less collateral ventilation, decreased elastic recoil pressure, early airway closure, and an unstable rib cage.[18]

Well-recognized triggers for ASA in children include viruses (e.g., respiratory syncytial virus, parainfluenza virus, adenovirus),[19] other infectious agents (*Mycoplasma, Chlamydia*),[20,21] inhaled allergens,[22,23] and inhaled irritants (particularly tobacco smoke).[24-26]

FATAL AND NEAR-FATAL ASTHMA

The lung pathology of children who have died of asthma shows smooth muscle hyperplasia of the bronchial and bronchiolar walls, thick tenacious plugs often occluding the airways, thickened basement membrane, variable degrees of mucosal edema, and denudation of bronchial and bronchiolar epithelium (Fig. 15-1).

A number of risk factors have been identified in children with fatal and near-fatal asthma including delay in seeking medical attention,[27-30] inadequate medical response,[27,30] underutilization of anti-inflammatory therapy,[27,29,31,32] overuse of metered-dose inhalers,[32,33] high denial scores and other psychosocial factors,[28-30,32,34] previous intensive care unit (ICU) admissions,[35] prior occurrence of a life-threatening event or seizures,[32,34] reduced perception of severe lung impairment,[35] and Alternaria exposure.[23] Although asphyxia due to suffocation is thought to be the most common cause of death,[36,37] drug therapy with resultant vasovagal

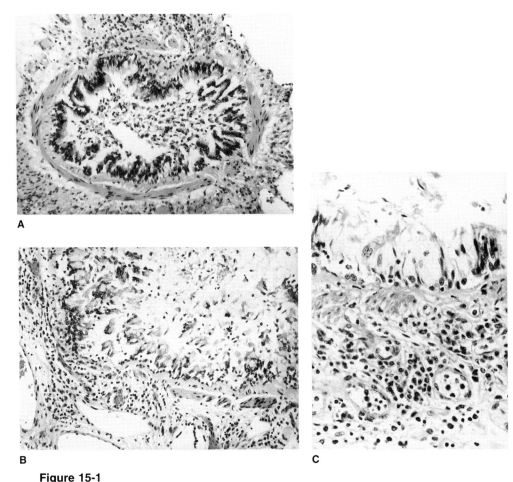

Figure 15-1
Airway pathology of a child who died from acute severe asthma. A. Cross-section of a membranous bronchiole shows smooth muscle hyperplasia, airway wall edema, mild inflammation, and a mucus plug in the lumen (original magnification ×50). B. A larger airway has similar features; in addition epithelial cell desquamation and basement membrane thickening are seen (original magnification ×50). C. Changes in this airway include extensive goblet cell hyperplasia and moderate inflammatory infiltrate (Original magnification ×100). (Courtesy of Claire Langston, M.D., Baylor College of Medicine)

reflexes,[33] cardiac arrhythmias,[38] and hypokalemia[39] have been implicated in some cases. Most disturbing, some children with fatal asthma have very mild disease and no prior identifiable risk factors.[40–42]

Specific programs have been developed to prevent death in children with life-threatening asthma. The best example is the "Red Alert Program,"developed by Sherman and Capen, which utilizes a comprehensive network of emergency medical services, school workers, extended family members, local physicians, emergency centers, and a referral center.[43] The network was designed to provide early, aggressive medical intervention and rapid access to care for children with life-threatening asthma who were enrolled in the program.

The program has demonstrated reduction in the number of hospitalizations and subsequent life-threatening events for high-risk patients.

ASSESSMENT

Management of ASA is highly dependent upon prompt recognition of acute symptoms so that appropriate action can be taken to reverse this process and prevent deterioration. Therefore, as part of chronic asthma management, caretakers should be given an action plan that provides specific practical instructions to identify early signs of worsening asthma, intensify therapy, and seek medical attention when appropriate. Examples of action plans are provided in the Expert Panel Report II.[11]

Children who develop serious exacerbations or fail to respond to home therapy should be evaluated in an emergency facility capable of managing pediatric emergencies. Although a functional assessment and a brief, focused history and physical examination are very important, treatment should be started as soon as an asthma exacerbation is recognized (see Management section below).

Essential information in the history that should be obtained includes 1) onset and duration of symptoms, 2) precipitating factors, 3) previous hospitalizations, especially ICU admissions and emergency department (ED) visits, particularly in the past year, 4) previous life-threatening events or seizures, and 5) current medication use, including time of last dose.

Several studies have validated the usefulness of clinical scoring systems, based on physical examination, in predicting which children will require hospitalization.[44–48] Although the scoring systems vary, measures of accessory muscle use, dyspnea, wheezing, heart rate, respiratory rate, cyanosis, level of consciousness, and pulsus paradoxus (PP) have been used to assess severity of illness.

As in adults, PP appears to be a useful and objective measure of acute asthma severity in children, especially when combined with other assessment tools. The magnitude of PP has direct relationship with increasing severity of illness and an inverse relationship with peak expiratory flow rate (PEFR).[49] There is also a direct correlation between PP and Pa_{CO_2} when the Pa_{CO_2} is high.[49,50] Children with ASA often have marked tachypnea that makes the measurement of changes in systolic blood pressure during the respiratory cycle somewhat difficult. Fortunately, timing is not necessary for accurate measurement.[49] The measurement is most conveniently made with a sphygmomanometer by inflating the blood pressure cuff until arterial occlusion is reached and then slowly deflating the cuff until Korotkoff's sound is first heard intermittently with a stethoscope. With further deflation, Korotkoff's sound can be heard continuously. The difference in the pressure between when the sound is first heard intermittently and when it is first heard continuously is the measurement of PP, with normal being less than 10 mm Hg. Pulsus paradoxus can also be demonstrated graphically with the arterial pressure tracing taken from an indwelling arterial line (Fig. 15-2), and can also be seen at times in the pulse oximetry tracing.

Figure 15-2

Arterial pressure tracing from a child with acute severe asthma demonstrating pulsus paradoxus. Intermittent decrease in systolic pressure of approximately 20 mm Hg corresponds to inspiration.

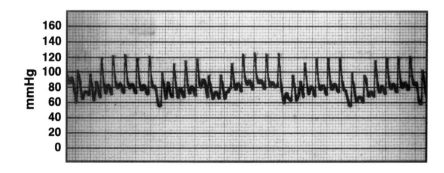

Spirometry, including PEFR and forced expiratory volume at 1 second (FEV_1), has been shown to reflect acute asthma severity in some studies,[45–51] but not in others.[44,52] The lack of improvement of PEFR after initial treatment may be a better predictor for hospitalization than the pretreatment measurement of PEFR.[46] Similar to spirometry, transcutaneous pulse oximetry alone has been demonstrated to be useful as a predictor of outcome in some studies[53,54] but not in others.[55] Geelhoed and colleagues demonstrated that an initial oxygen saturation of 91% or less predicted hospitalization as well as return visits in those children sent home from the ED.[53] In a subsequent study, the same group found that oxygen saturation predicted outcome better than PEFR, although both had value.[54]

Based on the above studies, a combination of physical examination, including pulsus paradoxus, spirometry, and pulse oximetry, should be used to determine asthma severity, response to treatment, and the need for hospitalization. In more severe cases, arterial blood gas measurements should be performed to assess more accurately oxygenation, ventilation and acid-base status.

In children with ASA, typical radiographic findings include hyperinflation and peribronchial thickening. Chest radiographs appear to have value for detecting other, more important findings, such as atelectasis, pneumonia, and air leak, in children requiring hospitalization but not in those needing only outpatient care. In children who presented to an ED with the first episode of wheezing, the diagnostic yield for chest films was low (5.7%).[56] In contrast, for children requiring hospitalization, the yield was higher (22% to 40%),[56,57] with atelectasis, consolidation, and pneumomediastinum identified most often.

MANAGEMENT

The goals of acute asthma treatment are to reverse the airflow obstruction rapidly and safely and to correct hypoxemia.[11] Since delay in seeking medical help is an important cause of death from asthma in childhood,[28,40,58,59] treatment should be initiated as early as possible, preferably at home.[60,61] Classic management of an acute asthma exacerbation consists of careful monitoring of the severity of symptoms and response to treatment and the administration of oxygen, bronchodilators, and corticosteroids.[11,60,62] A list of the most commonly used drugs for ASA with pediatric doses is given in Table 15-1.

General Supportive Measures

Children experiencing acute asthma attacks can be quite frightened, and it is important to provide care in a calm and reassuring manner and to avoid unnecessary painful procedures.[63]

Poor oral fluid intake, vomiting, and increased insensible fluid loss from the respiratory tract owing to hyperventilation may lead to the development of dehydration in children during an acute exacerbation.[62–64] Dehydration may contribute to formation of thicker, more viscous mucus which is difficult to expectorate.[65] Therefore, humidification of oxygen and correction of dehydration during an acute exacerbation are important.[62–64] However, it is critical to avoid overhydration because patients with asthma are prone to develop pulmonary edema as a result of high negative intrapleural pressures and increased antidiuretic hormone production.[66–68] Thus, once dehydration is corrected, patients should receive maintenance fluids only.

Pharmacotherapy

Oxygen   Since virtually all children with ASA are hypoxemic upon arrival to a hospital,[13,14] they should receive oxygen routinely and early in the course of disease to prevent the deleterious effects of hypoxemia. Humidified oxygen, supplied by nasal cannula or mask, should be administered to maintain an oxygen saturation above 92%.[63,64] Usually children who have mild hypoxemia tolerate nasal cannula better; masks are reserved for more severe cases. An oxygen flow rate of 2 to 4 L per minute by nasal cannula will provide an estimated 40% oxygen.[69] Simple masks with flow rates of 6 to 10 L per minute deliver 35% to 60%

Table 15-1
Pediatric Doses of Medications Used in the Management of Acute Severe Asthma

Medication	Route of administration	Dose	Frequency of administration
Albuterol	Inhalation Nebulized solution	0.15 mg/kg	Every 20 minutes for three doses, then every 1 to 6 hours, as needed
		0.3 mg/kg/hr	Continuous nebulization
	MDI	6 to 10 puffs	Every 20 minutes for three doses, then every 1 to 6 hours, as needed
Terbutaline	Intravenous	10 μg/kg given over 10 min	0.1 to 4.0 μg/kg/min continuous infusion
Prednisone	Oral	1 mg/kg	Two times a day
Prednisolone	Oral	1 mg/kg	Two times a day
Methyl-prednisolone	Intravenous	1 mg/kg	Every 6 hours
Ipratropium bromide	Inhalation Nebulized solution	250 μg	Every 20 minutes for three doses, then every 3 to 6 hours, as needed
Magnesium sulfate	Intravenous	25-75 mg/kg	Every 6 hours, as needed

oxygen.[69] If necessary, partial rebreathing or non-rebreathing masks can be used to deliver higher oxygen concentrations.[69]

Inhaled β_2 Agonists   Selective β_2 agonists, such as albuterol, are a cornerstone of acute asthma management since reversal of bronchospasm, a major factor in airway obstruction, is achieved through the stimulation of β_2-adrenergic receptors, which leads to smooth muscle relaxation within the airways. Inhaled β_2 agonists have replaced subcutaneous epinephrine as the treatment of choice for bronchodilation in children with ASA, owing to comparable efficacy, ease of administration, and lack of significant side effects.[70,71]

When first signs of an asthma exacerbation develop, such as increasing cough, decreasing activity level, chest discomfort or shortness of breath, patients should receive aerosolized albuterol. Albuterol given by nebulizer or metered dose inhaler (MDI) is preferred to oral administration because of a more rapid onset of action, greater potency, and fewer side effects.[70–73] If a nebulizer is being used, a unit dose of 2.5 mg (0.5 mL of 5mg/mL solution) should be given in 3 mL normal saline solution.[72] If an MDI is being used, the recommended initial dose is 2 to 6 actuations (commonly referred to as puffs). Waiting 5 minutes between inhalations allows initial improvement in airway obstruction and better deposition of the following doses of the medication.[73]

Recording PEFR before and after treatment is useful to assess the severity of the episode and the response to treatment. Children who improve with home bronchodilator therapy may repeat this treatment safely as frequently as every 4 hours.[11] Patients who require more frequent treatment, do not improve, or deteriorate after initial therapy should seek medical advice. It is likely that the degree of inflammation in the airways of these patients is significant enough to warrant initiation of systemic corticosteroid therapy.

Studies from a Toronto group have demonstrated that nebulized albuterol can be given more frequently and at higher doses than previously recommended.[74–76] In children with ASA receiving nebulized albuterol every 20 minutes, a dose of 0.15 mg/kg resulted in a more rapid and sustained improvement in FEV_1 values without any increase in side effects, compared to a dose of 0.05 mg/kg.[75] In a similar study using nebulized albuterol every hour, a dose of 0.3 mg/kg was more effective with no increase in side effects, compared to a dose of 0.15 mg/kg.[76]

Recently, asthma investigators have demonstrated that when equivalent doses are used, continuous albuterol nebulization (CAN) is superior to intermittent therapy in children.[77–79] In these studies, children receiving CAN achieved a higher FEV_1 more rapidly, and this response was sustained for a longer period of time. Other improved outcome measures of CAN therapy included shorter duration of therapy and a shorter hospital stay.[79] The safety of CAN therapy in children has also been well documented, with doses up to 0.3 mg/kg per hour or a fixed rate of 12 mg per hour administered for up to 72 hours without the development of cardiotoxicity or hypokalemia.[80,81] Transient and mild creatine phosphokinase (CPK)-MB isoenzyme elevation was noted in some patients, but no ECG changes indicative of myocardial ischemia or arrhythmia related to CAN therapy have been reported.

The technique for administration of albuterol by continuous nebulization is fairly simple (Fig. 15-3). Albuterol is mixed with normal saline and delivered into the chamber of a nebulizer via a standard syringe pump at a desired rate to maintain a constant level of solution in the nebulizing chamber.[79,81] The nebulizer is usually driven by 6 to 8 L per minute of oxygen flow.

Nebulized terbutaline, another β_2 agonist, has also been used to treat ASA in children. The recommended dose is 0.1 to 0.3 mg/kg given every 20 minutes for the first hour and then repeated every 2 to 6 hours, until the patient is stable.[82,83] Although terbutaline was the first agent given to children via continuous nebulization using the parenteral formulation,[84–86] albuterol has replaced terbutaline for both continuous and intermittent nebulization, since it is readily available as a nebulizer solution in the United States.[87]

Administration of β_2 agonists via an MDI with spacer has also been shown to cause significant bronchodilation both in younger and older children with ASA.[73,88,89] Several studies that compared metered dose inhalation and nebulization therapy, demonstrated that the MDI-with-spacer method was as effective as nebulization therapy.[90–94] The major advantage of the MDI with spacer is its low cost. Although concerns regarding

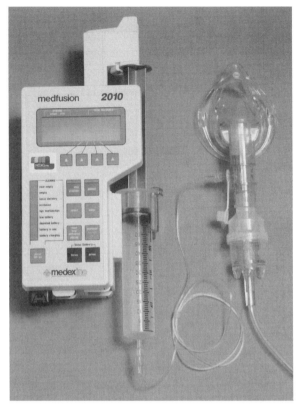

Figure 15-3
Apparatus for continuous nebulization of albuterol. A constant level of solution is delivered to the nebulizer by a standard infusion pump.

the complexity of instructions and the difficulty of administration have been raised, studies have shown that the MDI-with-spacer method can be used effectively, even in toddlers and older children with severe asthma.[95–97] Because one actuation of MDI provides 90 μg albuterol, 6 to 10 puffs every 20 minutes for 3 doses is recommended for ASA. Once the patient is stabilized, the same dose can be repeated every 1 to 4 hours, as needed.[83]

(R)albuterol (levalbuterol) is a recently developed form of albuterol currently only available in nebulization solution form.[97a] It appears to be at least as effective as conventional albuterol in terms of bronchodilation with fewer side effects in equivalent doses (1.25 mg levalbuterol = 2.5 mg albuterol).[97a,b] Further studies are required before recommending this medication for widespread use in treatment of pediatric acute asthma.

Adverse Effects of β Agonists Tremor is the most common side effect of β_2 agonists and can occur in as many as 65% of patients.[95,98] Tremor results from stimulation of skeletal muscle rather than the central nervous system.[99]

A major concern of β_2 agonist use in ASA has been their potential for cardiac toxicity. It is well recognized that epinephrine and isoproterenol, with their potent β_1-agonist activity, can cause tachycardia, arrhythmias, and even myocardial ischemia, especially when used parenterally.[95,100] Although not as potent, β_2 agonists have some intrinsic β_1 activity, which can be a potential problem when used at very high doses. Thus, monitoring of CPK-MB levels and ECGs is recommended in children receiving high doses of sympathomimetics.[100]

Albuterol and terbutaline can cause hypokalemia through stimulation of β_2 receptors which causes a shift of intracellular potassium to plasma, resulting in increased potassium delivery to kidneys and ultimately, loss in the urine.[95] The addition of corticosteroids to β_2 therapy may enhance this renal potassium loss.[98] Serum potassium should be closely monitored and hypokalemia should be corrected promptly since hypokalemia combined with hypoxemia and agents with potential cardiac toxicity may lead to fatal arrhythmias.

A relatively common complication of β_2-agonist therapy is paradoxical hypoxemia, especially if ASA is accompanied by atelectasis. This phenomenon may manifest as the inability of patients to wean from oxygen therapy during the recovery period of an exacerbation.[96,101] Since β_2 agonists are vasodilators as well as bronchodilators, they may increase blood flow to the areas of the lung that remain poorly ventilated, worsening V/Q mismatch.[96] In patients who are improving clinically but continue to require oxygen, decreasing the dose or frequency of albuterol therapy may be beneficial.

Headache, nausea, weakness, anorexia, and sleep disturbances are less common and less severe adverse effects of albuterol.[99]

Corticosteroids Used for more than 30 years, corticosteroids remain one of the mainstays of therapy for ASA in children. Given the important role inflammation plays in the pathogenesis of asthma, the use of corticosteroids with their broad anti-inflammatory properties is indicated for the treatment of ASA. Recent studies have demonstrated that nitric oxide, a putative marker of airway inflammation, decreased in children treated with corticosteroids during ASA, suggesting that corticosteroids suppress the inflammatory changes within the respiratory tract.[102,103]

In children with acute asthma treated with corticosteroids in an outpatient setting, most double-blind studies (5 of 7) have demonstrated that the administration of oral corticosteroids prevented hospitalization, reduced symptoms, and improved pulmonary function.[104-110] The beneficial effects of corticosteroids in infants and toddlers is less clear. One study demonstrated reduced admission rates,[111] while another showed no improvement in symptom scores.[112] A summary of these outpatient studies is shown in Table 15-2. Although dosages varied in different studies, a dose of prednisolone or prednisone, 1 to 2 mg/kg per day, administered orally in two divided doses, for 3 to 5 days, appears reasonable for management of acute asthma exacerbations in children in the outpatient setting. Although recommended in Expert Panel Report II, use of frequent, high-dose inhaled corticosteroids to prevent or treat asthma exacerbations in children is controversial.[11] Three of 4 double-blind, placebo-controlled studies showed beneficial effects and support this practice in pediatric age groups.[112a-d]

The beneficial effects of corticosteroids in the treatment of acute severe asthma in hospitalized children have also been well documented. There are four double-blind studies evaluating the efficacy of corticosteroids in the treatment of ASA in hospitalized children (Table 15-3).[113-116] In the earliest study, treatment with intravenous hydrocortisone, betamethasone, or dexamethasone resulted in significant improvement in arterial P_{O_2} in the first 24 hours of admission compared to placebo, although there was no difference in clini-

Table 15-2
Double-Blind Placebo Controlled Outpatient Studies of Corticosteroid Treatment of ASA in Children

Reference	Number of patients	Mean age, yrs	Dose and duration of therapy	Route	Improved outcome with steroids
Desphande[104]	44	10.5	Prednisolone 2 mg/kg, 1 mg/kg and 0.5 mg/kg once a day, for 3 days	PO	Yes
Harris[105]	41	12.0	Prednisone 30 or 40 mg, twice daily for 7 days	PO	Yes
Horowitz[106]	67	9.2	Prednisone 20 or 30 mg, single dose	PO	Yes
Shapiro[107]	28	8.1	Methylprednisolone 32 mg, first day tapered by 4 mg daily for 8 days	PO	Yes
Scarfone[108]	75	5.1	Prednisone 2 mg/kg, single dose	PO	Yes
Grant[109]	78	NA	Prednisone 2 mg/kg, single dose	PO	No
Wolfson[110]	88	9.4	Methylprednisolone 2 mg/kg, single dose	IV	No
Tal[111]	76	1.9	Methylprednisolone 4 mg/kg, single dose	IM	Yes
Webb[112]	38	0.8	Prednisolone 1 mg/kg, twice daily for 5 days	PO	No

cal scores or pulmonary functions.[113] In a subsequent study of children who were hospitalized in an asthma residential rehabilitation center and were experiencing an acute exacerbation, an oral dose of prednisone (2 mg/kg per day) was associated with a significant increase in PEFR and a decrease in the need for β_2-agonist nebulization treatments or injections.[114] In another study, an intravenous dose of methylprednisone, 1 mg/kg per dose, given every 6 hours, was associated with a significant improvement in forced expiratory flow (FEF) at 25% and 75% of vital capacity compared to the placebo group, which also had a higher incidence of asthma relapse within 4 weeks of dis-

Table 15-3
Double-Blind Placebo Controlled Inpatient Studies of Corticosteroid Treatment of ASA in Children

Reference	Number of patients	Mean age	Dose and duration of therapy	Route	Improved outcome with Steroids
Pierson[113]	45	12.0 yrs	Hydrocortisone 7 mg/kg or dexamethasone or betamethasone 0.3 mg/kg bolus once and 24-hour IV infusion	IV	Yes
Loren[114]	16	13.0 yrs	Prednisone 0.5 mg/kg, every 6 hours for 72 hours	PO	Yes
Younger[115]	49	9.5 yrs	Methylprednisolone 2 mg/kg once, followed by 1 mg/kg every 6 hours until discharge	IV	Yes
Daugbjerg[116]	123	9.3 mos	Prednisolone 4-6 mg/kg once, then 1.6-2.6 mg/kg once daily for 3 days or budesonide inhaled 0.5 mg every 4 hours for 3 days	PO	Yes

charge.[115] In a recent double-blind study, the use of oral prednisolone plus terbutaline, or inhaled budesonide plus terbutaline, was associated with earlier discharge compared with the use of terbutaline by itself.[116] By contrast, an early study in pediatric patients failed to show efficacy of hydrocortisone, 7 mg/kg per dose, given every 6 hours, but this study, although randomized, was not blinded.[117] Thus, most studies support the use of corticosteroids in the treatment of children hospitalized for ASA.

Although it is widely accepted that corticosteroids have a role in the treatment of children with ASA, little information is available on route, dose, frequency, and duration of therapy. A recent study demonstrated that oral and intravenous corticosteroids were equally effective in preventing hospitalization when used in the ED.[118] In another study conducted in an ED, nebulized dexamethasone was as effective as oral prednisone in the treatment of pediatric ASA; in addition, it was associated with more rapid clinical improvement, more reliable drug delivery, and fewer relapses.[119] No studies are available on the efficacy of different routes of administration in hospitalized patients. With regard to dose, in a double-blind study in children with ASA that compared a 30 mg/m^2 dose of methylprednisolone, given every 6 hours, with a 300 mg/m^2 dose, given every 6 hours, no difference in outcome could be demonstrated, suggesting that there is no advantage to the use of very high doses of corticosteroids.[120]

With regard to dosing frequency, in the only pediatric study evaluating the onset and duration of effect of corticosteroids in ASA, PEFR peaked at 4 to 6 hours, began to decline by 7 hours, and returned to baseline by 12 hours following administration of a single dose of oral prednisolone.[121] Thus, currently available data suggest that multiple daily dosing produces better results than single daily dosing if intermediate-acting steroid preparations are used. No other objective information is available on dosage and duration of therapy in children with ASA. Methylprednisolone, 1 mg/kg per dose, given intravenously every 6 hours, is recommended as the starting dose for children with ASA who require hospitalization.[11,115] Al-

though control studies are lacking, a duration of 3 to 5 days appears reasonable.

In summary, the majority of pediatric studies demonstrated that corticosteroids were effective in decreasing the hospitalization rates when given early to ambulatory children with acute asthma; in addition, they improved symptoms and lung function in children requiring inpatient care.

Side Effects of Corticosteroids   The most serious complication of corticosteroids is the development of prolonged muscle weakness when used in conjunction with nondepolarizing muscle relaxants. Other complications include hypokalemia, hyperglycemia, fluid retention and rarely, heart failure, if very high doses are used. Steroid induced acute psychosis has also been reported in children during short-term oral use.[121a] Suppression of the hypothalamic-pituitary-adrenal axis usually does not occur when corticosteroids are used for 5 days or less.[122,123] However, if the number of doses of short steroid bursts exceeds four in 1 year, patients should be considered to be at risk of developing adverse reactions from adrenal suppression associated with chronic corticosteroid administration.[123]

Anticholinergics   Although anticholinergic agents produce bronchodilation in children with ASA, they are less effective bronchodilators than β_2 agonists,[124,125] and therefore are not considered first-line drugs in treatment of ASA in children, but are reserved as adjunctive therapy to inhaled β_2 agonists. Anticholinergic agents most commonly used are atropine, ipratropium bromide (IB), and glycopyrrolate.[126] Currently IB is the only anticholinergic agent approved by the U.S. Food and Drug Administration as a bronchodilator because IB is associated with fewer systemic side effects when compared with aerosolized atropine and glycopyrrolate.[126,127]

Several studies have demonstrated that the combination of IB and nebulized β_2 agonists provided additive benefit for treatment of ASA in children, in terms of significant improvement in FEV_1, especially in severe cases.[128–131b] In contrast, some studies of children with mild exacerbations of asthma have failed to show additive effect of nebulized IB-albuterol combination.[132–134] This is thought to occur because in mild asthma, albuterol alone usually increases the FEV_1 to 90% to 95% of predicted values, leaving no room for IB to provide further benefit.[132] One recent important study in children with ASA (FEV_1 <35% of predicted) provided convincing evidence that administering nebulized IB at a dose of 250 μg every 20 minutes within the first hour of ED presentation, in combination with standard albuterol inhalation therapy, resulted in additional improvement in FEV_1 values and lower hospitalization rates when compared to albuterol by itself.[128] Following initial treatment, the recommended dose of nebulized ipratropium bromide is 250 μg, given every 3 to 6 hours.[124–126]

In view of these published data, it appears reasonable to use IB as adjunctive therapy to inhaled β_2 agonists in children with ASA, especially if they are not responding to standard therapy. Combining nebulized IB with more aggressive β_2-agonist therapies such as CAN is an interesting strategy that deserves to be studied. Finally, the development of more selective anticholinergic agents should further define the role played by these agents in the management of pediatric ASA.

Theophylline   Theophylline and aminophylline have long been considered one of the mainstays of treatment of ASA in children.[135,136] However, recent, well-designed studies have consistently shown that the addition of theophylline to standard therapy with nebulized albuterol and systemic corticosteroids, administered to patients who are either in the ED or have been admitted to the hospital, does not improve outcome in children with ASA.[137–141] Furthermore, adverse effects such as nausea, vomiting, headache, and palpitations were more common in the theophylline-treated groups.[139,141]

Considering these observations, it is clear that theophylline should not be used in routine management of acute asthma exacerbations in children. However, a recently published double-blind, placebo-controlled trial of 163 children with acute asthma unresponsive to conventional ther-

apy has shown that intravenous aminophylline led to significant improvement of FEV_1 and oxygen saturation, and prevented the need for intubation.[141a] Therefore, theophylline might be considered as an adjunctive drug in patients progressing to respiratory failure despite vigorous use of β_2 agonists and systemic corticosteroids.

Intensive Care Unit Management

Despite maximal pharmacologic therapy, a small percent of children with acute severe asthma may continue to deteriorate and require intubation and mechanical ventilation. Of all hospital admissions for pediatric asthma, 2.1% to 3.7% of patients require intensive care management, and of these, 24% to 33% require mechanical ventilation (0.7% to 0.8% of total hospital admissions for pediatric asthma).[142–145]

Intravenous β_2 Agonists   Intravenous β_2 agonists have been used in children with ASA who did not respond to inhaled β_2 agonists, based on the concept that nebulization may not deliver enough medication to severely obstructed airways to achieve sufficient airway smooth muscle relaxation. Therefore, systemic administration was necessary to produce a more effective bronchodilator response.[80,126,146]

Although intravenous β_2 agonists have traditionally been reserved for children who fail conventional therapy and face impending respiratory failure, recent data suggest that their use in the early management of ASA may also be beneficial. In a randomized double-blind study of 29 children presenting to an ED with ASA, Browne and colleagues examined the value of adding intravenous albuterol infusion to conventional therapy (oxygen, inhaled β_2 agonists, and intravenous corticosteroids).[147] An intravenous infusion of albuterol (15 μg/kg) over 10 minutes early in the course of an acute asthma attack resulted in more rapid recovery, as measured by clinical assessment scores and the need for inhaled β_2 agonists and oxygen. If the results of this study are confirmed, the use of intravenous β_2 agonists given by bolus may become a useful treatment option in the early management of ASA in children.

Although widely accepted and recommended by an expert panel, the use of intravenous β_2 agonists in hospitalized children with ASA who have failed conventional therapy and face impending respiratory failure has not been studied in prospective clinical trials. β_2 agonists, particularly albuterol and terbutaline, have replaced isoproterenol for continuous intravenous infusions, due to the cardiac toxicity of isoproterenol[100] and the suggestion in one retrospective study that albuterol is associated with more sustained decrease in Pa_{CO_2} and less tachycardia compared to isoproterenol.[146] Since albuterol is not available in parenteral form in the United States, terbutaline has become the drug of choice for intravenous infusions.[126,148,149] The recommended dose is an initial bolus of 10 μg/kg over 10 minutes followed by an infusion of 0.2 μg/kg per minute. The infusion can be increased by 0.1 μg/kg per minute every 30 minutes up to a maximum dosage of 4 μg/kg per minute. Patients on continuous IV β_2 agonist infusions should have serum potassium and CPK-MB levels and ECGs checked frequently.[146]

Mechanical Ventilation Mechanical ventilation becomes essential when children with ASA fail to respond to pharmacologic therapy. Although mortality rates as high as 38% have been reported in adults mechanically ventilated for asthma,[150] mortality rates are lower (0% to 5%) for children. However, mechanical ventilation in children with ASA is associated with significant morbidity, ranging from 15% to 82%.[144,151–153]

Limited information regarding the use of mechanical ventilation in children with ASA exists and much of it is derived from a few reported case series and reviews. Nonetheless, established principles of pediatric mechanical ventilation can be applied to children with respiratory failure from ASA.

Indications Although arterial blood gas measurements remain important factors in the detection of hypoxemia, hypercarbia, and respiratory and/or metabolic acidosis, they are not the sole indicators of respiratory failure and should be interpreted in the context of the clinical picture.[64,154,155] Failure to improve with maximal pharmacological therapy, altered mental status (lethargy or agitation), clinical deterioration and development of fatigue, hypoxemia (Pa_{O_2} <60 mm Hg) unrelieved by 100% oxygen, and rising Pa_{CO_2} are the indications for mechanical ventilation.[64,142–145]

Airway Management The patient should be stabilized with 100% oxygen administered via a face mask and bag. To diminish the risk of aspiration, the care giver should clear the patient's airway of oral secretions and empty the stomach by means of a nasogastric tube prior to intubation, if the condition of the patient allows for these maneuvers.[64] Intubation should be performed by the most experienced personnel available.[64,154] The orotracheal route should be considered in order to use the largest-diameter endotracheal tube possible, permitting easier suctioning of mucus plugs.[64,143–145] Pretreatment with atropine to minimize secretions is recommended.[144,145] For sedation, ketamine at a dose of 1 to 3 mg/kg is ideal because of its bronchodilating properties.[156–159] Morphine should be avoided because it may cause histamine release and increase the severity of bronchospasm.[64] Depolarizing muscle relaxants, such as succinylcholine (1 to 2 mg/kg) are often used to facilitate intubation owing to their rapid onset and short duration of action.

Institution of Mechanical Ventilation The goal of mechanical ventilation is to afford the fatigued respiratory muscles a rest and to provide adequate gas exchange until bronchospasm and airway inflammation are improved. Successful use of mechanical ventilation usually requires sedation and muscle relaxants in order to eliminate ventilator-patient asynchrony and improve chest wall compliance.[64,143–145]

Strategies utilizing either volume- or pressure-control modes of ventilation have been used in children with variable degrees of success and complication rates. No studies exist that demonstrate the superiority of either of these modes.

In the past, attempts to normalize Pa_{CO_2} levels with mechanical ventilation have required high airway pressures that often led to the development of air leak syndromes. Recognition that children can tolerate hypercapnia and acidosis if they are well oxygenated has led to the strategy of "controlled hypoventilation" or "permissive hypercapnia."[144,160] With this method, Pa_{CO_2} levels as high as 60 mm Hg are permitted, provided that adequate oxygenation and a pH of ≥ 7.20 can be maintained. The risk of barotrauma is decreased significantly because high plateau pressures are avoided. Some authors recommend the intermittent administration of sodium bicarbonate to keep blood pH above 7.20,[143,144,160] although there are theoretical considerations that this practice could actually worsen intracellular acidosis. Utilizing controlled hypoventilation, Dworkin and Kattan successfully managed 20 episodes of respiratory failure in 10 children with ASA with no deaths and little morbidity.[144]

Recently, pressure support ventilation without sedation and muscle relaxants has been used for management of four asthmatic children with respiratory failure.[160] Pressure support ventilation has potential advantages in that it decreases the inspiratory work of breathing, alleviating respiratory muscle fatigue; eliminates patient-ventilator asynchrony, thereby reducing the chances of air leak syndromes; and decreases hyperinflation by allowing active expiration.[160]

Complications   Potentially life-threatening complications, common to all children who require mechanical ventilation, include endotracheal tube obstruction with mucus plugs, misplacement of the endotracheal tube, air leak including tension pneumothorax, patient disconnect from the ventilator, and malfunction of the mechanical ventilator. All of these complications need to be considered and addressed immediately in any patient who deteriorates rapidly while receiving mechanical ventilatory support.[161,162]

Another serious complication of mechanical ventilation for ASA is prolonged paralysis or muscle weakness due to a synergystic effect of corticosteroids and nondepolarizing muscle relaxants.

For patients receiving these agents, muscle relaxants should be weaned daily to assess muscle strength and periodic bedside nerve stimulation studies should also be performed.[143]

A more common complication of mechanical ventilation is the development of intrinsic positive end-expiratory pressure (PEEP). Children with ASA are vulnerable to this problem because severe airways obstruction leads to long time constants in the lung and the need for prolonged expiration to empty alveoli. If expiratory times set by the ventilator are not long enough to allow the lungs to deflate, auto-PEEP will develop, with the potential to interfere with venous return and to cause hypotension. To prevent this complication, low ventilatory rates with high inspiratory flow rates should be used to provide low inspiration/expiration ratios and prolonged expiratory times.

The most common complication of mechanical ventilation in asthmatic children is atelectasis, which is often migratory (Fig. 15-4).[144,145] Atelectasis usually responds to conservative management, including frequent suctioning and removal of mucus plugs, use of chest physiotherapy as tolerated, and inhalation of bronchodilators. Refractory atelectasis may require flexible bronchoscopy to remove mucus plugs; however, this procedure may aggravate bronchospasm.[64]

Alternative Therapies

Although most children with ASA respond to conventional therapy, there remains a need to 1) develop new therapy to supplement routine management, 2) provide other strategies to avoid the need for mechanical ventilation, and 3) improve the outcome of the most severely ill patients with respiratory failure. A number of alternative therapies have been proposed that address these issues, including the use of magnesium sulfate, helium/oxygen, ketamine, inhalational anesthetics, and extracorporeal membrane oxygenation (ECMO).

Magnesium Sulfate   Magnesium sulfate has been advocated for treatment of ASA since the 1930s.[163] Suggested mechanisms of action include 1) antagonism of calcium translocation across cell

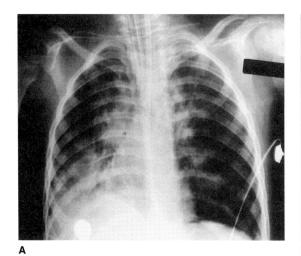

A

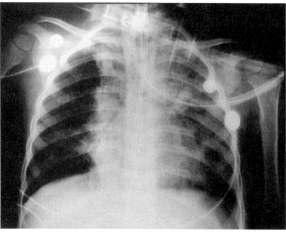

B

C

Figure 15-4

Migratory atelectasis in a child intubated and ventilated for acute severe asthma. A. Chest radiograph shows volume loss of the right lung with a shift of the mediastinum to the right. B. Repeat film taken 6 hours later shows re-expansion of the right lung but now there is volume loss of the left lung. C. Computed tomography of the chest following the chest radiograph of the same patient showing extensive atelectasis of the left lower lobe with leftward displacement of the heart.

membranes inhibiting smooth muscle contraction, 2) prevention of mast cell degranulation, and 3) reduction of acetylcholine release from cholinergic nerve endings.

Although controversy exists regarding its efficacy in adults with ASA, a recent, well-designed double-blind study in children with ASA suggested that an intravenous infusion of 25 mg/kg of magnesium sulfate added to conventional therapy in an ED setting is associated with more rapid improvement in pulmonary function and lower hospitalization rates.[164] These data coupled with other more anecdotal evidence of benefit[165] support the use of intravenous magnesium sulfate for the management of ASA in children.

Although a dose of 25 mg/kg up to 2 gm was used in the double-blind study,[164] others have recommended a dose of 50 to 75 mg/kg, administered as a slow IV bolus over 20 minutes, in order to obtain a serum magnesium level high enough (3 to 4 mg/dL) to achieve measurable bronchodilatation.[166,167]

Side effects of magnesium sulfate are generally mild and include transient sensation of warmth, flushing, nausea, vomiting, dry mouth, and malaise.[167] Slow infusion (>20 minutes) prevents alterations in pulse and blood pressure.[166] Loss of deep tendon reflexes, muscle weakness, and respiratory depression generally do not occur until serum magnesium levels exceed 12 mg/dL.[167]

Helium/Oxygen Mixture   When the diameters of the conducting airways narrow, there is a tendency for flow to become turbulent. This phenomenon is density dependent and is more likely to occur in the central airways where the cross-sectional area is small and the velocity is high. In more peripheral airways, flow is laminar because gas velocity rapidly decreases as the cross-sectional area increases. When airflow obstruction is not extreme, airway resistance is density independent in distal airways.

In patients with severe obstructive lung disease, the inhalation of helium, a low-density gas, may reduce the work of breathing by changing turbulent flow to more laminar flow, particularly if the major site of obstruction is in the central airways.[168] Based on this hypothesis, investigators have used heliox (helium/oxygen mixture: 80%/20%) for management of ASA with variable degrees of success.[169] Two recently published studies suggest that heliox is beneficial in adults presenting to the emergency room with ASA.[170,171]

A recent double-blind study of 18 children with ASA presenting to the ED reported that the inhalation of heliox for 15 minutes, in addition to CAN and IV methylprednisolone, significantly lowered pulsus paradoxus, increased PEFR, lessened the dyspnea index, and prevented the need

for mechanical ventilation.[172] In this study, heliox (80:20) was administered by a non-rebreathing face mask at a flow rate of 10 L per minute. Supplemental oxygen was provided via a nasal cannula at a flow rate of 2 L per minute to maintain oxygen saturations above 92%, if necessary. In contrast, a study of 11 children hospitalized for ASA failed to show improvement with adjunctive heliox therapy.[173]

In summary, although heliox inhalation may be beneficial in pediatric ASA patients unresponsive to conventional therapy, further studies are needed before this therapy can be routinely recommended.

Ketamine   Since the initial observation that ketamine decreased the airway resistance in a child with asthma during its use as an anesthetic,[174] ketamine has been advocated for the treatment of both children and adults with refractory acute severe asthma. Published information regarding the use of ketamine as an adjunct to conventional treatment of ASA in children is limited to case reports. Experience suggests that an initial intravenous bolus of 1.4 to 2.5 mg/kg of ketamine followed by an infusion of 0.2 mg/kg per hour may result in significant improvement in clinical symptoms and Pa_{CO_2} tensions.[156–159]

Side effects associated with ketamine include increased oral and tracheal secretions, cardiovascular stimulation, and increased intracranial pressure.[175,176]

Inhalation Anesthetics   Halothane, enflurane, and isoflurane are three commonly used inhalation anesthetics with bronchodilator effects.[175] As with ketamine, knowledge regarding the use of these agents in children with refractory ASA comes from a limited number of case reports. Review of these reports suggests that administration of these agents at concentrations of 0.5% to 1% via a vaporizer results in significant improvement in objective respiratory parameters, including decreased Pa_{CO_2}, increased lung compliance, decreased peak inspiratory pressure, and increased tidal volume.[177–180]

Complications and risks of using inhalation

anesthetics in refractory ASA include hypotension secondary to peripheral vasodilatation, myocardial depression, and arrhythmias.[64,175] Careful monitoring of blood pressure and ECG is essential, especially if the patient is acidotic, hypoxemic, or receiving theophylline.[64] These agents should only be administered under supervision of an anesthesiologist.

Extracorporeal Membrane Oxygenation In isolated cases of children with ASA who fail all standard and alternative treatment measures, ECMO has been tried experimentally, with encouraging results.[181] Thus, ECMO may be indicated for the pediatric patient who has not responded to maximal pharmacologic therapy and mechanical ventilation, and in whom a fatal outcome appears to be certain. Under any other circumstances, its use would appear to be unjustified.

CONCLUSIONS

Refinements in therapeutic strategies, such as the early outpatient use of oral corticosteroids to prevent hospitalization, have improved the outcome in children with acute asthma. Nonethelesss, ED visits and hospitalizations continue to account for the largest proportion of the direct health care costs of asthma. Global education and prevention programs have been developed to provide comprehensive guidelines to diagnose and manage asthma in hopes of reversing these trends. More focus is needed on identifying and addressing factors that contribute to disease management failure, such as poor compliance with treatment programs and inadequate access to continuing care.[182]

After an episode of acute asthma resolves, it is critical that patients be provided with a comprehensive plan to prevent future exacerbations. This plan should include 1) the identification and elimination of precipitating factors such as tobacco smoke, 2) the long-term use of anti-inflammatory therapy supplemented with bronchodilators as needed, and 3) a mechanism for ongoing and careful follow-up and asthma education. Further studies aimed at reducing asthma morbidity are needed.

REFERENCES

1. Centers for Disease Control and Prevention: Asthma mortality and hospitalization among children and young adults-United States, 1990–1993. *MMWR* 45:350, 1996.
2. Mitchell EA: International trends in hospital admission rates for asthma. *Arch Dis Child* 60:376, 1985.
3. Evans R, Mullally DI, Wilson RW, et al: National trends in the morbidity and mortality of asthma in the US-prevalence, hospitalization and death from asthma over two decades: 1965–1984. *Chest* 91:65S, 1987.
4. Jackson RT, Sears MR, Beaglehole R, et al: International trends in asthma mortality: 1970–1985. *Chest* 94:914, 1988.
5. Richards W: Hospitalization of children with status asthmaticus: A review. *Pediatrics* 84:111, 1989.
6. Anderson HR: Trends and district variations in the hospital care of childhood asthma: Results of a regional study 1970–1985. *Thorax* 45:431, 1990.
7. Gergen PJ, Weiss KB: Changing patterns of asthma hospitalization among children: 1979 to 1987. *JAMA* 264:1688, 1990.
8. National Asthma Education and Prevention Program: *Expert Panel Report: Guidelines for the Diagnosis and Management of Asthma.* Bethesda, National Institutes of Health, publ no 91-3642, 1991.
9. National Heart, Lung, and Blood Institute. *International Consensus Report on Diagnosis and Management of Asthma.* Bethesda, National Institutes of Health, publ no 92-3091, 1992.
10. National Heart, Lung, and Blood Institute and World Health Organization: *Global Initiative for Asthma.* Bethesda, National Institutes of Health publ no 95-3659, 1995.
11. National Asthma Education and Prevention Program: *Expert Panel Report II: Guidelines for the Diagnosis and Management of Asthma.* Bethesda, National Institutes of Health, publ no 97-4051, 1997.
12. Downes JJ, Wood DW, Striker TW, et al: Arterial blood gas and acid-base disorders in infants and children with status asthmaticus. *Pediatrics* 42:238, 1968.
13. Simpson H, Forfar JO, Grubb DJ: Arterial blood gas tensions and pH in acute asthma in childhood. *Br Med J* 3:460, 1968.
14. Weng TR, Langer HM, Featherby EA: Arterial blood gas tensions and acid-base balance in symp-

tomatic and asymptomatic asthma in childhood. *Am Rev Respir Dis* 101:274, 1970.

15. Nelson DR, Sachs MI, O'Connell EJ: Approaches to acute asthma and status asthmaticus in children. *Mayo Clin Proc* 64:1392, 1989.

16. Clancy RL, Cingolani HE, Taylor RR, et al: Influence of sodium bicarbonate on myocardial performance. *Am J Physiol* 212(4):917, 1967.

17. Steenbergen C, Deleeuw G, Rich T, et al: Effects of acidosis and ischemia on contractility and intracellular pH of rat heart. *Circ Res* 41(6):849, 1977.

18. Brugman SM, Larsen GL: Asthma in infants and small children. *Clin Chest Med* 16:637, 1995.

19. Zorarri ME, Busse WW: The role of respiratory infections in airway responsiveness and the pathogenesis of asthma. *Immunol Allergy Clin North Am* 10:449, 1990.

20. Gil JC, Cedillo RL, Mayagoitia BG, et al: Isolation of *Mycoplasma pneumoniae* from asthmatic patients. *Ann Allergy* 70:23, 1993.

21. Emre U, Roblin PM, Gelling M, et al: The association of *Chlamydia pneumoniae* infection and reactive airway disease in children. *Arch Pediatr Adolesc Med* 148:727, 1994.

22. Roux P, Smit M, Weinberg EG: Seasonal and recurrent intensive care unit admissions for acute severe asthma in children. *S Afr Med J* 83:177, 1993.

23. O'Hollaren MT, Yunginger JW, Offord KP, et al: Exposure to an aeroallergen as possible precipitating factor in respiratory arrest in young patients with asthma. *N Engl J Med* 324:359, 1991.

24. Weitzman M, Gortmaker S, Walker DK, et al: Maternal smoking and childhood asthma. *Pediatrics* 85:505, 1990.

25. Murray A, Morrison B: The effect of cigarette smoke from the mother on bronchial responsiveness and severity of symptoms in children with asthma. *J Allergy Clin Immunol* 77:575, 1986.

26. Martinez F, Cline M Burrows B: Increased incidence of asthma in children of smoking mothers. *Pediatrics* 89:21, 1992.

27. Fletcher HJ, Ibrahim SA, Speight N: Survey of asthma deaths in the Northern region, 1970–85. *Arch Dis Child* 65:163, 1990.

28. Martin AJ, Campbell DA, Gluyas PA, et al: Characteristics of near-fatal asthma in childhood. *Pediatr Pulmonol* 20:1, 1995.

29. Campbell DA, McLennan G, Coates JR: A comparison of asthma deaths and near-fatal asthma attacks in South Australia. *Eur Respir J* 7:490, 1994.

30. Sears MR, Rea HH, Fenwick J, et al: Deaths from asthma in New Zealand. *Arch Dis Child* 61:6, 1986.

31. Carswell F: Thirty deaths from asthma. *Arch Dis Child* 60:25, 1985.

32. Kravis LP, Kolski GB: Unexpected death in childhood asthma-a review of 13 deaths in ambulatory patients. *Am J Dis Child* 139:558, 1985.

33. Grubb BP, Wolfe DA, Nelson LA, et al: Malignant vasovagally mediated hypotension and bradycardia: A possible cause of sudden death in young patients with asthma. *Pediatrics* 90:983, 1992.

34. Strunk RC, Mrazek DA, Wolfson GS, et al: Physiologic and psychological characteristics associated with deaths due to asthma in childhood-a case controlled study. *JAMA* 254:1193, 1985.

35. Zach MS, Karner U: Sudden death in asthma. *Arch Dis Child* 64:1446, 1989.

36. McFadden ER: Fatal and near-fatal asthma. *N Engl J Med* 324(6):409, 1991.

37. Molfino NA, Nannini LJ, Martelli AN, et al: Respiratory arrest in near-fatal asthma. *N Engl J Med* 324(5):285, 1991.

38. Schoen FJ: Cardiac pathology in asthma. *J Allergy Clin Immunol* 80:419, 1987.

39. Kolski GB, Cunningham AS, Neimec PW: Hypokalemia and respiratory arrest in an infant with status asthmaticus. *J Pediatr* 112:304, 1988.

40. Robertson CF, Rubinfeld AR, Bowes G: Pediatric asthma deaths in Victoria: The mild are at risk. *Pediatr Pulmonol* 13:95, 1992.

41. Robin ED, Lewiston N: Unexpected, unexplained sudden death in young asthmatic subjects. *Chest* 96:790, 1989.

42. Saetta M, Thiene G, Crescioli S, et al: Fatal asthma in a young patient with severe bronchial hyperresponsiveness but stable peak flow records. *Eur Respir J* 2:1008, 1989.

43. Sherman JM, Capen CL: The red alert program for life-threatening asthma. *Pediatrics* 100:187, 1997.

44. Kerem E, Tibshirani R, Canny G, et al: Predicting the need for hospitalization in children with acute asthma. *Chest* 98:1355, 1990.

45. Kerem E, Canny G, Tibshirani R, et al: Clinical-physiologic correlations in acute asthma of childhood. *Pediatrics* 87:481, 1991.

46. Schuh S, Johnson D, Stephens D, et al: Hospitalization patterns in severe acute asthma in children. *Pediatr Pulmonol* 23:184, 1997.

47. Lulla S, Newcomb RW: Emergency management of asthma in children. *J Pediatr* 97:346, 1980.

48. Silver RB, Ginsburg CM: Early prediction of the

need for hospitalization in children with acute asthma. *Clin Pediatr* 23:81, 1984.

49. Galant SP, Groncy CE, Shaw KC: The value of pulsus paradoxus in assessing the child with status asthmaticus. *Pediatrics* 61:46, 1978.

50. Martell JAO, Lopez JGH, Harker JEG: Pulsus paradoxus in acute asthma in children. *J Asthma* 29:349, 1992.

51. Taylor MRH: Asthma: Audit of peak flow rate guidelines for admission and discharge. *Arch Dis Child* 70:432, 1994.

52. Ownby DR, Abarzua J, Anderson JA: Attempting to predict hospital admission in acute asthma. *Am J Dis Child* 138:1062, 1984.

53. Geelhoed GC, Landau LI, LeSouef PN: Predictive value of oxygen saturation in emergency evaluation of asthmatic children. *Br Med J* 297:393, 1988.

54. Geelhoed GC, Landau LI, LeSouef PN: Oximetry and peak expiratory flow in assessment of acute childhood asthma. *J Pediatr* 117:907, 1990.

55. Bishop J, Nolan T: Pulse oximetry in acute asthma. *Arch Dis Child* 66:724, 1991.

56. Gershel JC, Goldman HS, Stein EK, et al: The usefulness of chest radiographs in first asthma attacks. *N Engl J Med* 309:336, 1983.

57. Eggleston PA, Ward BH, Pierson WE, Et al: Radiographic abnormalities in acute asthma in children. *Pediatrics* 54:442, 1974.

58. Strunk RC: Death caused by asthma: Minimizing the risks. *J Respir Dis* 10(3):21, 1989.

59. Kikuchi Y, Okabe S, Tamura G, et al: Chemosensitivity and perception of dyspnea in patients with a history of near-fatal asthma. *N Engl J Med* 330(19):1329, 1994.

60. Stempel DA, Redding GJ: Management of acute asthma. *Pediatr Clin North Am* 39(6):1311, 1992.

61. Fergusson RJ, Stewart CM, Wathen CG, et al: Effectiveness of nebulised salbutamol administered in ambulances to patients with severe acute asthma. *Thorax* 50:81, 1995.

62. Stempel DA, Mellon M: Management of acute severe asthma. *Pediatr Clin North Am* 31(4):879, 1984.

63. Rubin BK, Marcushamer S, Priel I, et al: Emergency management of the child with asthma. *Pediatr Pulmonol* 8:45, 1990.

64. DeNicola LK, Monem GF, Gayle MO, et al: Treatment of critical status asthmaticus in children. *Pediatr Clin North Am* 41(6):1293, 1994.

65. Chopra SK, Taplin GV, Simmons DH, et al: Effects of hydration and physical therapy on tracheal transport velocity. *Am Rev Respir Dis* 115:1009, 1977.

66. Stalcup SA, Mellins RB: Mechanical forces producing pulmonary edema in acute asthma. *N Engl J Med* 297(11):592, 1977.

67. Baker JW, Yerger S, Segar WE: Elevated plasma antidiuretic hormone levels in status asthmaticus. *Mayo Clin Proc* 51:31, 1976.

68. Dawson KP, Fergusson DM, West J, et al: Acute asthma and antidiuretic hormone secretion. *Thorax* 38:589, 1983.

69. McPherson SP: *Respiratory Therapy Equipment*, 3d ed. St Louis, CV Mosby, 1985.

70. Edmunds AT, Godfrey S: Cardiovascular response during severe acute asthma and its treatment in children. *Thorax* 36:534, 1981.

71. Becker AB, Nelson NA, Simons FER: Inhaled salbutamol vs. injected epinephrine in the treatment of acute asthma in children. *J Pediatr* 102:465, 1981.

72. Oberkleid F, Mellis CM, Le Souef PN, et al: A comparison of a body weight versus a fixed dose of nebulised salbutamol in acute asthma in children. *Med J Aust* 158:751, 1993.

73. Perez-Yarza EG, Mintegui J, Garmiendia A, et al: Terbutaline sulfate turbuhaler in severe acute asthma. *Arch Dis Child* 67:1414, 1992.

74. Robertson CF, Smith F, Beck R, et al: Response to frequent low doses of nebulized salbutamol in acute asthma. *J Pediatr* 106(4):672, 1985.

75. Schuh S, Reider MJ, Canny G, et al: Nebulized albuterol in acute childhood asthma: Comparison of two doses. *Pediatrics* 86(4):509, 1990.

76. Schuh S, Parkin P, Rajan A, et al: High versus low dose frequently administered, nebulised albuterol in children with severe, acute asthma. *Pediatrics* 83(4):513, 1989.

77. Ba M, Thivierge RL, Lapierre JG, et al: Effects of continuous inhalation of salbutamol in acute asthma. *Am Rev Respir Dis* 135:A326, 1987. Abstract.

78. Montgomery VL, Eid NS: Low dose beta agonist continuous nebulization therapy for status asthmaticus in children. *J Asthma* 31(3):201, 1994.

79. Papo MC, Frank J, Thompson AE: A prospective, randomized study of continuous versus intermittent nebulized albuterol for severe status asthmaticus in children. *Crit Care Med* 21(10):1479, 1993.

80. Katz RW, Kelly HW, Crowley MR, et al: Safety of continuous nebulized albuterol for broncho-

spasm in infants and children. *Pediatrics* 92:666, 1993.

81. Craig VL, Bigos D, Brilli RJ: Efficacy and safety of continuous albuterol nebulization in children with severe status asthmaticus. *Pediatr Emerg Care* 12(1):1, 1996.

82. Kelly HW, McWilliams BC, Katz R, et al: Safety of frequent high dose nebulized terbutaline in children with acute severe asthma. *Ann Allergy* 64:229, 1990.

83. Murphy SJ, Kelly HW: Advances in the management of acute asthma in children. *Pediatr Rev* 17(7):227, 1996.

84. Moler FW, Hurwitz ME, Custer JR: Improvement in clinical asthma score and Pa_{CO_2} in children with severe asthma treated with continuously nebulized terbutaline. *J Allergy Clin Immunol* 81:1101, 1988.

85. Portnoy J, Aggarwal J: Continuous terbutaline nebulization for the treatment of severe exacerbations of asthma in children. *Ann Allergy* 60:368, 1988.

86. Moler FW, Johnson CE, Laanen CV, et al: Continuous versus intermittent nebulized terbutaline: Plasma levels and effects. *Am J Respir Crit Care Med* 151:602, 1995.

87. Buck ML: Administration of albuterol by continuous nebulization. *AACN Clin Issues* 6(2):279, 1995.

88. Benton G, Thomas RC, Nickerson BG, et al: Experience with a metered-dose inhaler with a spacer in the pediatric emergency department. *Am J Dis Child* 143:678, 1989.

89. Hickey RW, Gochman RF, Chande V, et al: Albuterol delivered via metered-dose inhaler with spacer for outpatient treatment of young children with wheezing. *Arch Pediatr Adolesc Med* 148:189, 1994.

90. Freelander M, VanAsperen PP: Nebuhaler versus nebuliser in children with acute asthma. *Br Med J* 288:1873, 1984.

91. Fuglsang G, Pedersen S: Comparison of nebuhaler and nebuliser treatment of acute severe asthma in children. *Eur J Respir Dis* 69:109, 1986.

92. Lin YZ, Hsieh KH: Metered dose inhaler and nebuliser in acute asthma. *Arch Dis Child* 72:214, 1995.

93. Ruggins NR, Milner AD, Swarbrick A: An assessment of a new breath actuated inhaler device in acutely wheezy children. *Arch Dis Child* 68:477, 1993.

94. Kerem E, Levison H, Schuh S, et al: Efficacy of albuterol administered by nebuliser versus spacer device in children with acute asthma. *J Pediatr* 123:313, 1993.

95. Sterling LP: Beta adrenergic agonists. *AACN Clin Issues* 6(2):271, 1995.

96. Kelly HW, Murphy S: Beta adrenergic agonists for acute, severe asthma. *DICP Ann Pharmacotherapy* 26:81, 1992.

97. Amirav I, Newhouse MT: Metered-dose inhaler accessory devices in acute asthma. *Arch Pediatr Adolesc Med* 151:876, 1997.

97a. Nelson HS, Bensch G, Pleskow WW, et al: Improved bronchodilation with levalbuterol compared with racemic albuterol in patients with asthma. *J Allergy Clin Immunol* 102:943, 1998.

97b. Gawchik SM, Saccar CL, Noonan M, et al: The safety and efficacy of nebulized levalbuterol compared with racemic albuterol and placebo in treatment of asthma in pediatric patients. *J Allergy Clin Immunol* 103:615, 1999.

98. Spangler DL: Review of side effects associated with beta agonists. *Ann Allergy* 62:59, 1989.

99. Reed CE: Adrenergic bronchodilators: Pharmacology and toxicology. *J Allergy Clin Immunol* 76:335, 1985.

100. Maguire JF, O'Rourke PP, Colan SD, et al: Cardiotoxicity during treatment of severe childhood asthma. *Pediatrics* 88(6):1180, 1991.

101. Connett G, Lenney W: Prolonged hypoxemia after nebulized salbutamol. *Thorax* 48:574, 1993.

102. Baraldi E, Azzolin NM, Zanconato S, et al: Corticosteroids decrease exhaled nitric oxide in children with acute asthma. *J Pediatr* 131:381, 1997.

103. Nelson BV, Sears S, Woods J, et al: Expired nitric oxide as a marker for childhood asthma. *J Pediatr* 130:423, 1997.

104. Deshpande A, McKenzie SA: Short course of steroids in home treatment of children with acute asthma. *Br Med J* 293:169, 1986.

105. Harris JB, Weinberger MM, Nassif E, et al: Early intervention with short courses of prednisone to prevent progression of asthma in ambulatory patients incompletely responsive to bronchodilators. *J Pediatr* 110(4):627, 1987.

106. Horowitz L, Zafrir O, Gilboa S, et al: Acute asthma. Single dose oral steroids in paediatric community clinics. *Eur J Pediatr* 153:526, 1994.

107. Shapiro GG, Furukawa CT, Pierson WE, et al: Double-blind evaluation of methylprednisolone versus placebo for acute asthma episodes. *Pediatrics* 71(4):510, 1983.

108. Scarfone RJ, Fuchs SM, Nager AL, et al: Controlled trial of oral prednisone in the emergency

department treatment of children with acute asthma. *Pediatrics* 92(4):513, 1993.

109. Grant CC, Duggan AK, De Angelis C: Independent parental administration of prednisone in acute asthma: A double-blind, placebo-controlled, crossover study. *Pediatrics* 96(2):224, 1995.

110. Wolfson DH, Nypaver MM, Blaser M, et al: A controlled trial of methylprednisolone in the early emergency department treatment of acute asthma in children. *Pediatr Emerg Care* 10:335, 1994.

111. Tal A, Levy N, Bearman JE: Methylprednisolone therapy for acute asthma in infants and toddlers: A controlled clinical trial. *Pediatrics* 86(3):350, 1990.

112. Webb MSC, Henry RL, Milner AD: Oral corticosteroids for wheezing attacks under 18 months. *Arch Dis Child* 61:15, 1986.

112a. Wilson NM, Silverman M: Treatment of acute, episodic asthma in preschool children using intermittent high dose inhaled steroids at home. *Arch Dis Child* 65:407, 1990.

112b. Svedmyr J, Nyberg E, Asbrink-Nilsson E, et al: Intermittent treatment with inhaled steroids for deterioration of asthma due to upper respiratory tract infections. *Acta Paediatr* 84:884, 1995.

112c. Garret J, Williams S, Wong C, et al: Treatment of acute asthmatic exacerbations with an increased dose of inhaled steroid. *Arch Dis Child* 79:12, 1998.

112d. Volovitz B, Bentur L, Finkelstein Y, et al: Effectiveness and safety of inhaled corticosteroids in controlling acute asthma attacks in children who were treated in the emergency department: A controlled comperative study with oral prednisolone. *J Allergy Clin Immunol* 102:605, 1998.

113. Pierson WE, Bierman W, Kelley VC: A double-blind trial of corticosteroid therapy in status asthmaticus. *Pediatrics* 54:282, 1974.

114. Loren ML, Chai H, Leung P, et al: Corticosteroids in the treatment of acute exacerbations of asthma. *Ann Allergy* 45:67, 1980.

115. Younger RE, Gerber PS, Herrod HG, et al: Intravenous methylprednisolone efficacy in status asthmaticus in childhood. *Pediatrics* 80:225, 1987.

116. Daugbjerg P, Brenoe E, Forchhammer H, et al: A comparison between nebulized terbutaline, nebulized corticosteroid and systemic corticosteroid for acute wheezing in children up to 18 months of age. *Acta Pediatr* 82:547, 1993.

117. Kattan M, Gurwitz D, Levison H: Corticosteroids in status asthmaticus. *J Pediatr* 96:596, 1980.

118. Barnett PLJ, Caputo GL, Baskin M, et al: Intravenous versus oral corticosteroids in the management

of acute asthma in children. *Ann Emerg Med* 29(2):212, 1997.

119. Scarfone RJ, Loiselle JM, Wiley JF, et al: Nebulized dexamethasone versus oral prednisone in the emergency treatment of asthmatic children. *Ann Emerg Med* 26:480, 1995.

120. Harfi H, Hanissian AS, Crawford LV: Treatment of status asthmaticus in children with high doses and conventional doses of methylprednisolone. *Pediatrics* 61(6):829, 1978.

121. Storr J, Barry W, Barrelle E, et al: Effect of a single dose of prednisolone in acute childhood asthma. *Lancet* 1:879, 1987.

121a. Dawson KL, Carter ER: A steroid-induced acute psychosis in a child with asthma. *Pediatr Pulmonology* 26:362, 1998.

122. Zora JA, Zimmerman D, Carey TL, et al: Hypothalamic-pituitary-adrenal axis suppression after short-term, high-dose glucocorticoid therapy in children with asthma. *J Allergy Clin Immunol* 77:9, 1986.

123. Dolan LM, Kesarwala HH, Holroyde JC, et al: Short-term, high-dose systemic steroids in children with asthma: The effect on the hypothalamic-pituitary-adrenal axis. *J Allergy Clin Immunol* 80:81, 1987.

124. Kelly HW, Murphy S: Should anticholinergics be used in acute severe asthma? *DICP Ann Pharmacother* 24:409, 1990.

125. Davis A, Vickerson F, Worsley G, et al: Determination of dose-response relationship for nebulized ipratropium in asthmatic children. *J Pediatr* 105(6):1002, 1984.

126. DeNicola L, Monem GF, Gayle MO, et al: Treatment of critical status asthmaticus in children. *Pediatr Clin North Am* 41(6):1293, 1994.

127. Nakagawa TA, Guerra L, Storgion SA: Aerosolized atropine as an unusual cause of anisocoria in a child with asthma. *Pediatr Emerg Care* 9(3):153, 1993.

128. Schuh S, Johnson DW, Callahan S, et al: Efficacy of frequent nebulized ipratropium bromide added to frequent high-dose albuterol therapy in severe childhood asthma. *J Pediatr* 126(4):639, 1995.

129. Naspitz CK, Sole D: Treatment of acute wheezing and dyspnea attacks in children under 2 years old: Inhalation of fenoterol plus ipratropium bromide versus fenoterol. *J Asthma* 29(4):253, 1992.

130. Reisman J, Galdes-Sebalt M, Kazim F, et al: Frequent administration by inhalation of salbutamol and ipratropium bromide in the initial manage-

ment of severe acute asthma in children. *J Allergy Clin Immunol* 81(1):16, 1988.

131. Beck R, Robertson C, Galdes-Sebalt M, et al: Combined salbutamol and ipratropium bromide by inhalation in the treatment of severe acute asthma. *J Pediatr* 107(4):605, 1985.

131a. Qureshi F, Pestian J, Davis P, et al: Effect of nebulized ipratropium on the hospitalization rates of children with asthma. *N Engl J Med* 339:1030, 1998.

131b. Zorc JJ, Pusic MV, Ogborn CJ, et al: Ipratropium bromide added to asthma treatment in the pediatric emergency department. *Pediatrics* 103:748, 1999.

132. Boner AL, De Stefano G, Niero E, et al: Salbutamol and ipratropium bromide solution in the treatment of bronchospasm in asthmatic children. *Ann Allergy* 58:54, 1987.

133. Storr J, Lenney W: Nebulized ipratropium and salbutamol in asthma. *Arch Dis Child* 61:602, 1986.

134. Fitzgerald JM, Grunfeld A, Pare PD, et al: The clinical efficacy of combination nebulized anticholinergic and adrenergic bronchodilators vs. nebulized adrenergic bronchodilator alone in acute asthma. *Chest* 111(2):311, 1997.

135. Goldberg P, Leffert F, Gonzales M, et al: Intravenous aminophylline therapy for asthma. *Am J Dis Child* 134:596, 1980.

136. Weinberger M: Theophylline: When should it be used? *J Pediatr* 122(3):403, 1993.

137. Needleman JP, Kaifer MC, Nold JT, et al: Theophylline does not shorten hospital stay for children admitted for asthma. *Arch Pediatr Adolesc Med* 149:206, 1995.

138. Carter E, Cruz M, Chesrown S, et al: Efficacy of intravenously administered theophylline in children hospitalized with asthma. *J Pediatr* 122(3):470, 1993.

139. Strauss RE, Wertheim DL, Bonagura VR, et al: Aminophylline therapy does not improve outcome and increases adverse effects in children hospitalized with acute asthmatic exacerbations. *Pediatrics* 93:205, 1994.

140. DiGiulio GA, Kercsmar CM, Krug SE, et al: Hospital treatment of asthma: Lack of benefit from theophylline given in addition to nebulized albuterol and intravenously administered corticosteroid. *J Pediatr* 122:464, 1993.

141. Bien JP, Bloom MD, Evans RL, et al: Intravenous theophylline in pediatric status asthmaticus. *Clin Pediatr* 34:475, 1995.

141a. Yung M, South M: Randomised controlled trial of aminophylline for severe acute asthma. *Arch Dis Child* 79:405, 1998.

142. Newcomb RW, Akhter J: Respiratory failure from asthma. *Am J Dis Child* 142:1041, 1988.

143. Stein R, Canny GJ, Bohn DJ, et al: Severe acute asthma in a pediatric intensive care unit: Six years' experience. *Pediatrics* 83(6):1023, 1989.

144. Dworkin G, Kattan M: Mechanical ventilation for status asthmaticus in children. *J Pediatr* 114:545, 1989.

145. Cox RG, Barker GA, Bohn DJ: Efficacy, results and complications of mechanical ventilation in children with status asthmaticus. *Pediatr Pulmonol* 11:120, 1991.

146. Bohn DJ, Kalloghlian A, Jenkins J, et al: Intravenous salbutamol in the treatment of status asthmaticus in children. *Crit Care Med* 12(10):892, 1984.

147. Browne GJ, Penna AS, Phung X, et al: Randomized trial of intravenous salbutamol in early management of acute severe asthma in children. *Lancet* 349:301, 1997.

148. Geller M: Acute management of severe childhood asthma. *AACN Clin Issues* 7(4):519, 1996.

149. Fuglsgang G, Pedersen S, Borgstrom L: Dose-response relationships of intravenously administered terbutaline in children with asthma. *J Pediatr* 114(2):315, 1989.

150. Scoggin CH, Sahn SA, Petty TL: Status asthmaticus. A nine-year experience. *JAMA* 238(11):1158, 1977.

151. Wood DW, Downes JJ, Lecks HI: The management of respiratory failure in childhood status asthmaticus. Experience with 30 episodes and evolution of a technique. *J Allergy* 42(5):261, 1968.

152. Simpson H, Mitchell I, Inglis JM, et al: Severe ventilatory failure in asthma in children. *Arch Dis Child* 53:714, 1978.

153. Simons FER, Pierson WE, Bierman CW: Respiratory failure in childhood status asthmaticus. *Am J Dis Child* 131:1097, 1977.

154. Jagoda A, Shepherd SM, Spevitz A, et al: Refractory asthma, part 2: Airway interventions and management. *Ann Emerg Med* 29(2):275, 1997.

155. Mountain RD, Sahn SA: Clinical features and outcome in patients with acute asthma presenting with hypercapnia. *Am Rev Respir Dis* 138:535, 1988.

156. Nehama J, Pass R, Bechtler-Karsch A, et al: Continuous ketamine infusion for the treatment of refractory asthma in a mechanically ventilated infant:

Case report and review of the pediatric literature. *Pediatr Emerg Care* 12(4):294, 1996.

157. Strube PJ, Hallam PL: Ketamine by continuous infusion in status asthmaticus. *Anaesthesia* 41:1017, 1986.

158. Rock MJ, De La Rocha SR, L'Hommedieu CS, et al: Use of ketamine in asthmatic children to treat respiratory failure refractory to conventional therapy. *Crit Care Med* 14(5):514, 1986.

159. L'Hommedieu CS, Arens JJ: The use of ketamine for the emergency intubation of patients with status asthmaticus. *Ann Emerg Med* 16(5):568, 1987.

160. Wetzel RC: Pressure support ventilation in children with severe asthma. *Crit Care Med* 24(9):1603, 1996.

161. Santiago SM, Klaustermeyer WB: Mortality in status asthmaticus: A nine year experience in a respiratory intensive care unit. *J Asthma Res* 17(2):75, 1980.

162. Mansel JK, Stogner SW, Petrini MF, et al: Mechanical ventilation in patients with acute severe asthma. *Am J Med* 89:42, 1990.

163. Rosello HJ: Sulfato de magnesia. *Prensa Med Argentina* 23:1677, 1936.

164. Ciarallo L, Sauer AH, Shannon MW: Intravenous magnesium therapy for moderate to severe pediatric asthma: Results of a randomized, placebo controlled trial. *J Pediatr* 129(6):809, 1996.

165. Pabon H, Monem G, Kissoon N: Safety and efficacy of magnesium sulfate infusions in children with status asthmaticus. *Pediatr Emerg Care* 10(4):200, 1994.

166. Monem G, Kissoon N, DeNicola L: Use of magnesium sulfate in asthma in childhood. *Pediatr Ann* 25(3):136, 1996.

167. Noppen M, Vanmaele L, Impens N, et al: Bronchodilating effect of intravenous magnesium sulfate in acute severe bronchial asthma. *Chest* 97(2):373, 1990.

168. West JB: *Respiratory Physiology—The Essentials,* 5th ed. Baltimore, Williams & Wilkins, 1995.

169. Barach AL: The therapeutic use of helium. *JAMA* 107(16):1273, 1936.

170. Manthous CA, Hall JB, Melmed A, et al: Heliox improves pulsus paradoxus and peak expiratory flow in nonintubated patients with severe asthma. *Am J Respir Crit Care Med* 151:310, 1995.

171. Kass JE, Castriotta RJ: Heliox therapy in acute severe asthma. *Chest* 107(3):757, 1995.

172. Kudukis TM, Manthous CA, Schmidt GA, et al: Inhaled helium-oxygen revisited: Effect of inhaled helium-oxygen during the treatment of status asthmaticus in children. *J Pediatr* 130:217, 1997.

173. Carter ER, Webb CR, Moffitt DR: Evaluation of heliox in children hospitalized with acute severe asthma. *Chest* 109(5):1257, 1996.

174. Betts EK, Parkin CE: Use of ketamine in an asthmatic child. *Anaesth Analg* 50(3):420, 1971.

175. Roy TM, Pruitt VL, Garner PA, et al: The potential role of anesthesia in status asthmaticus. *J Asthma* 29(2):73, 1992.

176. White PF, Way WL, Trevor AJ: Ketamine—its pharmacology and therapeutic uses. *Anesthesiology* 56:119, 1982.

177. O'Rourke PP, Crone RK: Halothane in status asthmaticus. *Crit Care Med* 10(3):341, 1982.

178. Revell S, Greenhalgh D, Absalom SR, et al: Isoflurane in the treatment of asthma. *Anaesthesia* 43:477, 1988.

179. Johnston RG, Noseworthy TW, Friesen EG, et al: Isoflurane therapy for status asthmaticus in children and adults. *Chest* 97:698, 1990.

180. Otte RW, Fireman P: Isoflurane anethesia for the treatment of the refractory status asthmaticus. *Ann Allergy* 66:305, 1991.

181. Nishiyama K, Kawai T, Niu S, et al: A case report of successful treatment using ECMO in severe status asthmaticus during open heart surgery. *Kyobu Geka—Japanese J Thoracic Surg* 42(12):1029, 1989.

182. Kattan M: Management of acute asthma: A continuing challenge. *J Pediatr* 129:783, 1996.

CHAPTER 16

ACUTE ASTHMA
IN PREGNANCY

Michael Schatz
Robert A. Wise

INTRODUCTION

Asthma complicates approximately 4% of pregnancies, making it one of the most common potentially serious medical problems to complicate pregnancy.[1] Episodes of acute asthma requiring emergency department (ED) visits or hospitalizations have been reported in 9% to 11% of pregnant women prospectively managed by asthma specialists.[2–4] However, hospitalizations for asthma exacerbations occurred in 42% to 46% of asthmatic women retrospectively identified from obstetric records.[5,6] Acute asthma may be associated with maternal hypoxia, which may lead directly to fetal hypoxia.[7] In addition, acute asthma and its treatment may be associated with dehydration, hypotension, hypertension, alkalosis, or hypocapnia, all of which may adversely affect fetal oxygenation by reducing uteroplacental blood flow.[7] Presumably through these mechanisms, acute asthma during pregnancy has been associated with adverse effects that range from fetal mortality to reduced intrauterine growth.[8,9] *Prevention* of episodes of acute asthma in theory will reduce the likelihood of these adverse outcomes. In addition, optimal *treatment* of acute asthma during pregnancy should reduce the maternal and fetal morbidity and mortality that is potentially associated with these episodes. Indeed, in two recent studies in which the asthma was managed by pulmonary or allergy specialists, acute episodes of asthma that were aggressively managed were not associated with increased maternal or fetal morbidity or mortality.[4,10]

This chapter reviews gestational pulmonary physiologic changes and the clinical interrelationships between asthma and pregnancy, and discusses general and specific information regarding the effects of asthma medications on pregnancy. Based on this information, prevention of acute episodes through optimal prophylactic and home management is also discussed. Finally, management of acute asthma during pregnancy, including assessment, emergency therapy, hospital management, and treatment of respiratory failure will be described.

PULMONARY PHYSIOLOGIC CHANGES DURING PREGNANCY

Pulmonary physiologic changes during pregnancy have been recently reviewed[11,12] and are summarized in Table 16-1. The most consistent and striking change in static lung volumes is the reduction in end-expiratory lung volume (functional residual capacity, FRC) and expiratory reserve volume (ERV). Beginning during the second trimester, the FRC falls progressively by about 10% to 25%. The reduction in ERV is accompanied by a compensatory increase in inspiratory capacity (IC) so that the vital capacity (VC) is preserved. The reduction in FRC is associated with a decrease in chest wall compliance during late pregnancy (both are likely due to the mechanical effects of the enlarging uterus compressing the abdominal compartment). This decrease in chest wall compliance

Table 16-1
Changes in Lung Functions with Pregnancy

Measure	Change with pregnancy
TLC	↓ ↔
VC	↑ ↔
FRC	↓
RV	↔ ↓
Lung compliance	↔
Chest wall compliance	↓
Total respiratory compliance	↓
Pa_{O_2}	↑
Pa_{CO_2}	↓
pH	↔
Minute ventilation	↑
Tidal volume (TV)	↑
Breathing rate (f)	↔
Airway conductance (raw)	↑
Closing volume (CV)	↑ ↔
Closing capacity (CC)	↔
FEV_1	↔
MVV	↔
PEFR	↔ ↓
Dl_{CO}, rest upright	↔
Dl_{CO}, rest supine	↓
Dl_{CO}, exercise	↔

KEY: ↑, increase; ↓, decrease; ↔, no change. When two symbols are given, it indicates a diversity of findings in different studies. The second symbol represents the most prevalent or most current finding.
SOURCE: With permission, from Wise.[11]

is thought to be offset by relaxin or other hormonal factors that also increase pelvic flexibility.[11]

Blood gases change substantially during pregnancy due to changes in ventilation. An increased Pa_{O_2} value (100 to 105 mm Hg) and a decreased Pa_{CO_2} (32 to 34 mm Hg) result from the 20% to 40% increase in gestational minute ventilation. This increase is the result of an increase in tidal volume (TV) with an unchanged respiratory rate and is attributed to the effects of increased serum progesterone, which stimulates respiratory center drive. The pH is maintained by renal compensation for the respiratory alkalosis by increased excretion of bicarbonate.

These blood gas changes have important specific implications for the assessment and management of acute gestational asthma. The hypocapnia and alkalosis of early acute asthma may be superimposed on the chronic (compensated or partially compensated) respiratory alkalosis of pregnancy, leading to increased hypocapnia and alkalosis. A given Pa_{O_2} value during pregnancy (e.g., 70 mm Hg) suggests more severe asthma than it would in a nonpregnant patient, since a pregnant patient starts with a higher normal value. Finally, a Pa_{CO_2} value of 35 mm Hg or more is consistent with respiratory failure during pregnancy.

Airway mechanics appear to change marginally or not at all during pregnancy. A slight increase in airway conductance has been reported during pregnancy, but most studies have shown no change in closing volume or closing capacity. In addition, no significant change in FEV_1, FEV_1/FVC ratio or flow rates at lower lung volumes have been reported during pregnancy. Thus, abnormalities of spirometry during pregnancy should be attributed to lung disease, not pregnancy. However, one study has reported that the FEV_1 and peak-expiratory flow rate (PEFR) are lower in pregnancy in a supine position compared with the seated position.[13] This suggests that women experiencing acute asthma should avoid the supine position. Other studies regarding PEFR during pregnancy have been conflicting; two studies have suggested a decrease in late pregnancy.[14,15] while two other studies[16,17] have reported no significant change in PEFR during pregnancy in normal women.

Most investigators have concluded that there is either no effect or a slight fall in the diffusing capacity for carbon monoxide (Dl_{CO}) during pregnancy. However, the normal increase in Dl_{CO} in the supine position is absent or diminished in pregnancy. One possible explanation for this is that the cardiac output normally rises in the supine position in nonpregnant women but falls in pregnant women as the result of uterine compression of the inferior vena cava.

Dyspnea, either a heightened sensation of breathing at rest or a sensation of breathlessness with exercise, occurs in 70% to 80% of pregnant women by 30 weeks gestation. The exact mechanism of this "physiologic" dyspnea is not certain, but it is generally attributed to either an increased drive to breathe or an increased work of breathing. A clinically important point is to differentiate this dyspnea of pregnancy from pathologic causes of gestational dyspnea. In this regard, numerous factors have been presented as indicators for pathologic dyspnea in pregnancy[11] including 1) history of cardiac or respiratory disease, 2) sudden onset or worsening of dyspnea, 3) respiratory rate greater than 20, 4) alveolar-arterial O_2 gradient greater than 25 mm Hg, 5) Pa_{CO_2} less than 30 mm Hg or greater than 35 mm Hg, 6) abnormal spirometry measurements, or 7) abnormal total lung capacity (TLC).

INTERRELATIONSHIPS BETWEEN ASTHMA AND PREGNANCY

Effect of Pregnancy on the Course of Asthma

Asthma may improve, worsen, or remain unchanged during pregnancy.[17a] Juniper and Newhouse have recently performed a systematic review and meta-analysis of the literature addressing the effect of pregnancy on the course of asthma.[18] They reviewed 14 original studies published since 1953. They concluded that the results of these studies were very inconsistent, but that three meta-analyses suggested that one third of women improve, one third worsen and one third stay the same during pregnancy. The variability in results among the studies may have been owing primarily to methodological differences, but differences in asthma severity among study populations may also play a role, since patients with severe asthma prior to pregnancy may be more likely to experience more severe asthma during pregnancy than patients with milder asthma.[19]

The mechanisms underlying these changes in asthma course during pregnancy remain unknown. Based on control data in nonpregnant women, as well as the generally observed postpartum reversion of asthma to the pre-pregnancy course, Juniper and Newhouse concluded that the changes in asthma course observed during pregnancy were more than just random fluctuations in the natural course of the disease.[18] There are a number of gestational physiologic changes that have the potential to directly or indirectly improve or worsen asthma, but the overall importance of any of these factors is unknown and may vary from individual to individual.[20] It has been demonstrated that women are usually (59% to 63%) concordant between successive pregnancies regarding their change in asthma course.[21] Thus, it appears that some of the responsible factors may remain constant in an individual from pregnancy to pregnancy, whereas other relevant changes may vary between pregnancies. Upper respiratory infections are likely the most common precipitants of severe gestational asthma.[20]

Several observations have been made regarding the course of asthma and the stage of pregnancy. Gluck and Gluck reported that the peak incidence of asthma flares occurred in the sixth month of gestation.[19] More recently, Stenius-Aarniala and colleagues reported that acute episodes of asthma were most likely to occur between gestational weeks 17 to 24.[4] Schatz and colleagues reported that symptoms in women whose asthma improved during pregnancy gradually decreased with advancing pregnancy, while symptoms peaked between 29 and 32 weeks gestation in women whose asthma worsened during pregnancy.[21] Both the Stenius-Aarniala and Schatz studies reported that, women with asthma tend to experience fewer symptoms or acute episodes during the last 4 weeks of pregnancy than during any other 4-week gestational period.[4,21] Finally, troublesome asthma during labor and delivery is extremely rare in prospectively managed asthmatic women.[21]

Outcome of Pregnancy in Asthmatic Women

Controlled studies that compared the outcome of pregnancy in patients with asthma to outcomes in concurrently followed nonasthmatic women have been recently reviewed.[9] Maternal asthma, especially when more severe or uncontrolled, may increase the risk of perinatal complications such as preeclampsia, perinatal mortality, preterm births, and low birthweight infants. In addition, severe asthma may be a cause of maternal mortality.[8]

Potential mechanisms that may explain the apparent increased perinatal risks in the pregnan-cies of asthmatic women include hypoxia and other adverse physiologic consequences of uncontrolled asthma, asthma medications, common sociodemo-graphic characteristics, and/or common pathoge-netic factors. The latter could include factors that predispose a patient to bronchial hyperreactivity as well as vascular and uterine muscle hyperreac-

Table 16-2
Potential Mechanisms of Increased Adverse Perinatal Outcomes Associated with Maternal Asthma

Hypothetical mechanism	Outcome	Supporting Data
Severely uncontrolled asthma	Perinatal mortality	"Severe" asthma during pregnancy has been associated with perinatal mortality,[9] while asthma managed by asthma specialists during pregnancy has not been associated with increased perinatal mortality.[2,3,28,35]
Moderately uncontrolled asthma	Intrauterine growth retarda-tion (IUGR)	Infants of mothers hospitalized during pregnancy for status asthmaticus weighed significantly less than infants of mothers who did not require emergency therapy for asthma;[3,79] lower maternal pulmonary function during pregnancy in asthmatic women was associated with an increased risk of IUGR.[80]
Medication	Preeclampsia	Incidence of preeclampsia increased in asthmatic subjects treated with *prednisone* in two studies,[10,35] *theophylline* in another.[28]
Medication	Prematurity	Incidence of preterm and low-birthweight infants increased in *corticosteroid*-dependent asthmatic subjects compared to non-corticosteroid-treated asthmatics or controls[5]
Medication	IUGR	Birthweight in infants of mothers treated with *prednisone* 10 mg daily throughout pregnancy (for pregnancy main-tenance) decreased compared to control infants.[36]
Common sociodemographic characteristics	Maternal smoking	Incidence of smoking in asthmatic versus nonasthmatic pregnant women increased[81-84]; maternal smoking associ-ated with increased perinatal mortality[85] prematurity[86] and low birthweight.[87]
Common sociodemographic characteristics	African-American	Prevalence of African-American asthmatic subjects in-creased[84,88]; incidence of low-birthweight infants of Afri-can-American mothers increased.[89]
Common pathogenetic factors	Preterm birth	Increased bronchial hyperreactivity demonstrated in 68% of women delivering preterm infants for no identifiable reasons;[90] increased incidence of preterm births in pa-tients with more severe asthma requiring corticosteroids[5]
Common pathogenetic factors	Preeclampsia	Vascular α-adrenergic hyperreactivity and β-adrenergic hy-poreactivity demonstrated in asthmatic subjects;[12] in-creased preeclampsia in patients with more severe asthma requiring corticosteroids;[9,35] endothelin and an-giotensin, which may be involved in preeclampsia,[91] are bronchoconstrictors[92,93]

SOURCE: Modified from Schatz et al.[12]

tivity (e.g., circulating mediators that act on smooth muscle or autonomic nervous system abnormalities). The data supporting these various mechanisms are summarized in Table 16-2. It is particularly difficult to differentiate the effects of corticosteroids used to treat more severe asthma from the effects of uncontrolled asthma itself or from associated extrapulmonary smooth muscle hyperreactivity in patients with more severe asthma. Although the precise mechanisms remain undefined, the lack of increased adverse fetal and infant outcomes in four prospective studies in which the asthma was managed by allergy or pulmonary specialists[9] supports the hypothesis that optimal control of asthma during pregnancy improves perinatal outcome.

USE OF ASTHMA MEDICATIONS DURING PREGNANCY

General Information[22]

A number of general principles apply to drug teratogenicity. The developmental insult will be dependent on the dose, route of delivery, duration of exposure, and precise gestational age at the time of exposure to the drug. The ultimate effect on the conceptus will also depend on the genetic make-up of the mother and the conceptus, and on the interaction with other possible environmental agents.

The conceptus is most susceptible to major organ malformations during the period of embryogenesis, from 4 to 10 completed weeks after the onset of the last menstrual period. When considering birth defects, it is important to be aware of the background risk factor. In the general population, major congenital malformations are identified in approximately 2% to 4% of all newborns. Another 2% may become apparent by the age of 1 year. Minor malformations occur in an additional 10% to 20% of children.

Genetic and chromosomal abnormalities probably account for approximately 25% of congenital defects. Approximately 1% of all birth defects are attributed specifically to medications.[1]

The cause of approximately 65% of congenital anomalies remains unknown. After 10 weeks of gestation, fully formed fetal organs continue to be susceptible to other effects of drugs taken by the mother, especially intrauterine growth and central nervous system development.

Information regarding the effects of drugs administered during pregnancy may come from several sources. Appropriately performed animal studies that do not reveal teratogenicity of an agent are reassuring, although animal studies showing adverse effects are harder to interpret due to species variability and dose considerations.[23] Case reports of human malformations must be considered, although the coincidental occurrence of a sporadic birth defect cannot be excluded. Most prospective cohort studies of asthma medications during pregnancy suffer from low statistical power, and retrospective case-control studies may be subject to recall bias.

Two large prospective studies have addressed the relationship between medication prescribed during early pregnancy (including asthma medications) and subsequent congenital malformations. The Collaborative Perinatal Project (CPP) was initially undertaken to identify factors during pregnancy or delivery that might be related to the risk of infant cerebral palsy or other adverse neurologic outcomes. The data were subsequently reorganized and reanalyzed to investigate the possible teratogenic role of drugs used in the first 4 lunar months of pregnancy.[24]

The final cohort included 50,282 women seen in 12 United States centers between 1959 and 1965 whose pregnancies lasted longer than 20 weeks gestation. Data from the study were presented as relative risks (i.e., the ratio of the malformation rate in exposed versus unexposed mother-child pairs) and statistical significance was tested. However, because of the complexities involved in such analyses, the authors warn that "none of the associations presented in this book should be regarded as anything more than hypothesis requiring independent confirmation.[24]" Conversely, lack of an association between a specific drug and congenital malformations cannot be taken as proof of safety because of sample-size considerations.

More recently, Briggs and colleagues have described the results of a surveillance study of Michigan Medicaid recipients involving 229,101 completed pregnancies conducted between 1985 and 1992.[25] The data were not considered to support an association between the drug and congenital defects in subjects receiving a number of asthma medications (see below). It is important to point out that these data have not been published in a peer-reviewed journal.

In 1979, the Food and Drug Administration (FDA) in the United States established five categories to describe a drug's potential to cause adverse effects during pregnancy (Table 16-3) and mandated that newly approved drugs introduced into this country after November 1, 1980 be classified into one of these categories in the package insert.[26] These categories are based on the results of animal studies, human data, and a consideration as to whether the benefit of use during pregnancy may outweigh the risk. Unfortunately, no asthma medication labeled to date meets the requirement for category A which states that "Adequate and well-controlled studies in pregnant women have failed to demonstrate a risk to the fetus in the first trimester of pregnancy and there is no evidence of a risk in later trimesters."

Specific Medications

The human gestational data for specific asthma medications, as well as their FDA pregnancy classifications and years of introduction into the United States, are summarized in Table 16-4. The choice of a specific medication for use in treating asthma during pregnancy should be based on 1) an evaluation of the available animal and human data with respect to the use of the drug during pregnancy, 2) the general efficacy of and necessity for the medication, 3) the route of administration (i.e., inhaled versus systemic), and 4) the length of time the drug has been in clinical use.[12] Based on these considerations, the Working Group on Asthma and Pregnancy of the National Asthma Education Program evaluated the information available up until 1993 and made recommendations regarding asthma drugs "preferred" for use

Table 16-3
FDA Pregnancy Categories

A	Controlled studies in pregnant women fail to demonstrate a risk to the fetus in the first trimester with no evidence of risk in later trimesters. The possibility of fetal harm appears remote.
B	Either animal-reproduction studies have not demonstrated a fetal risk but there are no controlled studies in pregnant women, or animal-reproduction studies have shown an adverse effect (other than a decrease in fertility) that was not confirmed in controlled studies in women in the first trimester and there is no evidence of a risk in later trimesters.
C	Either studies in animals have revealed adverse effects on the fetus (teratogenic or embryocidal effects or other) and there are no controlled studies in women, or studies in women and animals are not available. Drugs should be given only if the potential benefits justify the potential risk to the fetus.
D	There is positive evidence of human fetal risk, but the benefits from use in pregnant women may be acceptable despite the risk (eg, if the drug is needed in a life-threatening situation or for a serious disease for which safer drugs cannot be used or are ineffective).
X	Studies in animals or human beings have demonstrated fetal abnormalities or there is evidence of fetal risk based on human experience, or both, and the risk of the use of the drug in pregnant women clearly outweighs any possible benefit. The drug is contraindicated in women who are or may become pregnant.

during pregnancy.[1] These recommendations and other clinical implications of the data in Table 16-4 are described below. In the near future, information from ongoing clinical trials should become available to further inform treatment of asthma in pregnancy.[26a]

Bronchodilators   Inhaled β_2 agonists were recommended by the Working Group,[1] but the available data were considered insufficient to warrant recommending a specific inhaled β_2 agonist. Metaproterenol, terbutaline, and albuterol have been reported to be the most commonly used drugs, in recent studies.[10,25] Oral β_2 agonists were not generally suggested for use during pregnancy because of 1) limited data during early pregnancy, 2) potential inhibition of labor, and 3) increased side effects with little increased benefit in most subjects properly using inhaled β_2 agonists. However, if a systemic β_2 agonist is required, terbutaline was recommended by the Working Group due to the reassuring animal studies and the lack of adverse effects on uterine blood flow.[1]

A suspicion of an association of theophylline with congenital malformations has been raised in a report of three patients[27] and in the Michigan Medicaid study.[25] However, in the latter study, it is stated that other factors, such as the mother's disease, concurrent drug use, and chance may be involved.[25] In one additional study, preeclampsia was increased in patients receiving theophylline, but theophylline-treated patients in this study were also more likely than nontheophylline-treated subjects to experience asthma exacerbations and to require corticosteroids.[28] Theophylline was considered appropriate by the Working Group for use during pregnancy, but recommended current asthma practice in general and the above information suggests that theophylline should generally be reserved for patients not adequately controlled by cromolyn or inhaled corticosteroids.

Salmeterol has been introduced into the United States since the Working Group completed its report. Animal studies with salmeterol have not been reassuring[29] and there are no published human data. Salmeterol is not generally recommended for use during pregnancy in preference to older β_2 agonists, cromolyn, or inhaled corticosteroids (see below), but benefit-risk considerations may favor its continuation during pregnancy in patients with moderate or severe asthma who have demonstrated a very good therapeutic response prior to becoming pregnant. Based on recent efficacy data,[30–32] salmeterol may also be considered as an alternative to theophylline in pregnant patients not controlled on medium-dose inhaled corticosteroids (see below).

Prophylactic asthma medications   The Working Group recommended cromolyn for use during pregnancy, and beclomethasone was suggested as the inhaled corticosteroid of choice for gestational use because there is more published experience on its use during pregnancy than there is for other inhaled corticosteroids. A recent study from the Swedish Medical Birth Registry[100] (Table 16-4) suggests that budesonide could also be considered an inhaled corticosteroid of choice for use during pregnancy.

Four prophylactic medications have become available in the United States since the Working Group completed its report: nedocromil, montelukast, zafirlukast and zileuton. Animal studies with nedocromil have been reassuring,[29] but there are no published human data. It probably would not be chosen over cromolyn or inhaled corticosteroids for use during pregnancy in general, although the reassuring animal studies and inhalational route of delivery suggest that benefit-risk considerations might favor its continuation during pregnancy in patients responding well to it prior to pregnancy.

Animal studies have been reassuring for montelukast and zafirlukast but not for zileuton.[29] There are no human data for these drugs, and they are all oral medications. Zileuton cannot be recommended for use during pregnancy at this time, and montelukast and zafirlukast would only be considered in a patient with recalcitrant asthma who has shown a uniquely favorable response to one of these drugs prior to pregnancy.

Systemic corticosteroids   Systemic corticosteroids (prednisone, methylprednisolone, hydrocortisone) were recommended by the Working Group when indicated for the treatment of severe asthma during pregnancy.[1] However, the potential role of corticosteroids in contributing to adverse perinatal outcomes in the pregnancies of women with asthma warrants special consideration.

In a large case-control study of 20,830 infants with congenital malformations, the proportion of mothers who received oral corticosteroids was not significantly different than normal controls.[33] However, another recent case-control study found

Table 16-4

Data on the Safety of Asthma Medications During Pregnancy

Drug/yr introduced (U.S.)	FDA Class (see Table 1)	Human Data	
		Congenital Malformations (CM)	Other
Sympathomimetic bronchodilators			
Multiple		No increase in 448 patients[10]	No increase in preeclampsia, preterm or low birthweight (LBW) infants[10]
Systemic–Specific			
Epinephrine/pre-1938	±	Increased CM in 189 subjects in CPP[24]; 0/35 MM[25] (1.5 expected)	May inhibit labor[85]
Ephedrine/pre-1938	—	No increased CM in 373 subjects in CPP	...
Isoproterenol/1948	±	No increased CM in 31 subjects in CPP; 1/16 MM (0.7 expected)	...
Isothearine/1961	—	0/22 MM (1 expected)	...
Metaproterenol/1973	C	17/361 MM (15 expected)	May inhibit term labor[85]
Terbutaline/1974	B	7/149 MM (6 expected)	May inhibit term labor[85]; intravascular administration preserves or increases uteroplacental blood flow[85]
Albuterol/1981	C	48/1090 MM (43 expected)	May inhibit term labor[50]; no adverse effect of inhaled albuterol on fetal circulation[86]
Bitolterol/1985	C	...	...
Pirbuterol/1988	C	...	...
Salmeterol/1994	C	...	...
Theophylline/pre-1938	C	No increased CM in 193 subjects in CPP; severe unusual cardiac CM reported in 3 infants whose mothers received theophylline throughout pregnancy[27]; 68/1240 MM (53 expected); not increased in 429 subjects[10]	Neonatal symptoms of theophylline toxicity reported in 8 infants whose asthmatic mothers received theophylline at term[85]; may inhibit uterine contractions[85]; no increased risk of stillbirth in women receiving theophylline in the CPP[87]; increased[28] or decreased[88] preeclampsia; not independently related to preeclampsia, preterm or LBW infants in 429 subjects[10]
Anticholinergics			
Atropine/pre-1938	—	No increased CM in 401 subjects in CPP; 18/381 MM (16 expected)	
Ipratropium/1987	B	...	...
Cromolyn/1973	B	CM in 1.4% of 296 infants of asthmatics treated with cromolyn throughout their entire pregnancies[89]; 7/191 MM (8 expected); not increased in 243 subjects[10]	No perinatal mortality or prematurity in 296 infants of asthmatics treated with cromolyn throughout their entire pregnancies[89]; no increase in preeclampsia, preterm or LBW infants[10]
Nedocromil/1993	B	...	...
Antileukotriene drugs			
Montelukast/1998	B		
Zafirlukast/1996	B	...	...
Zileuton/1996	C	...	...
Corticosteroids			

Table 16-4

Data on the Safety of Asthma Medications During Pregnancy (Continued)

Drug/yr introduced (U.S.)	FDA Class (see Table 1)	Human Data Congenital Malformations (CM)	Other
Systemic/1950	+	No increased CM in 154 subjects in CPP; 11/236 prednisone MM (10 expected); 14/222 methylprednisolone MM (9 expected); not increased in 130 subjects[10]; not increased in 323 subjects in large case control study[33]; increased risk of oral clefts in case control study[34]	10 mg prednisone throughout pregnancy associated with lower infant birthweight,[36] but not 5–10 mg discontinued before 24 weeks[37,38]; increased preeclampsia,[35] preterm birth[5] or low birthweight infants[5]; independently associated with preeclampsia but not preterm or LBW infants in 130 subjects[10]
Inhaled			
Multiple		No increase in 149 subjects (137 beclomethasone)[10]	Not independently associated with preeclampsia, preterm births, or LBW infants in 149 subjects (137 beclomethasone)[10]
Beclomethasone/1976	C	No increase in CM in 45 pregnancies in 40 women (compared to general population figures)[90]; 16/395 MM (16 expected)	14% incidence of low birthweight in 43 infants from 42 mothers[90]; no decreased birthweight in infants of 14 mothers receiving beclomethasone vs. infants of 25 theophyl-line-treated mothers[91]
Flunisolide/1981	C	...	...
Triamcinolone/1984	C	...	No decreased birthweight in 15 infants of mothers receiving triamcinolone vs. infants of 25 theophylline treated mothers[91]
Fluticasone/1996	C	...	...
Budesonide/1997	C	No increase in 2014 subjects[100]	...

ABBREVIATIONS: 0, not classified and animal studies not reported; −, not classified but animal studies do not reveal teratogenicity; +, not classified, but animal studies do reveal teratogenicity; ±, Not classified, but teratogenicity suggested in some animal studies but not others.
CPP, Collaborative Perinatal Project[24]
SOURCE: with permission, modified from Schatz, et al.[12]

a significant association between first-trimester use of systemic corticosteroids and an increase in oral clefts (OR = 6.55, 95%; CI = 1.44 to 29.76).[34] The authors of this report concluded that the use of systemic corticosteroids during the first trimester should be restricted to life-threatening situations or diseases without any other safer therapeutic alternatives; severe asthma would certainly meet these criteria.

Increased incidences of preeclampsia[35] and preterm or low birthweight infants[5] have also been reported in the pregnancies of asthmatic women who required corticosteroids during pregnancy compared to nonsteroid-treated asthmatic women,

but one cannot differentiate a medication effect from the effect of severe asthma in these studies. Severe asthma did not confound the study of Reinisch and colleagues who reported a lower mean birthweight and an increased incidence of low birthweight in infants from mothers with prior pregnancy losses who received 10 mg of prednisone daily throughout gestation for pregnancy maintenance, compared to control infants from the same clinic.[36] However, subsequent reports using lower amounts of prednisone (5 to 10 mg) for shorter periods of time (<24 weeks gestation) did not confirm these results.[37,38] More recently, a multivariate analysis of the relationships of various medications, asthma severity, and demographic factors to adverse perinatal outcomes was conducted in 824 prospectively managed pregnant women with asthma.[10] In this study, oral corticosteroid use was independently associated with a doubling of the risk of pre-eclampsia, but was not associated with an increased risk of delivering preterm or low-birthweight infants. In summary, the available literature suggests that oral corticosteroids may increase the risk of oral clefts and pre-eclampsia and could decrease intrauterine growth. However, even if this is true, the data on the potential adverse effects of severe asthma suggest that patients who require prednisone for control of their asthma would still be at greater risk from their uncontrolled disease than from the lowest effective dose of prednisone.

OUTPATIENT MANAGEMENT OF GESTATIONAL ASTHMA

A major goal of outpatient management is the prevention of acute asthmatic episodes. Prevention of acute episodes potentially involves 1) reducing exposure or sensitivity to triggering factors, 2) optimizing pulmonary function with the lowest effective dose of medication, and 3) maintaining appropriate self-management behaviors and early contact with the physician if symptoms increase.

Reducing Exposure or Sensitivity to Triggering Factors

Complete information regarding antigen avoidance and irritant avoidance should be given to the patient. It is particularly important for a woman to discontinue smoking during pregnancy, since maternal smoking may adversely affect both respiratory disease and pregnancy.

Immunotherapy represents a means of reducing sensitivity to allergic triggering factors and may be appropriate in a selected group of allergic asthmatic patients. Abortions associated with systemic reactions following antigen immunotherapy have been reported,[39] and anaphylaxis during pregnancy due to other causes has been associated

with fetal mortality and morbidity.[12] However, aside from systemic reactions, allergen immunotherapy appears to be safe during pregnancy. Two studies of 121 pregnancies in 90 women[40] and 109 pregnancies in 81 women[41] receiving inhalant allergen immunotherapy reported no increase in abortions, fetal deaths, neonatal deaths, prematurity, toxemia, or congenital malformations in the treated patients in comparison to a non-treated pregnant allergic control group and to the general population.

Based on this information, it is recommended that allergen immunotherapy be carefully continued during pregnancy in patients who appear to be deriving benefit, are not prone to systemic reactions, and are at a maintenance dose or at least receiving a substantial dosage. A dose reduction of 20% to 50% may be considered to further decrease the risk of a systemic reaction. Benefit-risk considerations do not favor *beginning* immunotherapy during pregnancy for most patients, since 1) the patient's propensity for systemic reactions is undefined, 2) there is an increased likelihood of systemic reactions occurring during initiation of immunotherapy, 3) the clinical effect is usually delayed for at least several months, and 4) the degree of benefit to be achieved may be difficult to predict, especially in asthmatic patients.

Prophylactic Pharmacological Management

Data on the use of asthma medications during pregnancy reviewed above have led to certain specific recommendations for the pharmacologic management of asthma in pregnant women. Medications recommended for the outpatient management of mild, moderate, and severe chronic asthma are shown in Table 16-5. These recommendations are based on those of the National Asthma Education Program Report of the Working Group on Asthma and Pregnancy,[1] but have been updated to employ the terminology and recommendations of the National Asthma Education Program Expert Panel Report II.[42] Medications generally should be added one by one until adequate control is achieved. Effects of intermittent,

Table 16-5

Pharmacological Step Therapy of Chronic Asthma During Pregnancy[a]

Category	Frequency/Severity of Symptoms (Sx)	Pulmonary Function[b] (untreated)	Step Therapy
Mild Intermittent	Sx ≤ 2 times per week Nocturnal Sx ≤ 2/month Exacerbations brief (a few hours to a few days) Asymptomatic between episodes	≥80% Normal pulmonary function between episodes	Inhaled β_2 agonists as needed
Mild Persistent	Sx > 2 times per week but not daily Nocturnal Sx >2/month Exacerbations may affect activity	≥80%	Inhaled β_2 agonists as needed Inhaled cromolyn Substitute inhaled corticosteroids if not adequate
Moderate Persistent	Daily Sx Nocturnal Sx > 1/week Exacerbations affect activity	60–80%	Inhaled β_2 agonists as needed Inhaled corticosteroids Add oral theophylline[c]
Severe Persistent	Continual Sx Limited activity Frequent nocturnal symptoms Frequent acute exacerbations	<60%	Above + oral corticosteroids (burst for active symptoms, alternate day or daily if necessary)

[a]NOTE: Based on the recommendations of the National Asthma Education Program Report of the Working Group on Asthma During Pregnancy[1] and the Expert Panel Report II[42]

[b]NOTE: FEV$_1$ or PEFR based on the norm for the patient, which may be standardized norms or personal best

[c]NOTE: Consider inhaled salmeterol instead of or in addition to theophylline in patients not controlled on medium-dose inhaled corticosteroids

predictable exposures to allergens can be reduced or prevented by administration of cromolyn (two puffs) just before exposure and then every four hours during exposure.

A recent study reported that inhaled corticosteroids and, to a lesser extent inhaled cromolyn, reduced hospitalizations for asthma in general,[43] and recent data confirmed that inhaled corticosteroids reduced the occurrence of asthma exacerbations during pregnancy.[4,44] Pending additional data, beclomethasone or budesonide would generally be recommended as the inhaled corticosteroid of choice during pregnancy unless another specific inhaled corticosteroid appeared to be uniquely beneficial for the individual patient. As mentioned above, inhaled salmeterol may be considered as

an alternative to theophylline or high-dose inhaled corticosteroids in women not adequately controlled by medium-dose inhaled corticosteroids. As also discussed above, benefit-risk considerations favor the use of oral corticosteroids for the management of severe asthma during pregnancy; however, such patients must be monitored closely for the potential adverse effects of corticosteroids, especially hyperglycemia, preeclampsia, and intrauterine growth restriction.

Home Management of Asthma Exacerbations

When asthma exacerbations occur during pregnancy, one must maintain a high index of suspicion

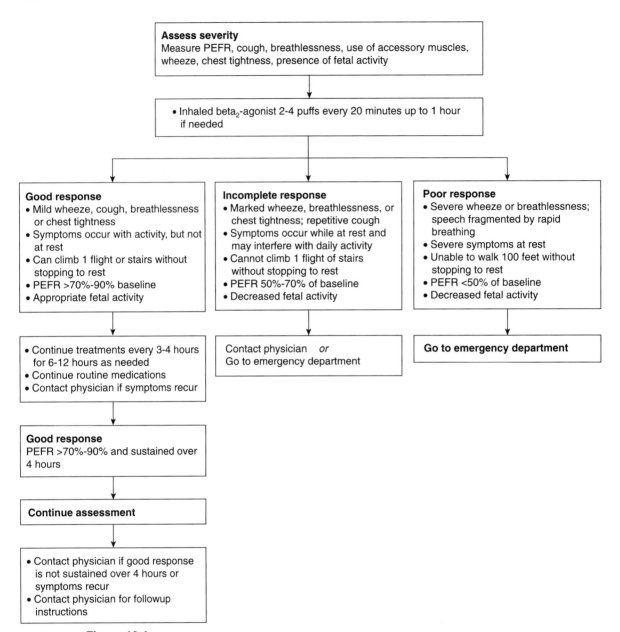

Figure 16-1

Flow chart of home management of acute exacerbations of asthma during pregnancy. PEFR% baseline refers to the norm for the individual, established by the clinician. This may be % predicted based on standardized norms or % of patient's personal best. (From National Institutes of Health[1]) for complicating bacterial respiratory infections, and particularly for bacterial sinusitis, which has been estimated to be six times more common during pregnancy than in non-pregnant patients.[1] Written action plans, prepared in advance with the asthma physician, help the patient to manage asthma exacerbations at home. Optimal home management involves 1) recognition of early indicators of an exacerbation, including symptoms and PEFR, 2) appropriate intensification of anti-asthma medications including, in many cases, systemic corticosteroids, 3) removal of or withdrawal from a relevant environmental trigger, if possible, and 4) prompt communication between patient and health care provider about any serious deterioration and its appropriate treatment.

The home management of asthma exacerbations during pregnancy is summarized in Figure 16-1. Patients receiving inhaled corticosteroids should also be advised to routinely increase their dose to at least four puffs, three to four times daily (beclomethasone or equivalent), when asthma exacerbations occur. Home PEFR determinations are an integral part of home management strategies. PEFR greater than 70% to 80% of personal best suggests that the exacerbation is being successfully managed. However, PEFR less than 50% of personal best in spite of therapy suggests that oral corticosteroids are indicated and/or the patient should seek emergency therapy. Oral corticosteroids should also be generally used if the patient requires 12 or more puffs of inhaled β_2 agonist in 24 hours. Oral corticosteroids are usually prescribed as prednisone, 40 to 60 mg daily (in one to three doses) for 3 to 5 days, and then tapered over the next 5 to 10 days.

MANAGEMENT OF ACUTE ASTHMA DURING PREGNANCY

Assessment

The management of acute gestational asthma begins with a proper assessment.[45–50] A brief history should attempt to ascertain the duration of the acute attack, the apparent precipitating event, the presence of upper respiratory infection (especially with fever and purulent mucus), current medication (especially theophylline and corticosteroids), and any prior history of respiratory failure or intubation. The physical examination should particularly attempt to identify features suggestive of severe asthma, including use of accessory muscles, diaphoresis, pulse paradoxus greater than 12, inability to lay down comfortably, pulse greater than 120 and respiratory rate greater than 30.

The first objective laboratory measurement that should be obtained is a PEFR or an FEV_1. Nowak and colleagues have shown that patients with an initial FEV_1 greater than 1 L or PEFR greater than 200 L per minute will have a Pa_{O_2} value greater than 60 mm Hg and a Pa_{CO_2} less than 42 mm Hg; initial blood gases may be deferred in such patients.[51] However, blood gases should be obtained in patients presenting with values worse than the above or in those not responding to therapy.

Pulse oximetry may be considered as a noninvasive alternative to blood gases when CO_2 retention appears unlikely. However, studies of the accuracy of oximetry and consideration of the oxyhemoglobin dissociation curve suggest that only an oximetry-determined O_2 saturation greater than 95% can be considered sufficient evidence of adequate oxygenation.[52]

A chest radiograph should not be obtained routinely, consistent with the recommended practice in nonpregnant patients with acute asthma.[53] However, a chest radiograph with a shielded abdomen does not constitute an increased risk during pregnancy[54] and should be obtained in patients in whom pneumonia, atelectasis, pneumothorax, or pneumomediastinum is suspected; in those not responding to therapy; and in those admitted to the hospital.[55] A baseline serum potassium level should be obtained since β_2 agonists and corticosteroids may lower serum potassium, and a baseline serum glucose concentration should be obtained to evaluate possible hypoglycemia (to which pregnant patients may be unusually susceptible,[56] particularly if not eating properly) or hyperglycemia (due to corticosteroids and/or pregnancy).

Emergency Therapy

The recommendations of the Working Group on Asthma and Pregnancy on emergency department (ED) management of acute gestational asthma are summarized in Figure 16-2. Supplemental oxygen (initially three to four L/min by nasal cannula) should be administered, adjusting Fi_{O_2} to maintain a Pa_{O_2} greater than 70 mm Hg and/or O_2 saturation by pulse oximetry greater than 95%.[1,48] Intravenous fluids (containing glucose if the patient is not hyperglycemic) should be administered, initially at a rate of at least 100cc per hour.

Inhaled β_2 agonists are the initial bronchodilators of choice for acute asthma in nonpregnant patients.[45,47,49,50] and information on the use of inhaled β_2 agonists during pregnancy (discussed above) suggests that this recommendation does not need to be altered during pregnancy. In addition, recent studies suggest that β_2 agonists administered by metered-dose inhaler (MDI) (e.g., four puffs MDI with spacer, waiting 1 minute between puffs) may be as effective and safe as nebulized bronchodilators.[45,57] Subcutaneous β_2 agonists would only be recommended for patients in whom inhalation treatment is not effective.

Three doses of inhaled β_2 agonists spaced every 20 to 30 minutes can be safely given as initial therapy to patients without coexistent cardiovascular disease. Thereafter, the frequency of administration varies according to the severity of the symptoms and occurrence of adverse side effects. In patients without cardiovascular disease, administration of β_2 agonists as frequently as every 1 to 2 hours is safe during periods of severe airflow obstruction.[1,49] It would also seem reasonable to administer one dose (500 μg in 2.5 cc) of nebulized ipratropium to patients who do not significantly improve after the first dose of albuterol, since recent data showed that its bronchodilatory effect

may be additive to that of inhaled β_2 agonists in the management of acute asthma.[58]

Parenteral corticosteroids should be administered along with initial therapy to patients on regular corticosteroids. In addition, intravenous corticosteroids should be utilized in patients with severe airflow obstruction (PEFR <200 L/min or FEV_1 <40% of predicted value) that persists after 1 hour of intensive β_2-agonist therapy.[1] There are no data on the pharmacokinetics of exogenous corticosteroids administered during pregnancy, and dosages of corticosteroids recommended for pregnancy generally are no different than those recommended for nonpregnant patients. Although there are insufficient data to determine the optimal dose of parenteral corticosteroids to be used in patients with acute asthma,[49] 1 mg/kg of methylprednisolone every 6 to 8 hours is recommended.[1]

Intravenous aminophylline is not generally recommended in the ED management of acute gestational asthma because it has been demonstrated that aminophylline does not provide additional benefit to optimal inhaled β_2-agonist therapy in the first 4 hours of treatment.[1,45] Moreover, when used in combination with intensive inhaled β_2-agonist therapy, intravenous aminophylline causes increased adverse side effects without providing additional bronchodilation.[1]

Patients who respond adequately to ED therapy (PEFR or FEV_1 > 60% to 70% of predicted value) may usually be discharged from the ED.[1,45] All patients who require more than a single inhaled β_2-agonist treatment should be discharged on a course of oral corticosteroids, as well as on inhaled corticosteroids.[44,45] Recommended doses of oral corticosteroids upon ED discharge are 30 to 60 mg per day of prednisone for 7 to 14 days.[45] Appropriate patient education with regard to the

---

FIGURE 16-2
Flow chart of emergency department management of acute exacerbations of asthma during pregnancy. Although therapies are often available in a physician's office, most acute severe exacerbations of asthma require a complete course of therapy in an emergency department. PEFR % baseline refers to the norm for the individual, established by the clinician. This may be % predicted based on standardized norms or % of patient's personal best. (From National Institutes of Health[1])

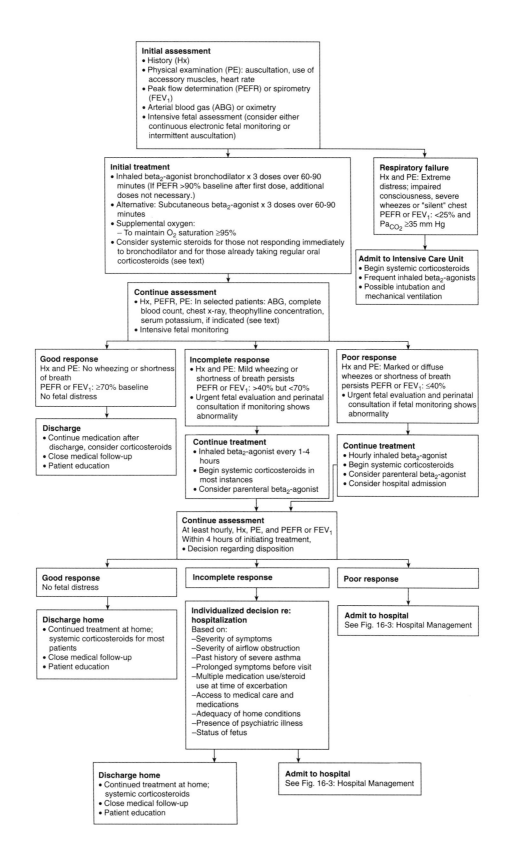

Initial assessment
- History (Hx)
- Physical examination (PE): auscultation, use of accessory muscles, heart rate
- Peak flow determination (PEFR) or spirometry (FEV_1)
- Arterial blood gas (ABG) or oximetry
- Intensive fetal assessment (consider either continuous electronic fetal monitoring or intermittent auscultation)

Initial treatment
- Inhaled beta$_2$-agonist bronchodilator x 3 doses over 60-90 minutes (If PEFR >90% baseline after first dose, additional doses not necessary.)
- Alternative: Subcutaneous beta$_2$-agonist x 3 doses over 60-90 minutes
- Supplemental oxygen:
  – To maintain O_2 saturation ≥95%
- Consider systemic steroids for those not responding immediately to bronchodilator and for those already taking regular oral corticosteroids (see text)

Respiratory failure
Hx and PE: Extreme distress; impaired consciousness, severe wheezes or "silent" chest
PEFR or FEV_1: <25% and Pa_{CO_2} ≥35 mm Hg

Admit to Intensive Care Unit
- Begin systemic corticosteroids
- Frequent inhaled beta$_2$-agonists
- Possible intubation and mechanical ventilation

Continue assessment
- Hx, PEFR, PE: In selected patients: ABG, complete blood count, chest x-ray, theophylline concentration, serum potassium, if indicated (see text)
- Intensive fetal monitoring

Good response
Hx and PE: No wheezing or shortness of breath
PEFR or FEV_1: ≥70% baseline
No fetal distress

Incomplete response
- Hx and PE: Mild wheezing or shortness of breath persists
PEFR or FEV_1: >40% but <70%
- Urgent fetal evaluation and perinatal consultation if monitoring shows abnormality

Poor response
Hx and PE: Marked or diffuse wheezes or shortness of breath persists PEFR or FEV_1: ≤40%
- Urgent fetal evaluation and perinatal consultation if fetal monitoring shows abnormality

Discharge
- Continue medication after discharge, consider corticosteroids
- Close medical follow-up
- Patient education

Continue treatment
- Inhaled beta$_2$-agonist every 1-4 hours
- Begin systemic corticosteroids in most instances
- Consider parenteral beta$_2$-agonist

Continue treatment
- Hourly inhaled beta$_2$-agonist
- Begin systemic corticosteroids
- Consider parenteral beta$_2$-agonist
- Consider hospital admission

Continue assessment
At least hourly, Hx, PE, and PEFR or FEV_1
Within 4 hours of initiating treatment,
- Decision regarding disposition

Good response
No fetal distress

Incomplete response

Poor response

Discharge home
- Continued treatment at home; systemic corticosteroids for most patients
- Close medical follow-up
- Patient education

Individualized decision re: hospitalization
Based on:
–Severity of symptoms
–Severity of airflow obstruction
–Past history of severe asthma
–Prolonged symptoms before visit
–Multiple medication use/steroid use at time of exacerbation
–Access to medical care and medications
–Adequacy of home conditions
–Presence of psychiatric illness
–Status of fetus

Admit to hospital
See Fig. 16-3: Hospital Management

Discharge home
- Continued treatment at home; systemic corticosteroids
- Close medical follow-up
- Patient education

Admit to hospital
See Fig. 16-3: Hospital Management

discharge treatment plan, especially concerning inhaler and spacer technique, and clear instructions for follow-up care are essential to preventing relapses.[45]

Clinicians may have a tendency to undertreat asthma in pregnancy, with possible adverse outcomes. In a recent study, 51 pregnant patients with acute asthma exacerbation presenting to emergency facilities were compared to age and disease severity matched control patients at the same facilities.[58a] Despite a similarity in duration of symptoms and PEFR between the two groups, pregnant women were less likely to be treated with corticosteroids in the emergency room and during a 2 week follow-up period were almost three times more likely to report an ongoing exacerbation of their asthma. The authors concluded that among women presenting to the emergency room with acute asthma, pregnant asthmatics were less likely to receive appropriate treatment with corticosteroids. While fetal and maternal risks of drug therapy must be carefully weighed, this study suggests undertreatment of asthma during pregnancy occurs and fails adequately to control symptoms.

Hospitalization

Ten to fifteen percent of non-pregnant patients presenting to the emergency room require hospital admission.[59] The following pulmonary function criteria for admission have been recommended: post-therapy FEV_1 less than 60% of predicted,[51] <2.0 L,[60,61] or post-therapy PEFR less than 300 L per minute. Other criteria for admission include initial respiratory failure (even with improvement), the presence of complications such as pneumonia, pneumothorax or cardiac arrhythmias, and repeat ED visits within 72 hours.[59] Certainly, criteria for admission of the pregnant asthma patient should be no less liberal, and the coexistence of uterine contractions or fetal distress with acute asthma also necessitates admission.

The recommendations of the Working Group on Asthma and Pregnancy[1] regarding the management of pregnant women who require hospitalization for asthma during pregnancy are summarized in Figure 16–3. When the pregnant asthma patient is hospitalized, both medical and obstetrical supervision is required. Patients in frank or impending respiratory failure ($Pa_{CO_2} > 35$ mm Hg) should be hospitalized in an ICU.

In the hospital, oxygen, inhaled β_2 agonists, and intravenous corticosteroids should be continued. Inhaled β_2 agonists should be administered continuously up to every 4 hours, depending on the severity and response. Nebulized ipratropium every 4 to 8 hours may be considered. Since recent studies suggested that intravenous magnesium sulfate (1 to 2 g) may be beneficial in acute severe asthma as an adjunct to inhaled β_2 agonists and intravenous corticosteroids,[62–64] magnesium sulfate could also be considered, especially in patients with coexistent hypertension or preterm uterine contractions, and intravenous aminophylline may be considered as well. When intravenous aminophylline has been used, pharmacokinetic studies during pregnancy[65–67] suggested that the loading dose recommendation for theophylline required no modification during pregnancy (5 mg/kg over 20 to 30 minutes), but the initial maintenance dose should be lower (0.5 mg/kg per hour). Studies have also suggested that protein binding of theophylline decreases during pregnancy such that there is an approximately 15% increase in free drug for any total drug concentration.[67,68] This suggests that a lower therapeutic range (8 to 12 μg/mL) than is usually recommended is appropriate during pregnancy.[1] Inhalation of heliox, a blend of oxygen and helium, has been reported to reverse hypercapnia and avert intubation in patients with severe status asthmaticus and impending respiratory failure; however, the use of heliox has not been reported in pregnant patients.[50] Similarly, inhaled anesthetic agents (ether, halothane, enflurane, isoflurane) have been reported to be effective in refractory cases,[45,69] but their use during pregnancy has not been reported.

Antibiotics should be utilized for hospitalized patients with purulent sputum containing polymorphonuclear leukocytes, or if pneumonia is documented on chest radiography. In addition, a high index of suspicion for sinusitis must be maintained, and sinus films should be considered in hospitalized asthma patients with substantial nasal

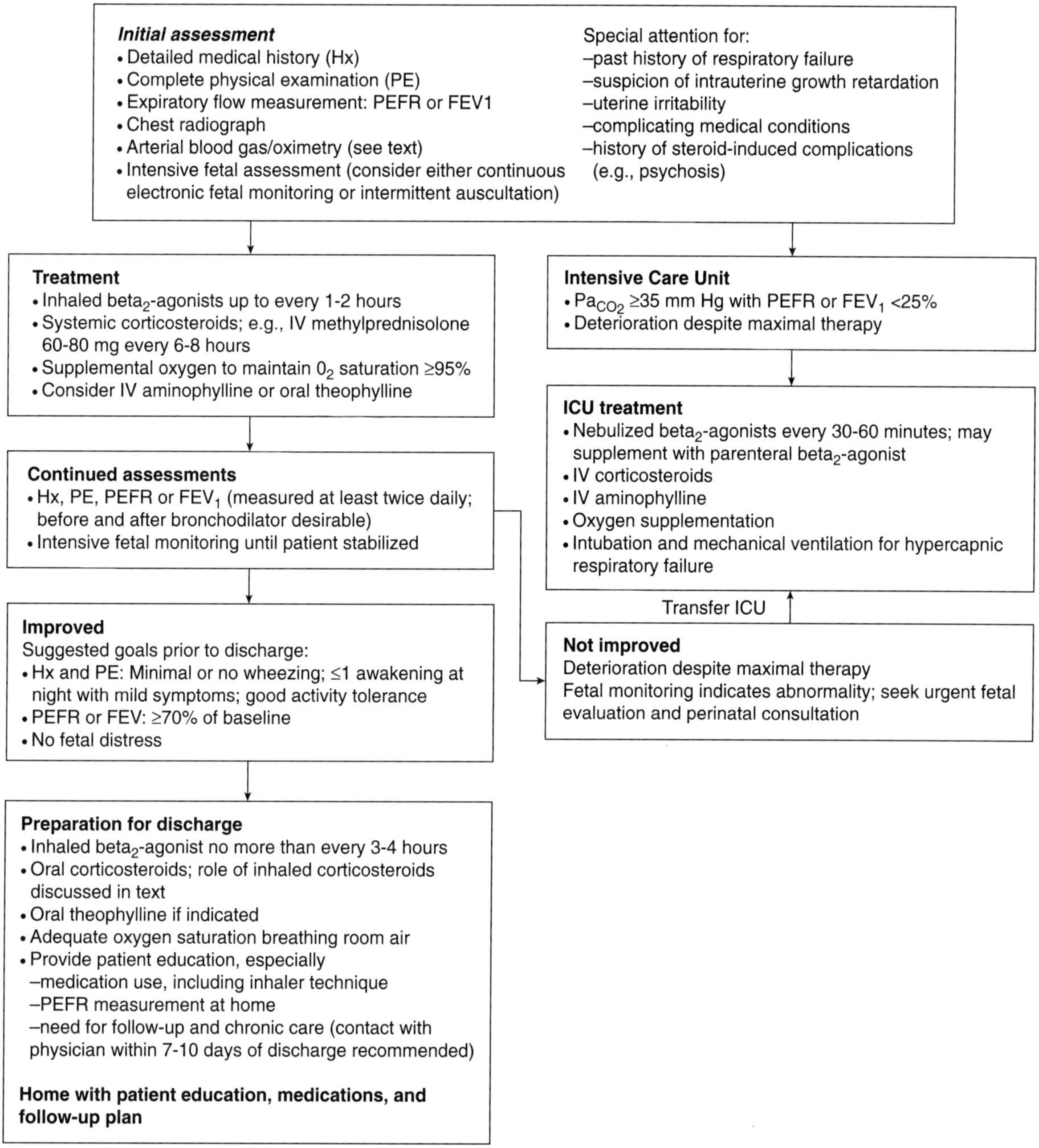

Initial assessment
- Detailed medical history (Hx)
- Complete physical examination (PE)
- Expiratory flow measurement: PEFR or FEV1
- Chest radiograph
- Arterial blood gas/oximetry (see text)
- Intensive fetal assessment (consider either continuous electronic fetal monitoring or intermittent auscultation)

Special attention for:
−past history of respiratory failure
−suspicion of intrauterine growth retardation
−uterine irritability
−complicating medical conditions
−history of steroid-induced complications
  (e.g., psychosis)

Treatment
- Inhaled beta$_2$-agonists up to every 1-2 hours
- Systemic corticosteroids; e.g., IV methylprednisolone 60-80 mg every 6-8 hours
- Supplemental oxygen to maintain O_2 saturation ≥95%
- Consider IV aminophylline or oral theophylline

Intensive Care Unit
- Pa_{CO_2} ≥35 mm Hg with PEFR or FEV$_1$ <25%
- Deterioration despite maximal therapy

Continued assessments
- Hx, PE, PEFR or FEV$_1$ (measured at least twice daily; before and after bronchodilator desirable)
- Intensive fetal monitoring until patient stabilized

ICU treatment
- Nebulized beta$_2$-agonists every 30-60 minutes; may supplement with parenteral beta$_2$-agonist
- IV corticosteroids
- IV aminophylline
- Oxygen supplementation
- Intubation and mechanical ventilation for hypercapnic respiratory failure

Transfer ICU

Improved
Suggested goals prior to discharge:
- Hx and PE: Minimal or no wheezing; ≤1 awakening at night with mild symptoms; good activity tolerance
- PEFR or FEV: ≥70% of baseline
- No fetal distress

Not improved
Deterioration despite maximal therapy
Fetal monitoring indicates abnormality; seek urgent fetal evaluation and perinatal consultation

Preparation for discharge
- Inhaled beta$_2$-agonist no more than every 3-4 hours
- Oral corticosteroids; role of inhaled corticosteroids discussed in text
- Oral theophylline if indicated
- Adequate oxygen saturation breathing room air
- Provide patient education, especially
 −medication use, including inhaler technique
 −PEFR measurement at home
 −need for follow-up and chronic care (contact with physician within 7-10 days of discharge recommended)

Home with patient education, medications, and follow-up plan

FIGURE 16-3

Flow chart of hospital management of acute exacerbations of asthma during pregnancy. PEFR % baseline refers to the norm for the individual, established by the clinician. This may be % predicted based on standardized norms or % of patient's personal best. (From National Institutes of Health[1]) congestion or postnasal drainage, even in the absence of purulent discharge. Based on the American Thoracic Society guidelines for the initial management of adults with community-acquired pneumonia[70] and on the organisms likely to cause sinusitis, intravenous cefuroxime is recommended initially for hospitalized pregnant asthmatic patients with suspected bacterial respiratory infections. Erythromycin should be included as part of initial therapy if *Mycoplasma pneumoniae*, *Chlamydia pneumoniae* or *Legionella* infection is suspected. After the first 24 to 72 hours, oral therapy with amoxicillin-clavulanate or cefuroxime may be substituted for intravenous cephalosporin therapy in most pregnant hospitalized asthmatic patients with pneumonia or sinusitis.

Respiratory Failure

Mechanical ventilation was required in 2.3% of 811 consecutive hospitalized, nonpregnant patients[71] and in 8% of nonpregnant patients presenting with acute asthma and hypercapnia (mean Pa_{CO_2}, 54 mm Hg).[72] The criteria for mechanical ventilation in nonpregnant patients include 1) Pa_{O_2} less than 60 to 65 mm Hg on maximum supplemental O_2, 2) uncompensated respiratory acidosis (Pa_{CO_2} greater than 55 mm Hg, pH $<$ 7.2) in spite of intensive therapy, 3) inability to clear secretions and protect the airway, 4) altered mental status, and 5) progressive fatigue of the respiratory muscles.[48,49,59,73] Although these criteria may also be applied to pregnant patients with asthma, it has been suggested that they should be mechanically ventilated at a lower level of hypercapnia (Pa_{CO_2} less than 45 mm Hg) since the normal Pa_{CO_2} of pregnancy is about 30 to 32 mm Hg.[73,74]

Because of airway narrowing due to hyperemia, intubation should be performed via an oral rather than a nasal route, usually using a smaller tube than would be used in the nonpregnant state.[48,73,74] The decreased FRC and increased oxygen consumption in pregnancy may lower oxygen reserve such that a short period of apnea at the time of intubation may be associated with a precipitous drop in Pa_{O_2}.[48,73,74] Therefore, pre-oxygenation of the pregnant asthma patient with 100%

oxygen is helpful before intubation, and cricoid pressure must be maintained to prevent gastric insufflation and subsequent aspiration before and during intubation.[48,73] When sedation and muscle paralysis are indicated, morphine sulfate and pancuronium bromide are recommended.[48]

Mechanical ventilation of the pregnant patient follows the same general principles as in nongravid patients.[48,73,74] In general, the minute ventilation should be adjusted to aim for a Pa_{CO_2} of 30 to 32 mm Hg, the normal level in pregnancy.[48,73,74] Strict attention to this detail is necessary to prevent hyperventilation and subsequent respiratory alkalosis, which can lead to reduced uterine blood flow and impaired fetal oxygenation.[73,74] It is reasonable to aim for the usual gestational Pa_{O_2} of greater than 95 mm Hg.[48]

Recent studies suggest that the major cause of complications from mechanical ventilation in patients with asthma, including shock, hypercapnia, and lung injury, results from dynamic hyperinflation and increased static lung pressure.[47,50,73] Thus, the presence and magnitude of intrinsic PEEP should be monitored in asthmatic patients who require mechanical ventilation. Intrinsic PEEP can be reduced by maximizing the expiratory time. This can usually be accomplished by using 1) small tidal volumes of 6 to 8 ml/kg,[45,73] 2) high-peak inspiratory flow rates (100 to 120 L/min)[47,73], 3) low respiratory rates,[73] such as 8 to 12 per minute,[45,47,50] and 4) use of the square flow inspiratory waveform, which minimizes inspiratory time.[47,50] Allowing Pa_{CO_2} to rise if adequate tidal volumes cannot be maintained at low distending pressures may be necessary for patients with severe asthma,[45,50,73] but this approach of controlled hypoventilation or permissive hypercapnia has not been assessed in pregnancy.[74] Weaning parameters should be the same as for nonpregnant patients, although it is recommended that pregnant patients maintain the lateral decubitus rather than supine position during weaning near term to minimize the inferior vena caval compression that is caused by the gravid uterus.[48]

Hypotension is a common complication when asthmatic patients are first put on mechanical ventilation. Most often this is the consequence of breath-stacking, causing intrinsic PEEP. However, tension pneumothorax, air embolism, and compression of the inferior vena cava by the gravid uterus must also be considered. Prompt diagnosis and treatment to prevent inadequate fetal-placental blood flow should be instituted. The use of α-adrenergic pressors are minimized because of the potential adverse effects on uterine perfusion. The presence and magnitude of intrinsic PEEP should be monitored regularly throughout the course of mechanical ventilation for status asthmaticus.

For patients responding poorly in spite of mechanical ventilation, alternatives reported during pregnancy included warm metaproterenol-saline solution irrigation and suction,[75] bronchoalveolar lavage,[76] and termination of pregnancy.[77,78] Obviously, consideration of emergent delivery by cesarean section is a difficult decision; however, depending on the gestational age of the fetus, it may be a reasonable consideration for a gravida with life-threatening refractory asthma.[48,77]

ASTHMA MANAGEMENT DURING LABOR AND DELIVERY

Fortunately, substantial asthma symptoms during labor in women whose asthma has been controlled during pregnancy are unusual. In one study, 90% of asthmatic women experienced no asthma symptoms during labor and, of those who did, only one half required treatment (4.1%, inhaled bronchodilators; 0.5%, intravenous aminophylline).[21] Nonetheless, it is suggested that daily prophylactic medications (e.g., cromolyn, inhaled corticosteroids, or theophylline) should be continued during labor. Asthma symptoms during labor that require therapy should be treated initially with inhaled β_2 agonists. If the patient's asthma responds poorly to inhaled β_2 agonists, intravenous methylprednisolone should be administered. For patients receiving regular corticosteroids, or who have received frequent courses during pregnancy, supplemental parenteral corticosteroids for the stress of labor and delivery are recommended as follows: 100 mg hydrocortisone intravenously at admission, followed by 100 mg intravenously every 8 hours for 24 hours or until the absence of complications is established.[1]

CONCLUSION

The most important goal regarding acute asthma during pregnancy is to prevent it by means of aggressive avoidance of triggers and appropriate prophylactic pharmacologic therapy. When increased asthma occurs, appropriate home management may prevent further deterioration. However, emergency treatment of acute asthma, hospitalization, or mechanical ventilation may be required. Optimal treatment of the severe exacerbations should prevent maternal death as well as minimize fetal morbidity and mortality.

REFERENCES

1. National Asthma Education Program Report of the Working Group on Asthma and Pregnancy: *Management of Asthma During Pregnancy*. National Institutes of Health, Publ No. 93–3279A, September, 1993.
2. Schatz M, Zeiger RS, Hoffman CP et al: Perinatal outcomes in the pregnancies of asthmatic women: A prospective controlled analysis. *Am J Respir Crit Care Med* 151:1170, 1995.
3. Jana N, Vasishta K, Saha SC, Khunnu B: Effect of bronchial asthma on the course of pregnancy, labour and perinatal outcome. *J Obstet Gynecol* 3:227–232, 1995.
4. Stenius-Aarniala BSM, Hedman J, Teramo KA: Acute asthma during pregnancy. *Thorax* 51:411–414, 1996.
5. Perlow JH, Montgomery D, Morgan MA, et al: Severity of asthma and perinatal outcome. *Am J. Obstet Gynecol* 167:963–967, 1992.
6. Mabie WC, Barton JR, Wasserstrum N, Sibal BM: Clinical observations on asthma in pregnancy. *J Mat Fet Med* 1:45–50, 1992.
7. Cousins L, Catanzarite VA: Fetal oxygenation, acid-base balance, and assessment of well-being in the pregnancy complicated by asthma or anaphylaxis, in Schatz M, Zeiger RS, Claman HN (eds): *Asthma and Immunologic Diseases in Pregnancy and Early Infancy*. New York, Marcel Dekker, 1998, p. 27.

8. Schatz M: Asthma and pregnancy. *Immunol Allergy Clin North Am* 16:893–916, 1996.

9. Schatz M: Interrelationships between asthma and pregnancy: A literature review. *J Allergy Clin Immunol* (Suppl) 103:5330–36, 1999.

10. Schatz M, Zeiger RS, Harden K, et al: The safety of asthma and allergy medications during pregnancy. *J Allergy Clin Immunol* 100:301–306, 1997.

11. Wise RA: Pulmonary function during pregnancy, in Schatz M, Zeiger RS, Claman HN (eds): *Asthma and Immunologic Diseases in Pregnancy and Early Infancy.* New York, Marcel Dekker, 1998, p 57.

12. Schatz M, Hoffman CP, Zeiger RS, et al: The course and management of asthma and allergic disease during pregnancy, in Middleton E, Reed CE, Ellis EF, et al (eds): *Allergy: Principles and Practices,* 5th ed. St. Louis, MO, CV Mosby 1998, p 938.

13. Norregaard O, Schultz P, Ostergaard A, et al: Lung function and postural changes during pregnancy. *Respir Med* 83:467, 1989.

14. Mokkapatti R, Prasad EC, Fatima V, Fatima K: Ventilatory functions in pregnancy. *Indian J Physiol Pharmacol* 35:237–240, 1991.

15. Puranik BM, Kurhade GA, Kaore SB, et al: PEFR in pregnancy: A longitudinal study. *Indian J Physiol Pharmacol* 39:135–139,1995.

16. Singh S, Singh KC, Sircar SS, Sharma KN: Airway functions in pregnant Indian women. *Indian J Physiol Pharmacol* 39:160–162, 1995.

17. Brancazio LR, Laifer SA, Schwartz T: Peak expiratory flow rate in normal pregnancy. *Obstet Gynecol* 89:383–6, 1997.

17a. Schatz M. Interrelationships between asthma and pregnancy: A literature review. *J Allergy Clin Immunol* 103(2 Pt 2):S330–336, 1999.

18. Juniper EF, Newhouse MT: Effect of pregnancy on asthma: A systematic review and metaanalysis, in Schatz M, Zeiger RS, Claman HC (ed): *Asthma and Immunological Diseases in Pregnancy and Early Infancy.* New York, Marcel Dekker, 1998, p 401.

19. Gluck JC, Gluck PA: The effects of pregnancy on asthma: A prospective study. *Ann Allergy* 37:164, 1976.

20. Schatz M: Asthma during pregnancy: interrelationships and management. *Ann Allergy* 68:123–133, 1992.

21. Schatz M, Harden K. Forsythe A, et al: The course of asthma during pregnancy, postpartum and with successive pregnancies: A prospective analysis. *J Allergy Clin Immunol.* 81:509, 1988.

22. Abrams RS, Hoffman CP: Use of medication during pregnancy and lactation: General considerations, in Schatz M, Zeiger RS, Claman HN (eds): *Asthma and Immunologic Diseases in Pregnancy and Early Infancy.* New York, Marcel Dekker, 1998, p 137.

23. Scialli AR, Lione A: Pregnancy effects of specific medications used to treat asthma and immunologic diseases, in Schatz M, Zeiger RS, Claman HN (eds): *Asthma and Immunologic Diseases in Pregnancy and Early Infancy.* New York, Marcel Dekker, 1998, p. 157.

24. Heinonen OP, Slone D, Shapiro S: *Birth Defects and Drugs in Pregnancy.* Littleton, Mass, PSG Publishing, 1977.

25. Briggs GG, Freeman Ra, Yaffe SJ: *Drugs in Pregnancy and Lactation,* 4th ed. Baltimore, Williams and Wilkins, 1994.

26. Content and format for labeling for human prescription drugs: Clarification of effective date. *Fed Register* 45:32550, 1980.

26a. Dombrowski M, Thom E, McNellis D. Maternal-fetal medicine units (MFMU) studies of inhaled corticosteroids during pregnancy. *J Allergy Clin Immunol* 103(2 Pt 2):S356–359, 1999.

27. Park JM, Schmer U, Myers TL: Cardiovascular anomalies associated with prenatal exposure to theophylline. *South Med J* 83:1487, 1990.

28. Stenius-Aarniala B, Riikonen S, Teramo K: Slow-release theophylline in pregnant asthmatics. *Chest* 107:642–647, 1995.

29. Huff BB (ed): *Physicians Desk Reference.* Oradell, NJ, Medical Economics Co, 1998.

30. Woolcock A. Lundback B, Ringdal N, Jacques LA: Comparison of addition of salmeterol to inhaled steroids with doubling of the dose of inhaled steroids. *Am J Respir Crit Care Med* 153:1481–1488, 1996.

31. Russell G, Williams DAJ, Weller P, Price JF: Salmeterol xinafoate in children on high dose inhaled steroids. *Ann Allergy Asthma Immunol* 75:423–428, 1995.

32. Pollard SJ, Spector SL, Yancey et al: Salmeterol versus theophylline in the treatment of asthma *Ann Allergy Asthma Immunol* 78:457–464, 1997.

33. Czeizel AE, Rockenbauer M: Population-based case control study of teratogenic potential of corticosteroids. *Teratology* 58:2–5, 1998.

34. Rodriguez-Pinilla E, Martinez-Frias ML: Corticosteroids during pregnancy and oral clefts: A case control study. *Teratology* 56:335–340, 1998.

35. Stenius-Aarniala R, Piirila P, Teramo K: Asthma

and pregnancy: A prospective study of 198 pregnancies, *Thorax* 43:12, 1988.

36. Reinisch JM, Simon NG, Karow WG, et al: Prenatal exposure to prednisone in humans and animals retards intrauterine growth. *Science* 202:436, 1978.

37. Lee F, Nelson N, Faiman C, et al: Low-dose corticoid therapy for anovulation: Effect on fetal weight. *Obstet Gynecol* 60:314–317, 1982.

38. Smith KD, Steinberger E, Rodriguez-Rigan LJ: Prednisone therapy and birth weight. *Science* 206:96, 1979.

39. Francis N: Abortion after grass pollen injection. *J Allergy* 12:559, 1941.

40. Metzger WJ, Turner E, Patterson R: The safety of immunotherapy during pregnancy. *J Allergy Clin Immunol* 61:268, 1978.

41. Shaikh WA: A retrospective study on the safety of immunotherapy in pregnancy. *Clin Exp Allergy* 23:857–860, 1993.

42. National Asthma Education and Prevention Program: Highlights of the Expert Panel Report 2: Guidelines for the Diagnosis and Management of Asthma. National Institutes of Health, February, 1997.

43. Donahue JG, Weiss ST, Livingston JM, et al: Inhaled steroids and the risk of hospitalization for asthma. *JAMA* 277:887–891, 1997.

44. Wendel PJ, Ramin SM, Barnett-Hamm C, et al: Asthma treatment in pregnancy: a randomized controlled study. *Am J Obstet Gynecol* 175:150–154, 1996.

45. Beveridge RC, Grunfeld AF, Hodder RV, et al: Guidelines for the emergency management of asthma in adults. *Can Med Assoc J* 155:25–37, 1996.

46. Cockroft DW: Management of acute severe asthma. *Ann Allergy Asthma Immunol* 75:83–89, 1995.

47. Corbridge TC, Hall JB: The assessment and management of adults with status asthmaticus. *Am J Respir Crit Care Med* 151:1296–1316, 1995.

48. Hollingsworth HM, Irwin RS: Acute respiratory failure in pregnancy. *Clin Chest Med* 13:723–740, 1992.

49. Leatherman J: Life-threatening asthma. *Clin Chest Med* 15:453–479, 1994.

50. Manthous CA: Management of severe exacerbatons of asthma. *Am J Med* 99:298–308, 1995.

51. Nowak RM, Tomlanovich MC, Sarkar DD, et al: Arterial blood gases and pulmonary function testing in acute bronchial asthma: Predicting patient outcome. *JAMA* 249:2043–2046, 1983.

52. Ries AL: Oximetry—Know thy limits. *Chest* 91:316, 1987.

53. Findley LJ, Sahn S: The value of chest roentgenograms in acute asthma in adults. *Chest* 80:535–536, 1988.

54. Swartz WM, Reichling BA: Hazards of radiation exposure for pregnant women. *JAMA* 239:1907–1908, 1978.

55. Hargreave FE, Dolovich J, Newhouse MT: The assessment and treatment of asthma: A conference report. *J Allergy Clin Immunol* 85:1098–1111, 1990.

56. Myers SA, Gleicher N: Physiologic changes in normal pregnancy, in Gleicher N (ed): *Principles and Practice of Medical Therapy in Pregnancy* 2d ed. Norwalk, Appleton and Lange, 1992, p 46.

57. Idris AH, McDermott MF, Raucci JC, et al: Emergency department treatment of severe asthma: Metered dose inhaler plus holding chamber is equivalent in effectiveness to nebulizer. *Chest* 103:665–672, 1993.

58. Lanes SF, Garrett JE, Wentworth CE, et al: The effect of adding ipratropium bromide to salbutamol in the treatment of acute asthma: A pooled analysis of three trials. *Chest* 114:365–372, 1998.

58a. Cydulka RK, Emerman CL, Schreiber D, Molander KH, et al: Acute asthma among pregnancy women presenting to the emergency department. *Am J Respir Crit Care Med* 160:887–892, 1999.

59. McDonald AJ: Asthma. *Emerg Med Clin North Am* 7:219–235, 1989.

60. Nowak RM, Pensler MI, Sarkar DD, et al: Comparison of peak expiratory flow and FEV₁ admission criteria for acute bronchial asthma. *Ann Emerg Med* 11:64–69, 1982.

61. Verbeek PR, Chapman KR: Asthma: Who to send home, when to hospitalize. *J Respir Dis* 7:15–31, 1986.

62. Bloch H, Silverman R, Mancherje N, et al: Intravenous magnesium sulfate as an adjunct in the treatment of acute asthma. *Chest* 107:1576–1581, 1995.

63. Skobeloff EM, Spivey WH, McNamara RM, Greenspan L: Intravenous magnesium sulfate for the treatment of acute asthma in the emergency department. *JAMA* 262:1210–1213, 1989.

64. Ciarallo L, Sauer AH, Shannon MW: Intravenous magnesium therapy for moderate to severe pediatric asthma: Results of a randomized, placebo-controlled trial. *J Pediatr* 129:809–814, 1996.

65. Carter BL, Driscoll CE, Smith GD: Theophylline clearance during pregnancy. *Obstet Gynecol* 68:555–559, 1986.

66. Frederiksen MC, Ruo TI, Chow MJ, Atkinson AJ: Theophylline pharmacokinetics in pregnancy. *Clin Pharmacol Ther* 40:321–328, 1986.

67. Gardner MJ, Schatz M, Cousins L, et al: Longitudinal effects of pregnancy on the pharmacokinetics of theophylline. *Eur J Clin Pharmacol* 32:289–295, 1987.

68. Connelly TJ, Rhuo TI, Frederiksen MC, Atkinson AJ: Characterization of theophylline binding to serum proteins in pregnant and non-pregnant women. *Clin Pharmacol Ther* 47:68–72, 1990.

69. Cohen NH, Eigen H, Shaughnessy TE: Status asthmaticus. *Crit Care Clinics* 13:459–476, 1997.

70. American Thoracic Society Statement: Guidelines for the initial management of adults with community-acquired pneumonia: Diagnosis, assessment of severity, and initial antimicrobial therapy. *Am Rev Respir Dis* 148:1418–1426, 1993.

71. Scoggin CH, Sahn SA, Petty TH: Status asthmaticus: A nine-year experience. *JAMA* 238:1158–1162, 1977.

72. Mountain RD, Sahn SA: Clinical features and outcome in patients with acute asthma presenting with hypercapnia. *Am Rev Respir Dis* 138:535–539, 1988.

73. Deblieux PM, Summer WR: Acute respiratory failure in pregnancy. *Clin Obstet Gynecol* 39:143–152, 1996.

74. Lapinsky SE, Kruczynski K, Slutsky AS: Critical care in the pregnant patient. *Am J Respir Crit Care Med* 152:427–455, 1995.

75. Schreier L, Cutler RM, Saigel V: Respiratory failure in asthma during the third trimester: Report of two cases. *Am J Obstet Gynecol* 160:80–81, 1989.

76. Munakata M, Abe S, Fujimoto S, Kawakami Y: Bronchoalveolar lavage during third-trimester pregnancy in patients with status asthmaticus: A case report. *Respiration* 51:252–255, 1987.

77. Gelber M, Sidi Y, Gassner S, et al: Uncontrollable life-threatening status asthmaticus–An indicator for termination of pregnancy by ceasarean section. *Respiration* 46:320–322, 1984.

78. Topilsky M, Levo Y, Spitzer SA, et al: Status asthmaticus in pregnancy: A case report. *Ann Allergy* 32:151–153, 1974.

79. Greenberger, Patterson R: The outcome of pregnancy complicated by severe asthma. *Allergy Proc* 9:539, 1988.

80. Schatz M, Zeiger RS, Hoffman CP, et al. Intrauterine growth is related to gestational pulmonary function in pregnant asthmatic women. *Chest* 98:389, 1990.

81. Dombrowski MR, Bottoms SF, Boike GM et al: Incidence of preeclampsia among asthmatic patients lower with theophylline, *Am J Obstet Gynecol* 155:265, 1986.

82. Minerbi-Codish I, Fraser D, Avnun L, et al: Influence of asthma in pregnancy on labor and the newborn. *Respiraton* 65:130–135, 1998.

83. Alexander S, Dodds L, Armson BA: Perinatal outcomes in women with asthma during pregnancy. *Obstet Gynecol* 92:435–440, 1998.

84. Demissie K, Breckenridge MB, Rhoads GG: Infant and maternal outcomes in the pregnancies of asthmatic women. *Am J Respir Crit Care Med* 158:1091–1095, 1998.

85. Cnattingus S, Haglund B, Meirik O: Cigarette smoking as risk factors for late fetal and early neonatal death. *Br Med J* 297:258–261, 1988.

86. Wisborg K, Henriksen TB, Hedegaard M, Secher NJ: Smoking during pregnancy and preterm birth. *Br J Obstet Gynecol* 103:800–805, 1996.

87. Ellard GA, Johnstoe FD, Prescott RJ, et al: Smoking during pregnancy: The dose dependence of birth weight deficits. *Br J Obstet Gyncol* 103:806–813, 1996.

88. Center for Disease Control: Asthma—United States 1980-87. *MMWR* 39:493–496, 1990.

89. Schoendorf KC, Hogue CJR, Kleinman JC, Rowley D: Mortality among infants of black as compared with white college-educated parents. *N Engl J Med* 326:1522–1526, 1992.

90. Bertrand JM, Riley SP, Papkin J, et al: The long term pulmonary sequelae of prematurity: The role of familial airway hyperreactivity and the respiratory distress syndrome. *N Engl J Med* 312:742, 1985.

91. Vinatier D, Monnier JC: Pre-eclampsia: physiology and immunological aspects. *Eur J Obstet Gynecol* 61:85–97, 1995.

92. Levin ER: Endothelins. *N Engl J Med* 333:356–363, 1995.

93. Millar EA, Nally JE, Thomson NC: Angiotensin II potentiates methacholine-induced bronchoconstriction in human airway both in vitro and in vivo. *Eur Respir J* 8:1938–1941, 1995.

94. Schatz M, Hoffman CP, Zeiger RS, et al: The course and management of asthma and allergic disease during pregnancy, In Middleton E, Reed CE, Ellis EF, et al (eds): *Allergy: Principles and Practices,* 3rd ed. St. Louis, CV Mosby, 1988.

95. Rayburn WF, Atkinson BD, Gilbert K, Turnbull GL: Short-term effects of inhaled albuterol on ma-

ternal and fetal circulations. *Am J Obstet Gynecol* 171:770–773, 1994.

96. Neff RK, Levitan A: Maternal theophylline consumption and the risk of stillbirth, *Chest* 97:1266, 1990.

97. Wilson J: Utilisation du cromoglycate de sodium au cours de la grossesse. *Acta Therapeutica* 8(supp): 45–51, 1982.

98. Greenberger PA, Patterson R: Beclomethasone di-proprionate for severe asthma during pregnancy. *Ann Intern Med* 98:478–480, 1983.

99. Dombrowski MP, Brown CL, Berry SM: Preliminary experience with triamcinolone acetonide during pregnancy. *J Mat Fet Med* 5:310–313, 1996.

100. Kallen B, Rydhstroem H, Aberg A. Congenital malformations after the use of inhaled budesonide in early pregnancy. *Obstet Gynecol* 93:392–395, 1999.

Chapter 17

ASTHMA AND ANESTHESIA

Héctor Litvan
Pere Casan

INTRODUCTION

As in other chronic illnesses patients with asthma can usually be anesthetized safely when surgery is required. Advances in asthma treatment and the evolution of anesthesia and postoperative care have allowed for safe administration of almost all types of anesthesia.[1] This is fortunate given the prevalence of asthma worldwide and the common need to anesthetize asthma patients.[2,3] The presence of bronchial hyperresponsiveness in other illnesses (e.g., COPD, bronchiectasis, rhinitis, and recent upper respiratory airway infections) increases the importance of this problem.[4]

As discussed in this chapter, patients with asthma are at risk of a number of respiratory complications during the perioperative period(s), the most important of which is acute bronchospasm and allergic drug reactions.[5] Although such episodes are relatively infrequent in the general population, they are more common in patients with a history of airway disease and can be life threatening.[6] In the general population, there are 1.6 episodes of intraoperative bronchospasm for every 1000 surgeries.[7] In patients with asthma, bronchospasm occurs in between 6.5%[1] and 7.1%[8] of cases, and in patients with COPD, bronchospasm occurs in 22% of cases, although most cases are not severe.[9] In children with asthma, Vener and colleagues found that 47 of 206 (22%) children developed perioperative bronchospasm.[10] In a study from the American Society of Anesthesiologists (ASA) database dealing with closed judicial claims, 32% of patients who had a respiratory mor-

bid event had a history of asthma and 11% had a history of COPD or active smoking.[11] In a retrospective analysis of 706 asthma patients who received either general or spinal anesthesia over a 20-year period in Rochester, Minnesota, Warner and colleagues[6] found that 1.8% of the patients developed bronchospasm (0.6% intraoperatively and 1.2% postoperatively). In this study, strict criteria were used to define asthma. Patients with other causes of bronchial hyperresponsiveness, such as COPD or recent upper respiratory tract infections, were excluded. Patients had well-controlled or mild asthma with only 54% reporting symptoms in the last year; 41% had received at least one medication for asthma during the last year. In the subgroup of patients reporting symptoms in the 30 days prior to surgery, the incidence of complications was higher (4.5%) than in asymptomatic patients (0.8%). Patients who had respiratory complications also had a higher ASA class risk (this classification system stratifies patients into five categories of risk, based on their preoperative physical condition, ranging from grade I for the healthy patient to grade V for the moribund patient).[12] At the authors' hospital, 277 episodes of bronchospasm in 15,963 anesthetic procedures (1.73%) have been reported.[13] Of these, 75 cases occurred during anesthesia (0.47%) and 202 in the immediate postoperative period (1.26%). In 42 patients (15% with bronchospasm, and 0.26% of the total number of patients) the episode was classified as severe. In almost all cases (94%), bronchospasm occurred after general anesthesia with tracheal intubation. At this same institution, in patients with severe asthma or with well-established COPD (FEV_1 < 40%), undergoing upper abdominal surgery, 36 (13%) developed severe bronchospasm during the intraoperative and 47 (17%) in the postoperative period.[14]

Shnider and Papper observed that bronchospasm episodes were more closely related to tracheal intubation (6.4%) than to the type of anesthetic used.[1] Indeed, there was no difference in incidence of bronchospasm between patients receiving general anesthesia without intubation (1.6% of cases) compared with regional blocks (1.9% of cases). Similarly, in the study by Warner and colleagues, bronchospasm occurred only in patients who were intubated.[6]

PREOPERATIVE EVALUATION

As part of risk stratification, asthma patients should be classified according to established criteria, such as those published by the National Institutes of Health[15,16] and the British Thoracic Society[17] (Table 17-1). This classification should be done in conjunction with the referring physician as close as possible to the date of the surgery, but allowing enough time to optimize patient stability. It is not surprising that patients with disease of lesser severity have better outcomes.[18] Additional factors to consider preoperatively are listed below.

1. *Triggering factors.* Specific attention should be paid to drug allergies and/or other phar-

Table 17-1
Classification of the Severity of Asthma[a]

Step 1:	Intermittent
	Intermittent symptoms (<1 time a week)
	Brief exacerbation (from a few hours to a few days)
	Nighttime asthma symptoms (<2 times a month)
	FEV_1 or PEF values = > 80% predicted
	PEF variability <20%
Step 2:	Mild persistent
	Symptoms (>1 time a week but <1 time per day)
	Exacerbation may affect activity and sleep
	Nighttime asthma symptoms (>2 times a month)
	FEV_1 or PEF values = > 80% predicted
	PEF variability 20%–30%
Step 3:	Moderate persistent
	Daily symptoms
	Exacerbations affect activity and sleep
	Nighttime asthma symptoms (>1 time a week)
	Daily use of inhaled short-acting β_2 agonist
	FEV_1 or PEF values (>60% and < 80% predicted)
	PEF variability >30%
Step 4:	Severe persistent
	Continuous symptoms
	Frequent exacerbations
	Frequent nighttime asthma symptoms
	Physical activities limited by asthma symptoms
	FEV_1 or PEF values (<60% predicted)
	PEF variability >30%

[a]NOTE: The presence of one of the features of severity is sufficient to place a patient in that category.
SOURCE: Modified from National Heart, Lung, and Blood Institute, World Health Organization.[15]

macological triggers that have precipitated asthma, and which may be potentially important in the perioperative period. Such medications include aspirin-related products, β-blockers, and antibiotics. The possibility of latex sensitivity should also be considered.

2. *Frequency of attacks.* Patients with frequent exacerbations are more likely to have exacerbations in the perioperative period.

3. *Elapsed time since last attack.* Recent exacerbations may predict greater bronchial hyperresponsiveness and the need for more aggressive pharmacotherapy.[19]

4. *Response to the current treatment.* Ideally, preoperative treatment achieves stability as defined by clinical and physiologic criteria. A patient with well-controlled asthma has little variability (day-to-day and morning-to-morning) in symptoms of cough, wheeze, and breathlessness, and peak expiratory flow rates (PEFR). They should sleep through the night, experience no deterioration in the early morning hours, be able to exercise without exacerbation, and have minimal need for short-acting rescue bronchodilators.

5. *Pulmonary function tests.* Whenever possible, objective assessment of pulmonary function should be obtained preoperatively. These tests should include spirometry with evaluation of response to bronchodilator, and determination of pulse oximetry saturation or arterial blood gas. Forced spirometry helps to assess the severity of airflow obstruction, whereas bronchodilator responsiveness is an indirect measure of airway hyperresponsiveness. Similarly, variability in PEFR correlates with airway hyperresponsiveness and the potential for perioperative complication. Rarely, if ever, is there a need to specifically measure bronchial hyperresponsiveness with methacholine or histamine challenge. To accurately assess the degree of airway obstruction, measurement of FEV_1 is preferable to PEFR, since PEFR is more affected by patient effort. In any event, frequent measurement of expiratory airflow at bedside aids in perioperative management.[20] Lung volume measurements are probably not required in most patients; however, identification of severe hyperinflated patients may help identify those at

greatest risk of intraoperative and postoperative dynamic hyperinflation. If measured, the finding of a low diffusing capacity for carbon monoxide (DLCO) should raise the suspicion of emphysema and the possibility of a more fixed form of airflow obstruction and chronic hypercapnia. Information on preoperative evaluation of pulmonary function that is beyond the scope of this chapter is available.[21,22]

6. *Recent airway infection.* Upper respiratory tract infection can increase airway resistance (Raw) and airway hyperreactivity in asthma patients.[23,24] Empy and colleagues showed a significant increase in Raw following histamine inhalation in patients with viral infection of the airways.[23] Seven weeks after infection, the patients demonstrated a normal response to the same stimulus. Ideally, elective surgery should be postponed for at least 2 to 3 weeks after upper respiratory tract infection.[21,22]

7. *COPD* Consideration should be given to the alternate diagnosis of COPD when there is a history of smoking. Patients with COPD have a higher incidence of postoperative complications, including acute or chronic ventilatory failure due to an imbalance between respiratory neuromuscular strength and respiratory system load.[25,26]

8. *Smoking* Beyond concerns of COPD, smoking increases bronchial hypersecretion and hyperresponsiveness, thereby further elevating airway resistance after tracheal intubation.[27] Smoking also increases the risk of acute infection of the airways, and the higher concentration of carboxyhemoglobin in smokers interferes with oxygen transport. In order to effectively diminish perioperative risk, patients should stop smoking at least 8 weeks prior to surgery. However, not smoking in the 48 hours before surgery decreases the carboxyhemoglobin and increases oxygen transfer to the tissues by shifting the oxyhemoglobin saturation curve to the right. In 1 week, motility of the bronchial cilia recovers and transport and elimination of secretions improves.[28]

9. *Type of surgery.* Proximity to the diaphragm, and the length and aggressiveness of the surgical procedure are important preoperative considerations. There are a higher percentage of

Table 17-2
Risk Factors for Respiratory Complications

- Recent airway infection
- COPD
- Smoking
- Region of surgery: thorax, upper abdomen
- Health status: age, obesity, undernourishment

SOURCE: Modified from Tisi[21]; Pedersen, et al[22]; Tarhan, et al[25]; Milledge, et al.[26]

respiratory complications after upper abdominal and thoracic surgery than, for instance, after surgery of the extremities. Emergency surgery has twice the complications of elective surgery, and procedures lasting more than 4 hours have more complications than shorter procedures.[29,30]

10. *Health status.* Advanced age and extremes of weight are also risk factors for pulmonary complication. Obesity, as may occur in patients receiving chronic oral corticosteroids, may cause restrictive pulmonary defect and increase the risk of postoperative atelectasis. Long-term steroids may also contribute to the development of obstructive sleep apnea which may manifest postoperatively, may increase the difficulty of oral intubation, and may cause respiratory muscle weakness. Severe malnutrition similarly may cause respiratory muscle weakness and interfere with cough and secretion clearance (see Table 17-2).

PREOPERATIVE PREPARATION

Asymptomatic Patients

Patients with asthma who are asymptomatic and are not taking asthma medication have no greater risk of respiratory complications in the perioperative period than do patients without asthma.[18] Asymptomatic asthma patients do not require preoperative preparation. Routine preoperative administration of systemic steroids to asymptomatic or very well-controlled patients has been questioned and is probably unjustified.[6] However, inhaled steroids and β_2-adrenergic agonist bron-

chodilators have been advocated before surgery in this patient group.[31] Parker and colleagues have recommended steroids if the FEV_1 is less than 80% of predicted,[32] a strategy that may help treat airway wall inflammation edema of the mucosa and minimize secretions.[33]

Patients who are asymptomatic because of appropriate pharmacotherapy should be continued on their usual medications during surgery.[31] It is important to remember that patients taking oral steroids (even in the past) or high-dose inhaled steroids may need stress doses of systemic steroids perioperatively to prevent adrenal insufficiency.

Symptomatic Patients

If surgery cannot be postponed for symptomatic patients, aggressive pharmacotherapy with inhaled β_2-agonists and intravenous corticosteroids should be initiated without delay[33,34] and continued in the intraoperative and postoperative periods. Inhaled bronchodilators may be delivered by nebulizer, MDI with spacer, or AMBU-type face mask (Fig. 17-1)[35]. Systemic steroids should also be adminis-

Figure 17-1
Commercially available MDI adapted to an AMBU mask; a practical solution for administration of $_2$-adrenergic agonists during the premedication.

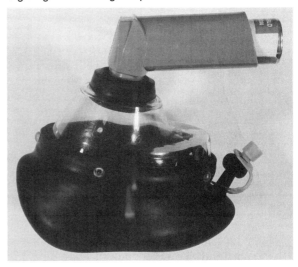

tered every 6 to 8 hours in the 24 hours prior to surgery, if possible, and continued in the postoperative period.[36] It may be useful to add intravenous anticholinergics (e.g., atropine, glycopyrrolate) to the list of anesthetic premedications that may be used to block muscarinic receptors in the tracheobronchial mucosa.[37] Inhaled ipratropium bromide has a slower onset of action, but it can be of help when administered in high doses, and it is extremely safe[34] (Chapter 10).

Whenever possible, the anesthesiologist should avoid airway stimulation (e.g., by using mask ventilation or regional nerve blockage). Using anesthetic agents with known bronchodilating action (such as propofol, ketamine, or sevoflurane) may also help.

CHANGES IN PULMONARY FUNCTION DURING ANESTHESIA:

Induction of general anesthesia decreases the respiratory muscle tone. The diaphragm moves cephalad lowering lung volumes, so that anesthesia and supine positioning reduce functional residual capacity (FRC) by about 20%.[38,39] Low lung volumes result in atelectasis and may worsen V/Q distribution.[40] In addition, tracheal intubation and introduction of dry, cold gases can trigger bronchospasm and impair clearance of airway secretions.[6,41]

General anesthesia also modifies the pulmonary circulation. Intrapulmonary shunt increases[42,43] and hypoxemia worsens acutely in 20% to 50% of patients in the immediate postoperative period.[44] In addition, many anesthetic drugs such as opioids and halogenated gases interfere with respiratory center function. There may be loss of drive to breathe and a decreased response to hypercapnia and hypoxemia.[45] Depression of the respiratory center in the postoperative period may be more important in asthmatic patients than those without asthma,[46] and can be potentiated by the residual effect of other drugs used during anesthesia. This may be particularly worrisome in the subgroup of patients with near-fatal asthma who already have diminished ventilatory response to hypercapnia and hypoxemia.[47]

Postoperative pain may alter the respiratory pattern. A fast and shallow pattern of breathing impairs cough and secretion clearance. Retained secretions diminish airway caliber and favor development of atelectasis and postoperative pneumonia. Changes in ventilatory pattern are usually transient, lasting for only a few hours. However, persistent fast and shallow breathing can occur in the setting of atelectasis, postoperative pulmonary edema, or when there is decreased diaphragmatic function after abdominal surgery.[48] Changes in pulmonary function are most pronounced during thoracic and upper abdominal surgery. Fewer changes occur in lower abdominal surgery and in surgeries involving the head or extremities.[49]

ANESTHETIC DRUGS AND BRONCHOMOTOR TONE

Airway smooth muscles are innervated by the parasympathetic nervous system. Cholinergic efferent fibers travel along the vagus nerve establishing synapses in the parasympathetic ganglia, located in airway walls. Stimulation of the vagus nerve releases acetylcholine from prejunctional postganglionic nerve endings. Acetylcholine binds to the M_3 muscarinic receptors found on smooth muscle cells of the airway, producing a contractile response. Acetylcholine also stimulates M_2 receptors in ganglia. These receptors create a negative feedback decreasing acetylcholine release and contractile response strength.[50] Drugs with a nonselective muscarinic effect can inhibit M_2 muscarinic receptors, and thereby worsen bronchoconstriction. Drugs not specifically cholinergic, such as some muscular relaxants or even nonselective anticholinergics such as atropine, can inhibit M_2 receptors and produce acetylcholine release in given circumstances. Opioids may also affect acetylcholine release and contractile strength.[51]

Barbiturates

Barbiturates have been the hypnotics of choice to induce anesthesia for more than 50 years.[52] Multiple studies of barbiturate action on bronchomotor tone have generated somewhat contradictory conclusions. Thiopental has been reported to induce bronchoconstriction by histamine release and therefore is thought to be contraindicated in patients with bronchial hyperresponsiveness,[53] contradicting the general claim that barbiturates are safe for most patients with asthma.[52,54] Also, data exist demonstrating that induction with barbiturates followed by tracheal intubation produced wheezing in approximately 50% of patients with a history of bronchial hyperresponsiveness, with more episodes occurring with thiobarbiturate (thiopental, thiamylal) (27%) than with oxybarbiturate (methohexital) (13%).[55] In this same study, thiopental produced wheezing in 16% of the patients who had no history of bronchial hyperresponsiveness.[55] However, experimental studies have shown that thiopental can inhibit vagal reflexes[56,57] and cause bronchodilation when used in higher concentrations.[58,59] Some authors link low-dose thiopental to bronchoconstriction and high-dose thiopental to bronchodilation.[60] At usual clinical doses, airway reflexes remain intact, so that bronchoconstriction may occur when the airway is stimulated.[1,61] The fact that thiopental also causes hyperalgesia (i.e., an increased pain response) is also a problem.

Smokers appear to be at greater risk of thiopental-induced bronchoconstriction than nonsmokers. Eames and associates compared Raw after anesthesia induction and tracheal intubation with propofol, thiopental or etomidate in 75 patients.[27] Propofol was associated with less of an increase in Raw compared with thiopental and etomidate.

Propofol

Propofol, an alkylphenol derivative with hypnotic and sedative effects, is one of the newer intravenous anesthetics. Due to its short action, bolus administration can be used to induce anesthesia; maintenance of anesthesia or sedation during regional anesthesia can be achieved through continuous infusion.[62,63] Similar to barbiturates, propofol causes respiratory center depression.[62] Propofol does not release histamine.[62] Indeed, propofol has been shown experimentally to decrease airway resistance clinically,[55,64,65] making it a useful agent for induction of anesthesia in asthma patients. In a study by Wu and colleagues, the effects of propofol were compared with thiopental in 37 healthy subjects.[66] After anesthesia induction and tracheal intubation, airway resistance was lower in the propofol group than in the thiopental group. Following the administration of isoflurane, an inhaled anesthetic that produces bronchodilation, airway resistance was not modified in the group induced with propofol, but it did decrease significantly in the group induced with thiopental. Thus, propofol protected the airways and produced a similar degree of bronchodilation as isofluorane.[66] Habre and colleagues studied changes in respiratory mechanics induced by propofol and halothane in children with and without asthma.[67] Results were similar in both groups, demonstrating that propofol is safe in children with asthma. The mechanism by which propofol produces bronchodilation is not known. It does not directly relax smooth muscle[68] nor interfere with calcium flow.[27]

Ketamine

Ketamine is a phencyclidine derivative with analgesic and dissociative anesthetic properties. It stimulates the central nervous system and maintains airway protective reflexes,[69] and can precipitate delirium and hallucinations during recovery from anesthesia. Ketamine minimally affects the respiratory center and relaxes bronchial smooth muscle by catecholamine release and antimuscarinic effects.[70] At higher concentrations, not used in the clinical setting, ketamine has a direct relaxing effect on bronchial smooth muscle and can inhibit vagal reflexes.[71] Experimentally, it is as effective a bronchodilator as halothane or enflurane.[71]

Ketamine is a sympathomimetic capable of increasing peripheral vascular resistance, arterial pressure, heart rate, and cardiac output. Thus, its use in hypovolemic patients with hemodynamic instability is recommended,[69] and its use is contraindicated in patients with pulmonary or intracranial hypertension. Ketamine is one of the drugs of choice for asthma patients undergoing emergency general anesthesia.[62]

Benzodiazepines

Benzodiazepines (diazepam, lorazepam, midazolam) are commonly used for sedation during regional anesthesia or to induce general anesthesia.[62] They do not increase airway resistance,[62] although bronchospasm has been described after administration of nebulized midazolam.[72,73] Respiratory depression induced by diazepam or midazolam can be more severe and prolonged in patients receiving opioids and in patients with severe COPD and hypercapnia, than in healthy subjects.[74,75]

Etomidate

Etomidate is a hypnotic imidazole derivative with minimal effects on hemodynamics or respiratory center function, making it an ideal drug in patients with hemodynamic instability.[75] Its use is limited by inhibition of cortisol synthesis at the adrenal level,[62] a condition reversed by vitamin C administration.[76] Etomidate is recommended in the induction of allergic patients because it does not release histamine.[77] However, as mentioned previously, etomidate does increase airway resistance after intubation compared to propofol.[27]

Halogenated Anesthetics

The potency of these powerful inhaled anesthetic agents is measured using minimum alveolar concentration (MAC), which is the concentration necessary to abolish the motor response to a painful stimulus in 50% of subjects.[78] Table 17-3 shows the most commonly used halogenated anesthetics and their effect on the bronchomotor tone. Halogenated anesthetics are effective bronchodilators[79,80] and have several mechanisms of action. They decrease motor tone by direct relaxation of the bronchial smooth muscle and they block the medullary arc reflex and the bronchoconstrictor stimulus of the anesthetic on the central nervous system.[81]

Effects on the bronchial smooth muscle tone are related to an increase in cyclic-AMP, a de-

Table 17-3
Bronchodilator Effects of Halogenated Anesthetics

Agent	MAC[a,b] %	Bronchodilator Effect <1 MAC	>1.5 MAC
Halothane	0.75	++	+++
Enflurane	2.0	+	+++
Isoflurane	1.15	+	+++
Desflurane	6.0	+	+++
Sevoflurane	2.0	+	+++

[a]NOTE: MAC of halogenated anesthetics and its bronchodilator effect at low and high MAC.
[b]ABBREVIATION: MAC, minimal alveolar concentration.
SOURCE: Modified from Warner, et al[84]; Shah and Hirshman[87]; Hirshman, et al.[90]

crease in free Ca^{++} in the cytoplasm of bronchial smooth muscle cells, and suppression of Ca^{++} flow across the cellular membrane, interfering with excitation-contraction coupling.[82,83] These effects take place only when the drug is administered by inhalation,[84] and not by vein.[85,86]

In vitro and in vivo, halothane, enflurane, and isoflurane diminish vagally mediated bronchoconstriction.[87] At low concentrations these anesthetics decrease the excitability of postsynaptic cholinergic parasympathetic receptors. At 1 MAC, halothane, enflurane, and sevoflurane decrease metacholine-induced bronchoconstriction.[88,89] At 1.5 MAC, halothane and isoflurane decrease ascaris antigen-induced bronchoconstriction[90,91] and, at concentrations greater than 1.7 MAC, halothane decreases acetylcholine release. Halogenated anesthetics do not inhibit mast cell mediator release. Histamine levels following antigenic stimulation are not affected by halothane.[92]

Halogenated anesthetics are the drugs of choice to achieve general anesthesia in asthma patients. Halothane has the greatest bronchodilating effect,[93] but it also has the greatest potential for drug intereactions (e.g., halothane can elevate theophylline levels). Isoflurane and sevoflurane are excellent alternatives.[94–96] Isoflurane, halothane, and sevoflurane have all been shown to have a more favorable effect on airway resistance in healthy intubated subjects compared to thiopental.[97] Both sevoflurane and desflurane are widely used due to their short duration of action. Because sevoflurane is a nonirritant gas, it is used for induction and maintenance of anesthesia in children with asthma.[97a] Since desflurane is an irritant, it should not be used for anesthesia induction, although it has been proven to be effective in maintaining anesthesia in asthma patients.[90] Because these gases have similar bronchodilating effects, agent selection is often based on nonrespiratory criteria such as potency, length of anesthetic effect, or effects on the cardiovascular system.

Because of their bronchodilating properties, some halogenated anesthetics, especially halothane and isoflurane, have been used to treat near-fatal asthma that was nonresponsive to conventional therapy.[98–101] However, when administered continuously during a prolonged period of time, halogenated anesthetics have produced serious side effects.[102,103]

Opioids

The main problem with opioids is that they can depress respiratory center function. Automatism and respiratory rate are decreased and apnea may occur at high dose. Opioids decrease the central response to hypoxemia and hypercapnia, even at low doses. Bronchomotor tone may also be affected by histamine release or by modulation of the cholinergic and noncholinergics receptors on peribronchial smooth muscle cells. Rosow and colleagues studied the histamine release induced by morphine (1 mg/kg) and fentanyl (50 μg/kg) in patients undergoing cardiac surgery.[104] They found that morphine increased plasma histamine up to 750%, but fentanyl, at equivalent doses, did not. Morphine-induced changes in histamine concentration were quite variable in this study, ranging from undetectable to values seen in some patients of anaphylactic reaction. There was also a convincing inverse correlation between peak levels of histamine and systemic vascular resistance and arterial blood pressure. Particular care must be taken in patients with severe allergies, who may

react to minimal increases in histamine concentration.[105]

Similar to morphine, meperidine induces histamine release, but its effects can be successfully blocked by prior administration of H_1 and H_2 histamine antagonists.[106,107] However, newer agents, such as alfentanyl, sulfentanyl, and remifentanyl, do not release histamine.

The importance of opioid-induced modulation of cholinergic and noncholinergic receptors on peribronchial smooth muscle cells is not yet clear. Zappi and colleagues[108] found that opioid agonists inhibited electrical muscle contraction in bovine tracheal (but not bronchial) preparations. On the other hand, opioid agonists inhibited contraction in bronchial preparations, suggesting that opioid receptors are not evenly distributed along the tracheobronchial tree. The clinical implications of these data are not yet clear, but some authors have suggested that opioids may prove to be useful in the treatment of asthma.[109]

Muscle Relaxants

Muscle relaxants are administered to facilitate tracheal intubation during induction of general anesthesia and to provide a quiet surgical field . There are two types of muscle relaxants: 1) depolarizing, which act by binding to acetylcholine receptor sites on the postjunctional neuromuscular membrane causing depolarization, and 2) nondepolarizing, which compete with acetylcholine at the neuromuscular junction to prevent depolarization of the postjunctional membrane.

These agents may cause bronchospasm as the result of 1) histamine release, especially d-tubocurarine, mivacurium, doxacurium, or high doses of atracurium, or 2) a cholinergic mechanism when they bind to the M2 muscarinic receptors on the tracheobronchial mucosa, especially pancuronium, atracurium, and mivacurium.[61,110]

Vetterman and colleagues studied the effects of different doses of several muscle relaxants in anesthetized dogs.[111] Vecuronium did not cause bronchoconstriction; however, high doses of atracurium did. The effects of atracurium were attributed to histamine release, a property not shared by the similar drug, cis-atracurium. Pancuronium demonstrated a biphasic response, with bronchoconstriction occurring at low doses and bronchodilation at high doses, likely due to different actions on the muscarinic receptors M_2 (inhibition at low doses) and M_3 (inhibition at high doses). In other studies, bronchospasm has been reported following administration of succinylcholine, possibly owing to its acetylcholine-like effect.[112,113] Nevertheless succinylcholine is frequently used to intubate patients with near-fatal asthma.

For ongoing paralysis, vecuronium, atracurium, or cis-atracurium are the drugs of choice, with little data supporting the use of one drug more than another. In one study, atracurium and vecuronium were associated with the same number of respiratory complications, although atracurium was associated with more hemodynamic alterations.[114] For more information on paralytic agents, including the risk of myopathy, see Chapter 14.

Cholinesterase Inhibitors

The cholinesterase inhibitors neostigmine, pyridostigmine, and edrophonium are used to reverse the effects of muscle relaxants. They can induce bronchial smooth muscle constriction by inhibiting the degradation of released acetylcholine at parasympathetic efferent endings. This effect can be prevented with anticholinergic drugs. However, the use of cholinesterase inhibitors is not recommended in asthma patients with recent exacerbation, even in the presence of anticholinergic therapy.

Anticholinergic Drugs

Anticholinergics drugs are muscarinic antagonists capable of relaxing bronchial smooth muscle. Atropine, glycopyrrolate, and scopolamine are drugs used frequently in anesthesia to prevent vagal reflexes and the muscarinic effects of anticholinesterase drugs. They are nonselective blockers, inhibiting both M_2 and M_3 muscarinic receptors.[50] Usual dosages are lower than those required to relax bronchial smooth muscle. At high doses, intravenous atropine produces neurological and car-

diovascular side effects (e.g., dry mouth, blurred vision, and tachycardia). However, glycopyrrolate is a good alternative. Ipratropium bromide by nebulization may also achieve some degree of bronchodilation.

Local Anesthetics

Intravenous lidocaine decreases the bronchospastic response to both nonspecific (citric acid) and specific stimuli (ascaris antigen).[115,115a] Additionally, bronchospasm induced by laryngoscopy may be prevented by pretreatment with intravenous lidocaine. No additional benefit appears to be conferred by use of inhaled lidocaine. Indeed, laryngospasm and bronchospasm may occur despite inhaled lidocaine when the airways are entered for purposes of intubation or bronchoscopy.[116,117] During anesthesia, lidocaine may be continued in order to diminish airway reflexes and to protect against arrhythmias. As bupivacaine by epidural or vein can be effective in decreasing responses to mucosal irritation, epidural bupivacaine is the anesthetic of choice for prolonged procedures.[118]

PREMEDICATIONS

Premedications are used to help patients arrive in the operating theater as calm and free of pain as possible. For this purpose, benzodiazepines (e.g., midazolam, lorazepam), H_1 histamine antagonists (e.g., hydroxyzine) and analgesics may all be indicated.[119] H_2 histamine blockers are often administered to protect the gastric mucosa. Interestingly, some authors suggest that H_1 histamine antagonists should be added to H_2 histamine antagonists, if H_2 antagonists are being administered to asthma patients to prevent the rare occurrence of bronchospasm triggered by predominance of H_1 receptors.[120] However, extensive experience suggests that H_2 blockers can be used safely in patients with asthma in the absence of H_1 blockade. The H_1 blockers diphenylhydramine and hydroxyzine are commonly used to achieve additional sedative effects.[121]

Inhaled agonists should be given within 1 hour of intubation. Kil and colleagues studied the prophylactic administration of inhaled bronchodilators in patients without asthma who were undergoing general anesthesia with tracheal intubation.[31] They demonstrated that both albuterol (360 mcg) and ipratropium bromide (72 mcg) were effective medications when given 1 hour before surgery. Each medication was associated with lower lung resistance after intubation compared with placebo.

As previously mentioned, patients who have been taking systemic steroids (either currently or in the past), or high doses of inhaled steroids, should be evaluated for stress dose steroid replacement. Hydrocortisone, 1 to 2 mg/kg every 8 hours by vein, is usually sufficient for this purpose, depending on patient status and type of surgery.[122]

Xanthine preparations may be continued up to the night of surgery (and continued after surgery) if blood levels do not exceed the therapeutic range.[123,124] However, xanthines are rarely used intraoperatively since they may interact with some anesthetic agents, are unlikely to confer added bronchodilation to inhaled agonists and halogenated anesthetics, and may promote arrhythmias.[125] Of additional concern is the potential for xanthines to cause gastroesophageal reflux, increasing the risk of aspiration of gastric contents during induction of anesthesia.[33]

INTRAOPERATIVE MONITORING

Monitoring during anesthesia depends on patient status, the type of surgery, and the anesthetic technique. In the low-risk patient receiving regional anesthesia, continuous electrocardiography, arterial blood pressure, and pulsed oximetry are sufficient. Monitoring low-risk patients receiving general anesthesia should also include measurement of end-tidal CO_2, body temperature and train-of-four electrical stimulation of muscles. Continuous monitoring of intraarterial blood pressure, central venous pressure and pulmonary arterial pressure, may be useful in high-risk patients. In addition, arterial cannulation allows serial blood samples for arterial blood gas determination. Additional monitoring may be needed in complex situations.[126] With regard to end-tidal CO_2 monitoring, it is important to note that expiratory airflow obstruction affects the shape of the CO_2 time curve due to uneven emptying of alveolar gas. The result is a loss of the normal expiratory plateau (Fig. 17-2).[127]

ANESTHETIC TECHNIQUE SELECTION

Blocking of nociceptive stimuli can occur by preventing progression of the stimulus through nerve pathways by local anesthetics (regional anesthesia) or by blocking perception of the stimulus by the central nervous system (general anesthesia). Each of these approaches are discussed below.

Regional Anesthesia

Regional anesthesia is intended to block nociceptive impulses by local anesthetics at the spinal cord

FIGURE 17-2
End-tidal CO_2 measurements in the normal state and in the setting of moderate and severe obstruction. Note the upsloping curve in patients with obstruction. (Modified from Good[127])

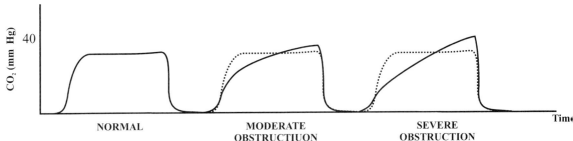

NORMAL   MODERATE OBSTRUCTIUON   SEVERE OBSTRUCTION   Time

(spinal or epidural blockade) or peripheral trunk levels, while the patient is awake, or lightly sedated, with spontaneous ventilation and without manipulating the airway. After blockade, a catheter is usually placed to administer drugs repeatedly or as a continuous perfusion in long procedures, and to maintain analgesia in the postoperative period. Local anesthesia of the peripheral nerves achieves analgesia and motor paralysis in the region of concern. This type of analgesia is mainly used in surgery of the extremities and head and neck.

Spinal blockade, subarachnoid or epidural, affects sensory, motor, and sympathetic nerve function. Sympathetic blockade causes vasodilatation, increased skin temperature in the blocked area, and arterial hypotension, depending on the level of blockage. Spinal anesthesia is used in surgery of the lower abdomen, perineum, and lower extremities. It is the technique of choice during childbirth,[128] but is rarely used in upper abdominal surgery. Some of the advantages and disadvantages of regional anesthesia are listed in Table 17-4.

In asthma patients, the main anesthetic priority should be the avoidance of airway manipulation. Regional anesthesia avoids laryngeal and tracheal manipulation, stimulation of airway reflexes, and the possibility of mechanical ventilator-induced auto-PEEP. The local anesthetics used are generally safe in asthma and with the use of a

catheter, regional analgesia can be maintained in the immediate postoperative period, comforting the patient and facilitating respiratory exercises.

The main limitation of regional anesthesia is that it can only be applied to the lower abdomen and extremities. There are also specific contraindications to regional anesthesia.[129] Depending on the level of motor blockade, FRC and expiratory reserve volume (ERV) decrease (at the T4 level), abdominal and intercostal muscle strength is reduced (at the T6 level), and productive cough is diminished.[130-132] In addition to arterial hypotension, sympathetic system blockade at a high thoracic level (the sympathetic pulmonary nerves arise from the spinal cord between T2 and T7[133]), can cause intraoperative bronchospasm through parasympathetic activity.[134,135]

The patient with asthma undergoing abdominal laparoscopy, which requires insufflating the abdomen with CO_2, warrants special consideration. Laparoscopy creates a pneumoperitoneum with pressurized CO_2. Abdominal pressure increases and the diaphragm moves cephalad, decreasing FRC and respiratory system compliance, favoring atelectasis and V/Q mismatch and shunting. Because of the high solubility of CO_2 and absorption through the peritoneum, Pa_{CO_2} levels may rise, particularly if regional anesthesia has decreased abdominal and intercostal muscle strength and the patient is in the Trendelenburg position. If bronchospasm occurs in this setting,

Table 17-4
Advantages and Disadvantages of Regional Anesthesia

Advantages	Disadvantages
Does not interfere with airway reflexes	Limited indications
Avoids endotracheal intubation and minimizes the chance of lung hyperinflation secondary to mechanical ventilation	Patient anxiety during procedure
Uses local anesthetics	Anesthetizes abdominal/intercostal muscles
Postoperative analgesia by catheter	Enhancement of parasympathetic system?

decreased respiratory reserve places the patient at risk for acute respiratory failure and the need for intubation. For these reasons, regional anesthesia should be reserved only for asymptomatic asthma patients undergoing laparoscopic surgery. In symptomatic patients, and in patients undergoing upper abdominal laproscopic procedures, general anesthesia is indicated.

General Anesthesia

Anesthesia Induction   For induction of anesthesia, drugs with known bronchodilating properties should be used, and drugs known to release histamine should be avoided. Propofol, benzodiazepines, etomidate, ketamine, and fentanyl are safe drugs for purposes of induction in asthma patients;[33,61] ketamine is preferred in emergency situations. Seroflurane appears to be particularly useful in children with asthma. Vecuronium has been reported to be the safest muscle relaxant;[110,113] complications have been reported with pancuronium, ciscuronium, rocuronium, and even atracrium or succinylcholine. Cis-atracurium, which does not release histamine, is an attractive alternative.

Tracheal Intubation   Irritation produced by the endotracheal tube is a major issue since it can cause an increase in airway resistance and bronchospasm even in patients without bronchial hyperresponsiveness.[55] In one study of healthy awake volunteers, intubation caused a 40% increase in airway resistance, possibly due to a parasympathetic-mediated bronchoconstrictive reflex induced by stimulation of the upper airway.[136] Indeed, intubation should be avoided in asthma patients whenever possible. Alternatives to intubation include ventilation with facial mask for short procedures or the use of a laryngeal mask airway (LMA), which allows for mechanical ventilation without tracheal intubation.[137,138] LMA has been successfully used for noninvasive mechanical ventilation during anesthesia and in the postoperative period.[139] The anesthesiologist should be aware that the LMA does not always produce an air-tight fit around the glottis, particularly at high airway

pressures, placing the patient at risk for gastric distension, vomiting, and aspiration of gastric contents.[140] For this reason, some authors do not recommend LMA in symptomatic asthma patients.[141] If tracheal intubation is needed in patients with bronchial hyperresponsiveness, deep anesthesia should be used in an attempt to abolish airway reflexes. It is useful to add sevoflurane during ventilation because this non-irritant gas has bronchodilating effects. If induction was achieved with a barbiturate or etomidate (both of which do not block airway reflexes), it is necessary to administer an opioid (e.g., fentanyl, alfentanyl, sulfentanyl or remifentanyl) to block nocioceptive stimuli from intubation and intravenous lidocaine should be considered before intubation to decrease airway reflexes.

Mechanical Ventilation   Tidal volume, inspiratory flow, and respiratory rate of the respirator should be adjusted to avoid lung overdistention and complications of pneumothorax and hypotension. To this end, expiratory time should be kept adequately long to allow for emptying of alveolar gas through narrowed airways. This can be achieved by choosing a high inspiratory flow rate and a low minute volume, insuring that excessive levels of auto-PEEP and plateau pressure do not develop. The use of a large-diameter endotracheal tube also decreases airway resistance and facilitates secretion clearance. For a detailed discussion of mechanical ventilation see Chapter 13.

Maintenance of Anesthesia   While surgery is being performed, a combination of a halogenated anesthetic with low doses of an opioid (e.g., fentanyl, remifentanyl) is usually adequate to maintain adequate anesthesia. Isoflurane has proven to be very effective owing to its bronchodilating effect, and to its having fewer hemodynamic effects than halothane. For short procedures or ambulatory surgery, sevoflurane and desflurane offer the advantage of faster elimination and minimal respiratory center depression in the postoperative period. A sustained intravenous propofol perfusion with low doses of opioids or opioids with lidocaine perfusion (1 to 3 mg/kg per hour), are other options.

Extubation If the patient is stable and breathing spontaneously, extubation following general anesthesia should be done when airway reflexes are still depressed, to avoid airway irritation during tracheal manipulation.[142] Intravenous lidocaine may provide additional protection before extubation. Extubation under deep anesthesia should be avoided in order to decrease the risk of reintubation and additional airway manipulation, particularly in patients who are difficult to intubate. The degree of muscle relaxation should be assessed. Anticholinesterases may cause bronchospasm and should be avoided.

BRONCHOSPASM

Acute bronchospasm in an anesthetized mechanically ventilated patient can be life threatening. It is usually signaled by an increase in airway resistive pressure and a drop in respiratory system compliance when air trapping and lung distension occur.[143,144] Depending on the depth of anesthesia and the severity of airflow obstruction, wheezes and accessory muscle use may occur, but these are unreliable markers of disease severity. Because F_{IO_2} is generally greater than 40% during general anesthesia, significant hypoxemia as assessed by pulsed oximetry is rarely seen. Changes in end-tidal CO_2 may occur with a sudden fall that may

be the precursor of pneumothorax or severe air trapping with diminished venous return and cardiac output.[145]

It is important to remember that conditions other than asthma may be responsible for changes in respiratory status (Table 17-5). Endotracheal tube kinking and mucus plugging should be considered when there is an increase in airway resistance, and an increase in plateau pressure may occur with right mainstem intubation, pneumothorax, pulmonary edema, and opioid-induced chest wall stiffness.

One of the most common causes of intraoperative bronchospasm is inadequate blockage of nocioceptive receptors.[120] When bronchospasm occurs it therefore follows that anesthesia should be deepened and adequate analgesia provided. Administration of halogenated agents, ketamine, propofol, and fentanyl may all be helpful. If bronchospasm persists, inhaled bronchodilators may be given by nebulizer or MDI with spacer. For detailed recommendations regarding bronchodilator use in mechanically ventilated patients see Chapter 11. Of note, few devices have been designed to facilitate bronchodilator administration during administration of anesthesia, often requiring the anesthesiologist to build devices with available spare parts. Two commercially available spacers for use during anesthesia are pictured in Figure 17-3.

A detailed discussion of the pharmacologic approach to acute bronchospasm can be found in Chapter 9. A few additional points deserve consid-

Table 17-5

Causes of Intraoperative Deterioration in Respiratory Status During Anesthesia and Mechanical Ventilation

• Bronchospasm	• Inadequate muscular relaxation
• Pulmonary hyperinsufflation	• Air entrapment, auto-PEEP
• Tracheal tube malposition	• Pneumothorax
• Tracheal tube kinking	• Gastric content aspiration
• Airway secretions	• Anaphylactic reaction
• Thoracic stiffness due to opioids	• Acute cardiogenic pulmonary edema
• Ventilator dysfunction	• Pulmonary thromboembolism

SOURCE: Modified from Gal[33]; Gold[59]; Hirshman[61]; Hirshman.[120]

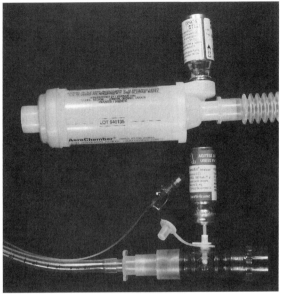

FIGURE 17-3
Commercially available spacers with tracheal tube connections that can be used during general anesthesia with mechanical ventilation. Top: AeroChamber; Bottom: Airlife.

eration in the anesthetized patient. First, β_2 agonists administered in the presence of halogenated anesthetics are particularly effective (and possibly synergistic) and safe.[146] Xanthines, on the other hand, should be used with extreme caution (if ever) during anesthesia, particularly since theophylline does not add to the effects of β_2 agonists combined with a halogenated agent.[147] Theophylline combined with halothane significantly increases the risk of cardiac arrhythmias, particularly in the setting of hypoxemia.[148] Theophylline combined with ketamine can induce grand mal seizures.[149] In addition, there is decreased hepatic metabolism of theophylline during anesthesia, increasing the risk of toxicity. The use of subcutaneous or intravenous β_2 agonists is restricted in the surgical arena due to the potential for arrhythmias, although epinephrine is indicated to treat anaphylactic reactions.

When bronchospasm persists, it may be useful to change from an anesthesia-type ventilator to an ICU-type ventilator with a low compliance circuit. A circuit with low compressible volume decreases the portion of tidal volume wasted in expanding the ventilator circuit, thereby allowing for a smaller set tidal volume to achieve the same effective tidal volume in the patient. This allows for lower minute ventilation and a longer exhalation time. As mentioned earlier, patients with severe airflow obstruction require longer exhalation times to avoid dangerous levels of lung hyperinflation, even if such a strategy elevates Pa_{CO_2}.

It is important to maintain close communication with the surgeon during such acute situations. In some circumstances, the surgeon may be able to interrupt maneuvers that stimulate cholinergic receptors.

IMMEDIATE POSTOPERATIVE PERIOD

In the immediate postoperative period, the patient with asthma is still at risk. In fact, the percentage of patients developing bronchospasm is higher in the immediate postoperative than intraoperative period,[150] requiring high-risk patients to be monitored in a ICU.

Patients with regional anesthesia are usually monitored in the postanesthesia care unit until regression of sensory and motor block occurs. The intensity of monitoring depends on the ASA class status, type of surgery, and events during anesthesia, but it must include ECG, arterial blood pressure, pulse oximetry saturation, and body temperature.

Analgesic drugs should be administered by catheter at a sufficient dose to produce analgesia without producing motor blockage, thus allowing, the patient to easily move and practice physical therapy excercises. Combination of low doses of local anesthetics with very low doses of fentanyl appears to be particularly useful in the postoperative period. Nonsteroidal anti-inflammatory agents should be avoided because of their potential to cause bronchospasm.[151,152]

Bronchodilating and anti-inflammatory medications should be restarted in all patients. Analgesics should be administered to allow the patient to take deep breaths and cough, to facilatate elimination of accumulated bronchial secretions. It has been widely shown that early physical therapy decreases respiratory complications,[153] making early ambulation important. Finally, other complementary steps should be kept in mind, such as adequate hydration and antiembolic prophylaxis.

CONCLUSION

Advances in the treatment of asthma and anesthetic technique allow for safe surgery in most cases. The risk of respiratory complications during anesthesia and surgery are directly related to the severity of asthma and stability of the patient at the time of operation, warranting, as possible, postponement of surgery in poorly controlled patients. Anesthetic risk is minimized by avoiding tracheal intubation, and by careful selection of anesthetic agents. When acute bronchospasm does occur under general anesthesia, a ventilator strategy that avoids lung hyperinflation by prolonging exhalation (even at the cost of hypercapnia) appears to minimize complications.

REFERENCES

1. Shnider SM, Papper EM: Anesthesia for the asthmatic patient. *Anesthesiology* 22:886–892, 1961.
2. Buist SA, Vollmer WM: Reflections on the rise in asthma morbidity and mortality. *JAMA* 13:1719–1720, 1990.
3. Weitzman M, Gortmaker SL, Sobol AM, Perrin JM: Recent trends in the prevalence and severity of childhood asthma. *JAMA* 268:2673–2677, 1992.
4. Gross NJ: Chronic obstructive pulmonary disease. Current concepts and therapeutic approaches. Chest 97(Suppl 2):19S–23S, 1990.
5. Geiger KK, Hedley-Whyte J: Preoperative and postoperative consideration, in Weiss EB, Stein M (eds): *Bronchial Asthma. Mechanisms and Therapeutics.* 3d ed. Boston, Little Brown, 1993, pp 1099–1113.
6. Warner DO, Warner MA, Barnes RD, et al: Perioperative respiratory complications in patients with asthma. *Anesthesiology* 85:460–467, 1996.
7. Olsson GL: Bronchospasm during anaesthesia. A computer-aided incidence study. *Acta Anaesthesiol Scand* 31:244–252, 1987.
8. Gold MI, Helrich MA: A study of the complications related to anesthesia in asthmatic patients. *Anesth Analg* 42:283–293, 1963.
9. Bishop MJ, Cheney FW: Anesthesia for patients with asthma. Low risk but not no risk (editorial). *Anesthesiology* 85:455–456, 1996.
10. Vener DF, Long T, Lerman J: Perioperative respiratory complications after general anesthesia in children with asthma (abstr.). *Can J Anesth* 41:A55, 1994.
11. Cheney FW, Posner KL, Caplan RA: Adverse respiratory events infrequently leading to malpractice suits. A closed claims analysis. *Anesthesiology* 75:932–939, 1991.
12. Pasternak LR: Preanesthesia evaluation of the surgical patient, in Barash PG (ed): *ASA Refresher Courses* vol 24. Philadelphia, American Society of Anesthesiologists, 1996, pp 205–219.
13. Litvan H: Complicaciones respiratorias postoperatorias, en *Formación Continuada de Anestesiología y Reanimación de Catalunya.* Fundación Europea de enseñanza en Anestesiología. 1998, pp 165–179.
14. Litvan H, Casas JI, Campos JM, Villar-Landeira JM: *Incidencia De Complicaciones Respiratorias En Pacientes Con Alto Riego Por Limitación Ventilatoria Severa.* VIII Congreso Luso-Espanhol de Anestesia e Reanimaçao. Oporto 1987, Libro de Actas.
15. National Heart, Lung, and Blood Institute, World Health Organization: *Global Initiative for Asthma. Global Strategy for Asthma Management and Prevention: Workshop Report.* Bethesda, National Institutes of Health, 1995.
16. Guidelines for the Diagnosis and Management of Asthma: Expert Panel Report II. Bethesda, National Institutes of Health, publ No 97-405, 1997.
17. British Thoracic Society: Guidelines and management of asthma. *Thorax* 48(Suppl.):S1–S24, 1993.
18. May HA, Smyth RL, Romer HC, et al: Effect of anaesthesia on lung function in children with asthma. *Br J Anaesth* 77:200–202, 1996.
19. Godart PH, Clark THJ, Busse WW, et al: Clinical assessment of patients. *Eur Respir J* 11(suppl 26):2S–5S, 1998.
20. Litvan H, Canet J, Balaña L, Sanchis J: Medidores simples de flujo espiratorio en la valoracion preoperatoria de la funcion pulmonar. *Rev Española Anest Rean* 31:41–143, 1984.
21. Tisi GM: Preoperative evaluation of pulmonary

function. State of the art. *Am Rev Respir Dis* 119:293–310, 1979.

22. Pedersen T, Eliasen K, Herriksen E: A prospective study of risk factors and cardiopulmonary complications associated with anesthesia and surgery: risk indicators of cardiopulmonary morbidity. *Acta Anaesthesiol Scand* 34:144–155, 1990.

23. Empy DW, Laitinen LA, Jacobs L, et al: Mechanisms of bronchial hyperreactivity in normal subjects after upper respiratory tract infection. *Am Rev Respir Dis* 113:131–139, 1976.

24. Tait AR, Knight PR: Intraoperative respiratory complications in patients with upper respiratory tract infections. *Can J Anaesth* 34:300–303, 1987.

25. Tarhan S, Moffit EA, Sessler AD, et al: Risk of anesthesia and surgery in patients with chronic bronchitis and chronic obstructive pulmonary disease. *Surgery* 74:720–726, 1973.

26. Milledge JS, Nunn JF: Criteria of fitness for anesthesia in patients with chronic obstructive lung disease. *Br Med J* 3:670–673, 1975.

27. Eames WO, Rooke GA, Wu RS, Bishop MJ: Comparison of the effects of etomidate, propofol and thiopental on respiratory resistance after tracheal intubation. *Anesthesiology* 84:1307–1311, 1996.

28. Dilworth JP, White RJ: Postoperative chest infection after upper abdominal surgery: an important problem for smokers. *Respir Med* 86:205–210, 1992.

29. Pedersen T, Viby-Mogensen J, Ringsted D: Anaesthetic practice and postoperative pulmonary complications. *Acta Anaesthesiol Scand* 36:812–818, 1992.

30. Garibaldi RA, Britt MR, Coleman RL, Reading JC, Pace NL: Risk factors for postoperative pneumonia. *Am J Med* 70:677–680, 1981.

31. Kil HK, Rooke GA, Ryan-Dykes MA, Bishop MJ: Effect of prophylactic bronchodilator treatment on lung resistance after tracheal intubation. *Anesthesiology* 81:43–48, 1994.

32. Parker SD, Brown RH, Darowski MJ, Hirshman CA: Time related decrease in airway reactivity by corticosteroids. *Anesthesiology* 71:A1077, 1989.

33. Gal TJ: Bronchial hyperresponsiveness and anesthesia: physiologic and therapeutic perspectives. *Anesth Analg* 78:559, 1994.

34. Rodrigo C, Rodrigo G: Inhaled therapy in nonintubated patients, in Hall JB et al (eds): *Acute Asthma: Assessment and Management.* New York, McGraw-Hill, 2000, pp. 161–178.

35. Rodrigo G, Rodrigo C: Metered dose inhaler sal-butamol treatment of asthma in the ED: Comparison of two doses with plasma levels. *Am J Emerg Med* 14:144–150, 1996.

36. Rubini F, Rampulla C, Nava S: Acute effects of corticosteroids on respiratory mechanics in mechanically ventilated patients with chronic airflow obstruction. *Am J Respir Crit Care Med* 149:306–310, 1994.

37. Gal TJ, Surratt PM: Atropine and glycopyrrolate effects on lung mechanics in normal man. *Anesth Analg* 60:85–90, 1980.

38. Froese AB, Bryan AC: Effects of anaesthesia and paralysis on diaphragmatic mechanics in man. *Anesthesiology* 41:242–255, 1974.

39. Hedenstierna G, Strandberg A, Brismar B, et al: Functional residual capacity, thoraco-abdominal dimensions and central blood volume during general anesthesia with muscle paralysis and mechanical ventilation. *Anesthesiology* 62:247–254, 1985.

40. Strandberg A, Tokics L, Brismar B, Lundquist H, Hedenstierna G: Atelectasis during anaesthesia and in the postoperative period: *Acta Anaesthiol Scand* 30:154–158, 1986.

41. Dosman JA, Hodgson WC, Cockcroft DW: Effect of cold air on the bronchial response to inhaled histamine in patients with asthma. *Am Rev Respir Dis* 144:45–50, 1991.

42. Tokics L, Hedenstierna G, Strandberg A, et al: Lung collapse and gas exchange during general anesthesia: Effects of spontaneous breathing, muscle paralysis, and positive end-expiratory pressure. *Anesthesiology* 66:157–167, 1987.

43. Fletcher R: Dead space during anaesthesia. *Acta Anaesthesiol Scand* 94(Suppl):46–50, 1990.

44. Canet J, Ricós M, Vidal F: Early postoperative oxygen desaturation. Determining factors and response to oxygen therapy. *Anesth Analg* 69:207–212, 1989.

45. Knill RL, Gelb AW: Ventilatory responses to hypoxia and hypercarbia during halothane sedation and anesthesia in man. *Anesthesiology* 49:244–251, 1978.

46. Hudgel DW, Weil JV: Depression of hypoxic and hypercapnic ventilatory drives in severe asthma. *Chest* 68:493, 1975.

47. Kikuchi Y, Okabe S, Tamura G et al: Chemosensitivity and perception of dysnea in patients with a history of near-fatal asthma. *N Engl J Med* 330:1329–1334, 1975.

48. Ford GT, Whitelaw WA, Rosenal TW, Cruse PJ, Guenter CA: Diaphragm function after upper ab-

dominal surgery in humans. *Am Rev Respir Dis* 127:431–436, 1983.

49. Schwieger I, Gamulin Z, Suter PM: Lung function during anesthesia and respiratory insufficiency in the postoperative period: Physiological and clinical implications. *Acta Anaesthesiol Scand* 33:527–534, 1989.

50. Hirshman CA, Bergman NA: Factors influencing intrapulmonary airway caliber during anesthesia. *Br J Anaesth* 65:30–42, 1990.

51. Belvisi MG, Stretton CD, Barnes PJ: Modulation of cholinergic neurotransmission in guinea-pig airways by opioids. *Br J Pharmacol* 100:131–137, 1990.

52. RJ Fragen, Avram MJ: Barbiturates, in Miller RD (ed): *Anesthesia*, 3d ed. New York, Churchill Livingstone, 1990, pp 225–242.

53. Adriani J, Rovenstein EA: The effect of anesthetic drugs upon bronchi and bronchioles of excised lung tissue. *Anesthesiology* 4:253–262, 1943.

54. Crunberg G, Cohen JD, Keslin J, Gassner S: Facilitation of mechanical ventilation in status asthmaticus with continuous intravenous thiopental. *Chest* 99:1216–1220, 1943.

55. Pizov R, Brown RH, Weiss YS, Baranov D, Hennes H, Baker S, Hirshman CA: Wheezing during induction of general anesthesia in patients with and without asthma. A randomized, blinded trial. *Anesthesiology* 82:1111–1116, 1995.

56. Bernstine ML, Berker E, Cullen M: The bronchomotor effects of certain intravenous barbiturates on vagal stimulation in dogs. *Anesthesiology* 18:866–870, 1957.

57. Skoogh BE, Holtzman MJ, Sheller JR, Nadel JA: Barbiturates depress vagal motor pathway to ferret trachea and ganglia. *J Appl Physiol* 53:253–257, 1982.

58. Harrison GA: The influence of different anesthetic agents on the response to respiratory tract irritation. *Br J Anaesth* 34:804, 1962.

59. Gold MI. Bronchospasm and asthma in the anesthestized patient. ASA Annual Refresher Course Lectures. 201:242–248, 1983.

60. Lenox WC, Mitzner W, Hirshman CA: Mechanism of thiopental-induced constricction of guinea pig trachea. *Anesthesiology* 72:921–925, 1990.

61. Hirshman CA: Perioperative management of the asthmatic patient. *Can J Anaesth* 38:R26–R32, 1991.

62. Reves JG, Glass PSA: Nonbarbiturate intravenous anesthetics, in Miller RD (ed): *Anesthesia*, 3d ed.

New York, Churchill Livingstone, 1990, pp 243–279.

63. Pedersen CM: The effect of sedation with propofol on postoperative bronchoconstriction in patients with hyperreactive airways disease. *Intensive Care Med* 18:45–46, 1992.

64. Pedersen CM, Thirstrup S, Nielsen-Kudsk JE: Smooth muscle relaxant effects of propofol and ketamine in isolated guinea-pig trachea. *Eur J Pharmacol* 238:75–80, 1993.

65. Conti G, Dell'Utri D, Vilardi V, et al: Propofol induces bronchodilation in mechanically ventilated chronic obstructive pulmonary disease (COPD) patients. *Acta Anaesthesiol Scand* 37:105–109, 1993.

66. Wu RSC, Wu KC, Sum DCW, Bishop MJ: Comparative effects of thiopentone and propofol on respiratory resistance after tracheal intubation. *Br J Anaesth* 77:735–738, 1996.

67. Habre W, Matsumoto I, Sly PD: Propofol or halothane anaesthesia for children with asthma: Effects on respiratory mechanics. *Br J Anaesth* 77:739–743, 1996.

68. Cheng EY, Mazzeo AJ, Bosnjak ZJ, et al: Direct relaxant effects of intravenous anesthetics on airway smooth muscle. *Anesth Analg* 83:162–168, 1996.

69. White PF, Way WI, Trevor AJ: Ketamine: its pharmacology and therapeutic uses. *Anesthesiology* 56:119–136, 1982.

70. McGrath JC, MacKenzie JE, Millar RA: Effects of ketamine on central sympathetic discharge and the baroreceptor reflex during mechanical ventilation. *Br J Anaesth* 47:1141, 1975.

71. Lundy PM, Gowdey CW, Colhoun EH: Tracheal smooth muscle relaxant effect of ketamine. *Br J Anaesth* 46:333–336, 1974.

72. McCormick ASM, Thomas VL: Bronchospasm during inhalation of nebulized midazolam (letter). *Br J Anaesth* 80:564, 1998.

73. Hodgson PE, Woods KM, Bromley LM: Administration of nebulized intranasal midazolam to healthy adult volunteers: a pilot study (abstr.). *Br J Anaesth* 73:719P, 1994.

74. Catchlove RFH, Kafer ER: The effects of diazepam on respiration in patients with obstructive pulmonary disease. *Anesthesiology* 34:14–18, 1971.

75. Gross JB, Zebrowski ME, Carel WD, et al: Time course of ventilatory depression after thiopental and midazolam in normal subjects and in patients

with chronic obstructive pulmonary disease. *Anesthesiology* 58:540–544, 1983.

76. Boidin MP, Erdman WE, Faithfull NS: The role of ascorbic acid in etomidate toxicity. *Eur J Anaesthesiol* 3:417, 1986.

77. Guldager H, Sondergaard I, Jensen FM, Col G: Basophil histamine release in asthma patients after in vitro provocation with althesin and etomidate. *Acta Anaesthesiol Scand* 29:352–353, 1985.

78. Eger EI, Saidman LJ, Brandstater B: Minimum alveolar anesthetic concentration: A standard of anesthetic potency. *Anesthesiology* 26:756–763, 1965.

79. Pavlin EG, Su JY: Cardiopulmonary pharmacology, in Miller RD (ed): *Anesthesia*, 3d ed. New York, Churchill Livingstone, 1990, pp 105–134.

80. De Souza G, de Lisser EA, Turry P, Gold MI: Comparison of propofol with isoflurane for maintenance of anesthesia in patients with chronic obstructive pulmonary disease: Use of pulmonary mechanics, peak flow rates, and blood gases. *J Cardiothorac Vasc Anesth* 9:24–28, 1995.

81. Brichant JF, Gunst SJ, Warner DO, Rehder K: Halothane, enflurane and isoflurane depress the peripheral vagal motor pathway in isolated canine tracheal smooth muscle. *Anesthesiology* 74:325–332, 1991.

82. Korenaga S, Tekeda K, Ito Y: Differential effects of halothane on airway nerves and muscle. *Anesthesiology* 60:309–318, 1984.

83. Yamakage M, Kohro S, Kawamata T, Namiki A: Inhibitory effects of four inhaled anesthetics on canine tracheal smooth muscle contraction and intracellular Ca^{++} concentration. *Anesth Analg* 77:67–72, 1993.

84. Warner DO, Vettermann J, Brichant JF, Rehder K: Direct and neurally mediated effects of halothane on pulmonary resistance in vivo. *Anesthesiology* 72:1057–1063, 1990.

85. Patterson RW, Sullivan SF, Malm JR, et al: The effect of halothane on human airway mechanics. *Anesthesiology* 29:900–907, 1968.

86. Meloche R, Norlander O, Norden I, Herzog P: Effects of carbon dioxide and halothane on compliance and pulmonary resistance during cardiopulmonary bypass. *Scand J Thorac Cardiovasc Surg* 3:69, 1969.

87. Shah MV, Hirshman CA: Mode of action of halothane on histamine-induced airway constriction in dogs with reactive airways. *Anesthesiology* 65:170–174, 1986.

88. Habre W, Wildhaber JH, Sly PD: Prevention of metacholine-induced changes in respiratory mechanics in piglets. A comparison of sevoflurane and halothane. *Anesthesiology* 87:585–590, 1997.

89. Brown RH, Mitzer W, Zerhouni E, Hirshman CA: Direct in vivo visualization of bronchodilation induced by inhalational anesthesia using high-resolution computed tomography. *Anesthesiology* 78:295–300, 1993.

90. Hirshman CA, Edelstein G, Peetz S, et al: Mechanism of action of inhalational anesthesia on airways. *Anesthesiology* 56:107–111, 1982.

91. Hirshman CA, Bergman NA: Halothane and enflurane protect against bronchospasm in an asthma dog model. *Anesth Analg* 57:629–633, 1978.

92. Hermens JM, Edelstein G, Hanifin JM: Inhalational anesthesia and histamine release during bronchospasm. *Anesthesiology* 61:69, 1984.

93. Dueck R, Young I, Clausen J, Wagner PD: Altered distribution of pulmonary ventilation and blood flow following induction of inhalation anesthesia. *Anesthesiology* 52:113–125, 1980.

94. Stirt JA, Berger JM, Sillivan SF: Lack of arrythmia of isoflurane following administration of aminophylline in dogs. *Anesth Analg* 62:568–571, 1983.

95. Mitsuhata H, Saitoh J, Shimizu R, et al: Sevoflurane and isoflurane protect against bronchospasm in dogs. *Anesthesiology* 81:1230–1234, 1994.

96. Katoh T, Ikeda K: A comparison of sevoflurane with halothane, enflurane and isoflurane on bronchoconstriction caused by histamine. *Anaesthesia* 41:1214, 1994.

97. Rooke GA, Choi JH, Bishop MJ: The effect of isoflurane, halothane, sevoflurane and thiopental/nitrous oxide on respiratory system resistance after tracheal intubation. *Anesthesiology* 86:1294–1299, 1997.

97a. Habre W, Scalfaro P, Sims C, Tiller K, Sly PD: Respiratory mechanics during sevoflurane anesthesia in children with and without asthma. *Anesth Analg* 89:1177–1181, 1999.

98. Schwartz SH: Treatment of status asthmaticus with halothane. *JAMA* 251:2688–2689, 1984.

99. Revell S, Greenhalgh D, Absalon SR, Soni N: Isoflurane in treatment of asthma. *Anaesthesia* 43:477–479, 1988.

100. Maltais F, Sovilj M, Goldberg P, Gottfried SB: Respiratory mechanics in status asthmaticus. Effects of inhalational anesthesia. *Chest* 106:1401–1406, 1994.

101. Gonzalez IJ, Mora ML, Abreu J, et al: Tratamiento

del Life threatening asthma con isoflurano *Ann Intern Med* 9:36–38, 1992.

102. Tanigaki T, Kondo T, Ohta Y, Yamabayashi H: Transient neuromuscular impairment resulting from prolonged inhalation of halothane and enflurane. *Chest* 98:1012–1013, 1990.

103. Echevarria M, Gelb AW, Wexler HR, Ahmad D, Kenefick P: Enflurane and halothane in status asthmaticus. *Chest* 89:152–154, 1986.

104. Rosow CE, Moss J, Philbin DM, Savarese JJ: Histamine release during morphine and fentanyl anesthesia. *Anesthesiology* 56:93–96, 1982.

105. Gal TJ: Physiologic and therapeutic concerns in anesthesia for patients with reactive airways. *Semin Anesth* 15:363–375, 1996.

106. Schachter M: The release of histamine by pethidine, atropine, quinine and other drugs. *Br J Pharmacol* 7:646–654, 1952.

107. Philbin DM, Moss J, Akins CW, Rosow CE, Kono K, Schneider RC, VeerLee TR, Savarese JJ: The use of H_1 and H_2 histamine antagonists with morphine anesthesia: A double blind study. *Anesthesiology* 55:292–296, 1981.

108. Zappi L, Song P, Nicosia S, Nicosia F, Rehder K: Inhibition of airway constriction by opioids is different down the isolated bovine airway. *Anesthesiology* 86:1334–1341, 1997.

109. Belvisi MG, Stretton CD, Verleden GM, et al: Inhibition of cholinergic neurotransmission in human airways by opioids. *J Appl Physiol* 72:1096–1100, 1992.

110. Onkanlami OA, Fryer A, Hirshman CA: Interaction of nondepolarizing muscle relaxants with M2 and M3 muscarinic receptors in guinea pig lung and heart. *Anesthesiology* 84:155–161, 1996.

111. Vetterman J, Beck KC, Lindahl SGE, Brichant JF, Rehder K: Actions of enflurane, isoflurane, vecuronium, atracurium and pancuronium on pulmonary resistance in dogs. *Anesthesiology* 69:688–695, 1988.

112. Fisher MM, Baldo BA: The incidence and clinical features of anaphylactic reactions during anesthesia in Australia. *Ann Fr Anesth Reanim* 12:97–104, 1993.

113. Fellini AA, Bernstein RL, Zauder HL: Bronchospasm due to suxamethonium. *Br J Anaesth* 35:657–659, 1963.

114. Caldwell JE, Lau M, Fisher DM: Atracurium versus vecuronium in asthmatic patients. A blinded, randomized comparison of adverse events. *Anesthesiology* 83:986–991, 1995.

115. Downes H, Gerber N, Hirshman CA: IV Lignocaine in reflex and allergic bronchoconstriction. *Br J Anaesth* 52:873–878, 1980.

115a. Decco ML, Neeno TA, Hunt LW, O'Connell EJ, et al. Nebulized lidocaine in the treatment of severe asthma in children: A pilot study *Ann Allergy Asthma Immunol* 82:29–32, 1999.

116. Downes H, Hirshman CA: Lidocaine aerosols do not prevent allergic bronchoconstriction. *Anesth Analg* 60:28–32, 1981.

117. McAlpine LG. Thomson NC: Lidocaine-induced bronchoconstriction in asthmatic patients. Relation to histamine airway responsiveness and effect of preservative. *Chest* 96:1012–1015, 1989.

118. Groeben H, Schwalen A, Irsfeld S, et al: High thoracic epidural anesthesia does not alter airway resistance and attenuates the response to an inhalational provocation test in patients with bronchial hyperreactivity. *Anesthesiology* 81:868–874, 1994.

119. Franssen C, Hans P, Brichant JF, Noirot D, Lamy M: Comparison between alprazolam and hydroxyzine as oral premedication. *Can J Anaesth* 40:13–17, 1993.

120. Hirshman CA: Airway reactivity in human. *Anesthesiology* 58:170–177, 1983.

121. Bilbault P, Boisson-Bertrand D, Duvivier C, Peslin R, Laxenaire MC: Influence de l'association propofol-alfentanil sur les resistances bronchiques du sujet asthmatique. *Ann Fr Anesth Reanim* 10:264–268, 1991.

122. Williams GH, Dluhy RG: Diseases of the adrenal cortex, in Wilson JD, Braunwald E, Isselbacher KJ, et al (eds): *Harrison's Principles of Internal Medicine*, 13th ed. New York, McGraw-Hill, 1994, pp1953-1979.

123. Siegel D, Sheppard D, Gelb A, Weinberg PF: Aminophylline increases the toxicity but not the efficacy of an inhaled beta adrenergic agonist in the treatment of acute exacerbations of asthma. *Am Rev Respir Dis* 132:283–286, 1985.

124. Littenberg B: Aminophylline treatment of severe acute asthma: A meta analysis. *JAMA* 259:1678–1684, 1988.

125. Tobias JD, Lubos KL, Hirshman CA: Aminophylline does not attenuate histamine-induced airway constriction during halothane anesthesia. *Anesthesiology* 71:723–729, 1989.

126. Standards for basic intraoperative monitoring. American Society of Anesthesiologists 56:670, 1991.

127. Good ML: Capnography: Uses, interpretation and

pitfalls, in Barash PG, Deutsch S, Tinker J (eds): *ASA Refresher Courses in Anesthesiology*, vol 18. Philadelphia, Lippincott, 1990, pp 175–193.

128. Ramanathan J, Osborne B, Sibai B: Epidural anesthesia in asthmatic parturients. *Anesth Analg* 70:S317, 1990.

129. Brown DL, Wedel DJ: Spinal, epidural and caudal anesthesia. in Miller RD (ed): *Anesthesia*, 3d ed. New York, Churchill Livingstone, 1990, pp 1377–1437

130. Sundberg A, Wattwil M, Arvill A: Respiratory effects of high thoracic epidural anaesthesia. *Acta Anaesthesiol Scand* 30:215–217, 1986.

131. Egbert LD, Tamersoy K, Deas TC: Pulmonary function during spinal anesthesia: the mechanism of cough depression. *Anesthesiology* 22:882–885, 1961.

132. Harrop-Griffiths AW, Ravalia A, Browne DA, Robison PN: Regional anaesthesia and cough effectiveness. A study in patients undergoing cesarean section. *Anaesthesia* 46:11–13, 1991.

133. Bonica JJ: Autonomic innervation of the viscera in relation to nerve block. *Anesthesiology* 29:793–813, 1968.

134. Wang CY, Ong GSY: Severe bronchospasm during epidural anaesthesia. *Anaesthesia* 48:514–515, 1993.

135. Eldor J, Frankel DZN, Barav E, Nyska M: Acute bronchospasm during epidural anesthesia in asthmatic patients. *J Asthma* 26:15–16, 1989.

136. Gal TJ, Suratt PM: Resistance to breathing in healthy subjects following endotracheal intubation under topical anesthesia. *Anesth Analg* 59:270–274, 1980.

137. Wilkins CJ, Cramp PGW, Staples J: Comparison of the anesthetic requirement for tolerance of laryngeal mask airway and endotracheal tube. *Anesth Analg* 75:794–797, 1992.

138. Taguchi M, Watanabe S, Asakura N, Inomata S: End-Tidal sevoflurane concentration for laryngeal mask airway insertion and for tracheal intubation in children. *Anesthesiology* 81:628–631, 1994.

139. Groudine SB, Lumb PD, Sandison MR: Pressure support ventilation with the laryngeal mask airway: a method to manage severe reactive airway disease postoperatively. *Can J Anaesth* 42:341–343, 1995.

140. Brimacombe J, Berry A: Incidence of aspiration with the laryngeal mask airway (Letter). *Br J Anaesth* 72:495, 1994.

141. Pothmann W, Fullekrug B, SchulteEsch J: Fiberoptische Befunde zum Sitz der Kehlkopfmaske. *Anaesthesist* 41:779–784, 1992.

142. Neelakanta G, Miller J: Minimum alveolar concentration of isoflurane for tracheal extubation in deeply anesthetized chidren. *Anesthesiology* 80:811–813, 1994.

143. Llorens J, Belda FJ, Company, Marti F: Monitorización de la mecánica ventilatoria, in Belda FJ, Llorens J (eds): *Ventilación Mecánica en Anestesia*. Madrid, Ediciones Arán, 1998, pp 131–151.

144. Pilbeam SP: Mechanical Ventilation, in Youtsey JW (ed): *Faculty Lectures Series in Respiratory Care*. St Louis, Mosby, 1986, pp 163–212.

145. Muchada R, Litvan H, Galan J, Barreiro G, Villar-Landeira JM, Cathignol D: Evaluación de la perfusión tisular mediante la monitorización simultanea del perfil hemodinámico no invasivo y la capnografía. *Rev Esp Anestesiol Reanim* 40:185–190, 1993.

146. Tobias JD, Hirshman CA: Attenuation of histamine induced airway constriction by albuterol during halothane anesthesia. *Anesth Analg* 60:587–602, 1981.

147. Tobias JD, Kobos KL, Hirshman CA: Aminophylline does not attenuate histamine induced airway constriction during halothane anesthesia. *Anesthesiology* 71:723–729, 1989.

148. Roizen MF, Stevens WC: Multiform ventricular tachycardia due to the interaction of aminophylline and halothane. *Anesth Analg* 57:738–741, 1978.

149. Hirshman CA, Krieger W: Ketamine, aminophylline induced decrease in seizure threshold. *Anesthesiology* 56:464, 1982.

150. Cohendy R. Joubert A. Eledjam JJ. Prefaut C: Le risque respiratoire en chirurgie generale chez l'adulte. *Rev Pneumol Clin* 47:10–20, 1991.

151. Haddow GR, Riley E, Isaacs R, McSharry R: Ketorolac, nasal polyposis and bronchial asthma: A cause for concern. *Anesth Analg* 76:420–422, 1993.

152. Szczeklik A: Analgesics, allergy and asthma. *Drugs* 32:148–163, 1986.

153. Christensen EF, Schultz P, Jensen OV, Egebo K, Engberg M, Gron I, Juhl B: Postoperative pulmonary complications and lung function in high-risk patients: a comparison of three physiotherapy regimens after upper abdominal surgery in general anesthesia. *Acta Anaesthesiol Scand* 35:97:104, 1991.

Chapter 18

CHRONIC ASTHMA

Kari J. Zahorik
William W. Busse

ESTABLISHING THE DIAGNOSIS

To optimally manage a patient with chronic asthma, one must first identify the patient who has the disease. According to updated guidelines from the National Institutes of Health (NIH) Expert Panel on the Treatment and Diagnosis of Asthma,[1] these patients may be divided into subsets of patients with mild, moderate, or severe persistent asthma. The main tools necessary to identify and classify patients include a thorough history, physical examination, and lung function testing.

Medical History

It is important, for chronic asthma care, to obtain a thorough initial history and then continue the initial assessment at every outpatient visit to establish a diagnosis and to monitor patient progress (Table 18-1).

The most common symptoms of asthma include cough, wheeze, dyspnea, and chest tightness. Often these symptoms vary diurnally and are worse at night or early in the morning. The nocturnal increase in asthma symptoms may be enough to awaken a patient from sleep[2–4] or result in daytime somnolence.[5] Symptom severity must also be assessed, and may be thought of in terms of clinical pattern, need for medication, medical interventions, response to therapy, and severity of airflow obstruction.[6] The clinical pattern includes the patient's subjective perception of severity and frequency of asthma symptoms, keeping in mind that patients with a history of severe exacerbations of asthma may have a significantly decreased perception of dyspnea.[6] This diminished perception may be due, in part, to the fact that during an acute rapid decrease in forced expired volume in 1 second (FEV_1), patients have been shown to perceive more severe dyspnea than when slower changes in FEV_1 occur, which may occur with the late asthmatic responses and more severe disease.[7] Diminished perception puts these patients at a much greater risk for severe episodes of asthma in the future, as well as for fatal asthma, because the degree of airway obstruction can be profound by the time significant dyspnea is perceived by the patient.[8]

Given the above subjective fallibility and patient-to-patient variability of symptoms, objective measures are helpful to establish asthma severity and include patient need for increased inhaled medications and/or oral corticosteroid bursts, emergency or urgent care visits, and the intensity of medical interventions required for acute episodes. Also, a single hospitalization for an asthma exacerbation within the past year is a risk factor itself, and recurrent hospitalizations and any life-threatening exacerbations that have required intubation secondary to respiratory failure and/or respiratory acidosis are important to note since they are associated with an increase in asthma morbidity and mortality.[6,9–13] A history of missed work or school, or a history of decreased daily activities also reflects disease severity. Records of daily peak expiratory flow rates are objective measures to determine the severity of airflow obstruction and to correlate with symptoms and response to ther-

Table 18-1
Key historical points

---

1. Is there a history of recurrent coughing, wheezing, dyspnea, and/or chest tightness?
    How many years has the patient had troubles with these symptoms?
    How frequently do they occur?
    How severe are these symptoms?
    How long do these symptoms last?
    Has any medication been used to treat the symptoms, and did it work?

2. Do any of the above symptoms vary diurnally?
    Is the patient awakened from sleep due to such symptoms?
    Do these symptoms result in daytime somnolence?

3. Are these symptoms worse
    During a certain time of the year?
    After exercise?
    In a specific environment (e.g., work vs. home, outdoors vs. indoors)?
    When around a particular animal?
    After exposure to irritants such as tobacco smoke or fumes?
    When the patient has a "cold"?

4. Are daily activities limited due to the symptoms?

5. Is the patient missing school or work?

6. Has the patient had emergency care or been hospitalized for the symptoms?
    What interventions were used, and what worked?
    Was the patient intubated?

7. Does the patient have or has the patient had any other associated conditions?
    Allergic rhinitis?
    Atopic dermatitis?
    Sinusitis?
    Nasal polyposis?
    GERD?[a]
    Pulmonary disease (e.g., BPD,[b] recurrent pneumonia)?

8. Is there a family history of atopic disease?

9. What is the patient's living environment?
    Tobacco smoke exposure?
    Pets?
    Rural or urban?
    Carpeting in the bedroom?

10. What is the patient's occupational or school environment?
    Fumes/other chemical exposures?
    Tobacco smoke?
    Animals?
    Unusual exposures?

[a,b]ABBREVIATIONS: GERD, gastroesophageal reflux disease; BPD, bronchopulmonary dysplasia

apy. The usefulness and limitations of home monitoring of peak flows will be addressed later.

To determine whether chronic asthma is adequately controlled, the history must also include questions about the factors that precipitated symptoms. Often patients have a pattern of exacerbations; monitoring the frequency and severity of these events at each visit is essential to properly assess and quantitate asthma control. Common exacerbators include exercise, respiratory infections, allergen exposure, weather changes, and irritants.

Bronchospasm with exercise usually presents as transient airflow obstruction (chest tightness, dyspnea, coughing and/or wheezing) following or during physical exertion.[14,15] Because even brief bursts of physical exertion can result in bronchial smooth muscle constriction,[15] exercise intolerance can range from wheezing while walking up a flight of stairs to increases in dyspnea following a normally tolerable distance run. This may lead to a cycle of exercise avoidance, decrease in conditioning, and diminished activities, which further decreases conditioning. This cycle can then become self-perpetuating. The syndrome of chronic exercise-induced asthma may exist in as many as 90% of patients with asthma,[16] and it is a component of asthma that may be seasonally or perennially exacerbated by allergens.[17] Patients must be asked if they avoid physical activities since exercise-induced bronchospasm is an important and treatable component of chronic asthma.

Finally, a patient may notice an increase in asthma symptoms at the beginning of a "cold," or along with symptoms of allergic rhinitis. Rhinovirus is the most commonly isolated virus during asthma exacerbations associated with viral upper respiratory tract infection.[18,19] Bronchial hyperresponsiveness increases with rhinovirus infections, especially in patients with allergies, reduced FEV_1,[20] or with severe viral symptoms.[21]

Social History

A social history can be helpful to discover whether a patient smokes or has exposure to smoke, whether animals are in their environment, and what other environmental exposures at work or home might contribute to their asthma.[22,23] For example, in families with children, day care or the start of the school year often results in new viral infections among household members, often causing increased asthma symptoms. At home, exposures to high levels of indoor allergens (i.e., cat dander, house-dust mites, or cockroaches) have been implicated in the development of asthma[24–26] and are commonly associated with episodes of acute wheezing.[27]

Smoking may play a role in the development of asthma in children whose parents or household members smoke[28–31] and in the persistence of asthma symptoms from childhood into adulthood.[32,33] Cigarette smoke is a known irritant and exposure to smoke can cause bronchoconstriction.[34,35] Furthermore, cigarette smoke exposure has been associated with increased in-hospital and post-hospitalization mortality in patients admitted with severe asthma.[10]

Five to ten percent of adults with asthma may also be affected by occupational exposures.[36] Western red cedar–wood dust, isocyanates, and soy beans are important occupational and environmental sensitizers.[37–40] Numerous other occupational and environmental exposures have been implicated in the morbidity and mortality of asthma[23,41] and are discussed further in the section on inducers and triggers. Finally, emotional states and stress should also be considered when evaluating chronic asthma control,[42] although their roles may not be easy to pinpoint or define.

Past Medical History

A past medical history of co-existing diseases is also important in the care of asthma. Atopic dermatitis is commonly the first manifestation of allergic disease and appears in 80% of children with chronic allergies prior to 3 years of age.[43] Furthermore, allergic rhinitis or hay fever not only increases the likelihood of developing chronic asthma[44,45] but can also be an important target in the treatment of chronic asthma symptoms. Wheezing, coughing, dyspnea, and responsiveness to methacholine challenge, for example, may be relieved or prevented by the use of topical nasal corticosteroids in patients with allergic rhinitis.[23,46,47]

Chronic sinusitis increases the severity of asthma and causes exacerbations. The mechanisms for this are not established, but may include the existence of a sinonasal-bronchial reflex. Asthma symptoms can improve with appropriate medical and/or surgical treatment of sinus disease.[48,49]

Finally, a history of nasal polyposis is associated with more severe asthma, especially in relation to aspirin sensitivity.[50]

Family History

The family history can provide helpful information in ascertaining the likelihood of asthma,[51,52] as well as determining the likely progression of the disease. The triad of asthma, allergies, and atopic dermatitis is often inherited alone or in combination; thus, a family history of one of these three diseases in parents or siblings is a risk factor for allergic diseases, including asthma.[53] The circumstances surrounding a history of severe asthma or a death in the family due to an asthma attack should be carefully investigated, since it may indicate a genetic predisposition to more severe life-threatening asthma[54] or a tendency toward noncompliance. Further, such an event may greatly affect the outlook a patient may have on his/her condition, and result in a heightened concern for minor symptoms or, conversely, in a feeling of nonchalance and a belief that the situation is not severe. The genetic linkage for atopy and asthma continues to be investigated[55,56] and no known "asthma gene" has been identified.

Physical Examination

A thorough and focused physical examination can give pertinent clues to the severity of chronic asthma. Observation of a patient during the initial interview is helpful, especially in the case of more severe asthma.[57] In mild, moderate, or severe chronic asthma that is partially controlled, patients often appear asymptomatic upon observation. In the context of chronic asthma management, acute symptoms are more likely to be observed if the patient is a new patient, noncompliant, has severe asthma, or has been receiving suboptimal care. The inability to speak in complete sentences, hoarseness, breathlessness, or paroxysms of coughing all indicate that the disease is not under good control. Of even more concern is the use of accessory muscles for breathing, paradoxical chest wall motion, hunched shoulders, or any chest deformity. If any of these are observed, the patient likely has severe respiratory compromise and needs immediate intervention. The management of acute asthma is discussed extensively throughout this textbook.

Examination of the lung fields may reveal wheezes, a prolonged expiratory phase, or decreased air movement. Wheezes may be high or low pitched (often referred to as *rhonchi*). In evaluating symptoms in never-, new-, and ex-smokers, investigators found that wheeze, not cough, was associated with positive skin tests,[58] a feature linked to asthma prevalence.[17,24-26] By comparison, in patients challenged with histamine or house dust–mite antigen, approximately 50% of patients did not wheeze despite evidence of marked airway obstruction as measured by pulmonary function testing.[59] Finally, wheezes may be produced by nonasthmatic conditions. Any narrowing of airway diameter, mucosal edema, internal or external compression, excessive secretions, or foreign body can lead to wheezing. Smoking, for instance, has been associated with adult onset of wheezing,[60] and wheezes may be elicited from a healthy subject upon auscultation of forced expiratory flow.[61] All of the above reiterates that auscultation of the lung fields by itself does not determine the presence or severity of asthma.

Co-existing upper airway disease (i.e., allergic rhinitis, viral infection, or sinus disease) contributes to asthma severity and airway hyperresponsiveness.[47,62,63] Allergic rhinitis is associated with pale, boggy nasal mucosa with clear, thin mucous drainage, an allergic crease in the nose, and/or allergic shiners, all of which indicate active upper airway allergic disease that may contribute to chronic asthma. Thick, discolored secretions in the nose and/or oropharynx warrant further investigation for sinusitis. The presence of nasal polyps strongly correlates both with sinusitis and asthma exacerbations.

Finally, examination of the skin can be helpful, particularly to identify co-existing conditions of asthma. The existence of atopic dermatitis increases the likelihood that a history of recurrent wheezing episodes are truly asthma. A primary historical feature of atopic dermatitis is significant pruritus that subsequently leads to chronic excoriation and lichenification. Often lichenification, particularly of flexural surfaces in older children and adults, is the only evidence of existing atopic dermatitis. Of patients with atopic dermatitis, 20% to 60% are estimated to also have asthma. Children with atopic dermatitis are more likely to develop asthma at an earlier age. In adults, a history of the rash, rather than the rash itself, may be the only evidence of disease, because the prevalence and the severity of atopic dermatitis decreases with increasing age.[64]

Pulmonary Function Testing

Pulmonary function testing is an integral part of the office visit, and essential to evaluate the existence and extent of airway obstruction in chronic asthma. The degree of airflow obstruction, as well as the reversibility of the obstruction, can be objectively measured. Spirometry provides a more precise measurement of airway function than peak flow readings, and spirometry can be used to detect abnormalities in lung function in patients as young as five years old.[1]

In chronic asthma, it is important to determine the degree of airflow obstruction and the extent of its reversibility. Two of the most important values are the forced vital capacity (FVC) and the FEV_1. The FVC measures the maximum volume of air forcibly exhaled after a maximal inhalation. The FEV_1 is the volume of air forcibly exhaled in the first second of exhalation. Airway obstruction causes a decrease in FEV_1, typically to less than 80% of the predicted normal. A decreased FEV_1/FVC for height, age, and gender is also an important indicator of airway obstruction.[65] Reference ranges are calculated using one of several established reference values. Clinic sites should choose reference values of lung functions that reflect the majority of their patient population. Equations may require input of age, height, and gender, and are often standardized for a specific ethnicity. It is important to take these nonvariable data into account when comparing a test result to the given normal.

Using spirometry, the primary indicator of reversibility is a 12%, and 200 mL or greater, improvement in FEV_1 or FVC, following the use of a short-acting β_2 agonist.[65] Examples of flow-time and flow-volume curves, and examples of flow-volume loops (normal and pathologic) are seen in Figures 18-1 and 18-2, respectively.

When interpreting pulmonary function results, evidence of other airway disease may be apparent. These diseases may confound the diagnosis and treatment of chronic asthma, and are important to recognize. A decreased FVC with a normal or high FEV_1/FVC ratio reflects restrictive lung disease. Such findings may occur, for example, in very obese individuals or in patients with interstitial lung disease. In addition, a flow-volume loop is often helpful to evaluate a patient for further pathology (Fig. 18-2). A flow-volume loop demonstrating severely limited flows during inspiration indicates the possibility of an extrathoracic obstruction such as vocal cord dysfunction, whereas a concave expiratory loop indicates small airway obstruction typical of both asthma and chronic obstructive pulmonary disease (COPD).[66] A measurement of diffusion capacity would be warranted to identify the presence of emphysema. When the diagnosis is uncertain, full pulmonary function testing is warranted to exclude alternative diseases that may contribute to patient disability.

Measurements of Bronchial Hyperresponsiveness

Measuring pulmonary functions following an airway challenge with histamine, methacholine, or physical activity may provide further information for the diagnosis and management of chronic asthma. Bronchoprovocation should be performed under the supervision of knowledgeable individuals and is not recommended as a standard office

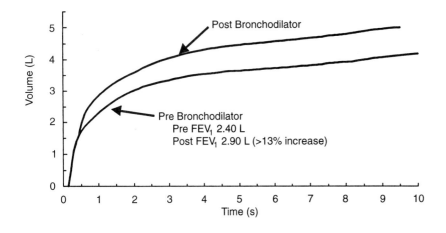

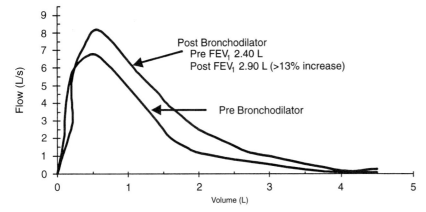

Figure 18-1

Flow-time and flow-volume curves. Curves show a >13% improvement in spirometry following use of a bronchodilator, consistent with airway reversibility (i.e., undertreated asthma). (From National Heart, Lung, and Blood Institute,[1] with permission.)

test for the untrained. Also, it is not recommended for patients with an FEV_1 of less than 65% of predicted normal. Testing for airway hyperresponsiveness can be useful when a patient reports recurrent asthma-type symptoms such as chronic cough, but does not demonstrate other symptoms or spirometry values consistent with asthma. In a case of asthma-induced cough, the positive predictive value of methacholine challenge was 74% whereas the negative predictive value was 100%.[67] Thus, a positive methacholine challenge can be a very helpful diagnostic tool, especially to *rule out* asthma as the cause for airway symptoms. Peak flow variability from AM to PM on home monitoring records has a significant association with positive responses to methacholine and may be considered a relatively simple and safe alternative to

methacholine challenge when evaluating new patients for the diagnosis of asthma.[68]

Other Tests

There are other tests that may be helpful in the assessment and diagnosis, as well as treatment, of chronic asthma. These include skin testing for inhalant hypersensitivity and radiographic views of the sinuses and chest. Skin testing is used both to establish atopy and to elicit specific aeroallergen sensitivity. Asthma is associated with a history of atopy, and thus objective evidence of atopy can be helpful in evaluating a new patient whose differential diagnosis list includes asthma.[69] It is helpful to establish specific aeroallergen sensitivities in patients in order to better manage and anticipate

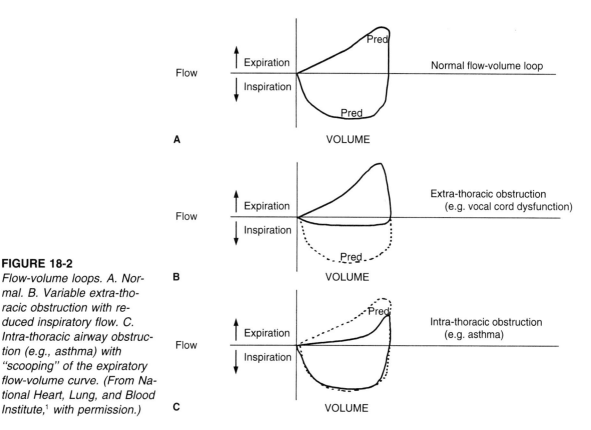

FIGURE 18-2

Flow-volume loops. A. Normal. B. Variable extra-thoracic obstruction with reduced inspiratory flow. C. Intra-thoracic airway obstruction (e.g., asthma) with "scooping" of the expiratory flow-volume curve. (From National Heart, Lung, and Blood Institute,[1] with permission.)

exacerbations of their disease. For example, specific aeroallergens such as Alternaria (linked to the development and severe exacerbations of asthma[70,71]) and house-dust mites (which peak in certain seasons[72]) are associated with perennial asthma. In vitro testing by radioallergosorbent tests (RAST) techniques may be used in place of skin testing. Both tests provide reliable information regarding the existence of allergen-specific IgE antibody.[73] Each, however, has its advantages and disadvantages. Skin testing is more sensitive and usually less expensive[23,74] and provides relatively fast and tangible results to the patient and physician. When patients have an extensive skin disease such as eczema, or when patients cannot stop antihistamine medications, skin testing is not feasible. In these instances, RAST testing provides a safe and specific alternative to skin testing, if specific allergen sensitivity is in question.[74] However, the results are not immediately available to

guide treatment and allergen avoidance. Finally, a serum IgE level may add validity to the diagnosis of asthma if no specific aeroallergen is demonstrated,[69] although this is not currently the standard of practice if the diagnosis can be made by the compilation of all other information. All testing for IgE sensitivity requires clinical correlation and interpretation.

A radiographic Water's view or computed tomography (CT) scan of the sinuses can aid in the management of chronic asthma, since a link between chronic sinus disease and asthma appears to exist. When symptoms compatible with sinusitis exist, these studies of the sinuses can provide very helpful and timely objective evidence of sinusitis, the treatment of which may be appropriate in the medical management of chronic asthma.

Finally, a chest radiograph can provide important information in the differential diagnosis of asthma. Further consideration of the radiographic

Table 18-2
Differential diagnosis of asthma-type symptoms

Adults and children	More commonly seen in adults	More commonly seen in children
More common • Rhinosinusitis (allergic or non-allergic) • GERD (with/without aspiration) • Vocal cord dysfunction • Extrathoracic obstruction —neoplasm (benign or malignant) —lymphadenopathy • Hyperventilation • Cardiac disease *Less common* • Allergic bronchopulmonary aspergillosis (ABPA) • Mechanical obstruction —tracheal stenosis —laryngeal or glottic web	• COPD (consider α-1 antitrypsin deficiency in younger adults) • Hypersensitivity pneumonitis • Medication-related effects —Angiotensin-converting enzyme inhibitor associated cough —β blocker use in asthmatics resistant to therapy • Pulmonary embolism • Pulmonary infiltrates with eosinophilia	• Foreign body aspiration • Viral bronchiolitis —respiratory syncytial virus —parainfluenza virus • Mycoplasma infection (esp >5 years old) Laryngotracheomalacia • Cystic fibrosis • Bronchopulmonary dysplasia (esp premature infant)

SOURCE: Modified from the NIH Guidelines.[1]

evidence of each disease in the differential diagnosis is beyond the scope of this chapter. A list of differential diagnoses to consider in the workup of asthma is provided in Table 18-2.

GOALS OF PERIODIC ASSESSMENT AND MANAGEMENT

Once the diagnosis of chronic asthma has been established, the primary goal of periodic outpatient asthma assessment is to recognize whether the goals of therapy are being achieved. According to the 1997 National Institutes of Health Guidelines,[1] the goals of asthma therapy are

- to prevent chronic and troublesome symptoms (nocturnal cough, activity or work limitations)
- to maintain near-normal pulmonary function
- to maintain normal activity levels (routine and exercise)

- to prevent recurrent exacerbations of asthma and minimize the need for urgent care/emergency department visits and hospitalizations
- to provide optimal pharmacotherapy with minimal or no adverse effects
- to meet the patient's and the family's expectations and thus provide satisfaction with asthma therapy

METHODS OF ASSESSMENT

To determine whether the goals of asthma therapy are being reached, the Expert Panel for the NIH Asthma Guidelines[1] recommended that the following six areas should be monitored and evaluated on a regular basis:

1. Signs and symptoms of asthma
2. Asthma exacerbations

3. Pulmonary function through spirometry and peak flow values
4. Pharmacotherapy
5. Quality of life/functional status
6. Patient-provider communication and patient satisfaction

Intermittent and mild persistent asthma that has been under control for a minimum of 3 months may be monitored every 6 months, whereas patients with uncontrolled mild, moderate, and severe persistent asthma, and who have difficulty with other issues, such as compliance or comprehension of disease, must be seen on a more frequent basis.[1]

Signs and Symptoms

The interval history, which elicits information similar to that of the initial history at the time of diagnosis, is extremely helpful to assess chronic asthma. Ongoing inquiries should include an assessment of daytime symptoms, nocturnal awakenings, and early morning asthma symptoms not responsive to β_2 agonists.[1] Patients experiencing any one of these features do not have adequate control of their asthma; thus, goals of treatment have not been met and chronic lung compromise is possible if control is not attained.

The NIH Expert Panel recommended that questions about symptoms should be divided into 'global' and 'recent' recall. The global questions should be general (i.e., "Has your asthma been better or worse since your last visit?").[1] Recent recall information should include a detailed history of the symptoms a patient has experienced during the previous 2- to 4-week period. This line of questioning addresses specific questions about the severity and frequency of recent symptoms and exacerbations, as discussed previously, and includes the three specific questions mentioned above.

Exacerbations

The apparent causal factors relating to exacerbations of asthma should be investigated. Often new information about the social history of the patient is helpful (e.g., "Are there new pets? Is the patient smoking or exposed to passive smoke? Has there been a change in the work environment?" and "Does the patient have any new hobbies?"). The action taken by a patient to treat the exacerbation, as well as the response to therapy should also be elicited. This can give the health care provider insight into the patient's understanding of asthma, and knowledge of whether an appropriate intervention occurred during exacerbations, both of which should be assessed and monitored in chronic asthma and are discussed below.

Pulmonary Function Testing: Spirometry and Peak Flow Measurement

Measures of pulmonary function are used not only to assist in the diagnosis of asthma, but to monitor the effectiveness of chronic therapy. In the outpatient clinic setting, spirometry provides a useful measurement of present airway function and also contributes to long-term assessment. For example, results from individual clinic visits can be compared in order to monitor changes in therapy or disease activity over time.

Home monitoring of peak flow readings can be a valuable tool in the evaluation of chronic asthma, particularly in patients with moderate to severe persistent asthma. There does not appear to be a substantial advantage of peak flow monitoring when compared to routine spirometry, in patients with mild intermittent or mild persistent asthma,[75] but in patients with more severe disease, home peak flow monitoring is extremely helpful. Home monitoring, in fact, substantially improved health outcome measures as reported in four separate studies examining the effectiveness of home asthma management programs which included peak flow monitoring.[76–79] Baseline values of peak expiratory flow rates (PEFR) need to be established for each patient, and all values should be compared to these rather than to "normal" numbers since expected values are not always specific to a patient's race or ethnicity, peak flow meters are not standardized, and peak flow values are considerably effort-dependent.

Once baseline peak flow values are established (i.e., personal best values), readings can be extremely helpful during exacerbations. Patients often cannot subjectively evaluate the extent of compromise in lung function. When peak flow values are assessed in comparison to baseline values, peak flow readings can provide an objective measure of acute disease severity and the need for therapy; they also reflect the effectiveness of treatment if measured before and after interventions are made.[80] Long-term records of peak flow values are helpful to identify early changes in lung function and to prevent rather than treat a major exacerbation. Peak flow variability over time is associated with bronchial hyperresponsiveness.[68] In one study of patients with severe asthma, fewer activity limitations were seen in patients who monitored their peak flow values and managed their treatment using guidelines based on peak flow values.[81] Finally, peak flow measurements are helpful to monitor the effectiveness of chronic therapy or changes made in a therapeutic regimen, as well as to evaluate the association between exacerbations and specific occupational or environmental exposures.[82]

The limitations of peak flow monitoring, particularly long-term monitoring, are primarily those of compliance. Patients often find such monitoring an inconvenience, or may have no plan of action that follows determination of peak flow values, thereby reducing the motivation to check PEFRs. Patients may also lack knowledge of the proper technique and/or interpretation of peak flow meter readings, which can also reduce their benefit. There is the potential for mechanical problems with the meters themselves, as well, which could result in faulty readings and comparisons. Finally, the usefulness of peak flow monitoring in patients with mild disease remains uncertain.[1,83,84] Nonetheless, monitoring of peak flow values can be extremely helpful for patients with more severe disease.

Monitoring Response to Pharmacotherapy

Chronic asthma pharmacotherapy needs to be monitored with regard to drugs used, response to therapy, side effects, and the patient's technique with inhaled medications. Inhaled corticosteroids such as fluticasone, for instance, improve quality of life scores related to health in patients with moderate asthma,[85] yet side effects or medication inconvenience may still decrease medication compliance. At each visit, it is not only important to have patients review what medications they use, but also to inquire regarding the frequency of medication use, both scheduled and PRN. It is helpful to find out how often patients require inhaled immediate-acting bronchodilators, since this information gives an indication about the level of asthma control on a daily basis. It is also important to ask how often patients miss taking prescribed medications per week, and the reasons for these missed doses. Questions in this area can include: "Are there problems getting the prescription filled? Are finances an issue?" and "Is the patient's schedule one that requires a different medication schedule?"

Inquiring about side effects that hinder medication compliance or interfere with the well- being of the patient is critical. Such side effects can range from agitation following use of short-acting β_2 agonists to oral candidiasis secondary to inhaled corticosteroid use, or any other symptom that a patient perceives as being related to asthma medication. If there is a question about medication use that cannot be resolved in the interview, a patient's pharmacy can provide additional data.[86]

Monitoring Patient-Provider Communication and Patient Satisfaction

There are few scientific methods to monitor patient-provider communication and satisfaction, but a recitation of the patients' understanding of their disease and their adherence to medications may be useful. In general, physicians tend to overestimate the use of inhaled corticosteroids by patients and underestimate inhaled short-acting β_2-agonist use.[87] Moreover, there exists a fear of corticosteroid use. These issues often go unrecognized and can lead to diminished effectiveness of asthma management. Simple changes in medication regimens, which have been proven to be as effective but may be more likely to be followed and tolerated by the patient, must be considered. For instance, one daily dose of 1000 μg of inhaled flunisolide versus 500 μg twice daily has been shown to be as effective in maintaining asthma control in patients with moderate well-controlled asthma, and does not result in a change in 24-hour serum cortisol excretion.[88] For some patients with unusual schedules (e.g., night-shift workers) or with a history of poor compliance, changes in the dosing schedule need to be considered.

There are several methods described to check adherence to medication regimens.[86] Assessment of adequacy of communication is particularly important to ensure proper use of medical care during changes in symptoms. To improve quality assurance in health care delivery, Wasserfallen and colleagues developed a rhinoconjunctivitis and asthma questionnaire that may be helpful to better evaluate disease severity, as well as to compare diseases between populations.[89] This sort of questionnaire could have a place in the assessment of patient-provider communication and satisfaction.

As in any effective relationship, lines of communication need to be established early and effectively. There are numerous potential obstacles to adequate disease management including 1) patient and family belief systems, 2) patient perceptions or denial of their disease, 3) comprehension of or fears regarding medications, 4) severity of disease, 5) literacy level, and 6) financial burdens of the illness and other limitations to health care access, to name but a few.[90] Physicians and other health care providers must keep in mind that if these obstacles are not elicited early on and management is not changed to resolve them, then it is unlikely that effective therapy will result.

MANAGEMENT OF CHRONIC ASTHMA

The keys to successful management of chronic asthma lie in control of factors which exacerbate the disease, in pharmacotherapy both to prevent symptoms and to treat exacerbations, and in patient education about both the disease and the rationale behind daily and rescue therapy interventions.

Controlling Factors That Exacerbate Asthma

Controlling factors that exacerbate asthma requires an understanding both by patients and physicians, as well as any other care providers, of what the exacerbating factors for each individual patient are. For simplicity, the factors that commonly exacerbate the disease can be divided into sensitizers (or provokers) and triggers. The sensitizers are those environmental factors that are thought to induce airway inflammation and can result in the establishment of asthma disease. Triggers cause bronchoconstriction, but not necessarily an increase in allergic inflammation, in sensitive airways (Table 18-3).

Table 18-3

Sensitizers (provokers) and triggers of chronic asthma

Sensitizers (provokers)
- Aeroallergens
    - Outdoor
        - Pollens
        - Molds
    - Indoor
        - Pets (esp. cats)
        - House dust mites
        - Cockroaches
        - Molds
        - Occupational exposures
- Viral respiratory infections

Triggers
- Exercise
- Upper airway inflammation
    - Allergic rhinitis
    - Bacterial or viral sinusitis
- Tobacco smoke
- Pollens
    - Occupational exposures
    - Cleaning supplies
- Gastroesophageal reflux disease
- Ambient temperature or humidity
- Strong emotions
- Severe/sudden reactions
    - aspirin and other NSAIDS
    - β-blocking medications
    - specific insect stings immunotherapy
    - sera-specific food allergens

Sensitizers (Provokers)   Inhaled aeroallergens are one of the primary sensitizers of chronic asthma symptoms and exacerbations.[17,22,24,24-26] To identify these factors, a physician must obtain a thorough history. In so doing, the physician may discover that symptoms occur during particular seasons or whether there are specific environmental factors either at work or at home, such as pets or mildewed walls that could be factors.. The next step following a physical examination is to perform skin testing or in vitro testing for specific IgE so that exposure to aeroallergen sensitizers can be determined and then controlled and/or avoided.

Ideally, only those antigens to which the patient is commonly exposed should be tested. In this way, assessing the relationship of positive tests to the patient symptoms is much more reliable, and guidelines for avoidance and treatment are clearer. For example, placing an extract of rabbit antigen in a panel of skin tests for a symptomatic patient who is not regularly exposed to a rabbit would be of no benefit, nor would it change the direction of treatment. Testing for house-dust mites, in contrast, is crucial to the assessment and management of chronic asthma in most regions of the United States, given their prevalence and association with asthma. A positive or negative test to important antigens can be very helpful in directing disease control, preventing exacerbations, and improving chronic treatment in a large number of asthma patients.[91]

Again, an in-depth interview to address home and work or school exposures is crucial to direct skin testing. Many occupational exposures are considered to be irritants or uncommon sensitizers. Nonetheless, the work environment has the potential to expose the patient to common inducers such as molds and pollens; thus, control measures both in the home and work environment must be addressed when forming a treatment plan.[23]

Occupational or regional environmental exposure to various airborne particles that are specific to work or living environment can induce atopy, bronchial hyperresponsiveness, and asthma.[23,40,82,92,93] These are distinct from the common aeroallergens discussed above and from the occupational exposures that act as triggers of bronchospasm (discussed below). When a particular work exposure is considered to be the primary inducer of a patient's chronic asthma, care must be taken to document findings that link the asthmatic response to the work environment. Physicians must maintain strict confidentiality in regard to these findings; working closely with the patient with the understanding that approaching an employer with even the suggestion that a work-related exposure could be potentially detrimental to the health of their employee may result in retaliation against the patient, including loss of employment.[1] Table 18-4 provides an example of the evaluation and management of presumed work-related asthma.

Viral respiratory infections are notorious for inducing asthma exacerbations. Rhinovirus, respiratory syncytial virus, and influenza viruses are the principal culprits.[20,94-96] Airway size seems to play a role in wheezing in infancy since infant airways are much smaller than adult airways and are more likely to be compromised by the inflammation caused by respiratory viruses.[30] Many infants who wheeze during or following a viral infection will not develop chronic asthma. However, if there is a family history of atopic disease that may predispose a child prone to wheezing to chronic childhood asthma, adjustments in the environment, such as avoiding tobacco smoke, animal dander, and house dust–mite exposure, should be instituted as a precautionary measure against the development of chronic asthma, which can start as early as in the first year of life.[1] For adults, prevention of increased disease severity secondary to respiratory viral infections should start with an influenza vaccination every autumn.[97]

Triggers   Triggers of asthma exacerbations are different from inducers in that they generally cause acute bronchoconstriction of the airways rather than inflammatory changes. Triggers usually act within minutes and cause bronchoconstriction via the immediate release of mediators from mast cells or other direct-acting events. In conjunction with chronic underlying inflammation, a trigger can cause a significant decrease in pulmonary

Table 18-4

Evaluation and management of presumed work-related asthma

Evaluation
1. Identify sensitizers and/or triggers at work
   Isocyanates, plant or animal materials, organic dust, ambient temperature or humidity
2. Identify coworkers with similar problems
3. Identify a pattern to the asthma:
   Symptoms improve at home or on vacation
   Symptoms may be immediate (≤1 hour), delayed, or nocturnal
   Symptoms may start following a high-level exposure
4. Document objective evidence of work-related airflow limitation:
   Record peak flow rates every 2 hours for ≥2 weeks at work and ≥1 week away from work
   Record when symptoms occur
   Record when specific exposures occur
   Record when rescue medication is used
5. Perform/Refer for further testing:
   Immunologic evaluation
   Full pulmonary function testing and/or bronchial challenge(s)

Management
1. Occupationally induced asthma:
   Recommend complete avoidance of exposure to sensitizing agent
2. Asthma exacerbations at work:
   Work with health care facilities on-site, and/or supervisors
   Discuss avoidance, ventilation, respiratory protection, or trigger-free environment

SOURCE: Modified from National Institutes of Health.[1]

function and should be considered an important factor in the prevention and control of chronic asthma.

One common trigger of bronchospasm is exercise. Patients often complain of activity or exercise intolerance.[16] Premedicating with a bronchodilator, 10 to 15 minutes prior to activity, can be quite helpful in these instances. This, however, is obviously impossible if a patient cannot tolerate short bursts of activity such as climbing stairs or walking short distances. This often requires more aggressive control of chronic inflammation. Some factors may need to be taken into account, such as weight and aerobic fitness, since they may play a role, as well. Patients should check peak flow rates when they feel short of breath following activity or exertion since this measurement can distinguish between poor fitness and bronchoconstriction.[80] Formal exercise testing using spirometry may be performed prior to and following exertion, if there is a suspicion of exercise-induced asthma.

Control of upper airway inflammation is important in the management of chronic asthma. Upper airway disease is associated with hyperresponsiveness of the bronchi.[47,62,63] It is helpful to manage both acute and chronic sinusitis and rhinitis. These disease processes can act as asthma triggers or inducers, and their treatment should be an integral part of chronic asthma management. Topical nasal corticosteroids reduce mucosal inflammation, and decrease lower airway bronchospastic symptoms and bronchial hyperresponsiveness.[23,46,47] Antibacterial treatment of bacterial sinusitis may also be necessary to effectively treat the inflamed upper airways,[98] and surgical treatment in chronic sinusitis may need to be considered for effective upper and lower airway management. For example, when the health-status scores of patients were examined 12 months after ethmoid sinus surgery, greater improvement in the scores of asthma patients over those without asthma was seen; both groups achieved near-predicted baseline scores, but the asthma patients started at a lower baseline score.[99]

Irritants are also common triggers of asthma. These include tobacco smoke, changes in ambient temperature, unvented fumes, fires, and strong odors. The NIH Expert Panel has recommended that asthma patients should not smoke or be exposed to environmental tobacco smoke.[1] The detrimental effects of smoking on healthy lung tissue are well known. Patients with a chronic and potentially life-threatening pulmonary disease such as asthma should not smoke; unfortunately, this advice is not followed by all asthma patients.[100] Numerous studies have shown that second-hand smoke exposure can be detrimental to patients with asthma, and that it acts as one of the primary precipitants of asthma in both adults and children.[34,35] Tobacco smoke has been considered "the most important environmental indoor irritant"[1] and exposure of adults to tobacco smoke has been associated with poorer pulmonary function, the need for more medication, and an increase in work absences.[34] Thus, control of first-hand and environmental tobacco smoke needs to be a major consideration in the assessment and management of chronic asthma.

Although airborne pollens may act as inducers of asthma through chronic exposure, resulting in inflammation, they also trigger bronchospasm. Avoiding animals to which a patient is sensitive, and staying indoors during days of high outdoor allergen counts are both appropriate precautionary measures. Some patients are sensitive to changes in ambient air temperature or humidity, and actions such as wearing a scarf to cover the mouth on cold days, or staying in air-conditioned buildings on particularly hot and humid days, may be effective.

Finally, other substances, including environmental pollutants, chemicals, fumes from gas, kerosene, or wood burning appliances, perfumes, and cleaning agents, are pulmonary irritants.[101] Avoiding these irritants, if possible, is helpful in asthma management. If not, better ventilation and/or use of protective masks may be considered. Avoiding the outdoors, particularly to exercise, on days when pollution is high can be helpful to prevent an acute asthma exacerbation.[102,103]

Gastroesophageal reflux disease (GERD) may also trigger asthma symptoms. GERD alone can cause cough due to upper airway irritation.[104,105] and may co-exist with asthma. Whether asthma itself is triggered during active GERD is unclear. However, studies have linked coughing and/or wheezing at night with GERD[1]; thus, appropriate medical or surgical treatment of GERD can decrease asthma symptoms.[106,107]

Other common miscellaneous triggers of bronchospasm include both cold and hot humid air, laughter, and emotional stimuli.[6] Since triggers are myriad, focus on causes of exacerbation in the individual patient is paramount in successfully managing chronic asthma.

Finally, there are triggers that can cause such severe bronchoconstriction that fatal reactions are a potential end-result. These include aspirin and other anti-inflammatory drugs, β-adrenergic antagonists, food additives (particularly metabisulfites), foods, anaphylaxis to stinging insects, or the administration of immunotherapy.[36] Aspirin and anti-inflammatory drugs have long been known to trigger severe asthma attacks,[108] and the sensitivity to these drugs is commonly associated with severe corticosteroid-dependent chronic asthma,[10] as well as recurrent nasal polyposis.[36]

Patients need information about where specific food and medication allergens are found. Sulfites, for example, are found in processed potatoes, shrimp, and dried fruit. Beer and wine may also be a source of sulfites. Aspirin may be "hiding" in combination over-the-counter cold remedies, and β blockers are common medications for both heart disease and chronic headaches. Patients, or their care givers, need to be taught to read food and drug labels and to look for specific allergens; physicians need to review all medications being used by each patient so that no potentially dangerous medications are being prescribed.

Skin testing may be necessary if there is a questionable history of an allergic reaction, or to discern what the allergen is in a mixture of foods and spices. However, caution should be taken since systemic symptoms may sometimes result from local skin testing. Desensitization may be undertaken for both insect and aspirin sensitivity. The success of the former is quite high,[109,110] and aspirin desensitization has worked as well. The latter, however, involves serious compliance and safety issues, and is not commonly undertaken or recommended except where the medication is needed for lifesaving circumstances (in cardiac disease, for instance), or in patients who have severe disease and traditional medical management has proven unsuccessful, uncommonly high doses of oral corticosteroids are being used, and/or repeated polypectomies and/or sinus surgeries are required.[49]

Pharmacotherapy

The goals of chronic asthma treatment, as put forth by the Expert Panel for the 1997 NIH Guidelines, are the same as those listed and discussed previously.[1] The medications used to treat chronic asthma, and to attain these goals, can be divided into quick-relief medications and long-term controllers. The quick-relief medications are used to relieve acute airflow obstruction, whereas long-term controllers are used both as long-acting bronchodilators and as medications to treat underlying and chronic airway inflammation, now identified as the 'root' of persistent asthma disease and its morbidity.[111] These medications are listed in Table 18-5.

Quick-relief, or rescue, medications include inhaled short-acting β_2 agonists and, to some degree, oral corticosteroids and anticholinergics. These medications are used on an "as-needed" basis to rapidly decrease reversible obstruction, regardless of the stimulant. Short-acting β_2 agonists and anticholinergics usually act within 30 minutes, whereas the onset of action of oral corticosteroids is approximately 4 to 6 hours. Albuterol, pirbuterol, bitolterol, and terbutaline are the primary short-acting β_2 agonists available and used in the United States. The anticholinergic used is ipratropium bromide. Oral corticosteroids include prednisone, prednisolone, and methylprednisolone. β_2 agonists act directly on airway receptors to relax smooth muscle, whereas anticholinergics act to inhibit cholinergic neuronal innervation which gives tone to airway smooth muscles. Corticosteroids have primarily anti-inflammatory properties. Anticholinergics are not particularly effective in asthma treatment and are most often used in combination with β_2 agonists for treatment of chronic obstructive lung disease. Although inhaled corticosteroids have mostly replaced oral corticosteroids for the treatment of chronic asthma, short courses of oral corticosteroids are important for the treatment of moderate to severe asthma exacerbations.[112,113]

In contrast, long-term control medications include a larger variety of medications that are used on a daily basis in order to maintain chronic asthma control. The first-line medications used as chronic controllers are inhaled corticosteroids which, unless used in very high doses, primarily act at a local level to relieve the chronic inflammation of persistent asthma.[114–116] Inhaled corticosteroids can prevent exacerbations of asthma that may lead to hospitalizations.[117] The regular use of inhaled corticosteroids can reduce airway hyperresponsiveness[118] and decrease the need for oral corticosteroids in chronic asthma control.[119,120] Peak expiratory flow rates improve, while nocturnal awakenings and β_2 agonist use decrease with regular use of an inhaled corticosteroid.[121] In addition to inhaled corticosteroids, long-term control medications include long-acting β_2 agonists, methylxanthines, leukotriene modifiers, and cromolyn and nedocromil sodium. The mechanism of action of each drug varies according to its class. Corticosteroids, and, to some degree leukotriene modifiers, have primarily anti-inflammatory effects,[122] whereas long-acting β_2 agonists and methylxanthines are used for their long-term bronchodilatory effects. Cromolyn sodium and nedocromil are thought to modify the inflammatory response.

Leukotriene modifiers are effective asthma therapy, but their role, or positioning in chronic asthma, has not yet been clearly defined. It has

Table 18-5

Quick-relief versus control medications

Quick-relief medications
    Short acting β_2 agonists
        Albuterol
        Bitolterol
        Pirbuterol
        Terbutaline
    Anticholinergics
        Ipratropium bromide

Control medications
    Inhaled corticosteroids
        Beclomethasone dipropionate
        Budesonide
        Flunisolide
        Fluticasone
        Triamcinolone acetonide
    Long-acting β_2 agonists
        Salmeterol

been suggested that they might be effective in special cases, such as in patients with aspirin sensitivity or in those who experience exercise-induced asthma.[123] It is important at this juncture to know that leukotriene modifiers may provide an additional tool in patients with special cases or poorly controlled asthma on traditional medications. However, in the 'Step-Care' therapy detailed below, leukotriene modifiers will not be discussed further due to the absence of long-term experience.

Comparable daily dose estimations for inhaled corticosteroids are shown in Table 18-6 since the Step-Care protocol for therapy refers simply to low, medium, and high doses. The specific medications used for the pharmacotherapy of acute asthma are discussed in detail elsewhere in this text; however, this chapter provides an approach to use when choosing a medication regimen to manage chronic asthma. To initiate therapy in adults and children more than 5 years old, two general approaches have been suggested by recent NIH Guidelines. A physician may either start with a high-dose regimen and "step down" to the minimal amount of medication eventually needed to control a patient's chronic asthma, or start with a lower dose of medications and "step up" therapy until control is attained.[1]

In order to establish the Step at which to initiate therapy, the physician must first decide upon the severity of the asthma (Table 18-7). Step 1 of therapy is for mild intermittent asthma, with exacerbations of symptoms occurring less than or equal to two times per week, persisting for hours or days, and with nocturnal symptoms occurring no more than twice a month. The patient must be free from symptoms and have no abnormalities on home peak flow monitoring in-between exacerbations. These patients require no routine medications, but do need inhaled short-acting β_2 agonists on an as-needed basis during exacerbations. Patients with exercise-induced asthma alone fall into this category.[1]

The next level, Step 2, in chronic persistent asthma therapy is for patients considered to have mild persistent asthma. These patients do not necessarily have symptoms on a daily basis, but do experience daytime asthma symptoms more than twice each week and nocturnal symptoms more than twice a month and are defined as having aggravations of their asthma that may affect their daily activities. Unlike mild intermittent asthma,

Table 18-6
Estimated comparable adult daily doses of inhaled corticosteroids

Medication	Low dose	Medium dose	High dose
Beclomethasone dipropionate	168-504 μg	504-840 μg	>840 μg
42 μg/puff	(4-12 puffs)	(12-20 puffs)	(>20 puffs)
84 μg/puff	(2-6 puffs)	(6-10 puffs)	(>10 puffs)
Budesonide	200-400 μg	400-600 μg	>600 μg
200 μg/puff	(1-2 inhalations)	(2-3 inhalations)	(>3 inhalations)
Flunisolide	500-1000 μg	1000-2,000 μg	>2000 μg
250 μg/puff	(2-4 puffs)	(4-8 puffs)	(>8 puffs)
Fluticasone	88-264 μg	264-660 μg	>660 μg
44 μg/puff	(2-6 puffs)	—	—
110 μg/puff	(2 puffs)	(2-6 puffs)	(>6 puffs)
220 μg/puff	—	—	(>3 puffs)
Triamcinolone acetonide	400-1000 μg	1000-2000 μg	>2000 μg
100 μg/puff	(4-10 puffs)	(10-20 puffs)	(>20 puffs)

SOURCE: Modified from the NIH Guidelines.[1]

Table 18-7
Stepwise approach to chronic asthma management

	Symptoms	Lung function
Step 1 *Mild intermittent*	Symptoms ≤2 times/week Asymptomatic between Exacerbations Exacerbations brief (hours to days) Intensity varies Nocturnal symptoms ≤2 Times/month	FEV_1 or PEFR ≥80% predicted PEFR variability <20%
Step 2 *Mild persistent*	Symptoms >2 times/week; <1 time/day Activity may be affected by exacerbations Nocturnal symptoms >2 times/month	FEV_1 or PEFR ≥80% predicted PEFR variability 20–30%
Step 3 *Moderate persistent*	Daily symptoms Daily use of inhaled rescue medication Exacerbations ≥2 times/week (may last days) Activity affected by exacerbations Nocturnal symptoms >1 time/week	FEV_1 or PEFR >60%–<80% predicted PEFR variability >30%
Step 4 *Severe persistent*	Continual symptoms Activity limited by symptoms Exacerbations frequent Nocturnal symptoms frequent	FEV_1 or PEFR ≤60% predicted PEFR variability >30%

SOURCE: Modified from the NIH Guidelines.[1]

daily anti-inflammatory medication is recommended for patients with mild persistent asthma. The drug of choice would be an inhaled low-dose corticosteroid, although cromolyn or nedocromil might be tried first in children; theophylline and leukotriene modifiers are other options, though not currently the treatments of choice.[1,124]

The third category, or Step 3, is for patients with moderate persistent asthma. These patients experience asthma symptoms and require the use of a short-acting β_2 agonist on a daily basis. They have significant exacerbations of their asthma which may last for several days, and can occur more than two times per week. Also, these patients are affected by nocturnal symptoms more than once per week, and daily activities are often altered due to their symptoms. Like patients under Step 2 care, these patients require daily anti-inflammatory medication. In this case, a medium dose of inhaled corticosteroid by itself, or a low-to-medium or medium-to-high dose inhaled corti-

costeroid with an added long-acting inhaled β_2 agonist, such as salmeterol, is recommended for daily therapy. The long-acting bronchodilator is usually added after a trial of inhaled corticosteroids by itself, and is particularly effective to control breakthrough nocturnal symptoms. Theophylline may be considered as an alternative to the inhaled long-acting β_2 agonist, but should not be used alone in this instance.[1]

The final and most intensive Step in chronic asthma therapy, Step 4, is for severe persistent asthma. Patients at this level of severity have daily persistent symptoms and restricted activities. Daytime and nocturnal exacerbations of their symptoms are very common. High-dose inhaled anti-inflammatory medications along with a long-acting inhaled β_2 agonist are the usual mainstay of therapy for these patients. In many cases, these patients require chronic oral corticosteroids for disease control. Theophylline and leukotriene modifiers may also be of use in these patients, but are not currently drugs of choice for chronic asthma maintenance at this level of severity.[1]

In all of the above Steps of therapy, inhaled short-acting bronchodilators are used on an as-needed basis. If their use increases, it usually indicates a change in the severity of disease or poor disease control, and the physician must re-evaluate whether the patient has been adequately treated. Despite some concerns, no detrimental effects have been shown with as-needed dosing of albuterol up to or more than four times per day,[125] but obviously this frequent rescue medication approach does not treat chronic inflammation, which is often the basis of the patient's exacerbation. Conversely, if a patient requires minimal to no rescue medication use, an indication of adequate control, the physician and patient may try to step down therapy in order to establish the minimal amount of therapy necessary for appropriate control. An additional note in regard to asthma severity and control is that patients with well-controlled asthma do not necessarily have mild asthma. For instance, a patient with severe persistent asthma may not have nocturnal symptoms if he/she is on high doses of inhaled corticosteroid and a long-acting β_2 agonist, but this does not change the definition of the level of disease severity.[126] This is important for both physicians and patients to keep in mind when assessing the potential severity or danger of a particular patient's disease.

There are some variations in the treatment of chronic asthma that require special consideration. Seasonal asthma, for instance, may be predictable and may relate to a particular aeroallergen sensitivity. In these cases, asthma exacerbations are predictable and the patient is essentially symptom-free during the rest of the year; consequently, the patient may be treated during their allergy season in the Step-Care approach discussed above, and may remain free of medications (or on as-needed bronchodilators for mild intermittent symptoms) during the other months of the year.[1]

Management of exercise-induced bronchospasm is less well defined. In patients with known persistent asthma, symptoms with exercise may indicate poor daily asthma control. A patient with persistent asthma should not have to limit activities due to asthma, except in the most severe cases, since there is usually an option to step up chronic therapy to improve exercise tolerance.[1] In the case of exercise-induced symptoms, for any patient, the use of the bronchodilator prior to exercise, rather than after exercise, may eliminate symptoms induced while exercising, although the patient may still use an inhaler for rescue if needed following their physical exertion. Pre-exercise use of cromolyn sodium or nedocromil may also be effective.

The management of asthma during pregnancy is worth mentioning as an important special situation occurring in chronic asthma management (see Chapter 16).

Education

When treating chronic diseases that require some self-monitoring and self-management, patient education is a key component for successful regulation of the disease; asthma is no exception to this rule.[127] In patients with near-fatal asthma, regular follow-up visits result in reduced morbidity and mortality. Despite the severity of near-fatal asthma, however, many patients continue to have poor compliance with follow-up visits.[12] Thus, educating patients when they are at the medical office would seem to be key in teaching patients about the significance of their disease and how to prevent future problems. Table 18-8 lists the key points pertaining to education that should be provided to each patient with chronic asthma.

Patients must understand that, much like hypertension, asthma can be a silent but deadly disease. Underlying inflammation must be appropriately treated on a daily basis to adequately manage the disease. Pictures and models are often helpful to illustrate the nature of inflammation and what smooth muscle constriction can actually do to the airways. Identification of specific inducers and triggers for each patient is very important for appropriate asthma management. Tobacco smoke and pet exposure tend to be key elements that can be altered in the environment to better control the asthma. One cannot assume that if a patient is

Table 18-8
Key points of patient education

1. Patients must understand that
    Asthma can be silent and deadly
    Inflammation requires daily control therapy
    Long-term controller medications are not for rescue

2. Models and pictures help demonstrate inflammation and bronchoconstriction

3. Identify/Discuss:
    Inducers
    Triggers
    Co-existing diseases which require therapy
    Environmental alterations for better asthma control:
        Tobacco smoke exposure (active or passive) reduction/elimination
        Pet removal or limited exposure
        House-dust mite precautions
        Indoor mold control
        Occupational adjustments
    Food allergen avoidance
    Medication avoidance
        Aspirin-sensitive patients
        β blocker medication

4. Consider professional counseling/referral for smoking cessation
    Long-term morbidity and mortality of smoking and asthma

5. Demonstrate inhaler use (with/without spacer device)

6. Observe/Adjust patient's technique of inhaler use

7. Review/Discuss:
    Long-term controller vs. rescue medications and appropriate use
        of each
    Peak flow measurement technique
    Peak flow and/or symptom diaries
    Patient's schedule and ability to take medications as prescribed
    Patient's ability to purchase medications prescribed

8. Provide an action plan
    Daily therapy
    Methods to monitor exacerbations
    Management of exacerbations acc. to symptoms or peak-flow
        measurements

9. Provide phone numbers/contacts for emergencies

known to be allergic to a pet that the patient will then automatically avoid or give away the pet, or that a patient with asthma will avoid exposure to tobacco. In fact, in one longitudinal cohort study, an increase in smoking was seen at all ages between 16 and 23 in asthma patients compared with healthy individuals.[100]

Patients who are allergic to pets should be instructed on how to avoid contact with them, particularly if there is a pet in the house, and even if compliance is questionable (e.g., keeping the pet out of the bedroom, and off of the bed and upholstered furniture). Although the evidence is somewhat confounding, washing the pet weekly, particularly a cat, may help reduce the allergic load of dander and saliva in the environment.[128,129] Ideally the pet should be removed from the daily environment.[1]

Patients who smoke or are exposed to smoke should be taught about the effect of smoking on their disease and how smoking affects long-term morbidity. Counseling by trained professionals improves long-term maintenance of smoking cessation.[130] Physicians and health care workers need to strongly consider referrals for such interventions in order to effectively promote smoking cessation of the patient and household members. Patients who have had recent asthma attacks tend to smoke less temporarily[100]; thus, this may be a key time for smoking cessation intervention.

There are many other interventions that may be discussed with patients, such as mattress and pillow covers, carpet removal from the bedroom for house-dust mite protection, and humidity control for both house-dust mite and mold control.[131,132] The report from the American Thoracic Society Workshop in 1995 provides a thorough guide to indoor allergen-exposure reduction for domestic and commercial settings, and is a useful reference for many questions on the effectiveness of air filtration systems and moisture control.[133] It is important to tailor education for each individual patient to more effectively control the disease.

Inhaled medications do not provide maximum therapeutic benefit unless properly administered. Demonstrating how to use inhalers, with or without spacer, depending upon the medications prescribed, and having the patients practice during each office visit is helpful to teach and monitor inhaler use. If a patient is to perform post-bronchodilatory spirometry, for instance, observing the patient taking the first actuation of medication and instructing on any adjustments offers a unique opportunity to evaluate and improve inhaler technique.

Patients should be taught which medications are chronic (long-term) controllers, which are res-

cue medications, and when it is recommended to use each one (e.g., prior to animal exposure). Each patient also needs an action plan (Figure 18-3). Each patient should have a plan to follow to facilitate the management of their asthma at home. This is particularly important for new patients or for returning patients when medication changes are made. The individual needs of each patient must be taken into account and some important considerations, among many, include the patient's schedule (is the patient a night shift worker?) and their ability to purchase and use medications.[90]

Many patients with chronic asthma are poor judges of the degree of their airflow obstruction[134,135] and need a method to objectively measure their asthma severity at home. The use of a peak flow meter, and how to use the information it provides, should be taught to each patient. Blank calendars or time lines to document peak flow values and concurrent subjective symptoms should also be provided. Each patient should be instructed where to record daily peak flow values, how to compare these to previous values and subjective symptoms, and what to do if these values change significantly. With this information, patients should be able to effectively self-monitor and initiate intervention therapy at the onset of an asthma exacerbation. At the very least, the patient would ideally have a record of pertinent objective and subjective information to provide the physician at the follow-up visit, or in an emergent situation.

All directions should be concisely and clearly stated and written, either for the patient or the care giver or guardian. Telephone numbers should be provided to obtain help at any hour of the day, whether from a clinic or from an on-call physician. The cost of emergency room visits and hospitalizations for poorly controlled asthma far exceeds the expense of a clinic visit and medications for daily asthma management.[136] Special considerations, such as those for parents or caretakers of very young, adolescent,[137–139] or geriatric patients, are beyond what will be discussed, but physicians and other health care providers should recall that there are often special needs for such patient populations that should be taken into consideration.

ASTHMA ACTION PLAN

Name:_____   Return to the Clinic:

Triggers: ☐ viral infections   ☐ exercise   ☐ irritants   ☐ cold air
         ☐ sinus infections   ☐ allergens   ☐ stress   ☐ change in
         temperature/humidity	

Rescue Medication: **dose:** **when the dose can be repeated:**	
GREEN ZONE PEAK FLOW: (80-100%) **medications:**	**Symptoms:** ·may range from none to occasional mild wheezing, coughing, or shortness of breath ·do not interfere with activity ·sleep is not disturbed
YELLOW ZONE PEAK FLOW: (50-80%) 1. Administer dose of rescue medication. 2. Repeat peak flow and/or reassess symptoms in 15 min. 3. If peak flow now in green zone, and/or symptoms reverse, follow regular schedule. 4. **If peak flow remains in yellow zone, and/or symptoms do not reverse, change medications to:** MAINTAIN THIS NEW SCHEDULE UNTIL YOU RETURN TO THE GREEN ZONE OR ARE FREE OF SYMPTOMS FOR 48 HOURS.	**Symptoms**: ·moderate wheezing, coughing, or shortness of breath ·may interfere with activity ·may cause nighttime awakenings for medication IF PEAK FLOWS CONTINUE TO DECLINE, OR SYMPTOMS WORSEN, CALL THE CLINIC AT (----------) AS SOON AS POSSIBLE AND MOVE TO THE RED ZONE PLAN
RED ZONE PEAK FLOW: (<50%) 1. Administer rescue medication. 2. **Notify the clinic (----------) as soon as possible.** 3. **Begin the following medication:**	**Symptoms:** ·moderate to severe coughing, wheezing or shortness of breath ·may have an increase in breathing rate, retractions of skin above the collar bone or between the ribs, paleness, blueness around the eyes or lips, and vomiting of mucus
24 HOUR EMERGENCY PHONE NUMBER: (----------)	

Signature:_____ Date:

FIGURE 18-3
Example of an action plan for patient management of their asthma at home.

CO-EXISTING CONDITIONS WHICH COMPROMISE TREATMENT

Some patients seem to have asthma that is refractory to standard therapy. In these cases, one must question the diagnosis. In the case of chronic cough or dyspnea, for instance, the possibility of allergic/nonallergic rhinosinusitis, GERD, vocal cord dysfunction, or other persistent upper airway irritation must be seriously considered.[67,140] Other diseases mimic asthma, including transient upper respiratory tract infections (especially *Mycoplasma*), allergic bronchopulmonary *aspergillosis* fungi, congestive heart failure, chronic obstructive pulmonary disease, mechanical airway obstruction, pulmonary infiltrates with eosinophilia, and other airway dysfunction (e.g., laryngeomalacia or tracheomalacia) (see Table 18-2). To evaluate each of these diseases in every patient is not productive; however, it is important to keep a working differential diagnosis in mind as one evaluates patients with apparent refractory chronic asthma.

CONSIDERATION FOR REFERRAL

The assessment and management of chronic asthma requires a detailed medical, social, and family history, and physical examination. The assessment and management of chronic asthma is also greatly enhanced by the addition of spirometry and skin testing to identify environmental allergies. Furthermore, significant time and effort to educate patients and teach proper home-monitoring and management of the disease are required. A 1991 study showed a significant difference in nocturnal awakenings and emergency department visits, and an improvement over previous medication usage if the patient was referred to an asthma specialist after the emergent visit rather than to a primary care physician.[141] Similarly, there were less emergency department visits and hospital admissions in patients who received regular outpatient care by an allergist compared to those followed by a general physician.[142] In light of these findings and the fact that the assessment and management of asthma takes very specific knowledge,

an investment in time and effort to evaluate, treat, and educate patients, referral to an asthma specialist should be considered under several circumstances.

Specialist referrals are warranted when 1) a patient is not responding to treatment or is not meeting the goals of therapy outlined, 2) if the patient requires more than two oral corticosteroid bursts in a year, or 3) has had a life-threatening asthma exacerbation. A specialist should also be consulted when a patient has other complicating medical conditions such as COPD, or when a patient has an unusual presentation or an uncertain diagnosis of asthma. If certain diagnostic tests are not available to a physician, the patient should be referred to a specialist, where appropriate tests may be obtained. The issues of education and medication compliance often require extra time, and

Table 18-9
When to consider referral to an asthma specialist

When . . .
- There is a history of a life-threatening asthma exacerbation
- The patient is not meeting the goals of asthma therapy
- There are atypical signs and/or symptoms or any problem in the differential diagnosis
- There are other complicating factors (e.g., sinusitis, GERD, polyposis, vocal cord dysfunction, COPD, aspirin sensitivity)
- Additional testing is necessary (e.g., skin testing, spirometry, methacholine challenge)
- The patient needs further education on issues such as medication compliance, allergen avoidance, and therapeutic complications
- Immunotherapy is being considered
- The patient has severe persistent asthma (Step 4 therapy), and consideration should be given for moderate persistent asthma (Step 3 therapy)
- The patient has steroid-dependent asthma, or required more than 2 oral corticosteroid bursts in one year
- The patient needs to confirm an environmental or occupational exposure as provoking or contributing to asthma

SOURCE: Modified from National Institutes of Health.[1]

patients who have trouble with these issues may benefit from a referral to a specialist who is appropriately staffed to manage such issues. There are other indications for a referral to an asthma specialist and Table 18-9 outlines those instances when the Expert Panel for the 1997 NIH Guidelines suggests a specialist referral or consult should be considered.[1]

CONCLUSION

The assessment and management of chronic asthma can be complicated. It involves a thorough history, physical examination, and, often, appropriate testing to establish the diagnosis, either alone or with coexisting disease processes such as upper airway inflammation, COPD, and GERD. Further investigation is often required to establish whether other diseases are masquerading as asthma. Once the diagnosis has been established, the physician and other health care providers must assess the level of asthma and co-existing disease severity in order to provide adequate treatment to the patient. The 1997 NIH Guidelines provide clear suggestions of the goals for chronic asthma treatment as well as the six areas to be monitored in the assessment of chronic asthma, in order to meet these goals. If these guidelines are followed and the patient continues to have poor control, further consideration into the etiology of refractory disease must be made, and a referral to or consultation with an asthma specialist, if not already done, should be considered. With this type of clinical action plan in mind, and with thorough education of the patient, who should have an action plan of their own to follow, the assessment and management of chronic asthma should be fairly clear, and ideally quite successful in the outpatient setting.

ACKNOWLEDGEMENT

The authors would like to thank Reitha Johnson for her assistance in preparing this manuscript.

REFERENCES

1. National Heart, Lung, and Blood Institute: *Expert Panel Report 2: Guidelines for the diagnosis and management of asthma.* Bethesda, National Institutes of Health, publ No 97-4051, 1997.
2. Martin RJ: Nocturnal asthma: circadian rhythms and therapeutic interventions. *Am Rev Respir Dis* 147:S25–S28, 1993.
3. Hetzel MR, Clark TJH: Comparison of normal and asthmatic circadian rhythms in peak expiratory flow rate. *Thorax* 35:732–8, 1980.
4. Quackenboss JJ, Lebowitz D, Krzyanowski M: The normal range of diurnal changes in peak expiratory flow rates. Relationship to symptoms and respiratory disease. *Am Rev Respir Dis* 140:232–30, 1991.
5. Vir R, Bhagat R, Shah A: Sleep disturbances in clinically stable young asthmatic adults. *Ann Allergy Asthma Immunol* 79:251–5, 1997.
6. Kleerup EC, Tashkin DP: Outpatient treatment of adult asthma. *West J Med* 163:49–63, 1995.
7. Turcotte H, Boulet LP: Perception of breathlessness during early and late asthmatic responses. *Am Rev Respir Dis* 148(2):514–8, 1993.
8. Kikuchi Y, Okabe S, Tamura G, et al: Chemosensitivity and perception of dyspnea in patients with a history of near-fatal asthma. *N Engl J Med* 330:1329–34, 1994.
9. Friday GA Jr., Khine H, Lin MS, Caliguiri LA: Profile of children requiring emergency treatment for asthma. *Ann Allergy Asthma Immunol* 78(2):221–4, 1997.
10. Marquette CH, Saulnier F, Leroy O, et al: Long-term prognosis of near-fatal asthma. *Am Rev Respir Dis* 146:76–81, 1992.
11. McFadden ER, Warren EL: Observations on asthma mortality. *Ann Intern Med* 127:142–147, 1992.
12. Ruffin RE, Latimer KM, Schembri DA: Longitudinal study of near fatal asthma. *Chest* 99:77–83, 1991.
13. Strunk RC: Identification of the fatality-prone subject with asthma. *J Allergy Clin Immunol* 83(2, Pt 1):477–485, 1989.
14. Mahler DA: Exercise-induced asthma. *Med Sci Sports Exerc* 25(5):554–561, 1993.
15. Gelb AF, Tashkin DP, Epstein JD, et al: Exercise-induced bronchodilation in asthma. *Chest* 87:196–201, 1985.
16. Anderson SD: Exercise-induced asthma: the state of the art. *Chest* 87(Suppl 5):191S–195S, 1985.

17. Brutsche M, Britschgi D, Dayer E, Tschopp JM: Exercise-induced bronchospasm (EIB) in relation to seasonal and perennial specific IgE in young adults. *Allergy* 50:905–9, 1995.

18. Nicholson KG, Kent J, Ireland DC: Respiratory viruses and exacerbations of asthma in adults. *Br Med J* 307:982–986, 1993.

19. Johnston SL, Pattemore PK, Sanderson G, et al: Community study of role of viral infections in exacerbations of asthma in 9-11 year old children. *Br Med J* 310:1225–1229, 1995.

20. Gern JE, Calhoun W, Swenson C, et al: Rhinovirus infection preferentially increases lower airway responsiveness in allergic subjects. *Am J Respir Crit Care Med* 155:1872–1876, 1997.

21. Grunberg K, Timmers MC, Smits HH, et al: Effect of experimental rhinovirus 16 colds on airway hyperresponsiveness to histamine and interleukin-8 in nasal lavage in asthmatic subjects *in vivo*. *Clin Exp Allergy* 27:36–45, 1997.

22. Newman-Taylor A: Environmental determinants of asthma. *Lancet* 345:296–299, 1995.

23. Bush RK: The role of allergens in asthma. *Chest* 101:378S–380S, 1992.

24. Shibasaki M, Emiko N, Kazunori T, Hitoshi T: Distribution of IgE and IgG antibody levels against house dust mites in school children, and their relation with asthma. *J Asthma* 34(3):235–242, 1997.

25. Boulet LP, Turcotte H, Laprise C, et al: Comparative degree and type of sensitization to common indoor and outdoor allergens in subjects with allergic rhinitis and/or asthma. *Clin Exp Allergy* 27:52–59, 1997.

26. Rosenstreich DL, Eggleston P, Kattan M, et al: The role of cockroach allergy and exposure to cockroach allergen in causing morbidity among inner-city children with asthma. *N Engl J Med* 336(19):1356–63, 1997.

27. Pollart SM, Chapman MD, Fiocco GP, et al: Epidemiology of acute asthma: IgE antibodies to common inhalant allergens as a risk factor for emergency room visits. *J Allergy Clin Immunol* 83:875–82, 1989.

28. Arshad SH, Hide DW: Effect of environmental factors on the development of allergic disorders in infancy. *J Allergy Clin Immunol* 90:235–41, 1992.

29. Frischer T, Kuehr J, Meinert R, et al: Maternal smoking in early childhood: a risk factor for bronchial responsiveness to exercise in primary-school children. *J Pediatr* 121:17–22, 1992.

30. Martinez FD, Wright AL, Taussig LM, et al: Asthma and wheezing in the first six years of life. *N Engl J Med* 332:133–8, 1995.

31. Ehrlich RI, Du Toit D, Jordaan E, et al: Risk factors for childhood asthma and wheezing. Importance of maternal and household smoking. *Am J Respir Crit Care Med* 154(3 Pt 1):681–8, 1996.

32. Strachan D, Butland BK, Anderson HR: Incidence and prognosis of asthma and wheezing illness from early childhood to age 33 in a national British cohort. *BMJ* 312:1195–99, 1996.

33. Coultas DB, Samet JM: Epidemiology and natural history of asthma, in Tinkelman DG, Naspitz CK (eds): *Childhood Asthma*. New York, Marcel Dekker, 1993; pp. 71–114.

34. Jindal SK, Gupta D, Singh A: Indices of morbidity and control of asthma in adult patients exposed to environmental tobacco smoke. *Chest* 106:746–9, 1994.

35. Leuenberger P, Schwartz J, Ackermann-Liebrich U, et al: Passive smoking exposure in adults and chronic respiratory symptoms (SAPALDIA Study). Swiss Study on Air Pollution and Lung Diseases in Adults, SALPALDIA Team. *Am J Respir Crit Care Med* 150:1221–8, 1994.

36. Cockroft DW, Kalra S: Outpatient asthma management. *Med Clin North Am* 80(4):701–18, 1996.

37. Lin FJ, Dimich-Ward H, Chan-Yeung M: Longitudinal decline in lung function in patients with occupational asthma due to western red cedar. *Occup Environ Med* 53(11):753–6, 1996.

38. Fuortes LJ, Kiken S, Makowsky M: An outbreak of napthalene di-isocyanate-induced asthma in a plastics factory. *Arch Environ Health* 50(5):337–40, 1995.

39. Piirila P, Estlander T, Keskinen H, et al: Occupational asthma caused by triglycidyl isocyanurate (TGIC). *Clin Exp Allergy* 27(5):510–14, 1997.

40. Anto JM, Sunyer J, Rodriguez-Roison R, Vasquez L: Community outbreak of asthma associated with inhalation of soya bean. *N Engl J Med* 320:1097–102, 1989.

41. Samet JM: Asthma and the environment: Do environmental factors affect the incidence and prognosis of asthma? *Toxicol Lett* 82/83:33–38, 1995.

42. Busse WW, Keicolt-Glaser JK, Coe C, et al: NHLBI workshop summary. Stress and asthma. *Am J Respir Crit Care Med* 151:249–52, 1995.

43. Leung DYM: Atopic dermatitis: The skin as a window into the pathogenesis of chronic allergic diseases, in Gern JE, Busse WW (eds): *Contemporary Diagnosis and Management of Allergic Diseases*

and Asthma. Philadelphia, Handbooks in Health, 1996, p 11.

44. Sporik R, Holgate ST, Platts-Mills TA, Cogswell JJ: Exposure to house-dust mite allergen (Der pI) and the development of asthma in childhood. A prospective study. *N Engl J Med* 323:502–7, 1990.

45. Larsen GL: Asthma in children. *N Engl J Med* 326:1540–5, 1992.

46. Foresi A, Pelucchi A, Gemma G, et al: Once daily intranasal fluticasone propionate (200mcg) reduces nasal symptoms and inflammation but also attenuates the increase in bronchial responsiveness during the pollen season in allergic rhinitis. *J Allergy Clin Immunol* 98:274–82, 1996.

47. Corren J, Adinoff AD, Buchmeier AK, Irvin CG: Nasal beclomethasone prevents the seasonal increase in bronchial responsiveness in patients with allergic rhinitis and asthma. *J Allergy Clin Immunol* 90:250–6, 1992.

48. Senior BA, Kennedy DW: Management of sinusitis in the asthmatic patient. *Ann Allergy Asthma Immunol* 77:6–19, 1996.

49. Stevenson DD, Hankammer MA, Mathison DA, et al: Aspirin desensitization treatment of aspirin-sensitive patients with rhinosinusitis-asthma: long term outcomes. *J Allergy Clin Immunol* 98:751–8, 1996.

50. Bush RK, Ashbury D: Aspirin-sensitive asthma, in Busse WW, Holgate ST (eds): *Asthma and Rhinitis.* Boston, Blackwell Scientific, 1995, pp 1429–1439.

51. Pirson F, Charpin D, Sansonetti M, et al: Is intrinsic asthma a hereditary disease? *Allergy* 46:367–71, 1991.

52. Rona RJ, Duran-Tauleria E, Chinn S: Family size, atopic disorders in parents, asthma in children and ethnicity. *J Allergy Clin Immunol* 99:454–60, 1997.

53. Dold S, Wjst M, von Mutius E, et al: Genetic risk for asthma, allergic rhinitis, and atopic dermatitis. *Arch Dis Child* 67:1018–1022, 1992.

54. Greisner WA 3rd, Settipane GA: Hereditary factor for nasal polyps. *Allergy Asthma Proc* 17(5):283–6, 1996.

55. Kauffmann F, Dizier M-H, Pin I, et al: Epidemiological study of the genetics and the environment of asthma, bronchial hyperresponsiveness, and atopy: phenotype issues. *Am J Respir Crit Care Med* 156:S123–S129, 1997.

56. Cookson, W: Atopy: A complex genetic disease. *Ann Med* 26(5):351–53, 1994.

57. Holleman DR, Jr, Simel DL: Does the clinical examination predict airflow limitation? *JAMA* 273(4):313–19, 1995.

58. Barbee RA, Halonen M, Kaltenborn WT, Burrows B: A longitudinal study of respiratory symptoms in a community population sample. Correlations with smoking, allergen skin-test reactivity and serum IgE. *Chest* 99:20–26, 1991.

59. Baumann UA, Haerdi E, Keller R: Relations between clinical signs and lung function in bronchial asthma: how is acute bronchial obstruction reflected in dyspnoea and wheezing? *Respir* 50:294–300, 1986.

60. Bodner C, Ross S, Douglas G, et al: The prevalence of adult onset wheeze: longitudinal study. *BMJ* 314(7083):792–3, 1997.

61. Meslier N, Charbonneau, G, Racineaux J-L: Wheezes. *Eur Respir J* 8:1942–8, 1995.

62. Rolla G, Colagrande P, Scappaticci E, et al: Damage of the pharyngeal mucosa and hyperresponsiveness of airway in sinusitis. *J Allergy Clin Immunol* 100:52–7, 1997.

63. Watson WT, Becker AB, Simons FE: Treatment of allergic rhinitis with intranasal corticosteroids in patients with mild asthma; effect on lower airway responsiveness. *J Allergy Clin Immunol* 91:97–101, 1993.

64. Middleton E Jr, Reed CE, Ellis E, et al (eds): *Allergy Principles and Practice,* 4th ed. St. Louis, Mosby-Year Book, 1993, p 1126.

65. American Thoracic Society: Lung function testing: selection of reference values and interpretive strategies. *Am Rev Respir Dis* 144:1202–18, 1991.

66. Barnes P, Grunstein MM, Leff AR, Woolcock AJ (eds): *Asthma.* Philadelphia, Lippincott–Raven, 1997, p 1282.

67. Pratter MR, Bartter T, Akers S, DuBois J: An algorithmic approach to chronic cough. *Ann Intern Med* 119(10):977–983, 1993.

68. Neukirch F, Liard R, Segala C, et al: Peak expiratory flow variability and bronchial responsiveness to methacholine. *Am Rev Respir Dis* 146:71–75, 1992.

69. Burrows B, Martinez FD, Halonen M, et al: Association of asthma with serum IgE levels and skin-test reactivity to allergens. *N Engl J Med* 320:271–7, 1989.

70. Halonen M, Stern DA, Wright AL, et al: Alternaria as a major allergen for asthma in children raised in a desert environment. *Am J Respir Crit Care Med* 155:1356–1361, 1997.

71. O'Hollaren MT, Yunginger JW, Offord KP, et al:

Exposure to an aeroallergen as a possible precipitating factor in respiratory arrest in young patients with asthma. *N Engl J Med* 324:359–63, 1991.

72. Nahm D-H, Park H-S, Kang S-S, Hong C-S: Seasonal variation of skin reactivity and specific IgE antibody to house dust mite. *Ann Allergy Asthma Immunol* 78:589–93, 1997.

73. Adinoff AD, Rosloniec DM, McCall LL, Nelson HS: Immediate skin test reactivity to food and drug administration-approved standardized extracts. *J Allergy Clin Immunol* 86:766–74, 1990.

74. Lehr AJ, Mabry RL, Mabry CS: The screening RAST: is it a valid concept? *Otolaryngol Head Neck Surg* 117:54–5, 1997.

75. Jones KP, Mullee MA, Middleton M, et al: Peak flow based asthma self-management: a randomized controlled study in general practice. British Thoracic Society Research Committee. *Thorax* 50:851–7, 1995.

76. Lahdensuo A, Haahtela T, Herrala J, et al: Randomized comparison of guided self management and traditional treatment of asthma over one year. *Br Med J* 312:748–52, 1996.

77. Ignacio-Garcia JM, Gonzalez-Santos P: Asthma self-management education program by home monitoring of peak expiratory flow. *Am J Respir Crit Care Med* 151:353–9, 1995.

78. Beasley R, Cushley M, Holgate ST: A self-management plan in the treatment of adult asthma. *Thorax* 44:200–4, 1989.

79. Woolcock AJ, Colman MH, Blackburn CR: Factors affecting normal values for ventilatory lung function. *Am Rev Respir Dis* 106:692–709, 1972.

80. Janson-Bjerklie S, Shnell S: Effect of peak flow information on patterns of self-care in adult asthma. *Heart Lung* 17:543–9, 1988.

81. Grampian Asthma Study of Integrated Care: Effectiveness of routine self-monitoring of peak flow in patients with asthma. *Br Med J* 308:564–7, 1994.

82. Chan-Yeung M: Assessment of asthma in the workplace. American College of Chest Physicians Consensus Statement. *Chest* 108:1084–117, 1995.

83. Sly PD, Cahill P, Willet K, Burton P: Accuracy of mini peak flow meters in indicating changes in lung function in children with asthma. *Br Med J* 308:572–4, 1994.

84. Malo JL, L'Archeveque J, Trudeau C, et al: Should we monitor peak expiratory flow rates or record symptoms with a simple diary in the management of asthma? *J Allergy Clin Immunol* 91:702–9, 1993.

85. Mahajan P, Okamoto LJ, Schaberg A, et al: Impact of fluticasone propionate powder on health-related quality of life in patients with moderate asthma. *J Asthma* 34(3):227–234, 1997.

86. Bender B, Milgrom H, Rand C: Nonadherence in asthmatic patients: is there a solution to the problem? *Ann Allergy Asthma Immunol* 79:177–86, 1997.

87. Van Ganse E, Leufkens HGM, Vincken W, et al: Assessing asthma management form interviews of patients and family physicians. *J Asthma* 34(3):203–9, 1997.

88. ZuWallack RL, Rosen JP, Cohen L, et al: The effectiveness of once-daily dosing of inhaled flunisolide in maintaining asthma control. *J Allergy Clin Immunol* 99:278–85, 1997.

89. Wasserfallen J-B, Gold K, Schulman KA, Baraniuk JN: Development and validation of a rhinoconjunctivitis and asthma symptom score for use as an outcome measure in clinical trials. *J Allergy Clin Immunol* 100:16-22, 1997.

90. Flaum M, Lum Lung C, Tinkelman D: Take control of high-cost asthma. *J Asthma* 34(1):5–14, 1997.

91. Gergen PJ, Turkeltaub PC: The association of individual allergen reactivity with respiratory disease in a national sample: data from the second National Health and Nutrition Examination Survey, 1976-1980 (NHANES II). *J Allergy Clin Immunol* 90:579–88, 1992.

92. Gautrin D, Infante-Rivard C, Dao T-V, et al: Specific IgE-dependent sensitization, atopy, and bronchial hyperresponsiveness in apprentices starting exposure to protein-derived agents. *Am J Respir Crit Care Med* 155:1841–47, 1997.

93. Pisati G, Baruffini A, Zedda S: Toluene di-isocyanate induced asthma: outcome according to persistence or cessation of exposure. *Br J Intern Med* 50:60–4, 1993.

94. Corne JM, Holgate ST: Mechanisms of virus induced exacerbations of asthma. *Thorax* 52:380–89, 1997.

95. Gern JE, Busse WW: The effects of rhinovirus infections on allergic airway responses. *Am J Respir Crit Care Med* 152:S40–S45, 1995.

96. Busse WW, Lemanske RF Jr, Stark JM, Calhoun WJ: The role of respiratory infections in asthma, in Holgate ST, Austen KF, Lichtenstein LM, Kay AB (eds): *Asthma: Physiology, Immunopharmacology, and Treatment*. London, Academic Press, 1993, pp 345–53.

97. Centers for Disease Control and Prevention: Pre-

vention and control of influenza. Recommendations of the Advisory Committee on Immunization Practices (ACIP). *MMWR* 42 (no. RR-6):1–14, 1993.

98. Gwaltney JM Jr, Scheld WM, Sande MA, Sydor A: The microbial etiology and antimicrobial therapy of adults with acute community-acquired sinusitis: a fifteen-year experience at the University of Virginia and review of other selected studies. *J Allergy Clin Immunol* 90:457–61, 1992.

99. Gliklich RE, Metson R: Effect of sinus surgery on quality of life. *Otolaryngol Head Neck Surg* 117:12–7, 1997.

100. Kaplan BA, Mascie-Taylor CGN: Smoking and asthma among 23 year-olds. *J Asthma* 34(3):219–226, 1997.

101. Ostro BD, Lipsett MJ, Mann JK, et al: Indoor air pollution and asthma, Results from a panel study. *Am J Respir Crit Care Med* 149:1200–6, 1994.

102. Abbey DE, Peterson F, Mills PK, Beeson WL: Long-term ambient concentrations of total suspended particulates, ozone, and sulfur dioxide and respiratory symptoms in a nonsmoking population. *Arch Environ Health* 48:33–46, 1993.

103. Koenig JQ, Covert DS, Marshall SG, et al: The effects of ozone and nitrogen dioxide on pulmonary function in healthy and in asthmatic adolescents. *Am Rev Respir Dis* 136:1152–7, 1987.

104. Irwin RS, Zawacki JK, Curley FJ, French CL, Hoffman PJ: Chronic cough as the sole presenting manifestation of gastroesophageal reflux. *Am Rev Respir Dis* 140:1294–1300, 1989.

105. Nelson HS: Gastroesophageal reflux and pulmonary disease. *J Allergy Clin Immunol* 75:337–9, 1984.

106. Harding SM, Richter JE, Guzzo MR, et al: Asthma and gastroesophageal reflux: acid suppressive therapy improves asthma outcome. *Am J Med* 100(4):395–405, 1996.

107. Perrin-Fayolle M, Gormand F, Braillon G, et al: Long-term results of surgical treatment for gastroesophageal reflux in asthmatic patients. *Chest* 96:40–5, 1989.

108. Spector SL, Wangaard CH, Farr RS: Aspirin and concomitant idiosyncrasies in adult asthmatic patients. *J Allergy Clin Immunol* 64:500–6, 1979.

109. Graft DF, Schuberth KC, Kagey-Sobotka A, et al: Assessment of prolonged venom immunotherapy in children. *J Allergy Clin Immunol* 80:162–9, 1987.

110. Hunt KJ, Valentine MD, Sobotka AK, et al: A controlled trial on immunotherapy in insect hypersensitivity. *N Engl J Med* 299:157–61, 1978.

111. Charlesworth EN: Late-phase inflammation: Influence on morbidity. *J Allergy Clin Immunol* 98:S291–7, 1996.

112. Scarfone RJ, Fuchs SM, Nager AL, Shane SA: Controlled trial of oral prednisone in the emergency department treatment of children with acute asthma. *Pediatrics* 92(4):513–8, 1993.

113. Chapman KR, Verbeek PR, White JG, Rebuck AS: Effect of a short course of prednisone in the prevention of early relapse after the emergency room treatment of acute asthma. *N Engl J Med* 324(12):788–94, 1991.

114. Lawrence M, Wolfe J, Webb DR, et al: Efficacy of inhaled fluticasone propionate in asthma results from topical and not from systemic activity. *Am J Respir Crit Care Med* 156:744–51, 1997.

115. Toogood JH, Frankish CW, Jennings BH, et al: A study of the mechanism of the antiasthmatic action of inhaled budesonide. *J Allergy Clin Immunol* 85:872–80, 1990.

116. Morrow-Brown H, Storey G, George WHS: Beclomethasone dipropionate: a new steroid aerosol for the treatment of allergic asthma. *Br Med J* 1:585–590, 1972.

117. Donahue JG, Weiss ST, Livingston JM, et al: Inhaled steroids and the risk of hospitalization for asthma. *JAMA* 277(11):887–91, 1997.

118. Booms P, Cheung D, Timmers MC, et al: Protective effect of inhaled budesonide against unlimited airway narrowing to methacholine in atopic patients with asthma. *J Allergy Clin Immunol* 99:330–7, 1997.

119. Noonan M, Chervinsky P, Busse WW, et al: Fluticasone propionate reduces oral prednisone use while it improves asthma control and quality of life. *Am J Respir Crit Care Med* 152(5, pt.1):1467–73, 1995.

120. Lacronique J, Renon D, Georges D, et al: High-dose beclomethasone: oral steroid-sparing effect in severe asthmatic patients. *Eur Respir J* 4:807–12, 1991.

121. Chervinsky P, van As A, Bronsky EA, et al: Fluticasone propionate aerosol for the treatment of adults with mild to moderate asthma. The Fluticasone Propionate Asthma Study Group. *J Allergy Clin Immunol* 94:676–83, 1994.

122. Laitinen LA, Laitinen A, Haahtela T: A comparative study of the effects of an inhaled corticosteroid, budesonide, and a β_2-agonist, terbutaline, on

airway inflammation in newly diagnosed asthma: a randomized, double-blind, parallel-group controlled trial *J Allergy Clin Immunol* 90:32–42, 1992.

123. O'Byrne PM, Israel E, Drazen JM: Antileukotrienes in the treatment of asthma. *Ann Intern Med* 127:472–80, 1997.

124. Galant SP, Lawrence M, Meltzer EO, et al: Fluticasone propionate compared with theophylline for mild-to-moderate asthma. *Ann Allergy Asthma Immunol* 77(2):112–8, 1996.

125. Apter AJ, Reisine ST, Willard A, et al: The effect of inhaled albuterol in moderate to severe asthma. *J Allergy Clin Immunol* 98:295–301, 1996.

126. Cockroft DW, Swystun VA: Asthma control versus asthma severity. *J Allergy Clin Immunol* 98:1016–8, 1996.

127. Côté L, Cartier A, Robichaud P, et al: Influence on asthma morbidity of asthma education programs based on self-management plans following treatment optimization: *Am J Respir Crit Care Med* 155:1509–1514, 1997.

128. Klucka CV, Ownby DR, Green J, Zoratti E: Cat shedding of Fel d I is not reduced by washings, Allerpet-C spray, or acepromazine. *J Allergy Clin Immunol* 95:1164–71, 1995.

129. de Blay F, Chapman MD, Platts-Mills TAE: Airborne cat allergen (Fel d I): environmental control with the cat in situ. *Am Rev Respir Dis* 143:1334–9, 1991.

130. Wahlgren DR, Hovell MF, Meltzer SB, et al: Reduction of environmental tobacco smoke exposure in asthmatic children. A 2-year follow-up. *Chest* 111(1):81–8, 1997.

131. Hill DJ, Thompson PJ, Stewart GA, et al: The Melbourne House Dust Mite Study: Eliminating house dust mites in the domestic environment. *J Allergy Clin Immunol* 99:323–9, 1997.

132. Wickman M: Prevention and nonpharmacologic treatment of mite allergy. *Allergy* 52:369–73, 1997.

133. American Thoracic Society: Achieving healthy indoor air: Report of the ATS workshop: Santa Fe, New Mexico, Nov. 16–19, 1995. *Am J Respir Crit Care Med* 156:S33–S64, 1997.

134. Kendrik AH, Higgs CMB, Whitfield MJ, Laszlo G: Accuracy of perception of severity of asthma: Patients treated in general practice. *Br Med J* 307(6901):422–4, 1993.

135. Apter AJ, Affleck G, Reisine ST, et al: Perception of airway obstruction in asthma: sequential daily analyses of symptoms, peak expiratory flow rate, and mood. *J Allergy Clin Immunol* 99:605–12, 1997.

136. Smith DH, Malone DC, Lawson KA, et al: A national estimate of the economic costs of asthma. *Am J Respir Crit Care Med* 156:787–93, 1997.

137. Gern JE, Schroth MK, Lemanske RF: Childhood asthma: older children and adolescents. *Clin Chest Med* 16(4):657–70, 1995.

138. Price JF: Issues in adolescent asthma: what are the needs? *Thorax* 51(S1):S13–S17, 1996.

139. Weinstein AG: Clinical management strategies to maintain drug compliance in asthmatic children. *Ann Allergy Asthma Immunol* 74(4):304–10, 1995.

140. McFadden ER Jr, Zawaski DK: Vocal cord dysfunction masquerading as exercise-induced asthma. A physiologic cause for "choking" during athletic activities. *Am J Respir Crit Care Med* 153:942–7, 1996.

141. Zeiger RS, Heller S, Mellon M, et al: Facilitated referral to asthma specialist reduces relapses in asthma emergency room visits. *J Allergy Clin Immunol* 87:1160–8, 1991.

142. Mahr TA, Evans R 3d: Allergist influence on asthma care. *Ann Allergy* 71(2):115–120, 1993.

INDEX

Page numbers followed by t and f refer to tables and illustrations respectively.

NOTES

NOTES

NOTES

NOTES

NOTES

NOTES

NOTES

NOTES